THIS BOOK BELONGS TO

NAME: _____

PAGER: _____

PHONE: _____

EMAIL: _____

MEDICINE: SURVIVAL GUIDE   ISBN: 978-0-9890657-5-7

Copyright © 2020 by Jacob Mathew, Jr. D.O. FACOI FACP CHSE FAWM

All rights reserved. No part of this publication may be reproduced, distributed, or transmitted in any form or by any means, including photocopying, recording, or other electronic or mechanical methods, without the prior written permission of the publisher, except in the case of brief quotations embodied in critical reviews and certain other noncommercial uses permitted by copyright law. For permission requests, write to the publisher, addressed "Attention: Permissions Coordinator," at the address below. Every attempt has been made to cite all figures used in this book. The writer takes no ownership of such images and as such has referenced them to the appropriate owners. If any errors are found, please contact the publisher at the address below. The publisher is not responsible (as a matter of product liability, negligence, or otherwise) for any injury resulting from any material contained herein. This publication contains information relating to general principles of medical care that should not be construed as specific instructions for individual patients. Manufacturers' product information and package inserts should be reviewed for current information, including contraindications, dosages, and precautions. The author has made every effort to use sources believed to be reliable to provide information that is accurate and compatible with the standards generally accepted at the time of publication. Because medical science is continually advancing, our knowledge base continues to expand. Therefore, as new information becomes available, changes in procedures become necessary. We recommend that the reader always consult current research and specific institutional policies before performing any clinical procedure. To the maximum extent permitted under applicable law, no responsibility is assumed by the publisher for any injury and/or damage to persons or property, as a matter of products liability, negligence law or otherwise, or from any reference to or use by any person of this work.

NOTICE

Medicine is an ever-changing, rapidly advancing field. Standard safety precautions must be followed, and allowances must be made for new discoveries, drugs, and changes to standards of care. Though every effort has been made to ensure that the information in this book is accurate and up to date, readers are advised to verify for themselves, relying on their experience and knowledge of their patient to determine if the recommendations made are actually the best for their individual patient. Reviews have been performed to confirm the accuracy of the information presented in this book and often describe generally accepted practices, or "pearls". The author is not responsible for errors or omissions or for any consequences from application of the information in this book and make no warranty, expressed or implied, with respect to the currency, completeness, or accuracy of the contents of the publication. Furthermore, readers are encouraged to confirm the information contained herein with other sources. Neither the author nor the Department of Medicine assume any liability for any injury and/or damage to persons or property arising from use of this handbook. Some drugs and medical devices presented in this publication have Food and Drug Administration (FDA) clearance for limited use in restricted research settings. It is the responsibility of health care providers to ascertain the FDA status of each drug or device planned for use in their clinical practice. When prescribing medication, health care professionals are advised to consult the product information sheet (the manufacturer's package insert) accompanying each drug to verify, among other things, conditions of use, warnings, and side effects, and identify any changes in dosage schedule or contraindications, particularly if the medication to be administered is new, infrequently used, or has a narrow therapeutic range. Unless otherwise stated, all medications are for the non-pregnant, non-breast feeding adult who has reasonable liver and renal function living in the USA. The publisher has made every effort to trace copyright holders for borrowed material. If there is any information that may have inadvertently been overlooked, the publisher will be pleased to make the necessary arrangements as soon as possible.

Previous editions copyrighted 2020, 2019, 2018, 2017, 2016, 2015, 2014, 2013

10 9 8 7 6 5 4 3 2 1

For details on ordering additional copies, contact the publisher through Amazon.

Printed in the United States of America

Fourth Edition

Library of Congress Control Number: 2019910140

Medicine
Survival Guide

4th Edition

Jacob Mathew, Jr. DO FACOI FACP CHSE FAWM

PREFACE

I am excited to present to you the renamed "Medicine: Survival Guide" which acts as the fourth edition of the popular Internal Medicine: Intern Survival Guide series. I have taken the feedback I have received from many of you who have been gracious enough to purchase the book to make this edition even better than the past works. As always, please email me (drjacobmathewjr@gmail.com) if you have any suggestions for future editions. No matter your background, I hope you find it helpful and that it continues to allow you to provide the best care possible for your patients.

Jacob Mathew Jr. DO

CONTENTS

Wards

Lab Shorthand	11
Common Scenarios	11
Accidental Needle Stick	12
Declaring Patient Deceased	13
Discharging Patients	15
Code Status	16

Dermatology

Topical Steroids	19
Acne	19
Common Skin Conditions	25
Skin Biopsy	26

Gastroenterology

Approach to abdominal pain	29
Ascites	29
Gallbladder Disorders	33
Cirrhosis	35
Irritable Bowel Syndrome	40
Constipation	41
Colon Cancer	43
Diarrhea	44
Diverticulitis	52
Dysphagia	53
GI Bleed	54
Acute Pancreatitis	60
Bowel Obstruction	66
GERD	67

Quick ACLS

Primary and Secondary ABCD Survey	80
Asystole	80
Bradycardia	80
Pulseless Electrical Activity	81
VFib/Pulseless VTach	82
Tachycardia	82

Infectious Disease

Reading Microbiology Report	86
Susceptibility Interpretation	88
Empiric Antibiotic Regimen	88
Fever of Unknown Origin	103
Cellulitis	105
Clostridium Difficile	107
Meningitis	112
Urinary Tract Infections	116
Pyelonephritis	120
Sepsis	121
Bacterial endocarditis	127
Pneumonia	129
Surgical Site Infections	137

Cardiology

How to Read an ECG	140
Heart Failure	150
Coronary Artery Disease	167
Stress Testing	172

Chest Pain & ACS 176
UA/NSTEMI 188
STEMI 194
Murmurs 203
Cardiomyopathy 205
Hypotension 205
Hypertension 207
Resistent Hypertension 219
Aortic Stenosis 219
Atrial Fibrillation 221
Pacemakers 229

Endocrinology

Adrenal Incidentaloma 235
Osteoporosis 236
Sexual Dysfunction 241
Diabetes Mellitus 244
Insulin Management 260
Diabetic Ketoacidosis (DKA) 267
Hyperosmolar Nonketotic Coma 275
Hypoglycemia 277
Hyperthyroidism 277
Hypothyroidism 281
Pituitary Incidentaloma 284
Steroids 285
Thyroid Nodule 286
Vitamin D Deficiency 288

Geriatrics

Dementia 292
Mild Cognitive Impairment 301
End of Life Management 301

Hematology/Oncology

The CBC 304
Anemia 305
Breast Cancer Screening 313
Blood Transfusion 314
Screening for Bleeding Disorders 324
Disseminated Intravascular Coagulation 326
Elevated INR 327
Hemolytic Anemia 328
Heparin-Induced Thrombocytopenia 328
Neutropenia 331
Neutropenic Fever 332
Supportive Care of Cancer Patients 339
Venous Thromboembolism 340

Ophthalmology

Eye Pain 352
Conjunctivitis 353
Corneal Abrasion 357

Radiology

CXR 360
Abdominal Film 366
Echocardiography 367

Musculoskeletal

Back Examination 376
Knee Examination 378
Knee Effusion 386
Leg/Ankle/Foot Pain Differential 388
Shoulder Examination 391

Neurology

- Neurological Exam 404
- Syncope 407
- Altered Mental Status 411
- Concussion 413
- Headaches 417
- Migraine Headaches 421
- Parkinson's Disease 427
- Sensory/Motor Deficits 429
- Seizure 430
- Unresponsive Patient 438
- Stroke 439
- Transient Ischemic Attack 454
- Vertigo 456

Pulmonology/Critical Care

- Cough 462
- Dyspnea 463
- Interpretation of PFT's 465
- Asthma 472
- COPD 480
- Interstitial Lung Diseases 490
- Hypoxia 494
- Supplemental Oxygen 495
- Pleural Effusion 496
- Solitary Pulmonary Nodule 499
- Pulmonary Hypertension 501
- Hemodynamic Monitoring in the ICU 503
- ARDS 523
- Intubation 504
- Ventilator Review 517
- Extubation Criteria 516
- Anaphylaxis 525
- Shock 526

Nephrology

- Acid Base Physiology 531
- Acute Kidney Injury 536
- Chronic Kidney Disease 543
- Polyuria 547
- Glomerular Disease 551
- Nephrolithiasis 553

Otolaryngology

- Allergic Rhinitis 557
- Rhinosinusitis 559
- Pharyngitis 560
- Epistaxis 564
- Hearing Loss 565

Rheumatology

- Gout 570
- Approach to Joint Pain 573
- Monoarthritis 574
- Polyarticular Arthritis 575
- Common Rheumatologic Labs 578

Psychiatry

- Capacity 582
- Delirium 582
- Insomnia 587
- Sedation of the Violent Patient 589
- Depression 590
- Alcoholic Patient 599
- PTSD 601
- Anxiety Disorder 602

Perioperative Care

Perioperative Management of Warfarin .607
Bridging Anticoagulation........................610
Perioperative Evaluation 616
Surgical Site Infections...........................137

Toxicology

Alcohol Withdrawal.................................630
Urine Drug Testing 635
Overdose...637

Women's Health

Abnormal Uterine Bleeding 641
Polycystic Ovarian Syndrome (PCOS)..643
Menopause 644
Contraception 645
Emergency Contraception.....................651
Menorrhagia 652

Urology

Hematuria..656
BPH..657
Testicular Pain 658
Overactive Bladder.................................659
Urinary Incontinence 661

Nutrition/Diet

Inpatient Diets 664
Body Weight Calculations 666
Labs Associated with Nutrition 666
Hyperlipidemia 667
Hypertriglyceridemia..............................672

Nutritional Requirements.......................674

Fluids

Fluid Calculations...................................677
IV Fluids 678

Pain Management

Pain Management 681
Conversion Factors for Opioids 687

Formulas 690
Electrolytes...692
Abbreviations...711
Appendix 713
Index 723

WHAT / WHO	DEPARTMENT	PHONE NUMBER

WARDS

Lab Shorthand 11
Common Scenarios 11
Accidental Needle Stick 12
Declaring Patient Deceased 13
Discharging Patients 15
Code Status 16

LAB SHORTHAND

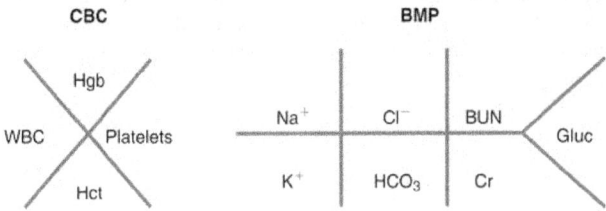

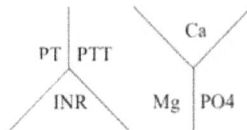

Others

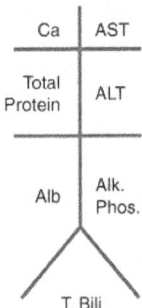

pH / PaCO2 / PaO2 / HCO3 / O2 Sat / Base Excess
7.35-7.45 / 35-45 mmHg / 80-100 mmHg / 21-27 mEq/L / 95-98% / +/-2 mEq/L

COMMON SCENARIOS

- **Alcohol withdrawal** - see page 630
- **Altered mental status** – see page 411
- **Chest pain** - see page 176
- **Fever**
    - *Fever is defined as T>100.4F for at least one hour or any temperature above 101F*
    - At nighttime, it is safest to assume a fever is infectious in etiology and consider broad spectrum treatment if necessary; day team coverage can always narrow down if necessary.

- If giving antibiotics, confirm allergies, then you should always perform a FFWU (see page 103) to include cultures (blood, sputum, urine)
- If patient is already on antibiotics, consider broadening
  - Rule out non-infectious causes like medications, NMS, or SS (see page 599)
  - For high fevers being treated (or known source), consider treating with Tylenol. If infectious in etiology, however, consider avoiding Tylenol (masking).
  - For FUO, see page 103
- **Hyperglycemia** - see page 260
- **Hypertension** - see page 218
- **Hypoglycemia** - see page 277
- **Pain management** - see page 681
- **Shortness of breath**
  - Get a full set of vitals to determine if the patient is subjectively SOB or if they have a low oxygen saturation.
  - The big 3 tests of dyspnea
    - ECG
    - ABG
    - Portable CXR
  - If the patient has a low oxygen saturation, administer O2:
    - Nasal cannula→venti mask→non-rebreather→NIPPV→intubation (if the patient requires NRB/NIPPV/Intubation then MICU should be notified)
    - Remember in general, CPAP should be used for **hypoxia** and BiPAP for **hypercapnia** or **mixed hypoxia/hypercapnia**.
    - See page 495 for supplemental oxygen options and page 520 for BiPAP vs CPAP
  - Pulmonary causes of SOB:
    - Obstructive (COPD, asthma, foreign body), pneumothorax, pneumonia, aspiration, ILD, pleural effusions, DAH, PE
    - Cardiovascular causes of SOB: ACS, cardiac arrhythmia (e.g. AFib, VT), pulmonary HTN, cardiac tamponade, acute decompensated HF
    - Non-pulmonary and non-cardiac causes of SOB: anemia, metabolic acidosis, carboxy/sulph/met-Hgb, diaphragmatic paralysis (e.g. in ALS), abdominal HTN
  - Additional tests to consider include CBC, RFP, D-dimer, CT PE, troponin and BNP
- **Seizure** – see page 430
- **Stroke** – see page 439

ACCIDENTAL NEEDLE STICK

- **General**
  - Confirm that all identified personnel go to the ER for proper initial treatment per protocol
  - Obtain source patient information from nurse
  - Can call National Clinicians' Post-Exposure Prophylaxis Hotline, PEPline: 1-888-448-4911
- **Examination**:
  - <u>Puncture</u>: clean wound with alcohol-based agent (viricidal to HBV, HCV, and HIV)
  - <u>Skin</u>: soap+water
  - <u>Mucosa</u>: flush with copious amounts of water and irrigate eyes with saline or water
- **Labs**
  - Lab order exists for needle stick, otherwise:
    - HIV AB/RB (rapid) with gold tube
    - HepB surface Ag

- HepB Core IGM
- Hep C surface Ab
- Syphilis RPR
- ALT
    - Tests for source patient
        - Rapid test HIV
- **Treatment**
    - <u>HIV positive source / exposee negative</u> - Truvada+raltegravir within 1-2 hours of exposure x 1 month
    - <u>Hepatitis B</u>
        - HBIG if exposed nonresponder to vaccine or unvaccinated
        - HepB vaccination only if vaccination response unknown or no vaccination on record
    - <u>HCV</u>
        - Post-exposure prophylaxis not recommended
- **Follow up**
    - Notify nurse involved of above results so treatment can be d/c or continued as necessary

DECLARING PATIENT DECEASED

- You will be informed by nurse that patient has passed away and needs to be declared.
- Be prepared to encounter the family at bedside; explain that you need to examine the patient and that they may stay and that the body can stay in the room as long as the family needs
- **Diagnosis is based on 4 areas:** [1]
    - Meeting prerequisites
    - Performing the clinical examination
    - Using ancillary testing if necessary
    - Consideration for organ donation
- **Knowledge of the proximate cause**
    - Intoxication
    - Metabolic abnormalities
    - ↓Temp
- **Bedside Examination:**
    - <u>Clinical Criteria Required:</u>
        - Clinical and/or imaging evidence of CNS destruction
        - Absence of drug intoxication (i.e. EtOH)
        - Absence of severe electrolyte abnormalities
        - Core temperature >32C
        - They cannot be declared dead until 4-5 half-lives of the suspected substance have passed. Note that substances we give patients such as paralytics, benzos, sedatives, etc. also fall under this category.
    - Exam:
        - Brainstem function (check for reflexes: pupillary, oculocephalic, oculovestibular)
        - Absent motor reflexes
        - Absent cough on tracheal suction
        - Observe for spontaneous breathing or movements
        - Auscultate for heart tones
        - Assess for response to pain by pinching fingernail or skin while auscultating (sternal rub can be done as well)
- **All above are present**

- o Apnea Test
    - Preoxygenate then disconnect from ventilator
    - Absence of response for 10 minutes with PaCO2>60 (or >20 change from baseline) and arterial PH <7.2 confirms
- o Repeat clinical exam second time to confirm no changes
- **Not all criteria present but brain death still suspected...**
    - o Ancillary Testing
        - An isoelectric EEG for 30 minutes with the machine set at high gain.
        - SSEP and BAEP (absence of evoked potentials)
        - MRA/CTA (absence of intracranial blood flow)
        - Carotid angiography to document lack of flow (**gold standard**)
        - Transcranial Doppler
- **Note time, offer condolences, and ask family if they would like an autopsy.**
    - o Inform them of benefits of autopsy (will help in the education of house staff and may identify incidental inherited diseases and thus benefit surviving family). The autopsy will not interfere with an open casket funeral; there is the option of limited autopsy, and costs are covered by the hospital.
    - o Also ask if the patient was an organ donor, if so, ask nurse to call donor hotline and obtain organ donor # (required for electronic registration)
    - o Contact the chaplain if family wishes
- **Call or page attending physician!**
- **Paperwork**
    - o EMR
        - Death Note
        - Discharge Summary
    - o Checklist (front only)
    - o Death summary (paper form)
        - **Time and date of death**
        - Hospital dx
        - Need to note immediate cause of death.
            1. **Cannot** use the following:
                - Cardiac Arrest
                - Respiratory Arrest
                - Failure to Thrive
                - Cardiopulmonary Arrest
                - Respiratory Failure
                - Multi Organ – System Failure
            2. **Can** use the following:
                - Bronchopneumonia
                - AMI/ACS
                - Intracerebral hemorrhage
                - Liver failure
                - Pulmonary Embolism
                - Coagulopathy
                - CHF
                - Metastasis
        - Total # of HD's
        - Describe exam
        - Mention that the family, chaplain and attending were informed
        - Note if autopsy is requested by family
        - Determine of organ donation will be performed
- **Death requiring autopsy/medical examiner (family request; death <24 hrs. of admission)**

- o Contact the local medical examiner
  - Leave a message if after business hours
- o Have the following information ready:
  - Time on arrival to hospital (Check T-System à Event Log)
  - Time of death
  - PMHx
  - Hospital course
  - Home address
  - DPOA/Wife/Husband name and contact #
  - Ask if they will examine patient in hospital, or if okay to take patient to morgue
- **Input case into online local health system (if applicable)**

DISCHARGING PATIENTS

1. The following items are necessary to discharge a patient:
   - o Discharge Summary: typically, the intern completes e-Discharge form, arranges follow-up, and completes prescriptions; the upper resident will dictate/type a complete discharge summary with the following elements:
     - Date of admission
     - Date of discharge
     - R1, R2/3, attending on discharge
     - **Admitting diagnoses (i.e. what the patient had prior to coming to the hospital)**
     - **Discharge diagnoses (i.e. what the patient was diagnosed with during this hospital stay only) → first should always be the admitting diagnosis**
     - Procedures
     - Consults
     - Brief history of present illness
     - Hospital course
     - Physical exam (same length as a SOAP note)
     - Discharge medications:
       1. New
       2. Changed (any prehospital medications with dose/frequency changes)
       3. Unchanged (any prehospital medications to be continued without changes)
       4. Stopped (any prehospital medications that should be stopped)
     - Pending studies/labs
     - Outpatient workup needed (i.e. anemia workup, repeat CT chest, etc.)
     - Disposition (i.e. where the patient is going)
     - Diet
     - Code status
     - Activity
     - Home health/PT/wound care (if applicable)
   - o Follow-up
     - Note that all discharge summaries should be completed and signed within 24 hours of the patient's discharge. This is to ensure proper physician communication during this important transition of care.
2. **Patient Discharge Instructions** (printed from e-Discharge system)
3. **Prescriptions** (either printed from e-Discharge system and signed, or handwritten)
   - o Narcotics require security Rx, either from the resident or attending
   - o All Medi-CAL prescriptions need to be on security paper (ask Chiefs for this paper)
4. **D/C home, D/C IV order**

5. Notify patient's PMD of discharge or schedule a post-discharge appointment with them in IMS clinic with a member of your team
6. If the patient needs a primary care doctor, try to see them yourself, set them up with a member of your team, or verbally communicate with whomever they are intended to establish care.

CODE STATUS

- Discussion[2,3]
  - Beginning
    - Establish an appropriate setting for the discussion
      - I'd like to talk with you about possible health care decisions in the future.
      - I'd like to review your advance care planning. Would you like your daughter to be here with you?
      - I'd like to discuss something I discuss with all patients admitted to the hospital
    - Ask the patient and family what they understand
      - What do you understand about your current health situation?
      - Tell me about how you see your health.
      - What do you understand from what the doctors have told you?
    - Find out what they expect will happen.
    - Discuss a DNR order, including context
      - If you should die despite all of our efforts, do you want us to use "heroic measures" to bring you back?
      - How do you want things to be when you die?
      - If you were to die unexpectedly, would you want us to try to bring you back?
    - Respond to emotions.
    - Establish and implement the plan.
- Options
  - Full Code
    - **Do** everything (CPR, Intubation if necessary)
  - DNR-Comfort Care Arrest
    - Do everything until pt. goes into Cardiac or Respiratory Arrest.
    - Pt receives treatment **INCLUDING resuscitative efforts** if necessary until they experience C/R Arrest. Once an arrest is confirmed, all resuscitative and treatment efforts are withdrawn, and Comfort Care alone is initiated. May continue respiratory assistance (O2) and IV medications, etc. that have been a part of the patient's ongoing treatment for underlying disease.
  - DNR-Comfort Care
    - Pt receives any care that eases pain and suffering in the final days of life, but **NO RESUSCITATIVE EFFORTS** to save or sustain life.
    - **Do:** Suction airway, administer O2, Position for comfort, splint or immobilize, control bleeding, provide pain medication, provide emotional support, given antibiotics, Contact other appropriate health care providers.
      - **Do Not:** administer chest compressions, insert artificial airway, administer resuscitative drugs, defibrillate or cardiovert, provide respiratory assistance (other than those listed under DO category), initiate resuscitative IV or Initiate cardiac monitoring

Bibliography

[1] Wijdicks EF. The diagnosis of brain death. N Engl J Med. 2001 Apr 19;344(16):1215-21.

[2] Mills, Crystal. "Night Call Survival Guide."

[3] Von Gunten, Charles F. "Discussing Do-Not-Resuscitate Status."THE ART OF ONCOLOGY: WHEN THE TUMOR IS NOT THE TARGET. Journal of Clinical Oncology, Vol 19, No 5 (March 1), 2001: pp 1576-1581

DERMATOLOGY

Topical Steroids 19
Acne 19
Common Skin Conditions 25
Skin Biopsy 26

DERMATOLOGY

TOPICAL STEROIDS

Corticosteroid potency chart (in order of popularity)

Generic	Brand	Uses
High Potency (Class I, II)		
Fluocinonide 0.05% cream, ointment	Lidex	
Clobetasol 0.05% cream, ointment, solution	Temovate	
Clobetasol 0.05% foam	Olux	
Medium Potency (Classes III, IV, V) – *avoid using for more than 10 days*		
Triamcinolone 0.1% cream, ointment	Aristocort	
Hydrocortisone valerate 0.2% cream, ointment	Westcort	
Triamcinolone 0.025% cream; 0.015% spray	Aristocort	
Desonide 0.05% ointment	DesOwen	
Desonide 0.05% lotion	DesOwen	
Low Potency (Classes VI, VII)		
Hydrocortisone 1% cream	Westcort	Sensitive skin; eyelids; face; scrotum; intertriginous areas
Desonide 0.05% cream	DesOwen	
Fluocinolone 0.01% solution	Synalar	
Betamethasone 0.05% lotion	Bataloan	

Adapted from Steroids. Portland (OR): National Psoriasis Foundation; 1998.

Treatment Formulations

Formulation	Description / Indication
Cream	Water based; low occlusion risk; No greasy feel; best for hairy intertriginous areas and wet lesions
Ointment	Preferred for dry or scaly lesions; areas with thicker skin such as palms and soles, ↑skin hydration; avoid in intertriginous areas; considered to be the most potent
Lotion	Oil-in-water emulsion; good for scalp lesions

ACNE

- **Definition**[4]
  - Common skin disease characterized as a chronic inflammatory dermatosis composed of open and closed comedones (blackheads and whiteheads) and inflammatory lesions.
- **Overview**
  - Acne vulgaris is the most common of all skin disorders.
  - It is a chronic inflammatory process that affects the pilosebaceous unit
  - D/t recessive sebum production secondary to androgen stimulation
- **Physiology**
  - The primary lesion of acne vulgaris is the microcomedone
  - The closed comedo (whitehead) is the first visible acne lesion
  - The open comedo (blackhead) is a 0.1- to 3.0-mm noninflammatory lesion that looks like a black dot
- **Etiology**
  - The prevalent bacterium implicated in the inflammatory phase of acne is *Propionibacterium acnes (P acnes)*
- **Types and Progression**
  - Comedones (blackheads or whiteheads) → papules/pustules +/- inflammation → nodules/cysts (refer to Derm)
- **Grades/Classification**

- Grade 1 / Mild - Open and closed comedones (blackheads or whiteheads) with few inflammatory papules and pustules. The more oil builds up, the more likely it is that bacteria will multiply and lead to inflammatory acne. Acne is also considered to be "mild acne" if someone only has a few pimples, or only has small ones.
- Grade 2 / Moderate - Inflammatory lesions present as a small papule with erythema.
- Grade 3 / Moderately Severe - Numerous papules and pustules, and occasional inflamed nodules, also on chest and back
- Grade 4 / Severe - a lot of papules and pustules, as well as nodules on their skin. These nodules are often reddish and painful. The acne may lead to scarring.

- **DDx**
    - Rosacea (generally older than are acne patient)
    - Perioral dermatitis (most commonly in young adult women, clinically it is characterized by a combination of eczematous and acneiform features)
    - Hidradenitis suppurative, bacterial folliculitis, drug-induced acne, miliaria

Acne Treatment Options

Class	Options	Indication
Topical Retinoids	tretinoin (0.025-0.1% in cream, gel, or microsphere gel vehicles) (*Pregnancy Category C*)	Help address the development and maintenance of acne; monotherapy for primarily comedones acne
	adapalene (0.1% cream/gel/lotion, 0.3% cream (*Pregnancy Category C*)	S/E: peeling, dryness, erythema, irritation
	tazarotene (0.05%, 0.1% cream, gel or foam) (*Pregnancy Category X*)	
Topical Antibiotics	Clindamycin 1% solution or gel Erythromycin 2% cream, gel, lotion, pledget	Effective overall tx for mild/moderate **and should always be combined with benzoyl peroxide**
	Dapsone 5-7.5% applied BID for 6-12 months	Dapsone has no ↑ risk in G6PD deficiency pts. Best for pts with inflammatory acne.
Oral Antibiotics	Doxycycline 20mg BID or 40mg/d Minocycline ER 1mg/kg Azithromycin TMP-SMx	Effective for moderate/severe acne; good for those patients unresponsive to topical ABx
		Macrolides should be limited to pregnancy or young kids (<8) due to risk for bacterial resistance
Wash	Benzoyl Peroxide 5%	Decrease risk for bacterial resistance developing
		S/E: irritation, staining, dermatitis
Hormonal Agents	Spironolactone, OCP (w/ estrogen), Flutamide	Effective as alternative tx options
Salicylic Acid	0.5-2% strength 1-3x/d as tolerated	Leave on vs wash off preparations

- **Treatment (gels preferred over other vehicles)** [5,6]
    - Mild-moderate:
        - Use topical antibiotics (clindamycin and erythromycin) and benzoyl peroxide gels (2%, 5%, or 10%).
            - Best combined with benzoyl peroxide-erythromycin gels.
            - Benzoyl peroxide is effective in the prevention of bacterial resistance and is recommended for patients on topical or systemic antibiotic therapy
            - Always combine topical Abx with benzoyl peroxide

- Tretinoin cream (Retin-a 0.01% gel, 0.025% gel/cream, 0.1% cream qHS) + clindamycin lotion (1% applied nightly or twice daily) + OTC BPO (5% twice daily)
- Combination benzoyl peroxide topical clindamycin (BenzaClin) +/- Topical Retinoid
- Topical retinoids (retinoic acid, adapalene, tazarotene) require detailed instructions regarding gradual increases in concentration from 0.01% to 0.025% to 0.05% cream/gel or liquid.
  - Mild irritation may occur at the start of treatment (1-2 weeks)
  - Use pea-sized dose to apply thin layer to affected areas
  - Apply every other day for first 2-4 weeks (apply to face for 60 min then wash off), then apply a gentle, non-comedogenic moisturizer
- **Adapalene (Differin 0.1% cream, 0.3% gel qHS)** + clindamycin/BPO combination
- If not responsive after 3 months...
  - Add doxycycline (50-100 mg orally once or twice daily)
- Moderately Severe:
  - Add PO ABx to the above regimen. Limit duration to 3-4 months and always combine with topical retinoid!
    - Doxycycline, 50-100 mg twice daily, tapered to 50 mg/d as acne lessens.
    - Minocycline is most effective, 50-100 mg/d (beware risk for DRESS)
    - Use of oral isotretinoin in moderate acne **to prevent scarring** has become much more common and is effective.
      - Topical dapsone 5% recommended for inflammatory acne
  - Doxycycline + tretinoin cream + OTC BPO wash
  - Doxycycline + adapalene/BPO combination
  - If not responsive after 3 months...
    - refer to dermatology for Accutane
  - Topical dapsone 5% BID a good option for **inflammatory acne in patients who cannot tolerate benzoyl peroxide+Abx combination**. Be aware of patients with G6PD deficiency however trials did not suggest ↑ risk.
  - **Post inflammatory dyspigmentation** is best treated with azelaic acid
- Severe Acne
  - Indicated for: cystic or conglobate acne or for any other acne refractory to treatment.
  - Precautions:
    - Concurrent tetracycline and isotretinoin may cause pseudotumor cerebri
    - Determine blood lipids, transaminases (ALT, AST) before therapy.
  - Isotretinoin, 0.5-1 mg/kg given in divided doses with food.
    - Most patients clear within 20 weeks with 1 mg/kg.
    - Recent studies suggest that 0.5 mg/kg is equally effective.
  - **Photodynamic Therapy (PDT)**
    - MOA: With exposure to the visible spectrum of light and in the presence of oxygen, the activated photosensitizer then generates reactive oxygen species and may induce selective phototoxicity of the targeted sebaceous units.
    - Emerging treatment option for all stages of acne (inflammatory and non-inflammatory), still considered off-label
    - An additional therapy option the standard acne regimen for patients with mild acne who are not responding to topical retinoids and benzyl peroxide, or in patients with moderate acne who cannot tolerate or do not respond to oral antibacterial or hormonal therapies
    - S/E: transient hyperpigmentation, erythema, swelling
- Post Inflammatory Dyspigmentation
  - Add azelaic acid

- o Hormonal
  Suspect in females with irregular periods with cyclic acne
  - Topical retinoin + combined OCP (must contain estrogen; options include Yaz, Yasmine. Avoid Sronyx)
    - OCP: ethinyl estradiol/ norgestimate, ethinyl estradiol/norethindrone acetate/ferrous fumarate, ethinyl estradiol/drospirenone, and ethinyl estradiol/drospirenone/levomefolate
  - If not responsive after 3 months...
    - add Aldactone
  - If not responsive after 3 months...
    - reassess

Acne Treatment by Severity

Severity	Almost Clear	Mild	Moderate	Severe
First Line Treatment	Benzoyl Peroxide -or- Topical Retinoid -or- Topical combination therapy (BP+TPAx/retinoid)	Benzoyl Peroxide plus Topical Retinoid (start 1-2x/week then ↑ to daily as tolerated)	Topical Combination tx > BP+TABx > BP + TR > TR+BP+TABx -or- Oral Abx (Doxy) +TR+BP	Oral Abx (Doxy)+BP+TR -or- Isotretinoin (if risk of scarring high)
Second Line Treatments (if failure after 3 months)	Benzoyl Peroxide plus Topical Retinoid	Add TR or BP (if not on already) -or- PO Abx (doxycycline) + BP + TR	Consider alternative combination therapy -or- PO Isotretinoin -or- Add combined OCP or PO Spironolactone (females)	Consider PO isotretinoin

Maintenance Therapy
> Tretinoin or adapalene or BP daily
> OCP in women with acne options: must contain levonorgestrel such as Mirena (second line would be norgestimate such as Ortho-Tri cyclin)

ABx = antibiotic TABx = topical antibiotic BP = benzoyl peroxide OCP = oral contraceptive TR = topical retinoid

Pharmacologic Treatment of Acne

Name	Indication	Dosage	S/E
Topical Retinoid			
Adapalene	Mild/moderate	• Cream, lotion (0.1%) • Gel (0.3%) • Adapalene/benzoyl peroxide (Epiduo) gel (0.1%/2.5%)	• Local erythema • peeling • dryness • pruritus • stinging
Tazarotene	Mild/moderate	Cream, gel (0.05%, 0.1%)	
Tretinoin (Retin-A)	Mild/moderate	• Cream (0.025%, 0.1%) • Gel (0.01%, 0.025%, 0.05%) • Microsphere gel (0.04%, 0.1%)	
Combination (Adapalene/Benzoyl Peroxide) Epiduo	Moderate	• Adapalene 0.3% • Benzoyl Peroxide 0.025%	
Topical Antibiotics			
Clindamycin	Mild/moderate	• Foam, gel, lotion, solution (1.0%) • Clindamycin/benzoyl peroxide (BenzaClin) gel (1%/5%, 1.2%/2.5%) • Clindamycin/tretinoin gel (Veltin, Ziana; 1.2%/0.025%)	Local erythema, peeling, dryness, pruritus, burning, oiliness
Erythromycin	Mild/moderate (can be considered in pregnancy)	• Gel, solution, ointment (2%) • Erythromycin/benzoyl peroxide (Benzamycin) gel (3%/5%)	
Other Topicals			
Benzoyl Peroxide	Mild/moderate	Bar, cream, gel, lotion, pad, wash (2.5% to 10%)	
Dapsone	Mild/moderate	Gel (Aczone, 5%)	
Oral Antibiotics			
Advised not to use for longer than 3 months			
Doxycycline/ Minocycline	Moderate	50-100mg/d or BID	Photosensitivity, esophagitis, hepatotoxicity
Erythromycin	Moderate	250-500mg BID or QID	GI sx
Isotretinoin			
Isotretinoin	Severe	0.5 to 1.0 mg per kg per day for about 20 weeks, or a cumulative dose of 120 mg per kg (see comment to right)	Patients with moderate acne may respond to lower dosages (0.3 mg per kg per day) and experience fewer adverse effects.

COMMON SKIN CONDITIONS

- **Acne** *(see above)*
- **Seborrheic Dermatitis**[7]
  - Characterized by redness and scaling and occurring in regions where the sebaceous glands are most active, such as the face and scalp
  - Management
    - First-line:
      - Clobetasol 0.05% TID/QID
      - Desonide 0.05% cream on face 2-3x/week
      - Ketoconazole topical 2% shampoo; lather can be used on face and chest during shower.
      - Ketoconazole topical 2% to face 2/3x/week
    - Alternative
      - 1% or 2.5% hydrocortisone cream
      - In more resistant cases → clobetasol propionate, 2% ketoconazole cream, 1% pimecrolimus cream, and 0.03% or 0.1% tacrolimus ointment
      - Pimecrolimus, 1% cream, is very beneficial
- **Atopic Dermatitis**
  - Overview
    - Dry skin and pruritus; consequent rubbing leads to increased inflammation and lichenification and to further itching and scratching: *itch-scratch cycle*.
    - Eczema is the itch that rashes
    - Predilection for the flexures, front and sides of the neck, eyelids, forehead, face, wrists, and dorsa of the feet and hands
  - Labs
    - Cultures to include bacterial (staph), viral (HSV), IgE, ↑eos, HSV antigen
  - Management
    - Dilute bleach baths (may ↓ severity after 6 weeks)
    - Topical steroids:
      - Corticosteroids
      - Pimecrolimus
      - Tacrolimus
    - Baseline therapy of dryness with emollients
    - Oral and topical antibiotics to eliminate *S. aureus*
    - Hydroxyzine 10-100mg QID to suppress pruritus
    - UVA-UVB phototherapy
- **Stasis Dermatitis**
  - Often due to chronic venous insufficiency
  - Symptoms
    - Pain (aching, cramping, heaviness, ↓ w/walking)
    - Edema
    - Venous dilation
    - Erythema & serosanguinous seepage
    - Brawny discoloration
    - Ulcerations most often seen at the medial malleoli
  - Treatment
    - Sequential compression therapy
    - Elevation (20-30m TID to QID)
    - Impact of intermittent pneumatic devices is unclear
    - ASA improves ulcer healing process

DERMATOLOGY

- **Perioral Dermatitis**
  - Age of Onset: 16-45 years; can occur in children and the old.
  - Females predominantly
  - 1- to 2-mm erythematous papulopustules on an erythematous background irregularly grouped, symmetric.
  - Perioral distribution with rim of sparing around the vermilion border of lips
  - Management:
    - *Topical*:
      - Metronidazole, 0.75% gel two times daily or 1% once daily; erythromycin, 2% gel applied twice daily.
      - Avoid topical glucocorticoids
    - *Systemic*
      - Minocycline or doxycycline, 100 mg daily until clear, then 50 mg daily for another 2 months or Tetracycline, 500 mg twice daily until clear, then 500 mg daily for 1 month, then 250 mg daily for an additional month.

SKIN BIOPSY

Biopsies for different conditions[a]

Indication	Clinical presentation	Possible diagnosis	Biopsy technique
Diagnosis	Rashes or blisters involving dermis	Drug reaction, cutaneous lymphoma, deep tissue infection, erythema multiforme, Kaposi sarcoma, lupus erythematosus, pemphigoid, pemphigus, vasculitis	Partial/perilesional punch
	Processes Involving the subcutis	Erythema nodosum, panniculitis	Elliptical excision; saucerization
Diagnosis and treatment	Atypical moles and pigmented lesions	Dysplastic nevi, malignant melanoma	Elliptical excision, saucerization, punch for 1- to 4-mm lesions with 1- to 3-mm margins

- **Procedure**
  - Shave
    1. Obtain consent.
    2. Clean skin.
    3. Anesthetize skin.
    4. Superficial shave:
       - For macular or raised nonsuspicious lesions, hold blade parallel to the skin and shallowly remove a thin disk or the lesion itself, if raised
    5. Saucerization:
       - For pigmented lesions, measure a 1- to 3-mm margin before shaving
       - Anesthetize, creating a wheal to make the lesion easier to shave and squeeze skin between the thumb and forefinger of the nondominant hand to further elevate the lesion.

- Hold blade at a 45-degree angle to the skin, bend or bow the blade depending on the width of lesion, and remove a disk of tissue well into the subcutaneous fat
- If a nidus of pigment remains after saucerization, a punch or elliptical biopsy must be performed, and the sample sent in the same specimen container.
- Use a hemostatic agent or electrocautery and wipe clean.

6. Dress with petrolatum and instruct the patient to keep the area moist and covered for at least one week to minimize scarring.
7. Cauterization with **Drysol**

Bibliography

[4] Zaenglein, A. L., Pathy, A. L., Schlosser, B. J., Alikhan, A., Baldwin, H. E., Berson, D. S., ... Bhushan, R. (2016). Guidelines of care for the management of acne vulgaris. Journal of the American Academy of Dermatology, 74(5), 945–973.e33. doi:10.1016/j.jaad.2015.12.037
[5] Titus et al. "Diagnosis and Treatment of Acne." Am Fam Physician. 2012;86(8):734-740.
[6] Leyden et al. "Why Topical Retinoids Are Mainstay of Therapy for Acne." Dermatol Ther (Heidelb): 25 APR 2017.
[7] Wolff K, Johnson R, Saavedra AP. *Fitzpatrick's Color Atlas and Synopsis of Clinical Dermatology, 7e.* New York, NY: McGraw-Hill; 2013
[8] Alguire PC, Mathes BM. Skin biopsy techniques for the internist. J Gen Intern Med. 1998;13(1):47

GASTROENTEROLOGY

Approach to abdominal pain 29
Ascites 29
Gallbladder Disorders 33
Cirrhosis 35
Irritable Bowel Syndrome 40
Constipation 41
Colon Cancer 43
Diarrhea 44
Diverticulitis 52
Dysphagia 53
GI Bleed 54
Acute Pancreatitis 60
Bowel Obstruction 66
GERD 67
Peptic Ulcer Disease 69
Elevated liver Associated Enzymes 71
Non-Alcoholic Fatty Liver Disease 75

GASTROENTEROLOGY

APPROACH TO ABDOMINAL PAIN

Immediate Approach
- Characterize pain: Location, acute or chronic, constant or intermittent, relation to eating, associated sxs such as fever, nausea, vomiting, dysuria, change in bowel habits
- Previous abd surgeries?
- <u>Labs</u>: CBC, BMP, UA, LFTs, lipase, hCG, lactate, low threshold to evaluate for AAA w/ bedside US & ACS w/ EKG

Differential Diagnosis of Abdominal Pain[9]

Right Upper Quadrant[10]	Epigastric	Left Upper Quadrant
Cholecystitis	Peptic ulcer disease	Splenic infarct
Cholangitis	Gastritis	Splenic rupture
Pancreatitis	GERD	Splenic abscess
Pneumonia/empyema	Pancreatitis	Gastritis
Pleurisy/pleurodynia	Myocardial infarction	Gastric ulcer
Subdiaphragmatic abscess	Pericarditis	Pancreatitis
Hepatitis	Ruptured aortic aneurysm	Subdiaphragmatic abscess
Budd-Chiari syndrome	Esophagitis	
Right Lower Quadrant	**Periumbilical**	**Left Lower Quadrant**
Appendicitis	Early appendicitis	Diverticulitis
Salpingitis	Gastroenteritis	Salpingitis
Inguinal hernia	Bowel obstruction	Inguinal hernia
Ectopic pregnancy	Ruptured aortic aneurysm	Ectopic pregnancy
Nephrolithiasis		Nephrolithiasis
Inflammatory bowel disease		Irritable bowel syndrome
Mesenteric lymphadenitis		Inflammatory bowel disease
Typhlitis		
Diffuse Nonlocalized Pain		
Gastroenteritis		
Mesenteric ischemia (↑lipase, amylase)		
Bowel obstruction		
Irritable bowel syndrome		
Peritonitis		
Diabetes		
Malaria		
Constipation		
IBD		
Familial Mediterranean fever		
Metabolic diseases		
Psychiatric disease		

ASCITES

- **Pathophysiology**[11]
  - Cirrhosis and portal hypertension lead to nitrous oxide (NO) development which causes splanchnic vasodilation. The dilation leads to:
    1) Arterial under filling causing the heart to respond by ↑CO and ↑plasma volume. To do this, it:

GASTROENTEROLOGY

- a. Stimulates renin-angiotensin-aldosterone system→renal Na and water retention is then caused. This retention is a part of what causes ascites.
- 2) Increase in the splanchnic pressure (hepatic sinusoids and vessels) which ↑ lymph accumulation. That accumulation of lymph is what causes ascites to develop.
- 3) 3 most common causes of ascites in the US are (1) cirrhosis (2) malignancy and (3) heart failure
- Clinical signs and symptoms
  - Medium/large volume ascites can be detected on physical exam generally by:
    - Distended abdomen
    - shifting dullness
    - fluid wave
    - bulging flanks
    - Abdominal pain may be due to hepatic congestion (in CHF) or hepatitis d/t EtOH or Budd-Chiari (portal vein thrombosis). Can also be concerning for SBP in acute cases esp. if coexistent fever.
    - Flank dullness to percussion
    - Chronic stigmata: palmar erythema, peripheral wasting, gynecomastia, spider angiomata
- Staging
  - 1: ascites is only detectable with US
  - 2: ascites is moderate with some abdominal distention; treat with diuretics and 2g sodium restriction
  - 3: massive ascites with marked abdominal distention; treat as above with diuresis, Na restriction, therapeutic paracentesis, and consider TIPS
- Hospitalized Patients[12]
  - 2012 American Association for the Study of Liver Diseases guidelines recommend diagnostic paracentesis in all patients who are hospitalized with cirrhosis and ascites to evaluate for spontaneous bacterial peritonitis (SBP).
  - Paracentesis within 1 day of hospital admission is associated with lower inpatient mortality and fewer readmissions.
- Workup
  - New onset: needs diagnostic paracentesis to determine cause (even if admitted for other reason). Can be therapeutic and diagnostic.
    - Send ascitic fluid for:
      1. Cell count and differential
      2. Albumin (also send serum albumin)
      3. Total protein (<1g/dl increases risk of SBP)
         - Optional:
           - Culture in blood culture bottles
           - Glucose
           - LDH
           - Amylase
           - Gram stain
           - Cytology
           - AFB
  - If you suspect ascites but none is apparent on physical exam, get an abdominal ultrasound to detect fluid and mark ascites for paracentesis
    - Add Doppler to evaluate the portal vein for patency, masses, and LAD
  - Looking for infected ascites is part of the workup in a patient with cirrhosis and fever/leukocytosis/altered mental status.
    - PMN>250

GASTROENTEROLOGY

Differential Diagnosis based on SAAG value

SAAG	
High gradient ≥ 1.1 g/dl	**Low gradient < 1.1 g/dl**
Fluid is coming from the liver sinusoid due to a high pressure and volume gradient	Albumin levels in serum are nearly equal to the ascitic fluid. Denotes ascites is from extra-hepatic source
• Etiology: Portal HTN	• Nephrotic syndrome
• Cirrhosis (often low ascitic total protein level <2.5)	• Peritoneal carcinomatosis (high ascitic total protein)
• Alcoholic hepatitis	• Pancreatic ascites
• RCHF (elevated ascitic total protein ≥2.5)	• Tuberculous peritonitis
• pHTN	• Biliary ascites
• Budd-Chiari syndrome	• Collagen vascular disease serositis
• Massive hepatic metastases	• Infection
• Veno-occlusive disease	• Malignancy
• Portal vein thrombosis	
• Fatty liver of pregnancy	

- **Etiologies**
  - Classification by serum ascites albumin gradient (SAAG= serum albumin – ascites albumin)
    >95% accuracy

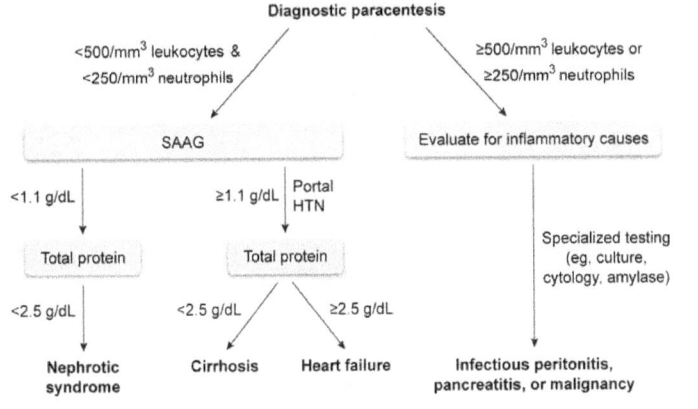

Figure. Flow chart in the evaluation of ascites

Child-Turcotte-Pugh Scoring[13]

Assesses the prognosis (and priority/need for liver transplantation) of chronic liver disease and cirrhosis

	1 point	2 point	3 point
Ascites	Absent	Nontense	Tense
Encephalopathy	Absent	Grades 1-2	Grades 3-4
Bilirubin (mg/dl)	<2.0	2-3	>3.0
Albumin (mg/dl)	>3.5	2.8-3.5	<2.8
Pt (sec over normal)	1-3	4-6	>6
Classification			
Score	Class	1-5-yr survival	
5-6	A	95%	

7-9	B	75%
10-15	C	50%

MELD Na Score[14,15]

Used with CP score to determine priority for liver transplantation
MELD-Na = MELD Score - Na - 0.025 x MELD x (140-Na) + 140

MELD-Na Score	90-day mortality
<17	<2%
17-20	3-4%
21-22	7-10%
23-26	14-15%
27-31	27-32%
≥32	65-66%

- **Treatment**
  - See staging above
  - Salt restriction
  - Fluid restriction (free water <1L/d)
  - Therapeutic Paracentesis
    - Indicated in Stage 2 ascites and above
    - Large volume paracentesis (LVP) is defined as removing ≥5L at one time.
      1. The most common complication is paracentesis-induced circulatory dysfunction (PICD).
      2. Treatment: 50g of 25% albumin for first **5L** removed then another 25g for next 5L not to exceed 100g of albumin). It should be given **during** LVP.
  - Diuretic Sensitive
    - Consider therapeutic paracentesis if tense ascites noted (will req 5L removal)
      1. Large volume paracentesis (≥5L) should be combined with albumin 6-8g per L removed
    - SAAG > 1.1
      1. **If Na < 120 mEq/L**
         - Fluid restriction
         - Hypertonic Saline
         - Vasopressin Receptor Antagonists
      2. **If Na >120 mEq/L**
         - Lasix (40mg, BID in AM and at 3pm; max 160mg), spironolactone 100mg (max 400mg), salt restriction (<2g/day)
           - Increase diuretics q1w with maintenance of the 40:100 ratio to maintain normokalaemia. If ↓K, then avoid Lasix and give spironolactone alone.
         - Max spironolactone: 400mg; max furosemide: 160mg
         - **If hypotension develops, administer Midodrine and consider TIPS or liver transplantation**
      3. Cease alcohol if applicable
    - SAAG < 1.1
      1. **Not due to cardiac or intrinsic liver pathology**
      2. Do not respond to salt restriction and diuretics
    - Start referral for liver transplant
    - Avoid NSAIDs
  - Diuretic Resistant/Refractory Ascites
    - Unresponsive to sodium restriction and high dose diuretics (>400mg spironolactone; furosemide 160mg) or ascites that reoccurs after paracentesis
    - Options

1. Serial therapeutic paracentesis
2. Liver transplant
3. **TIPS**[16]
   - Indications
     - Acute bleeding refractory to endoscopic therapy
   - Workout prior to referral for a TIPS includes:
     - CBC, T&C, Coombs, BMP, LFT, Coag panel
     - Doppler US liver to ensure portal and hepatic veins are patent
     - TTE to evaluate pulmonary pressures and R heart function
   - Contraindications include CHF, severe TR, severe PHTN, active hepatic encephalopathy, severe liver failure, and polycystic liver disease.
- Spontaneous Bacterial Peritonitis (see page 39)

GALLBLADDER DISORDERS

- **Types**
  - Cholecystitis
  - Cholelithiasis
  - Choledocholithiasis
  - Cholangitis
- **Cholecystitis**
  - Types (most common)
    - Calculous (gallstone) - obstruction of the cystic duct by gallstone
    - Acalculous cholecystitis - occurs as a result of bile stasis and gallbladder ischemia that can be complicated by enteric bacterial infection in critically ill patients and associated with higher rate of mortality than in calculous causes
  - Risk Factors
    - Gallstones
    - EtOH
    - In acalculous specifically, factors include trauma, shock, burns, sepsis, TPN and/or prolonged fasting, cardiac and aortic surgery, and vasculitis.
  - Clinical presentation
    - RUQ/epigastric abdominal pain, nausea and vomiting, fever.
    - Murphy's sign (inspiratory arrest on deep palpation of the RUQ).
    - Systemic inflammatory markers such as fever, leukocytosis, ↑CRP are highly suggestive of acute cholecystitis.
  - Diagnostics
    - ↑WBC
    - May or may not have abnormal liver function tests.
    - RUQ ultrasound shows thickened gallbladder wall, pericholecystic fluid, and sonographic Murphy sign.
    - HIDA (hepatobiliary iminodiacetic acid scan-most sensitive, can be used when the symptoms suggest cholecystitis, but sonogram is normal.
  - Treatment
    - NPO, IV fluids, IV antibiotics with gram-negative and anaerobic coverage (monotherapy with a beta-lactam or beta-lactamase or combination therapy with a third-generation cephalosporin plus metronidazole)
    - General surgery consult → cholecystectomy
      - Emergent cholecystectomy is indicated and suspected gallbladder perforation or emphysematous cholecystitis (infection of the gallbladder wall with gas-forming organism such as *Clostridium perfringens*).
    - *Surgical candidates*

- Early laparoscopic cholecystectomy within 24 hours of hospital admission was shown to be superior to the conservative approach concerning morbidity and cause.
- Had conversion rate that was lower in duration of hospital stay therefore shorter[17]
- For acalculous cause, cholecystostomy and/or cholecystectomy advised
- Non-surgical candidates
    - Patients were deemed high risk for surgery and who respond to antibiotics can be reassessed at a later time to determine if there surgical risk is decreased.
    - In patients who are not good candidates for cholecystectomy and do not respond to antibiotics, percutaneous cholecystostomy tube or endoscopic drainage can be pursued for calculous cholecystitis.
    - In acalculous causes, when neither cholecystostomy nor cholecystectomy can be performed, direct ERCP with GB drainage can be attempted to assist decompression.
- **Cholelithiasis**[18]
  - General
    - Types of stones
      - Most are cholesterol
      - Pigment gallstones - seen in hemolysis, cirrhosis, chronic biliary infection.
      - Black pigment stones can be seen in chronic hemolysis.
      - Brown pigment stones typically develop an obstructed and infected bile ducts.
  - Risk factors - genetic, age > 50, obesity, pregnancy, medications (OCPs, octreotide, ceftriaxone, HRT in post-menopausal women), prolonged TPN, rapid weight loss, diseases of terminal ileum which resulted in decreased resorption of bile acids.
    - Obesity increases bile stasis and cholesterol saturation.
    - Rapid weight loss – such as after bariatric surgery, occurs from decreased caloric intake→bile stasis, while lipolysis increases cholesterol mobilization→secretion into the gall bladder. This results in bile supersaturation with cholesterol → gall stone formation
  - Complications
    - Acute cholecystitis
    - Chronic cholecystitis
    - Choledocholithiasis
    - Acute cholangitis
    - Acute biliary pancreatitis
    - Empyema-gallbladder
    - Choledochoduodenal fistula
    - Gallbladder perforation
  - Clinical Presentation
    - Can be asymptomatic or symptomatic.
    - Biliary colic - episodic right upper quadrant/epigastric abdominal pain with or without radiation to scapula. Associated with nausea. Precipitated by fatty foods. Symptom onset more than an hour after eating or in the late evening at night also very strongly suggests biliary pain.
  - Diagnosis
    - RUQ ultrasound - can show gall stones greater than 5 mm. Should be performed after fasting for at least 8 hours to ensure distended bile filled gallbladder.
  - Treatment
    - Asymptomatic - no treatment unless:
      - Porcelain gall bladder, gall stones >3mm, gall bladder polyp >1 cm, pts with primary sclerosing cholangitis, gall bladder adenomas or polyps > 1cm in size or anomaly of pancreatic duct drainage.
    - Symptomatic
      - Cholecystectomy recommended
  - Prevention

- Healthy lifestyle and food, physical activity and maintenance of normal body weight not only prevent gall stones bur also reduce the risk of symptoms due to gall stones.
- In specific situations that are associated with rapid weight loss (such as bariatric surgery) temporary ursodeoxycholic acid ≥ 500 mg per day until stable is an evidence based prevention of gall stones.
- **Choledocholithiasis**
  - Defined: gall stone in the common bile duct.
  - Cause - stones in the common bile duct migrate from the cystic duct to the gallbladder. Less commonly, primary duct stones forming the duct due to biliary stasis.
  - Complications - obstruction of CBD with bile stones→bile flow disruption→jaundice
  - Clinical presentation
    - Can be asymptomatic or present with RUQ/epigastric pain, jaundice, pruritus, nausea.
  - Diagnosis/Diagnostics
    - ↑Bilirubin, RUQ ultrasound may show dilated bile duct > 6 mm and stones within the common bile duct.
    - MRCP and ERCP are both recommended as highly accurate test for identifying CBD stones among patients with an intermediate probability of disease.
  - Treatment
    - ERCP and stone extraction followed by cholecystectomy within 6 weeks if no contraindication
    - Removing the gallbladder does not completely eliminate the risk of bile duct stones, as stones can remain or recur after surgery.
- **Acute cholangitis**
  - Defined - obstruction of the common bile duct, usually by gallstone or may be due to malignancy, biliary stricture, infection.
  - Clinical presentation - Fever, RUQ abdominal pain, jaundice (Charcot's triad), altered mentation, shock (Reynold's Pentad) .
  - Diagnosis/Diagnostics
    - RUQ ultrasound,
    - ERCP
    - Percutaneous transhepatic cholangiogram if ERCP cannot be performed
  - Treatment
    - IV antibiotic therapy
    - Urgent ERCP with sphincterotomy with or without biliary stent.

CIRRHOSIS

- **Pathophysiology**[19]
  - Prolonged period of persistent liver inflammation, extracellular matrix remodeling and persistent deposition of collagen in the liver tissue leading to fibrosis.
  - This fibrosis together with focal hyperplasia and proliferation of hepatocytes eventually disrupts the hepatic architecture leading to regenerative nodules seen on imaging/biopsy.
- **Types**[20,21]
  - Compensated – disease stage that precedes complications. No ascites, encephalopathy, or variceal bleeds. Can be sub divided into those with or without *varices*, and those with or without *portal hypertension*.
  - Decompensated – first occurrence of *complications* such as: encephalopathy, variceal bleeds (see page 39), hepatorenal syndrome, ascites present.

GASTROENTEROLOGY

- *Early complications*- ascites, edema, GE varices
  - Should have screening EGD for varices
    - **Variceal Prophylaxis**
      - <u>Cirrhosis without varices</u> = no BB; EGD q2-3y or q1y if decompensated
      - <u>Small nonbleeding varices</u> = no BB; EGD q1-2y if compensated and yearly if decompensated
      - <u>Medium/Large varices</u> = EVL or BB; q1y EGD
      - <u>Small varices with red whale sign or decompensated cirrhosis</u> = BB with yearly EGD
- *Late complications* – jaundice, coagulopathy, bacterial infections, recurrent bleeding, hepatic encephalopathy, refractory ascites, or evidence of HRS; should be considered for immediate liver transplant.
  - Often evidence of loss of function → ↑INR, ↓PLT, jaundice, ↓albumin
- **Etiologies**
  - Alcoholism
  - Hepatitis C
  - AIH
  - NASH
  - Inherited: Hemochromatosis, Wilson, Alpha-1
  - Hepatitis B
- **History**
  - Known cirrhosis? AST/PLT >2 indicative of likely cirrhosis (Lok index; Bonacini score)
  - Melena?
  - Any new recent medications (i.e. narcotics, NSAIDS, blood thinners)
  - Infectious symptoms?
- **Physical Exam**
  - If non-acute: look for palmar erythema, spider angioma
  - Fluid wave
  - HJR
  - Clubbing
  - Muscle wasting
  - Hepatosplenomegaly
  - Flap test (for asterixis)
- **Labs/Work-up**
  - LFTs: ↑bilirubin, ↑PT/INR, ↓albumin, +/- ↑AST/ALT (AST>ALT late), ↑ALP
    - INR not representative of true bleeding risk; correcting does not ↓risk
  - H/H
    - Anemia likely 2/2 to splenomegaly, hemolysis, IDA, bone marrow suppression, folate deficiency
    - Neutropenia in setting of hypersplenism
    - Thrombocytopenia due to hypersplenism, EtOH toxicity, ↓TPO production
  - CMP
    - Sodium (↓ level suggests HRS; level due to ↑ADH)
  - ↑Ferritin due to release from hepatocytes
  - RUQ US with portal flow
    - Evaluate liver size, echotexture, r/o HCC, check for ascites, establish patency of vasculature
    - Portal flow of ≥10 mmHg a strong predictor of progression to decompensation
  - Paracentesis (diagnostic with 2-3L removal to r/o infection; do therapeutic only if non-septic appearing; see *Ascites* section on page 32 for more details)
  - FibroScan or FibroSure to assess for fibrosis
  - EtOH
  - HCV Ab, HBs Ag, anti-HBs, HBeAg, HCV genotype

- o Antinuclear or Anti-smooth muscle Ab (r/o AIH)
- o NH3/Ammonia – only obtain in patients with encephalopathy of unknown etiology (no known cirrhosis) or ALF due to Tylenol
- **Prognostic Tools**
  - o Overview
    - Scoring mechanisms prognosticate survival over a longer time scale--months to years--rather than days to weeks.
    - They are not useful for prognosticating acute complications in the cirrhotic patient.
  - o Child-Pugh Score - used to broadly summarize functional status in the non-acute setting.
  - o MELD - prognosticates mortality over a *three-month course*.
  - o CLIF – the only acute prognosticating score tool; mostly used in the ICU to assess the likelihood of improving clinical status with continued intervention.
- **Complications**
  - o Acute on Chronic Liver Failure – rapid onset of failure of the liver/extra hepatic organs (including kidneys) due to acute decompensation with concurrent ascites, encephalopathy, GI bleed, and/or bacterial infxn.
    - Most commonly occurs in those with prior history of decompensation
    - High short-term mortality (1 month)
  - o PHTN → Ascites, variceal hemorrhage, and portal vein thrombosis (high suspicion if fever, abdominal pain, lower extremity edema) → tx with anti coag
  - o Infection → might not mount fever or leukocytosis
  - o ↑INR → does not respond to Vitamin K
  - o SBP
  - o Hepatorenal syndrome (look for ↓Na)
  - o Variceal hemorrhage
    - Screening[22]
      - All patients diagnosed with cirrhosis should have screening EGD.
      - If initial endoscopy shows no varices, then re-evaluation can be done in 2-3 years
    - Grading
      - Small (<5mm) → Repeat endoscopy q1-2y
      - Large (>5mm) → Repeat endoscopy in 1 year
      - Presence of 'red whale' or 'spots' is considered high risk for bleeding events. Other high-risk features include alcohol abuse, decompensated liver failure. These patients should also have repeat endoscopy on a **yearly** basis
    - Prophylaxis
      - Nonselective BB (propranolol, nadolol), see below for dosing
      - Endoscopic variceal ligation (EVL) in combination with BB is best
  - o Hepatic encephalopathy
    - Graded by West Haven criteria or GCS

Encephalopathy Grading	
Grade 0	Abnormal psychometric tests but no obvious abnormalities in consciousness, personality, or behavior
Grade 1	Trivial lack of awareness, short attention span, reversed day-night sleep cycle
Grade 2	Lethargy, disorientation, personality change, inappropriate behavior
Grade 3	Somnolence to semistupor, confusion, response to noxious stimuli preserved
Grade 4	Coma; no response to noxious stimuli

- Precipitating Causes
  - Drugs (benzodiazepines, sedatives, narcotics, not using lactulose)

- ↓Volume (bleeding, diarrhea, vomiting, diuretics)
- ↑Nitrogen (GIB, constipation, ↑protein)
- ↓K, MetAlk
- ↓O2 ↓gluc
- Infection (PNA, UTI, SBP)
- Shunting (surgical, thrombosis, malignancy)
- Labs
    - Ammonia level not helpful, diagnosis is clinically based
    - CMP
    - LFT
    - Cx
    - UDS
- **Management**[23]
    - Compensated Cirrhosis
        - Nonselective B-blocker
            - Choices
                - Propranolol 20-40mg PO BID and increase by 20mg/BID steps q2-3d until target HR of 55-60, SBP>90)
                    - Max dose: 320mg/d for compensated, 160mg/d for decompensated
                - Nadolol 20-40mg PO/d and increase by 20mg/d q2-3d until HR of 55-60, SBP>90)
                    - Max dose: 160mg/d for compensated, 80mg/d for decompensated
                - Carvedilol 6.25mg/d and increase after 3d to BID dosing
                    - Max dose: 12.5mg/d
            - May held prevent first bleeding or rebleeding of oesophageal varices
        - Vasopressor: midodrine 7.5mg PO TID to ↑BP, improve renal perfusion, convert from diuretic resistant to sensitive
    - Pain
        - Avoid NSAIDs
        - Tylenol at max 2g/d
    - Ascites
        - Diuretics started with minimal or moderate volume ascites
            - Start with Spironolactone 50mg/d QAM (or divided BID up to 400mg/d)
                - Morning doses will ↓ need for PM urination
                - If $U_k \geq 60$ mEq/L → ↑dose of spironolactone
            - Add Lasix 20mg/QAM for each 50mg/d of spironolactone if further diuresis requested, max 160mg/d
                - Increasing AM dose will be more effective than a BID/split dose
                - If $U_{Na} \leq 20$ mEq/L → ↑dose of Lasix
        - Newer data suggests potentially benefit of albumin in those with persistent ascites despite diuresis (albumin 40g 2x/week for 2 weeks then 40g/w for 18 months total) *(ANSWER study)*
    - DVT Prophylaxis
        - If no active bleed present, okay to use enoxaparin or heparin for PLT>50k
    - Decompensated/Ascites (see separate section on page 29)
        - ↓sodium diet (≤2g)→compliance leads to ↓diuretics and ↓ascites
        - 2 L fluid restriction (if Na ≤ 125)
        - Lasix 40mg and spironolactone 100mg
        - Lack of response to above → TIPS or therapeutic paracentesis
    - Encephalopathy
        - Stop sedatives
        - Lactulose (start at 25cc/1-2h until 2 BM then maintain at 10-30g/BID to QID to have 2-3 BM (↓absorption of NH3)

- Use enema if patient obtunded
- Consider combination of lactulose+PEG 4L PO/NG over 4h
- Alternatives:
  - Rifaximin 550mg BID (broad spectrum against G+, G-, and anaerobes to ↓ production of NH3)
    - *Not routinely used, but can be considered: neomycin 1-2g/d divided)*
  - *Alternative: metronidazole 250mg BID*
- Limit protein intake to 1.2-1.5 g/kg/d, ↑vegetable intake if persistent encephalopathy
- Diet: limit weight loss to ≤1 kg/d (or if mild edema present, then limit is 0.5kg/d)
- Bacterial Peritonitis[24]
  - *Spontaneous*: acute ascites infection
  - *Secondary*: rare; one of two causes include perforated viscus (consider if 2+ organisms on cx) vs. walled abscess without perforation. 2/2 bacterial translocation (*E.coli, s. viridans, s. aureus*). Causes include perforated organ, appendicitis, cholecystitis, mesenteric ischemia, etc.
  - Use **Runyon's** criteria to distinguish between secondary and spontaneous bacterial peritonitis.
  - Inoculate a blood culture vial with the ascitic fluid, and send it for fluid culture
    - Diagnosed when ascitic PMN count is ≥ 250 with symptoms of fever, abdominal pain, general malaise, loss of appetite, nausea, and/or vomiting.
  - Treat with cefotaxime 2g IV daily + albumin @ 1.5 g/kg on admission and 1 g/kg on day 3
    - Alternative to cefotaxime is Augmentin 1.2g QID x5 days
  - Upon discharge, should take secondary prophylaxis for life (Ciprofloxacin 500mg/d)
- Variceal bleed
  - *Acute Bleed*
    - Initial Management
      - Give octreotide and prophylactic antibiotics immediately for 4-7d (see below)
      - Fluid resuscitation (0.9NS) ideally through large bore (18G) x2
        - Aggressive hydration can be detrimental as it may increase portal pressures
      - CBC, T&C with consideration of blood transfusion to keep HGB 7-9
      - INR to ensure correction of concomitant coagulopathy (i.e. FFP)
        - Transfusion of FFP may lead to decrease coagulation in up to 1/3 of cirrhotics[25]
      - PLT to ensure treatment of thrombocytopenia
      - PPI (IV vs. PO) not very helpful except to prevent ulcers s/p banding
      - Nonselective beta blocker (propranolol 20mg BID or nadolol 40mg daily) after patients are hemodynamically stable (SBP>90). Avoid in patients with refractory ascites.
      - IV Octreotide 50mcg IV bolus f/b 25-50mcg/hr. infusion x3-5d
      - IV ABx (Ceftriaxone 1g q24h x7d; alternatives: IV ciprofloxacin 750mg/week or PO norfloxacin 400mg BID x 7d)
    - Upper Endoscopy (within 12 hours of admission)
      - Controlled with above interventions? Stop
      - Uncontrolled with above interventions? Balloon tamponade → TIPS (see page 33)
        - Balloon tamponade can be utilized in patients who do not respond to endoscopic therapy (should not be maintained for more than 24 hours) but rather as an adjunct to TIPS vs. repeat endoscopy
    - TIPS

- *Indications:* ↑ hepatic venous pressure gradients, ↑↑pHTN (>20 mmHg) or a Childs B or C cirrhotic who is still bleeding after banding.

Figure. Management flow chart for suspected variceal hemorrhage

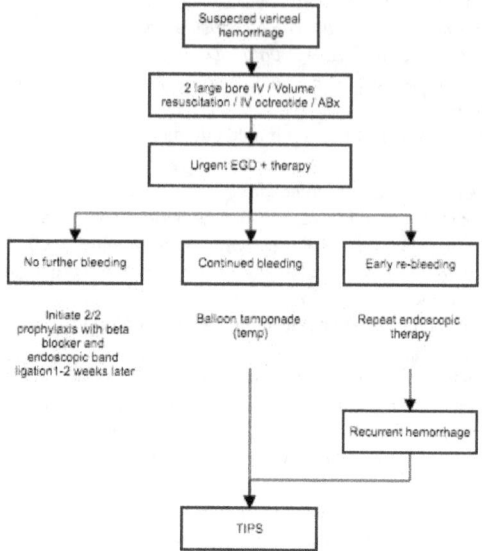

- Vaccinations: Hepatitis A, B, and pneumonia
- Screening: EGD for varices once, r/o HCC with US q6m
- HRS
    - Due to reflex renal vasoconstriction
    - Diagnosis is based on exclusion of other potential causes of renal failure. Major criteria include ↓GFR, absence of shock physiology, volume depletion, and nephrotoxic drugs. UA should show no proteinuria or obstructive uropathy. Minor criteria include a urine volume <500cc/d and urine sodium <10 mmol/L.
    - Types 1 and 2
        - Type 1
            - Treatment includes:
                - Stopping diuretics
                - Volume challenge with IV albumin @ 1g/kg or 1-1.5L of normal isotonic saline
                - Consider initiating midodrine, octreotide
        - Type 2
            - Usually due to refractory ascites, see separate management of refractory ascites

IRRITABLE BOWEL SYNDROME

- **Types**[26,27,28]
    - IBS-C, IBS-D, IBS-M, IBS-U
- **Diagnosis**
    - *ROME III guidelines:*

- Recurrent abdominal pain for at least 3d/month in the last 3 months that started at least 6 months ago associated with 2+ of the following:
    1) Improvement with defecation
    2) Onset associated with Δ in frequency of stool
    3) Onset associated with Δ in form of stool
    4) Not associated with a structural cause
- **Treatment**
    - Consider, overall a diet low in FODMAP (fermentable oligosaccharides, disaccharides, monosaccharides, and polyols) can decrease IBS symptoms
    - IBS-M
        - Mixture of *Lactobacillus* and *Bifidobacterium spp* appx 20-40 billion CFU/d for 4-6 weeks
        - Soluble fiber of 15g/d
        - Dicyclomine (40mg/QID x2w), Hyoscyamine (10mg QID x 4w), Peppermint Oil (200-500mg x 4w)
        - TCA (Amitriptyline 10-75mg/d x12w)
        - Rifaximin
    - IBS-D
        - Loperamide
        - Alosetron
        - Eluxadoline 75mg/100mg BID
    - IBS-C
        - Polyethylene glycol
        - Linaclotide 290 mcg/d
        - Tenapanor 50 mg b.i.d.
        - Lubiprostone

CONSTIPATION

- **Types**: Functional (see below) and Secondary (medication or 2/2 condition)
- **Definition**[29]
    - Must include two or more of the following:
        - Straining during at least 25 percent of defecations
        - Lumpy or hard stools in at least 25 percent of defecations
        - Sensation of incomplete evacuation for at least 25 percent of defecations
        - Sensation of anorectal obstruction/blockage for at least 25 percent of defecations
        - Manual maneuvers to facilitate at least 25 percent of defecations (e.g., digital evacuation, support of the pelvic floor)
        - Fewer than three defecations per week
- Avoid PO agents if pt. is impacted or obstructed (KUB & DRE can assess this)
- Rule out secondary causes:
    - Hypothyroidism
    - Neurologic disorders (i.e. PD, MS, spinal cord injury, amyloidosis, DM, ↑Ca, low fiber intake)
- PE involves confirming good sphincter tone exists, and relaxation possible when prompted
- **Indications for Endoscopy**
    - Age older than 50 years with no previous colorectal cancer screening
    - Before surgery for constipation
    - Δ in stool caliber
    - Heme-positive stools Iron deficiency anemia

GASTROENTEROLOGY

- Obstructive symptoms
- Recent onset of constipation
- Rectal bleeding
- Rectal prolapse
- Weight loss

- **MOA of Laxatives**
  - Osmotic agents (i.e. lactulose, MiraLAX, sorbitol) promote secretion of water into the lumen of the colon and stimulate movement of the bowel. Onset is typically from 12 to 96 hours.
  - Fiber/bulk agents (i.e. Citrucel, Fibercon, and psyllium/Metamucil) - hold water in stool, increase stool weight, increase colonic distension, and improve frequency of bowel movements. Onset is typically from 12 to 72 hours.
  - Stimulant laxatives (i.e. bisacodyl/Dulcolax, Senokot) - increase intestinal motility and colonic secretions. Onset with oral formulations is six to ten hours, possibly up to 24 hours. The onset with rectal suppositories is 15 to 60 minutes.
  - Stool softeners (i.e. docusate) - improve the interaction of water and solid stool.
  - Saline laxatives (i.e. magnesium hydroxide, magnesium citrate, and oral sodium phosphate) - draw water into intestines and colon by osmosis to increase motility. Onset is 30 minutes to eight hours (magnesium hydroxide), one to three hours (oral sodium phosphate), and 30 minutes to six hours (magnesium citrate). The onset of sodium phosphate enema (e.g., Fleet, etc.) is usually within one to five minutes.

- **Mainstay Treatment**
  (1) Senna Docusate (2) MiraLAX/Lactulose (3) Laxatives
  - ↑exercise, ↑dietary fiber (25-30g), adequate H2O, bulk laxatives (psyllium, methylcellulose)
  - MOM 30 ml PO Q 12 hours prn constipation
    - Caution in pts with renal dysfunction
  - MgOH
  - Magnesium Citrate 8 oz. (240 ml) bottle PO
    - Caution in pts with renal dysfunction d/t risk of ↑Mg
  - Senna 1-2 tabs HS + docusate 100-240 mg PO bid

- **If no BM by day 3**
  - Give Fleet enema or Bisacodyl suppository PR
    - Fleet's caution in pts with renal dysfunction or CHF
  - Avoid all the above in dialysis patient's d/t hyper MG and PO4
  - Mineral Oil enema
  - Psyllium indicated for chronic constipation and those on opiates
  - Lactulose 30 ml PO
  - Bisacodyl 10 mg PO/PR
    - Not for chronic use d/t risk of ↓K and ↑Na
    - Good for those on opiates
  - Dulcolax suppository PR x1
    - Causes contraction of intestine by stimulating mesenteric plexus
  - Glycerin Suppository PR x1
  - Colace 100mg PO daily

- **Opiate-Induced Constipation (OIC)**
  - Use traditional laxatives as above, if no response after ≥2 then use peripherally acting mu-opioid receptor antagonists (naldemedine, naloxegol)

Chronic Constipation[30]		
Medication	Indication	Considerations
Linactolide 72 or 145 mcg/d	Chronic idiopathic constipation IBS-C	Take on empty stomach

GASTROENTEROLOGY

Lubiprostone 8-24 mcg BID	Chronic idiopathic constipation IBS-C	Not effective in those taking methadone
Plecanatide 3-6 mg/d	Chronic idiopathic constipation	No drug interactions
Psyllium 10 g/d	Chronic constipation	
Polyethylene glycol 17 g/d	Chronic constipation	
Lactulose 20 g/d	Chronic constipation	
Senna 17 mg/d	Chronic constipation	
Bisacodyl 10 mg/d	Chronic constipation	
Prucalopride 1-2 mg/d	Chronic constipation	
	OIC	
Naldemedine 0.2 mg/d	OIC	
Naloxegol 12.5-25 mg/d	OIC	
Methylnaltrexone >PO 450 mg/d >SQ 12 mg QOD	OIC	Empty stomach Avoid with opiate antagonists

COLON CANCER

- **Screening**
    o Normal population with no history of familial colon cancer should start at age 45 with a colonoscopy, repeated every 10 years through age of 75 if life expectancy is 10 years or more
    o Screening is discouraged for those >85
    o If family history of colon cancer (diagnosis before age 60) or 2+ family members who have biopsy showing high grade dysplasia should receive screening start at 40 (10 years before normal population) or 10 years from diagnosis (whichever is earlier)
        - Repeat colonoscopies will occur at 5-year intervals
    o Repeat in 3 years if:
        - 3 or more adenomas of any size are found
        - 2 or more adenomas >1cm in size are found
        - Any adenoma that is villous or high grade in dysplasia
        - Can return to 5-year intervals if repeat shows no abnormalities

Screening Options for CRC[31]

Method	Advantages	Disadvantages
Colonoscopy	• Ability to detect and remove polyps • Visualizes the entire colon	• Requires comprehensive bowel preparation • Takes 20 to 30 minutes plus recovery time • Patient may not drive or return to work if sedation is given
CT Colonoscopy	• 10-15 min • Noninvasive • No sedation • Can drive and work same day	• Same bowel prep req'd • Radiation • May miss small polyps • + test → colonoscopy
FIT	• At home • Safe • No diet affects	• Required yearly • + test → colonoscopy
Flex Sigmoid	• Safer than colonoscopy • 10 minutes • May still drive and go to work same day	• Req bowel prep • Only distal 1/3 of colon seen • +test → colonoscopy
FOBT	• At home • Easy • Convenient	• Yearly • Diet Δs • +test → colonoscopy
FIT-DNA	• At home • Safe • Convenient • No dietary Δs	• Expensive • +test → colonoscopy • Requires repeat testing q3y

Follow-up Guidelines

Number/Size/Histopathology	Surveillance Colonoscopy
Hyperplastic polyps	10 yrs.
1-2 small (<1cm) tubular adenomas with no high-grade dysplasia	5 yrs.
3+ adenomas	3 yrs.
High grade dysplasia	
Villous features	
Any adenoma of 1cm or larger	

DIARRHEA

- Acute[32,33]
  - Defined: <2 weeks
  - Etiology
    - Appearance of the stool: blood (inflammatory or invasive ulceration), mucus (IBS), or oil (malabsorption).
    - Infectious (viral, bacterial, parasitic)
    - Food exposure (onset 12h to 10d after eating)
    - Medications antibiotics, alcohol, illicit drugs, laxatives, magnesium-containing antacids, digoxin, quinidine, colchicine.
    - Ischemia (RF: HTN, DM, chronic AFib, HLD)
    - Proctitis and rectal discharge suggest gonorrhea, syphilis, lymphogranuloma venereum, and herpes simplex
    - History of gastrectomy, vagotomy, intestinal resection (short gut syndrome).

GASTROENTEROLOGY

Etiologies To Consider with Acute Diarrhea

Clinical Presentation	Potential Causes to Consider
Vomiting primarily (little diarrhea)	Viral gastroenteritis
	Rotavirus
	Norwalk
	Preformed toxin (staph, B. cereus, clostridium perfringens)
	Enterotoxin (vibrio, ETEC, klebsiella, Aeromonas)
Noninflammatory diarrhea (acute watery diarrhea without fever/dysentery)	Can be caused by all pathogens (bacterial, viral, parasitic) but most commonly performed toxin causers (bacillus, staph aureus, clostridium) and enterotoxin causers (vibrio, ETEC, klebsiella)
Inflammatory diarrhea (invasive GI, gross blood in stool)	Shigella, Salmonella, Campylobacter, EHEC, Vibrio, Yersinia, C. diff, entamoeba
Chronic diarrhea (≥14d)	Evaluate for parasites
	Consider Cyclosporacyetanesis
	Crypto
	E. histolytica
	Giardia
Systemic sx	Listeria
	Brucella
	Toxoplasma
	Vibrio
	HepA
Fever predominant	Shigella
	Salmonella
	Entamoeba
	Campylobacter
	Yersinia
Abdominal pains predominant	C. diff
	EHEC
	Rotavirus, Norovirus
	Salmonella, Campylobacter

Bacterial Causes of Diarrhea

Etiology	Incubation Period	Signs/Sx	Duration	Associated Foods	Labs	Clinical Features & Treatment
Salmonella	1-3d	Diarrhea, fever, abdominal pain, vomiting (if associated with HA, constipation, malaise, chills, myalgias consider Typhoid)	4-7d	Contaminated eggs, poultry, unpasteurized milk or juice, cheese, contaminated raw fruits and veggies	+/- fecal WBCs	Supportive care. ABx are not indicated unless Typhoid during which use TMP-SMX or gentamycin
Shigella	1-2d	Abdominal cramps, fever, diarrhea. Stool may have blood+mucous	4-7d	Food or water contaminated with fecal material; often person to person	Stool cx +fecal WBCs	Supportive care; TMP-SMX if organism is susceptible; Fluoroquinolone x3d
B cereus (preformed)	1-8h	↑↑↑vomiting + diarrhea no fever	1d	Reheated fried rice causes vomiting or diarrhea.	Food and stool can be tested for toxin. - fecal WBCs	Acute onset, severe nausea and vomiting lasting 24 hours. Supportive care.
S.aureus	1-8h	Sudden onset of severe nausea and vomiting. Abdominal cramps. Diarrhea and fever may be present	1-2d	Unrefrigerated or improperly refrigerated meats, potato, and egg salads, cream pastries	Normally a clinical diagnosis; stool, vomitus, and food can be tested for toxin - fecal WBCs	Abrupt onset, intense nausea and vomiting for up to 24 hours, recovery in 24–48 hours. Supportive care.
Vibrio parahaemolyticus	2-48h	Watery diarrhea, abdominal cramps, nausea, vomiting	2-5d	Undercooked or raw seafood, such as fish, shellfish	Stool cx, vibrio requires special media - fecal WBCs	Supportive care. ABx recommended if severe (i.e. Tetracycline 500mg QID x3d)

Bacterial Causes of Diarrhea

Etiology	Incubation Period	Signs/Sx	Duration	Associated Foods	Labs	Clinical Features & Treatment
Yersinia enterocolitica	1-2d	Appendicitis-like symptoms (diarrhea, vomiting, fever, and abdominal pain); primarily in older children/young adults. May have scarlatiniform rash	1-3w	Undercooked pork, unpasteurized milk, contaminated water	Stool, vomitus or blood cx +/- fecal WBCs	Supportive care, usually self-limiting
Listeria monocytogenes	9-48h for GI sx; 2-6w for invasive disease	Fever, muscle aches, and nausea or diarrhea.	Variable	Fresh soft cheeses, unpasteurized milk, inadequately pasteurized milk, ready-to-eat deli meat	Blood or cerebrospinal fluid cx; stool cx not helpful	Supportive care
ETEC	1-3d	Watery diarrhea, abdominal cramps, some vomiting	3-7d	Water or food contaminated with human feces	Stool cx; ETEC requires special lab techniques. - fecal WBCs	Supportive care; Abx rarely indicated
EHEC (including E.coli O157:H7)	1-8d	Severe diarrhea, often bloody, abdominal pain and vomiting	5-10d	Undercooked beef, unpasteurized milk and juice	Stool cx; O157:H7 requires special media and reporting to local agencies. +fecal WBCs	Supportive care, monitor renal function, H/H, and PLT closely; if ABx necessary then TMP-SMX 160-800mg BID x3d

Bacterial Causes of Diarrhea

Etiology	Incubation Period	Signs/Sx	Duration	Associated Foods	Labs	Clinical Features & Treatment
Clostridium perfringens	8-16h	Watery diarrhea, nausea, abdominal cramps, fever rare	1-2d	Meats, poultry, gravy, or dried precooked foods	Stools can be tested for enterotoxin	Supportive care
C. jejuni	2-5d	Diarrhea, cramps, fever, and vomiting, diarrhea may be bloody	2-10d	Raw and undercooked poultry, unpast. Milk, contaminated water	Routine stool cx; campy req. special agar +fecal WBCs	Supportive care; early in dz course can use FLQ
Norwalk	1-2d	Nausea, vomiting, watery large-volume diarrhea, rare fever	24-60h	Poorly cooked shellfish; ready-to-eat foods touched by infected workers	Clinical dx; negative bacterial cx; negative fecal leukocytes. - fecal WBCs	Supportive care Bismuth sulfate
Rotavirus	1-3d	Vomiting, watery diarrhea, low-grade fever. Temporary lactose intolerance	4-8d	Fecally contaminated foods	ID of virus in stool immunoassay. - fecal WBCs	Supportive care
Cryptosporidium	7 days	Cramping, abdominal pain, watery diarrhea, fever and vomiting may be present	Days to weeks	Contaminated water, veggies	Must be specifically requested	Supportive care
E. histolytica	2-3d to 1-4w	Bloody diarrhea, frequent bowel movements	Months	Fecal-oral	Examination of stool for cysts and parasites	Metronidazole
Giardia	1-4w	Acute or chronic diarrhea, flatus, bloating	Weeks	Drinking water from other sources	Examination of stool for O&P. +/- fecal WBCs	Metronidazole

- Symptoms
  - Nocturnal diarrhea suggests infectious or inflammatory cause
  - Admit patients with:
    1. Severe diarrhea with dehydration
    2. Bloody diarrhea
    3. Fever
    4. Duration > 2 days
    5. With abdominal pain in elderly (r/o mesenteric ischemia)
- **Red Flags That Require Prompt Evaluation**
  - Inflammatory diarrhea: fever (> 38.5°C), WBC ≥ 15,000/mcL, bloody diarrhea, or severe abdominal pain
  - Passage of six or more unformed stools in 24 hours
  - Profuse watery diarrhea and dehydration
  - Frail older patients
  - Immunocompromised patients (AIDS, post transplantation)
  - Exposure to antibiotics
  - Hospital-acquired diarrhea (onset following at least 3 days of hospitalization)
  - Systemic illness
- Labs
  - Stools for markers of inflammation (leukocytes, guaiac)
    1. Stool cultures positive in < 3%; therefore, initial symptomatic treatment is given for mild symptoms
  - Bacterial cultures
  - Ovocytes and Parasites (O&P) (in patients who have traveled recently)
  - C. difficile toxin (in patients with recent institutionalization and/or antibiotic or chemotherapy exposure)
  - Campylobacter, microsporidia, Isospora, and cryptosporidia. Also consider Giardia antigen.
- Management
  - Treat electrolyte abnormalities with IV or PO rehydration (sports drinks)
  - Avoid antimotility agents if suspecting infectious cause (febrile dysentery)
  - Stop newly started medications
  - Antibiotics are not recommended in nontyphoid Salmonella, Campylobacter, Aeromonas, Yersinia, or Shiga-toxin producing E coli infection except in severe disease. When indicated, consider treatment below:
    1. *Empiric Regiments*
       - Fluoroquinolones (e.g., ciprofloxacin 500 mg BID, ofloxacin 400 mg, or levofloxacin 500 mg once daily) for 1–3 days
       - Trimethoprim-sulfamethoxazole, 160/800 mg twice daily orally
       - Doxycycline, 100 mg twice daily orally
       - Metronidazole 250mg QID x7d for giardiasis
       - For Traveler's Diarrhea: Azithromycin, 1000 mg single dose or 500 mg daily for 3 days
- **Chronic**[34]
  - Definition – loose stools for more than 1 month
  - History
    - Onset – congenital, acute, gradual onset
    - Continuous or intermittent pattern
    - Duration
    - Recent travel, other sick family members, ingestion of contaminated water
    - Stool characteristics – watery, bloody, fatty
      1. Small frequent bowel movements with tenesmus and bleeding suggest proctitis

GASTROENTEROLOGY

    2. Larger volume stools that are less frequent suggest a small bowel source
    3. Steatorrhea suggest fat malabsorption or fat maldigestion
- Concomitant incontinence?
- Abdominal pain? More suggestive of IBS, IBD,

Differential diagnosis of chronic diarrhea based on stool osmolar gap

Classification | **Causes** | **Clinical Symptoms**

Stool Osmolarity → stool analysis by calculating

$$(\text{Measured Stool Osmolarity} - 2([Na]+[K]))$$

1. Verify stool osmolarity makes sense (never lower than plasma osmolarity; suspect water contamination if it is lower)
2. Calculate gap by comparing actual to calculated above
3. Gap>50→osmotic
   - Upon fasting if symptoms improve, then likely ingestion of lactose or gluten → can do hydrogen breath test to r/o lactose intolerance
4. Gap<50→secretory
   - Stool O&P, colonoscopy to r/o microscopic colitis, urine metanephrine, TSH, ACTH

Classification	Causes	Clinical Symptoms
Osmotic	Lactase deficiency Medications: antacids, lactulose, sorbitol, olestra Gluten or FODMAP diet intolerance Factitious: magnesium-containing antacids or laxatives (Mg, PO4, SO4) Ischemic enteritis Injury 2/2 radiation tx	• Abdominal distention • Flatulence
Secretory	Hormonal: Zollinger-Ellison syndrome (gastrinoma), carcinoid, VIPoma, medullary thyroid carcinoma, adrenal insufficiency Laxative abuse: cascara, senna Medications Bowel resection SIBO Pancreatic insufficiency (w/ steatorrhea) Microscopic colitis (no steatorrhea)	• High-volume (> 1 L) watery diarrhea leading to dehydration • Electrolyte imbalance
Inflammatory conditions	Inflammatory bowel disease Cancer with obstruction and pseudo diarrhea Radiation colitis GI malignancies Collagenous colitis	• Abdominal pain • Fever • ↓Weight • Hematochezia • Pus • ↑stool wt. (>200g)
Malabsorption	Small bowel: celiac disease, Whipple disease, tropical sprue, eosinophilic gastroenteritis, small bowel resection, Crohn disease Pancreatic insufficiency: chronic pancreatitis, cystic fibrosis, pancreatic cancer Bacterial overgrowth	• ↓ weight • Osmotic diarrhea • Steatorrhea • Nutritional deficiencies
Motility	IBS Post-surgical DM, thyroid Caffeine/EtOH	
Steatorrhea	Pancreatic exocrine insufficiency s/p Bariatric surgery Liver dz Celiac sprue Whipple's disease	

- Differential
  - *Osmotic*
    1. Stool volume ↓ with fasting

2. ↑ stool osmolar gap (see below)
3. Often due to medications, lactose intolerance, or factitious intake
- *Secretory*
    1. Large volume stools despite fasting (symptoms @ night)
    2. Normal stool osmolar gap (see below)
    3. Can be from myriad of causes to include hormone induced, malabsorption, and from medications
- *Inflammatory*
    1. Patients will often have a fever, hematochezia, and abdominal pain
    2. Common causes include UC, Crohn's, microscopic colitis, radiation colitis
    3. Look for leukocytes in stool
- *Malabsorption*
    1. Look for weight loss, abnormal metabolic panel, ↑ fecal fat (>10g in 24h)
    2. Common causes include pancreatic insufficiency, SIBO, scleroderma, celiac, Crohn's
- *Motility*
    1. Often associated with recent abdominal surgery, IBS, DM, or ↑thyroid
- *Others*: chronic idiopathic secretory diarrhea, microscopic colitis, fecal incontinence, iatrogenic diarrhea, IBS, autonomic neuropathy (in diabetic patients), and factitious diarrhea
o Exam
- Rash (c/w IgA deficiency)
- Thyroid mass (hypothyroidism)
- Ascites (cirrhosis)
- Fistulas (IBD)
o Labs
- **Testing is indicated in the presence of alarm features**
- CBC, CMP, LFTs, Ca, PO4, albumin, TSH
- **Infectious** → CBC with leukocytosis (eosinophilia→neoplasm, eosinophilic colitis, parasitic infection, allergies, collagen disorder)
- INR, ESR, and C-RP should be obtained in most patients
- Fecal calprotectin to exclude Crohn's, fecal lactoferrin can be used as a surrogate for fecal leukocytes
- Fecal leukocytes (inflammatory diarrhea)
- *Clostridium difficile* toxin
- **Malabsorption**
    1. Obtain serum folate, B12, iron, vitamin A and D, prothrombin time.
    2. Consider hydrogen breath testing or dietary removal of lactose/carbohydrates if suspecting lactose insufficiency.
    3. Consider fecal elastase or chymotrypsin for fat malabsorption (i.e. pancreatic d/o)
- 24-hour stool collection for weight and quantitative fecal fat
    1. Stool weight < 200–300 g/24 h excludes diarrhea and suggests a functional disorder such as irritable bowel
    2. Stool weight > 200 g/24 hours confirms diarrhea
    3. Stool weight > 1000–1500 g/24 hours suggests secretory diarrhea, including neuroendocrine tumors
    4. Fecal fat > 10 g/24 hours indicates a malabsorption syndrome
- R/O **Celiac**→ ↑ALP; vitamin A, B_{12}, D, K deficiencies; iron level (deficiency expected), serum albumin (often low), anti-transglutaminase ab (IgA)
- R/O **microscopic colitis** → ↑ESR, +ANA
- Screening → folate, Fe, 25-hydroxyvitamin D

GASTROENTEROLOGY

- o Imaging
  - Imaging is mostly indicated in patients with steatorrhea (r/o pancreatic dz) and secretory or inflammatory diarrhea
    1. Evaluate for strictures, fistulae, and diverticula.
    2. Degree of inflammation if IBD suspected
  - CT enterography – consider as initial evaluation method for suspicion of Crohn's
- o Procedures
  - Consider colonoscopy to r/o CRC in patients with altered bowel habits +/- BRBPR
  - Small bowel disorders can be evaluated with MR Enterography or video capsule endoscopy.
  - Breath tests for carbohydrate malabsorption and SIBO
- o Treatment
  - Bulk Forming: Psyllium 1-2 tsp BID-TID
  - Imodium 4 mg PO Q 4 hours x 16 hours (Max=16 mg in 24 hours)
    - Don't give with blood in stool or fever
  - Lomotil 2.5-5 mg PO TID-QID (Max=20mg in 24 hours)
    - Avoid in Hepatic failure or cirrhosis

DIVERTICULITIS

- **Classification**[35]
  - o Hinchy's Criteria (mortality)
    - Stage 1 (<5%) – small confined, pericolic or mesenteric abscess
    - Stage 2 (<5%)– larger abscesses often combined to pelvis
    - Stage 3 (13%)– perforated diverticulitis due to diverticular rupture → peritonitis
    - Stage 4 (43%)– free rupture leading to fecal contamination
- **Diagnosis**
  - o Computed tomography (CT) is recommended as the initial radiologic examination.
  - o High sensitivity (approximately 93 to 97%)
  - o Specificity approaching 100%
  - o Look for diverticula, inflammation of pericolic fat, bowel-wall thickness > 4mm, abscess formation
- **When to Hospitalize**
  - o Outpatient therapy reasonable with 7-10 days of PO Ciprofloxacin + Metronidazole
  - o Admit it:
    - No PO intake
    - Pain requiring narcotics
    - Sx failure to improve after outpatient tx
- **Treatment**
  - o NPO
  - o NG tube if obstruction or ileus present
  - o Repeat CT if sx do not improve in 72 hrs.
  - o Perform colonoscopy 2-6 weeks post recovery to rule out atypical colorectal carcinoma in patients with no documented colonoscopy in past 3 years.
- **Surgical consult if:**
  - o Stage 4 / Peritonitis
  - o Treatment does not respond to medical management in 72 hrs.
  - o Perforation
  - o Abscess
  - o Fistula
  - o Repeated attacks (2+)
  - o Sepsis

- o Approach
  - First operation - the diseased colonic segment is drained, and a diverting ostomy (usually a transverse colostomy) is created proximally.
  - Allows for fecal diversion and drainage of infection.
  - During the second operation, the diseased colon is resected, and a primary anastomosis of the colonic segments is performed.
  - The ostomy is reversed during the third and final operation to reestablish bowel continuity. The three-stage procedure is rarely performed and should be considered only in critical situations in which resection cannot be performed safely
  - Percutaneous Drainage
  - Bowel rest and broad-spectrum ABx if abscess <4cm and Hinchey Stage 1
  - CT-guided percutaneous drainage if >4cm (Stage II)

Treatment Regimen for Diverticulitis (5-7days)	
Medication	Dosage
Oral	
Metronidazole and a quinolone	Metronidazole — 500 mg q 6 to 8 hr.
	Ciprofloxacin — 500–750 mg q 12 hr.
Metronidazole and trimethoprim–sulfamethoxazole	Metronidazole — 500 mg q 6 to 8 hr.
	TMP/SMX — 160/800 mg q 12 hrs.
Amoxicillin–clavulanate	Amoxicillin–clavulanate — 875 mg q 12 hr.
IV	
Metronidazole and a quinolone	Metronidazole — 500 mg q 6 to 8 hr.
	Ciprofloxacin 400 mg q 12 hr.
Metronidazole and a third-generation cephalosporin	Metronidazole — 500 mg q 6 to 8 hr.
	Ceftriaxone — 1–2 g q 24 hr.
Beta-lactam with a beta-lactamase inhibitor	Beta-lactam with a beta-lactamase inhibitor (e.g., ampicillin–sulbactam — 3 g q 6 hr.)

- **Complications**
  - o Abscess
  - o Fistula
  - o Obstruction
  - o Peritonitis
  - o Stricture
- **Follow-up**
  - o Colonoscopy 6 weeks after acute process to r/o cancer and IBD

DYSPHAGIA

- **Defined**[36,37,38,39] – any type of difficulty with moving food and/or liquid from mouth into stomach
- **Phases**
  - o Oral preparatory – food stays in mouth, forming bolus
  - o Oral transit – tongue elevates against the palate
  - o Pharyngeal – bolus passes into esophagus, nasal cavity blocked
  - o Esophageal – bolus enters the esophagus and upper esophageal sphincter closes
- **Signs/Symptoms** – aspiration (coughing, trouble clearing throat), residue remaining in oral cavity, prolonged time to chew and swallow, SOB, odynophagia, globus
- **Etiologies**
  - o Oropharyngeal typically from neurologic (likely if dysphagia to solids and liquids; seen in 67% of strokes, MS, MG, ALS, PD), structural (zenker, osteophytes) or myogenic pathology (to include tumors), most common seen in nursing home residents.

- Patients have difficulty with drooling, cannot begin their swallow, and feel food is stuck in neck
  - Esophageal can be due to direct disorders of the esophagus, mechanical obstruction (ring, web, stricture, cancer, EE), altered esophageal motility (spasm, scleroderma, achalasia), mechanical (LAE, substernal thyroid), iatrogenic (pill, malnutrition), infectious (candida)
    - Patient will complain of food getting stuck after swallowing, typically progresses from liquids only to then including solids
- **ROS and History** – h/o tobacco use, h/o stroke, head injury, dysphagia to solids+liquids
- **Alarm Symptoms** – weight loss, anemia, progressive symptoms, hematochezia, dysarthria, hoarse voice.
- **Assessment**
  - Bedside swallow evaluation – typically performed by nurse or SLP. Assess for mental status, speech quality, posture (able to sit upright?), respiratory status, oral trial
  - Videofluoroscopic Swallow Study – also termed modified barium swallow, considered the gold standard for swallow assessments. Patient given various consistencies of barium to swallow creating a video of liquids/solids passing from oral cavity through the pharynx to the esophagus.
  - Fiberoptic Endoscopic Evaluation of Swallowing (FEES) – scope passed through nares and held in pharynx above tongue to view pharynx and larynx. Performed by SLP. Does not allow for visualization of oral phase, may miss periods of aspiration.
  - CT neck/chest- if concern for neoplasm
  - Manometry – perform if concern for mechanical obstruction that cannot be found on imaging, esp. if high suspicion for achalasia.
- **Diagnosis**
  - Use assessments as above
  - Solid and liquid dysphagia (neuromuscular)
    - *Intermittent* – think DES if patient has CP
    - *Progressive* – think achalasia or scleroderma
  - Solid dysphagia only (mechanical)
    - *Intermittent* – think lower esophageal ring
    - *Progressive* – peptic stricture (if patient has GERD) or carcinoma (if older)
- **Management**
  - Diet modification
  - Postural changes
  - Swallow maneuvers
  - PEG tube placement

GI BLEED

- **Classification**[40]
  - Upper (above ligament of Treitz)
  - Lower (below ligament)
- **History**
  - Prior bleeds, diverticular disease, prior GI or aortic surgery, trauma, coagulopathy, medications (ASA, NSAIDs, anticoagulants, steroids, antiplatelet medications), liver disease, alcohol abuse, renal insufficiency, poor cardiac output, hypertension, hypotension, recreational drugs (cocaine, amphetamines), rectal foreign objects (sexual activity or used to disimpact), history of STDs
- **Etiology**
  - Upper GI Bleeds (UGIB):

- Peptic ulcer disease (H. pylori or NSAIDs)
- Portal hypertensive gastropathy
- Varices
- Mallory-Weiss tear
- Erosive esophagitis (especially alcoholics)
- Vascular malformations
- Dieulafoy's lesion (an abnormally large submucosal artery located in the proximal stomach)
- Neoplasm
- Note that gastritis is not a cause of bleeding (possibly occult blood loss but not acute bleeding)
  - Lower GI Bleeds (LGIB):
    - Diverticular disease
    - Hemorrhoids
    - Solitary rectal ulcer syndrome
    - Ischemic colitis
    - Infectious colitis
    - Inflammatory bowel disease (IBD)
    - Angiodysplasia
    - Neoplastic disease
    - Post polypectomy bleeding
    - NSAID ulcerations
    - CMV ulcerations (immunosuppressed)
    - Portal hypertensive colopathy and rectal varices (cirrhosis)
- **Clinical Signs and Symptoms**
  - Suggestive of UGIB: nausea, vomiting, hematemesis, melena, epigastric pain, liver disease, EtOH abuse, NSAID use, peptic ulcer disease, syncope, coffee-ground emesis
  - Suggestive of LGIB: hematochezia (BRBPR), diarrhea, diverticulosis, colon cancer
    - Risk factors for adverse outcomes (recurrent bleeding, need for intervention, or death) in patients presenting with presumed acute lower gastrointestinal bleeding include ↓BP, tachycardia, ongoing hematochezia, an age of more than 60 years, a creatinine level of more than 1.7 mg per deciliter, and unstable or clinically significant coexisting conditions.
- **Physical Exam**
  - Vital Signs:
    - Tachycardia (at 10 % volume loss)
    - Orthostatics (at 20% volume loss)
    - Hypotension (at 30% volume loss)
  - Pallor, stigmata of liver disease, localized abdominal tenderness
  - Rectal:
  - Stool may appear bright red, maroon, black and tarry, or brown
    - Look for evidence of hemorrhoids or fissures
    - No guaiac necessary if concern of acute bleed. Guaiac should be used for colon cancer screening and workup of iron deficient anemia of unclear etiology not for acute hemoglobin drops.
      - 1 cc of blood loss will result in a positive guaiac; 50 cc of blood loss results in melena. Therefore, if recent bleeding you will find it without a guaiac
- **Admission vs. Outpatient Therapy**[41]
  - **The Glasgow Blatchford score** has the highest accuracy for predicting the need for hospitalization for his gastrointestinal bleed.
    - The Glasgow Blatchford Bleeding Score is determined by **nine factors**:
      - hemoglobin level
      - blood urea nitrogen level

- initial systolic blood pressure
- sex
- heart rate of 100/min or less
- presence of melena
- recent syncope
- history of hepatic disease
- History of heart failure.
    - The results of this study cannot be applied to inpatients who develop upper gastrointestinal bleeding.
    - A score of ≤1 on the Glasgow Blatchford bleeding score identified a low-risk patient who could be directed to outpatient management of the upper gastrointestinal bleeding. *(NICE 2012)*
  - Other risk scores (nonvariceal)
    - AIM65
    - Rockall
    - https://dshung.shinyapps.io/UGIB_App_USA/
  - Other discharge from ER criteria:
    - BUN <18.2 mg/dL, Hg >13 g/dL (men) or 12 g/dL (women), systolic BP ≥110 mmHg, pulse <100 bpm, and no history of melena, syncope, cardiac failure, liver disease. *(ACG 2012)*
- **Diagnostics**
  - ECG - R/o ACS 2/2 to severe anemia in patients with risk factors.
  - EGD – see below
- **Labs**
  - CBC
    - HCT generally ↓ by 2-3 points and the HGB ↓ by 1 point for every 500cc of blood lost.
    - Initial value should be considered until crystalloid fluid resuscitation complete
    - After bleeding ceases, the HCT may continue to ↓ for up to 6h, and full equilibration may require 24h.
    - Follow CBC q6-8h while active bleeding present
  - Chemistry panel, type and cross, liver function tests, iron panel, reticulocyte count
    - BUN disproportionately elevated from Cr suggests an upper GI source (30:1)
  - INR
    - If elevated, consider phytonadione (Vitamin K) 10mg IM daily if INR > 2.0
  - Consider fecal leukocytes/stool culture/C. diff/SSPC if infectious or inflammatory cause suspected
  - TROP if age>45 or hx CAD
  - H. pylori[42]
    - in a patient with a bleeding peptic ulcer, a negative rapid urease test or histology is not sufficient to rule out H. pylori infection, and a second test is warranted such as **H. Pylori serology**
    - The sensitivity of the rapid urease test can be reduced up to 25% in patients who have taken a proton pump inhibitor (PPI) or bismuth within 2 weeks of testing or antibiotic therapy within 4 weeks.
    - The sensitivity of the urea breath test and stool antigen test, like that of the rapid urease test, is reduced by medications that affect urease production. (fecal or urea breath test 2 weeks after cessation of PPI)
- **Nursing Orders**
  - Type and cross for 2-4 U
  - NPO 8 hours before procedure (clears allowed up to 2 hours before procedure)
- **Management**[43,44]
  - Approximately 70-80% of all GI bleeds stop spontaneously.

- Transfuse platelets if count <50k or if impaired function d/t ASA or Plavix use
- DDAVP 0.3 mcg/kg IV q12h if uremia present
- Endoscopy within 24 hours
- FFP to maintain INR <1.8 (EGD safe for INR <2.5)
- Maintain HGB >8 if no active ischemia

Treatment Regimen for UGIB (5-7days)

Acid Suppression
Protonix 80mg IV load then 40mg IV BID and then switch to PO daily regimen <u>72h</u> after EGD for low risk lesions
Alternative: Pantoprazole (Protonix) 80mg IV load, then 8mg/hr. IV continuous drip x 72 hrs. if a drip is desired

Prokinetic agent
Erythromycin 3mg/kg IV over 20-30m can be given 30-90m prior to endoscopy to aid in viewing if large blood burden suspected

Variceal Bleeding / Portal Hypertension Present
- Octreotide 100mcg bolus f/b 50-100mcg/h continuous infusion for 3-5 days after endoscopy *(AASLD '07)*
- For advanced cirrhosis or variceal bleed, antibiotic prophylaxis with Ceftriaxone (Rocephin) 1g IV every 24 hrs.

Antiplatelet
- Consider stopping ASA (for 1-7 days; resume after 1 week) unless required for secondary prophylaxis
- Dual therapy patients should have all except ASA stopped unless catheterization was recent (90 days)

GI bleed management based on location

Upper GI Bleed

- **Initial Management**
  - NPO except medications
  - Place NG tube if etiology unclear
  - Do not give the patient sucralfate or antacids until after EGD, as they will interfere with the endoscopy

Threshold	Population
≤9	Age>65 ASCAD UA/NSTEMI/STEMI Respiratory Disease Symptomatic
<8	Other

  - Blood transfusions if HGB<8 (restrictive strategy vs 9 showed better outcomes in regard to morbidity and mortality however if patient has underlying unstable CAD, age>65, or respiratory disease goal should be 9)
  - Correct any coagulopathies (FFP if INR > 1.5; keep platelets > 50)
  - Medications: see table above
- **Endoscopy**
  - *Timing of EGD:* ≤12h if high risk patient; if unstable patient needs to stabilize first. Otherwise, within 24 hours.
  - Results of EGD:
    - *Forrest 1A/B or 2A (active bleed, non-bleeding vessel):* requires endoscopic therapy with IV PPI bolus and infusion
    - *Forrest 2B (adherent clot):* can consider endoscopic therapy, still do IV PPI bolus and infusion
    - *Forrest 2C or 3 (flat spot, clean base):* no endoscopic therapy required; oral PPI
  - 72-hour admission, NPO after endoscopy, IV PPI

Lower GI Bleed

- **Determine Stability**
  - Unstable: shock index >1 *(calculated as HR/SBP)*
  - Stable: categorize then based on major or minor by Oakland score
- **Risk Factors:** male sex, age>70, intestinal ischemia, ↓BP, need for transfusion
- **Differential:**
  - If elderly, consider Angiodysplasia/AVM (3-15%), diverticulosis (20-40%), ischemic colitis (12-16%), malignancy
  - All ages: hemorrhoids (outlet bleeding), fissure, colitis (infectious, radiation), C. diff, IBD, intussusception, vasculitis, NSAID induced
- Correct any coagulopathies (FFP if INR > 1.5; keep platelets > 50)
- NPO except medications for at least 8 hours prior to colonoscopy (fluids are 2 hours prior)
- IV fluids (crystalloid)
- PPI IV/PO BID (pantoprazole 40 mg IV/PO BID)
- **Colonoscopy prep:** 1st choice for initial evaluation of LGIB
  - For colon prep in setting of LGIB, GoLYTELY 800 cc/hour (or Colyte) via NG tube. Start with 4L PM prior to procedure and give additional 4L approximately 5 hours before planned procedure in AM (4L total)[4,5]
  - Give 1x Dulcolax 10mg the day before procedure
  - Optional magnesium citrate
  - Have versed and fentanyl held at bedside for procedure
  - Reglan 10mg IV 30min prior to and 2 hours after starting the prep.
  - Do not do PO prep when trying to clear bleeding.
- **Radiographic Imaging**
  - Consider in patients who continue to have significant bleeding despite colonoscopy
  - Options include
    - CT angiography (preferred method; bleeding ≥0.3cc/min; 79-100% SENS)
    - Tagged RBC scan (bleeding as low as 0.1 cc/min can be detected)

GI bleed management based on location

Upper GI Bleed	Lower GI Bleed

- **Discharge**
  - Can be discharged same day if no high-risk features (clean ulcer base, no comorbid conditions)
  - Patients that should be monitored for 72 hrs.
    - Comorbid conditions (heart failure, recent cardiovascular or CVA, chronic alcoholism, or active cancer)
    - Hemodynamically unstable
    - Endoscopic finding of high-risk stigmata:
      - Active bleeding
      - NBVV
      - Adherent clot
  - Home PPI once daily after 72h from procedure

Obscure Bleed (unknown source)
- Push enteroscopy – can reach proximal 150cm portion of the small bowel; may ↑ dx yield by 35%
- Video capsule endoscopy – req 2L of polyethylene glycol f/b overnight fast; can also be used to look for Crohns, malabsorption disorders, polyposis surveillance. C/I in known SBO or LBO.
- Double-balloon enteroscopy – can reach the upper 2/3 from above or lower 1/3 from below of colon
- Intraoperative enteroscopy – dx yield ↑ by 60-88%; risks include serosal tear, avulsion, HF, RF

ACUTE PANCREATITIS

- **Clinical Signs and Symptoms**
    - Constant, epigastric tenderness ± radiation to back, nausea/vomiting, relief with bending forward
    - Gallstone pancreatitis more likely to present as abrupt in onset, with radiation to back
    - Alcoholic pancreatitis more likely to present as dull pain that increases with time
- **Etiologies**
    - Gallstones (AST>3x ULN)
    - Alcohol
    - Hypertriglyceridemia → in the absence of gallstones +/- h/o EtOH then consider TG (concerning if >1000)
    - Biliary sludge
    - Blunt trauma
    - Hypercalcemia
    - Family history of pancreatic diseases
    - Autoimmune diseases
    - Medications: pentamidine, azathioprine, 6-mercaptopurine, thiazide diuretics, sulfonamides, valproic acid, estrogens, tetracyclines
    - Malignancy (hypercalcemia)
    - Infections: mumps, CMV, HIV, E. coli
    - Scorpion sting
    - Mechanical: post-ERCP, sphincter of Oddi dysfunction, pancreatic divisum, malignancy, perforated peptic ulcer
    - Miscellaneous: cystic fibrosis, genetic mutations
- **Physical Exam**
    - Hypovolemia, abdominal tenderness, guarding, ↓ bowel sounds, signs of retroperitoneal hemorrhage (Cullen's and Turner's signs)
- **Diagnosis**
    - **2 of the 3 criteria required:**
        - Clinical Presentation c/w disease (i.e. abdominal pain, epigastric or LUQ, constant with radiation to back, chest, or flanks)
        - Imaging evidence on CT, US, or MRI
        - Biochemical lab evidence of amylase or lipase > 3x ULN. Lipase is preferred, amylase nml in 1/5 of patients.
    - Diagnostic imaging is reserved for patients in whom the diagnosis is unclear or do not improve clinically with supportive care within 48-72 hrs.

Staging of Acute Pancreatitis		
Mild	Moderate	Severe
No organ failure	Local complications	Persistent organ failure (>48 hours) as defined by *Marshal Score*
No local complications	+/-	
	Transient organ failure (<48 hours)	

Local complications include necrosis, peripancreatic fluid collections
Organ failure includes shock (SBP<90), PaO2<60, renal failure (SCr>2 after hydration), GIB (>500cc lost/24 hours)

- **Labs:** amylase, **lipase**, liver function tests, calcium, chemistry panel, C-reactive protein Increase in ALT **to ≥ 3x the baseline** is more specific for pancreatitis 2/2 gallstones but levels <3x cannot be excluded
    - Amylase

- A sensitive diagnostic method if patient presents within hours of the onset of pain. Returns to normal faster than lipase.
- Normal in 1/5 of patients with pancreatitis
- Non pancreatic sources of amylase include salivary glands, lung CA, ovaries, and fallopian tubes.
- Amylase levels tend not to be as high in alcoholic pancreatitis as in nonalcoholic forms.
- Elevated in the first 4-12 hours of diagnosis and returns to normal in 3-5 days
- **Not favored**
  - Lipase
    - \>3x ULN
    - **Is a more sensitive and specific test**. It is made only in the pancreas and stomach.
    - Non pancreatic elevation may be seen if the bowels are inflamed and the lipase is reabsorbed after being properly secreted from the pancreas.
    - Note that renal insufficiency and inflammation/perforation of small bowel can lead to elevated amylase/lipase levels without active pancreatitis.
    - Degree of amylase and lipase elevation does not correlate with severity.
  - Others
    - C-RP: >150 @ 48 hours is indicative of severity
    - Procalcitonin
    - Antithrombin III
- **Imaging**
  - Transabdominal ultrasound
    - Should be performed in all patients in the early assessment period
    - The most sensitive way of evaluating the biliary tract in acute pancreatitis
    - R/o choledocholithiasis and cholelithiasis
  - Contrast-enhanced CT (PO and IV) is used to *diagnose* as well as to *determine potential complications.*
    - Indications:
      - 72-92 hours after presentation in patients who are clinically deteriorating or have severe pancreatitis (necrosis, pseudocyst, abscess)
      - If initial diagnosis is in doubt
  - MRCP if you have high suspicion for choledocholithiasis
  - ERCP if concomitant cholangitis present or suspicion for ascending cholangitis
- **Risk Stratification**
  - The most useful predictors of severe disease are elevations at admission and during the following 24 to 48 hours of the following (sick patient → severe course expected; notify ICU):
    - HCT (>44%) or rising
    - BUN (>20 mg/dL) or rising
    - SCr (>1.8 mg/dL)
    - Systemic inflammatory response syndrome
  - Imaging findings that are concerning (signs of ARDS):
    - Pleural effusion
    - Pulmonary infiltrates
    - Multiple or extensive extra pancreatic collections
  - Scoring Systems: *Assessment of severity*
    - APACHE-III (threshold is ≥8)
    - RANSOM (threshold is ≥3)

		SCORING
Age > 55	HCT > 10% decrease	<3 = 1%
BG > 200	Ca < 8	3-4 = 15%
WBC > 16	Base Deficit > 4	5-6 = 40%
LDH > 350	BUN > 5	>7 = 100%
ALT > 250	Fluid sequestration > 6L	
	PPO2a < 60	

  - BISAP (helps with triage)
    - Within 24 hours of presentation:
      - Factors

- BUN >25
- GCS <15
- Evidence of SIRS
- Age >60
- Pleural effusions on CXR
- Calculation
  - 3 points = 5.3% death
  - 4 points = 12.7% death
  - 5 points = 22.5% death
- CT Severity Index
  - Combination of the sum of the necrosis score and points assigned to five grades of findings on CT. The index ranges from 0 to 10, with higher scores indicating a greater severity of illness
- **Classification (Atlanta Classification)**
  - Mild – absence of organ failure, local, or systemic complications
  - Moderate Severe – transient organ failure (recovers in 48h) or local/systemic complications
  - Severe – persistent organ failure for >48h that may involve one or more organs; mortality has high as 25%
- **Management**[46,47,48,49,50]
  - Rest the pancreas and support as necessary
  - Fluids[51]
    - *Amounts*
      - Initial
        - 20 cc/kg of LR should be given over 30 minutes followed by 3 cc/kg/hr. for 8-12 hours if patient is hypotensive.
          - On average, you will give about 7-12L in the first 12 hours.
            - Otherwise, more conservative approach is 1-2L fluid bolus followed by 250-300 cc/hr. for additional 1-2L (total 3-4L given) in first 24/h
              - Monitor volume status every 6 hours via UOP goal of >0.5cc/kg/hr.
        - Infusion of large volumes of NS → development of a hyperchloremic metabolic acidosis→ important factor contributing to pathologic zymogen activation and severity of pancreatitis
        - Monitor the HCT and BUN in the first 12-24 hours, decreases in both are signs that you are giving enough fluids
      - Maintenance:
        - First 12-24 hours: 250-500cc/hr. of LR on average
        - Use decreasing BUN as a marker to monitor every 6 hours to determine if hydration is adequate
      - Total: 70kg person will often require at least 6L
      - More aggressive based on severity markers below
        - BUN: Serial monitoring of BUN to determine fluid resuscitation effectiveness
          - Accurate predictor of in-hospital mortality during first 24 hours
        - HCT (elevation is specifically associated with pancreatic necrosis)
        - ↑SCr as noted below
    - *Type*
      - Crystalloids can be chosen initially however:
        - **LR is fluid of choice**
        - **NS advised only in patients with hypercalcemia**
        - Colloids (pRBC) if HCT < 25%
        - Albumin if albumin level <2 g/dL

Figure. Fluid management of acute pancreatitis

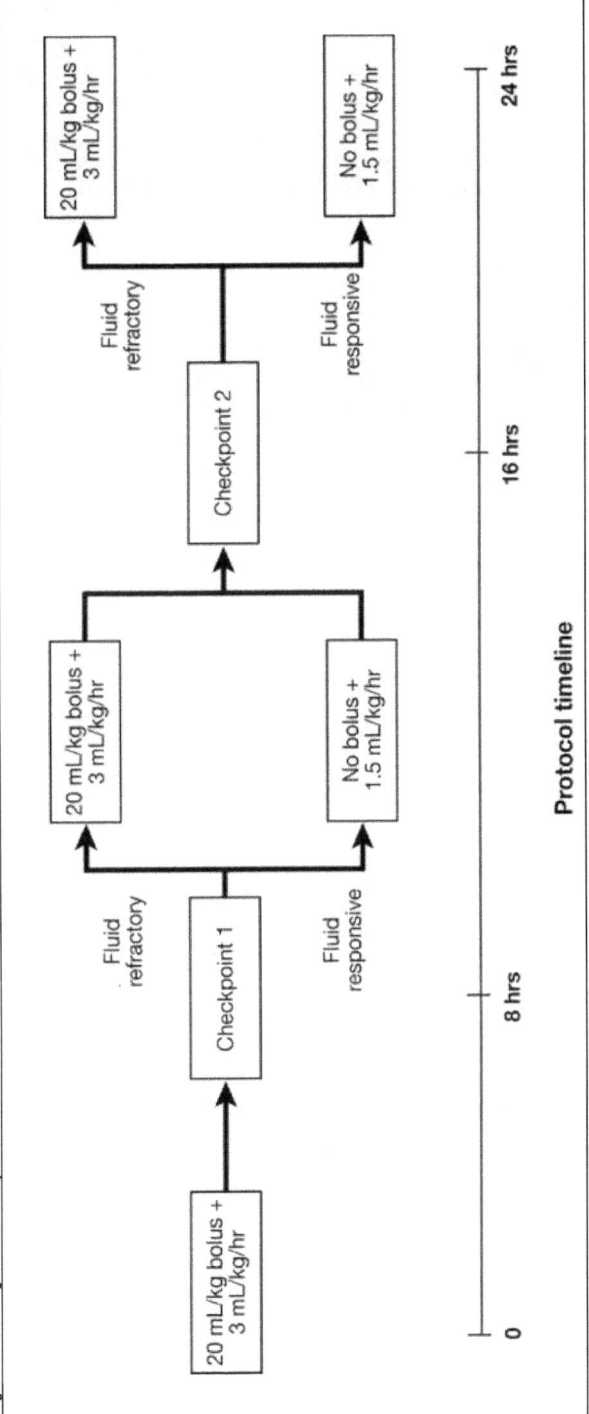

GASTROENTEROLOGY

- Monitoring
  - UOP at least 0.5cc/kg/hr. → some studies suggest goal of 1 cc/kg/hr. in first 24 hours
  - Bladder pressures[52]
    - Intraabdominal hypertension can be worsened by fluid resuscitation. Defined as steady-state pressure within the abdominal cavity which is $\geq$12 mmHg.
    - Grades:
      - 1: 12-15 mmHg
      - 2: 16-20 mmHg
      - **3: 21-25 mmHg**
      - **4: >25 mmHg**
    - Risks for ICH/ACS:
      - Increased intra-abdominal volume (GI tract dilatation: gastroparesis and gastric distention, ileus, volvulus)
      - Ascites or hemoperitoneum
      - Decreased abdominal wall compliance (2/2 abdominal surgery, especially with tight abdominal closures)
      - Obesity
      - Sepsis, severe sepsis, and septic shock
      - Severe acute pancreatitis
      - Massive fluid resuscitation
      - Major burns (with or without abdominal eschars)
      - Complicated intra-abdominal infection
    - Levels >20 are suggestive of abdominal compartment syndrome
    - Treatment
      - Monitoring (transvesicular technique for at least 4 hours until IAP/IAH/ACS <12 for at least 24 hours)
      - Ultrafiltration
      - Diuretics
      - NG tube if suspecting ileus
      - Endoscopic decompression
      - Limit fluids by using colloids or hypertonic solutions (often in burn patients)
      - Remove any restrictive eschars
      - HOB @ 20 degrees, avoid prone positioning
      - Luminal decompression with rectal tube placement
      - Percutaneous drainage of ascites
      - NM blockade if ventilated to relax abdomen
      - Open abdominal decompression (last resort)
  - Serial ICUP for BUN, SCr, albumin
  - Serial H/H for HCT levels
  - MAP>65
  - Routine CVP not necessary, if present, goal 8-12
- Feeds
  Data suggest that <u>early</u> enteral nutrition helps stimulate the gut and maintain its protective barrier, thus reducing bacterial overgrowth and preventing bacterial translocation and sepsis. Enteral nutrition is typically withheld during initial resuscitation. Enteral feeding may have benefits that could decrease length of stay, such as reduced intestinal permeability, improved gut motility, and reduced infection of pancreatic necrosis.
  - If mild and patient has no nausea or vomiting, PO is allowed with **low fat diet** (within 24 hours of admission)
  - If symptomatic, NPO until improved (pain-free, hungry)

- Typically start enteral feeding by day 3, solid foods advanced by day 5
- Enteral nutrition (NG) for necrotizing pancreatitis unless ileus present (then TPN)
  - NJ shows no ↓ risk of worsening of condition
- Repletion of **electrolytes**
- **NGT** to suction only if protracted nausea and vomiting to prevent aspiration not to help pancreas as previously believed
- Antibiotics
  - Treat infections if clinically suspected
    - ABx only indicated in sterile or infected pancreatitis necrosis (pt presents with fever and ↑WBC)
      - Prior to which a CT guided biopsy for cultures is required
    - No clear studies have shown a benefit to prophylactic ABx however if significant sterile necrosis (>30%) present, some treat with ABx for 14 days
      - ABx to consider imipenem 500mg q6h, combination of cipro 750mg BID + metronidazole 500mg TID or cefuroxime 1.5g TID then 250mg BID
  - Fevers initially are expected secondary to inflammatory response
  - FNA if suspicious for infection (↑WBC, fevers 10-14d out from dx, tachycardia, **peripancreatic gas on imaging**)
- Pain control: meperidine (morphine in theory causes spasm of sphincter of Oddi; no evidence in humans and most feel clinically safe), or PCA (20-50mcg of fentanyl with 10m lockout)
- **Complications**
  - If patient is >40 YO, **pancreatic tumor** should be considered as a cause in the DDx
  - Acute pancreatic fluid collection (APFC), pseudocyst (>4 weeks after diagnosis), necrosis, cholangitis, abscesses, ARDS, renal failure, sepsis, shock
    - Necrosis/Necrotizing Pancreatitis - is 2/2 to ischemia; try to prevent with substantial fluid resuscitation on admission. Diagnosed when >30% of the gland is affected by necrosis. May not be present on initial contrast-enhanced CT, may consider repeat CT after 1 week (look for non-enhancing regions).
      - Percutaneous aspiration of necrosis with Gram stain and culture should be performed if there are ongoing signs of possible pancreatic infection such as sustained leukocytosis, fever, or organ failure.
      - There is no role for *prophylactic antibiotics* in necrotizing pancreatitis, only indicated in confirmed infected necrosis
        - Consider starting broad-spectrum antibiotics in a patient who appears septic while awaiting the results of Gram stain and cultures → if cultures are negative, the antibiotics should be discontinued to minimize the risk of developing opportunistic or fungal superinfection.
        - Risk of infection (bacterial translocation) based on severity of necrosis
          - <30% necrosis = 22.5% chance of infection
          - >50% necrosis = 46.5% chance of infection
      - Repeated fine-needle aspiration and Gram stain with culture of pancreatic necrosis may be done every 5–7 days in the presence of persistent fever.
      - Repeated CT or MRI imaging should also be considered with any change in clinical course to monitor for complications (e.g., thromboses, hemorrhage, and abdominal compartment syndrome).
      - SCr of ≥ 1.8 within 48 hours of admission has 35x more likelihood for development of necrosis. Good marker for organ injury
    - Debridement only indicated if evidence of infection, sterile necrosis should not be taken to the OR
  - DIC (PLT<100,000, Fibrinogen <1g/L, ↑aPTT, ↑PT)
  - If suspicion for concomitant cholangitis, obtain ERCP

- o If suspicion for choledocholithiasis, obtain MRCP
- **Prognosis**
  - o Outcomes depend on whether disease is interstitial versus necrotizing
    - Interstitial mortality rate < 1%
    - Necrotizing (defined as necrosis of 30% of the gland seen on CT) mortality rate 10-30% mortality risk with a 70% complication risk
  - o Scoring systems: Ranson, Glasgow, Apache II (none are completely accurate)

BOWEL OBSTRUCTION

- **Presentation**[53]
  - o Abdominal pain, crampy, diffuse, episodic in nature
  - o Depending on location → more proximal = vomiting is bilious, more distal = feculent vomiting
- **Etiology**
  - o Small
    - Adhesions
    - Hernia
    - IBD
    - GSI
    - Cancer (lymphoma, adenocarcinoma, polyp)
  - o Large
    - Cancer
    - Diverticulitis
    - Sigmoid volvulus
- **Types**
  - o Complete – passage of neither flatus nor stool, more vomiting
  - o Partial – can pass flatus; colicky; peristaltic rushes
  - o Pseudo obstruction (Ogilvie's)
- **Diagnosis**
  - o Capsule imaging
  - o KUB
  - o CT with oral and IV contrast
- **Treatment**
  - o NPO
  - o IVF - Provide IV fluids (nothing is being absorbed by the stomach!) → monitor by watching HR and UOP
  - o NG if needed: In presence of severe nausea and vomiting, use NG tube with intermittent suctioning to gravity
  - o Serial Abdominal Exams
  - o If patient does not clinically respond, or, shows signs of ischemia then proceed directly to surgery
    - If surgery required, preoperative ABx:
      1. Tazobactam-Piperacillin 3.375g IV q6h
      2. Ampicillin-Sulbactam 3g IV q6h
  - o Avoid medications that ↓ bowel motility:
    - Opioids
    - Anticholinergics
    - CCB
  - o **Ogilvie's**
    - Most common in hospitalized or institutionalized men >60

- Symptoms: nausea, vomiting, abdominal distention, CT imaging with dilation without e/o obvious obstruction
- Treat underlying cause (trauma, electrolytes, infection, post-operative, chemotherapy, neurologic)
- Replete all electrolytes (look for low K and Mg)
- Discontinue opiates, anti-cholinergics, sedatives
- IV fluids only, NPO, place NG tube, have rectal tube to gravity with flushes
- Serial KUB q12-24h
- Prone positioning with left and right lateral decubitus positions q1h
- Neostigmine unless bradycardic or hx of bronchospasm in patients who fail above treatment after **24-48 hours or cecal diameter >12cm**
    1. Hold atropine at bedside
    2. Keep on telemetry during and 30min after administration
    3. Have bedpan ready

GERD

- **Definition**: a condition which develops when the reflux of stomach contents causes troublesome symptoms and/or complications.
- **Diagnosis**[54,55]
    - A presumptive diagnosis of GERD can be established in the setting of typical symptoms of heartburn and regurgitation. Empiric medical therapy with a proton pump inhibitor (PPI) is recommended in this setting.
- **Causes of GERD**
    - PUD
    - Motility disorder (achalasia, DES)
    - Reflux Hypersensitivity
    - Nonerosive Reflux Disease
    - Eosinophilic Esophagitis
- **Associated Symptoms**
    - Chronic cough, laryngitis, and asthma have an established association with GERD on the basis of population-based studies.
- **Red Flags**[56]
    - Age>50
    - Dysphagia or odynophagia
    - FHx of GI malignancy
    - Unintended ↓wt.
    - Recurrent vomiting
    - Sx > 5 yrs. or <6 mo.
    - Epigastric mass
- **Diagnostics**
    - Barium radiographs - should not be performed to diagnose GERD
    - EGD
        - The principal use of endoscopy in suspected GERD is the evaluation of treatment failures, presence of red flags.
        - Poor evidence for screening for Barrett's esophagus or malignancy in chronic GERD
        - Consider in patients unresponsive to BID therapy for 5-6 weeks
        - Repeat endoscopy is not indicated in patients without Barrett's esophagus in the absence of new symptoms.
    - Manometry – done by GI if patient does not respond to be BID therapy and has no EGD evidence of erosive disease

GASTROENTEROLOGY

- o Ambulatory impedance-pH
  - To evaluate patients with a suspected esophageal GERD syndrome who have not responded to an empirical trial of PPI therapy, have normal findings on endoscopy, and have no major abnormality on manometry.
  - PPI therapy withheld for 7 days
  - Wireless pH monitoring has superior sensitivity to catheter studies for detecting pathological esophageal acid exposure because of the extended period of recording (48 hours) and has also shown superior recording accuracy compared with some catheter designs
- **Labs**
  - o Screening for *Helicobacter pylori* infection is not recommended in GERD patients.
- **Treatment/Management**
  - o Pharmacotherapy
    - Anti-secretory therapy is highly recommended in patients to obtain symptomatic relief and those with evidence of esophagitis
      - PPI (A 4-8-week course of PPIs is the therapy of choice for symptom relief and healing of erosive esophagitis) with concurrent lifestyle modification
        - Omeprazole 20 mg PO daily
        - Pantoprazole 40 mg PO daily
        - Esomeprazole 20 mg PO daily
      - H2 therapy
        - Cimetidine 800 mg PO at bedtime
        - Ranitidine 300 mg PO at bedtime
        - Famotidine 40 mg PO at bedtime
      - PPI>H2 blocker
        - There are no major differences in efficacy between the different PPIs.
        - Understand risks of long-term PPI therapy (i.e. CKD, osteoporosis, CAP, C.diff)
          - o Long term therapy, consider DEXA scan, calcium supplementation, H. pylori screening
        - Traditional delayed release PPIs should be administered 30–60 min before meal for maximal pH control.
        - PPI therapy should be initiated at **once a day dosing**, before the first meal of the day.
          - o For patients with partial response to once daily therapy, tailored therapy with adjustment of dose timing and/or twice daily dosing should be considered in patients with night-time symptoms, variable schedules, and/or sleep disturbance.
          - o In patients with partial response to PPI therapy, increasing the dose to **twice daily therapy** or switching to a different PPI may provide additional symptom relief
        - If esophagitis is noted, consider BID therapy
          - o In patients with just symptoms but no pathology, can try PRN therapy or short-term use
          - o Pharmacokinetics recommend BID dosing however all trials have been with once daily dosing
        - There is no evidence of improved efficacy by adding a nocturnal dose of an H2RA to twice-daily PPI therapy.
        - Side Effects: HA, diarrhea, abdominal pain, CKD, pneumonia, fractures, osteoporosis, ↓Mg, *C.diff*, ↓VB12, dementia.
          - o Chronic PPI therapy may lead to ↑ # of hyperplastic polyps in the gastric fundus
  - o Non-Pharmacologic

- Weight loss
- Elevate head shortly after eating if laying down
- Avoid late night meals
    - Surgery
        - Surgical therapy is a treatment option for long-term therapy in GERD patients.
        - Preoperative ambulatory pH monitoring is mandatory in patients without evidence of erosive esophagitis. All patients should undergo preoperative manometry to rule out achalasia or scleroderma-like esophagus.
- **Duration of Therapy**
    - Long-term therapy should be titrated down <u>to the lowest effective dose</u> based on symptom control.
        - If you cannot wean them off, consider switching to H2 blocker
    - Consider on-demand therapy for those with no evidence of esophagitis previously; those who did resolve try long term on-demand therapy have high risk for return of erosive disease
    - Chronic PPI therapy ↑ risk for *C.difficile,* PNA, and development of osteoporosis (>7 yrs. of PPI use). Theory behind these adverse causes is unknown but suspected to be due to ↓ absorption of Ca by PPI.

PEPTIC ULCER DISEASE

- **Pearl**[57]
    - *H. pylori* important to tx d/t risk for gastric cancer and MALT lymphoma along with it being the most common cause of most ulcers
- **Alarm Symptoms**
    - Unexplained weight loss
    - Want to rule out gastric cancer (look for dysphagia as well) or vomiting d/t blockage of the pylorus
    - New onset sx in pt >45 YO
    - Bleeding
    - Iron deficiency anemia (see page 305)
    - Progressive dysphagia
    - Odynophagia
    - Recurrent emesis
    - Family history of GI cancer
- **Etiology of PUD**
    - H. pylori
        - One of the most common causes of PUD and functional dyspepsia
        - Should test in patients on chronic NSAIDs, unexplained IDA, and ITP via urea breath testing or stool antigen
    - NSAIDs
    - ZE syndrome
- **Types**
    - Gastric - Food ↑pain and not relieved with antacids
    - Duodenal - Food relieves pain (worse on empty stomach), is relieved with antacids as well.
- **Symptoms**
    - Symptoms of ulcers are caused by presence of acid without food or other acid buffers
    - Dyspepsia (pain in upper abdomen, fullness, early satiety, bloating, and nausea
    - Nighttime pain may be due to circadian rhythm increasing acid production

GASTROENTEROLOGY

- o NUD – upper abdominal IBS, sx are similar to dyspepsia that last for 12+ weeks, likely functional in nature, when EGD done no ulcer is found, patients are often **not** responsive to PPI's
- o GERD – heartburn, mid chest pain, occurs after meals and worse with lying down
- **Diagnosis**
  - o Endoscopy reserved for pts not responding to empiric PPI, have red flag symptoms, or those with new symptoms and ≥60. For diagnosis to be accurate, patients must be off PPIs for at least 2 weeks, and bismuth and antibiotics should be held for 4 weeks to avoid false-negative results.
    - R/O *H. pylori*: Bx obtained x3 at antrum and incisura angularis, urease testing, CLOtest, fecal antigen
    - Should be done only after off PPI for 2 weeks or 24 hours after H2 blocker
    - May obtain biopsies at duodenum to r/o celiac if necessary
  - o For those patients who do not require immediate endoscopy, **"test and treat"** for *H.pylori* advised along with counseling to avoid smoking, alcohol, and NSAIDs.
    - For diagnosis, patients must be off PPIs for at least 2 weeks, and bismuth and antibiotics should be held for 4 weeks to avoid false-negative results.
      - Acute *H.pylori* diagnosis via:
        - Urea breath test
          - o Best used after tx to confirm eradication as it is only positive in current infections
        - Stool antigen testing
      - Do not choose AB testing as this cannot differentiate between acute and chronic disease.
- **Treatment**[58]
  - o Pharmacotherapy
    - Patients without *H.pylori* should be treated with a PPI for 2 months
      - PPI options
        - Can chose from any PPI
        - Daily doses of **lansoprazole from 20 to 40 mg** produced better healing results (rabeprazole was the best but cost may be too high to use)
    - All four H2 receptor antagonists (cimetidine, ranitidine, famotidine, and nizatidine) are associated with healing rates of 70 to 80 percent for duodenal ulcers after four weeks, and 87 to 94 percent after eight weeks of therapy
      - Split dose, evening, and nighttime therapy are all effective.
      - Cimetidine, ranitidine, and famotidine are approved for gastric ulcer healing in the United States
    - Stop all NSAIDs
- **H. pylori Treatment**[59]

GASTROENTEROLOGY

H.pylori Treatment Options			
Triple-Therapy	Lansoprazole 30mg BID + Clarithromycin 500mg BID + Amoxicillin 1 g BID	10-14 days	Reserved for patients with **no** previous history of macrolide exposure who live where clarithromycin resistance among H. pylori isolates is low.
Quadruple-Therapy	PPI BID (consider lansoprazole) + Bismuth (525 mg four times daily) + Two antibiotics (e.g., metronidazole 250 mg four times daily and tetracycline 500 mg four times daily)	14 days	N/A

- o Sequential
    - May improve eradication rates, especially with clarithromycin resistant strains.
    - This 14-day regimen involves:
        1) Amoxicillin (1 g twice daily) for five days
        2) PPI (twice daily)
        3) clarithromycin (500 mg twice daily)
        4) metronidazole 500 mg twice daily
- o Confirming Eradication/Treatment
    - After **4 weeks** from the last dose, urea breath test or stool antigen testing should be performed to **confirm successful treatment**
    - If treatment failed, consider testing spouse as infection is transferred via saliva.

ELEVATED LIVER ASSOCIATED ENZYMES

- **General**[60,61]
    - o Include AST, ALT, ALKP, and bilirubin
    - o Mild elevation is defined as less than 5x the ULN
    - o ALT is more specific than AST
    - o The predominant pattern of enzyme alteration (hepatocellular v. cholestatic v mixed) *Calculate R factor (ALT/ALT ULN) / (ALKP/ALKP ULN) to help distinguish*[62]
        - **AST/ALT ratios**
            - Understand that AST>ALT is most common in EtOH associated causes however in cirrhosis this pattern also develops
            - ALT>ALT more common in hepatocellular injuries (non-EtOH)
        - **"Hepatocellular"** – AST, ALT (ALT/ALKP > 2.2), R factor >5
            - Often seen with ↑bilirubin and jaundice
            - Consider viral hepatitis and toxin exposure (drugs, herbs, EtOH)
        - **"Cholestatic"** – ALKPH, GGT (ALT/ALKP < 2.2), R factor <2
        See next section for full chart
            - ALKP is suggestive of biliary obstruction or intrahepatic cholestasis
            - Liver US to look for bile duct dilatation, r/o chronic liver disease
            - GGT to confirm biliary origin
            - Medications (ACEi) can cause isolated elevations (https://livertox.nih.gov)
            - R/o metastatic malignancy (esp. pancreatic cancer)
            - R/o infiltrative diseases
        - **"Biliary"** – TBILI, DBILI, IBILI

- IBILI – hemolysis
  - Unconjugated or indirect
  - Hemolysis (H/H, smear, LDH, haptoglobin, reticulocyte count)
  - DDx: Gilbert's (clinical dx), Criggler-Najjar
- DBILI
  - Conjugated or direct
  - Usually sign of liver disease as normally elevated bilirubin can be excreted quickly
  - R/O viral hepatitis, toxic injury, shock liver, AIH (+smooth muscle AB, normal saturation), hemochromatosis (↑iron saturation)
  - Normal AST/ALT but elevations in DBILI and ALKP are suggestive of cholestatic drug reaction, PBC, PSC
  - DDx: Dubin-johnson, Rotor's
- **Synthetic function**
  - albumin - made by liver, ↓ with liver failure
  - PT/INR – increase due to ↓ synthesis of liver-derived coagulation factors (I, II, V, VII, X). Remember PT is affected by warfarin and ↓vitamin K
- **History**
  - Exposure to hepatotoxins
  - Alcohol (>3 drinks/d in men; >2 drinks/d in women), medications, supplements, herbs
    - www.livertox.nih.gov
  - RF for viral hepatitis (IVDA, blood transfusion <'92, travel)
  - Job: industrial chemicals
- **Pathology**
  - Indicates inflammation +/- injury to hepatocytes resulting in leakage of contents into plasma
- **Differential**
  - *Always rule out:*
    - Viral hepatitis
    - Hemochromatosis (not common in high ALT/AST levels)
    - AIH
    - NAFLD

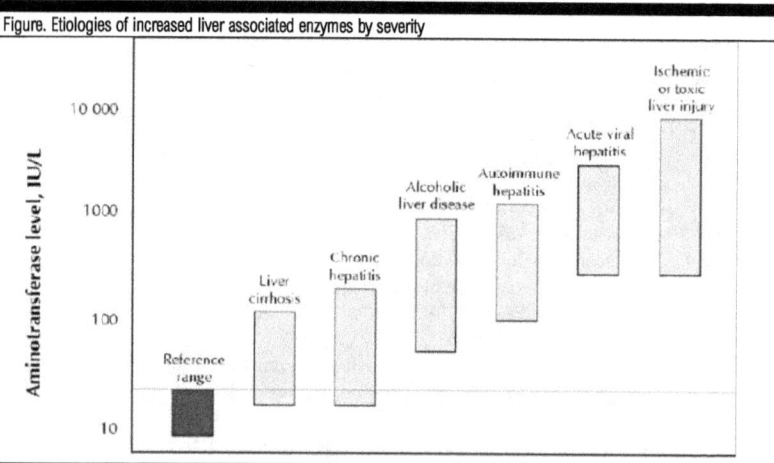

Figure. Etiologies of increased liver associated enzymes by severity

(1) Magnitude of enzyme alteration in the case of aminotransferases

Marked: >10x ULN
- Toxin/Medication
  - EtOH
  - Tylenol
  - Herbal
  - Statin
  - Glucophage
- Ischemia / Shock (TBILI< 34 µmol/L, and ALT/LDH ratio < 1)
- Thrombosis
  - Budd-Chiari
  - Portal vein
- Acute viral hepatitis
  - A/B/D/E
  - Less common: CMV, EBV, HSV
- AIH

Moderate: 5–10x ULN
- Medications
- Chronic viral hepatitis
- **NAFLD** (evidence of metabolic syndrome (increased waist circumference, elevated blood pressure, lipid pattern of high serum triglyceride levels and low serum high-density lipoprotein levels, elevated blood glucose levels or evidence of insulin resistance) See page 75 for more information.
- Wilson's (check ceruloplasmin)
- Alpha-1 antitrypsin (early onset emphysema, family history)
- PBC
- PSC

Mild: < 5x ULN

ALT elevation > than AST is more specific for liver origin (AST elevations can also be caused by thyroid disease, celiac disease, hemolysis, and muscle disorders)
- Hepatitis (anti-HCV and HBsAg)
- Alcohol (AST:ALT >2)
- Hemochromatosis (transferrin saturation, ferritin)
- Autoimmune: ANA, anti-smooth muscle
- Medications
- Congestive hepatopathy 2/2 right sided heart failure
- Celiac' s disease
- NAFLD (2/2 DM +/- obesity)

(2) Rate of change (increase or decrease over time)
(3) Course of alteration (e.g., mild fluctuation v. progressive increase).

Causes of Liver Enzyme Elevation				
Cause	AST	ALT	ALKP	Bili
NAFLD	ALT>AST (<5x)		Nml	Nml/Direct
Alcoholic Liver Disease	AST>ALT 2:1 (<5x)		Nml	Nml/Direct
Drug-Induced Liver Injury (i.e. Tylenol)	↑↑↑ (10x)	↑↑↑ (10x)	Nml	Nml
Chronic Hepatitis B/C	ALT>AST (<5x)		Nml	Nml
Acute Viral Hepatitis	ALT>AST (10x)		Nml	Nml
Hereditary Hemochromatosis	ALT>AST (10x)			
Autoimmune Hepatitis	ALT>AST (10x)		Nml	Nml
Wilson Disease	ALT>AST (10x)		Nml	Nml
Hemolytic	Nml		Nml	Indirect

- **Labs/Work-up**
  - Serial LFTs with GGT
  - Lipid panel (NAFLD)
  - A1c (NAFLD)
  - CBC (MCV>100 more suggestive of thyroid or alcohol cause)
  - Alpha-1
  - Viral panel
    - Hepatitis A: IgM anti-HAV
    - Hepatitis B: HBsAg, IgM anti-HBc, IgG anti-HBc, HBsAg, anti-HBe, HBeAg
    - Hepatitis C: anti-HCV, HCV RNA
    - Hepatitis D: anti-HBs, anti-HDV
    - Hepatitis E: anti-HEV
    - Others
      - CMV
      - EBV
      - HSV
  - Others to consider
    - Anti-smooth muscle (AIH)
    - Anti-mitochondrial (PBC)

Hepatitis Panel Evaluation								
	HBsAg	HBeAg	IgM anti-HBc	IgG anti-HBc	Anti-HBs	Anti-HBe	HBV DNA
Early Acute	+	+	+				+++
Late Acute	+	+	+	+			
Window			+				+
Recovery				+	+	+	Likely +
Chronic carrier	+			+			
Acute on chronic	+	Likely +	+	+			
Vaccinated					+		
Immune 2/2 past infection				+	+		

USMLEWorld

The presence of HBeAg is indicative of ongoing infection/viral replication

  - RUQ US with Doppler flow
  - Toxicology screen
    - APAP
  - Consider ceruloplasmin, iron panel (Fe, TIBC, ferritin)
  - Anti-smooth muscle AB
  - Functional labs:
    - Coagulation panel
    - PLT (CBC)
    - Fractionated bilirubin
    - Albumin
- **Fulminant Hepatic Failure**
  - Encephalopathy (order NH3)
  - Cerebral edema
  - ↑INR, ↑Lactate, PO4
  - Shock
  - Ascites
- **Treatment of statin-induced liver enzyme elevation**[63]

- o Commonly only see elevations 2-3x ULN
- o Direct relationship seen between the dose of statin and elevation of AST/ALT
- o Statins appear to be associated with a very low risk of true and serious liver injury
- o Some cases may see spontaneous resolution without discontinuation of the offending medication (unsure of physiology, could be tolerance vs adaptation)
- o Options include decreasing dose, changing statin, or discontinuing therapy.
- **Physical Exam**
  - o Temporal and proximal muscle wasting
  - o Ascites
  - o R pleural effusion
  - o ↑JVP
  - o Hepatic encephalopathy
  - o Dupuytren's contractures
  - o Testicular atrophy

NON-ALCOHOLIC FATTY LIVER DISEASE

- **General**[64]
  - o Most common cause for mild liver enzyme elevations
  - o Second most common cause of liver transplant
  - o It is thought to be the hepatic consequence of **systemic insulin resistance** and the metabolic syndrome characterized by obesity, dyslipidemia, and type 2 diabetes mellitus.
  - o **Diagnosis of exclusion** must exclude significant alcohol use or other conditions that could cause liver damage.
- **Subtypes**
  - o NAFL (non-alcoholic fatty liver) - steatosis, **without inflammation**, in at least 5% of hepatocytes.
  - o NASH (non-alcoholic steatohepatitis) - constellation of features that include steatosis, lobular and portal **inflammation**, and liver cell injury in the form of hepatocyte ballooning. Worse prognosis with development to cirrhosis in 15% of patients.
- **Evaluation**
  - o Labs
  Up to 30% of patients have elevated serum ferritin and autoantibodies, including ANA, ASMA, and AMA.
    - Hepatitis panel (2-3x ULN ↑ of AST/ALT)
    - ANA
    - Albumin
    - BMI (from vitals)
    - PLT
    - Anti-smooth muscle AB
    - Anti-mitochondrial AB
    - Iron panel (mild elevations expected due to inflammation)
    - Alpha-1 anti-trypsin
    - Ceruloplasmin
  - o Procedures
    - US – the best way to diagnose hepatic steatosis but cannot differentiate between the subtypes (steatosis vs. steatohepatitis)
    - Liver biopsy is the only way to diagnose and stage (assess the degree of steatosis)
    - *Indications*
      - ▫ Before starting therapy
      - ▫ To confirm diagnosis

- Non-invasive testing
    - NAFLD fibrosis score / Fibroscan - can be used to identify patients who may have fibrosis or cirrhosis (**without the need for biopsy**) and can help direct the use of liver biopsy in patients who would benefit from prognostication and potential treatment. Based on patient age, body mass index, hyperglycemia, platelet count, albumin, and ratio of aspartate aminotransferase to alanine aminotransferase. Accessed from: http://nafldscore.com
- Treatment
    - It is pivotal to determine which patients are at high risk of progression to advanced disease. The presence of fibrosis on imaging or biopsy is a high risk.
    - The first step in managing patients who have NAFLD is to treat components of the metabolic syndrome, including obesity, dyslipidemia, and type 2 diabetes.
    - Pharmacotherapy
        - **Pentoxifylline** and **obeticholic acid** improve fibrosis
        - **Vitamin E**, probiotics, thiazolidinediones, and obeticholic acid improve neuroinflammation associated with NASH
        - **Metformin** recommended in those with T2DM
        - Poor evidence to support use of statins

Bibliography

[9] Baudendistel TE, Sandhu A. Chapter 31. Abdominal Pain. In: Henderson MC, Tierney LM, Jr., Smetana GW. eds. The Patient History: An Evidence-Based Approach to Differential Diagnosis New York, NY: McGraw-Hill; 2012.

[10] Silen W. (2012). Chapter 13. Abdominal Pain. In D.L. Longo, A.S. Fauci, D.L. Kasper, S.L. Hauser, J.L. Jameson, J. Loscalzo (Eds), Harrison's Principles of Internal Medicine, 18e. Retrieved April 29, 2012

[11] Runyon, Bruce. Management of Adult Patients with Ascites due to Cirrhosis: An Update. AASLD Practice Guidelines. 2009

[12] Rosenblatt R et al. Early paracentesis in high-risk hospitalized patients: Time for a new quality indicator. Am J Gastroenterol 2019 Dec; 114:1863.

[13] Cheung et al. 2MM. 2013.

[14] Bambha et al. "Model for End-stage Liver Disease (MELD)" UpToDate.com

[15] Kim WR, Biggins SW, Kremers WK, Wiesner RH, Kamath PS, Benson JT, Edwards E, Therneau TM. Hyponatremia and mortality among patients on the liver-transplant waiting list. N Engl J Med. 2008 Sep 4;359(10):1018-26. PMID: 18768945

[16] Rifai et al. "Bleeding esophageal varices: Who should receive a shunt?" Cleveland Clinic Journal of Medicine. 2017 March;84(3):199-201.

[17] Gutt CN, Encke J, Köninger J, et al. Acute cholecystitis: early versus delayed cholecystectomy, a multicenter randomized trial (ACDC study, NCT00447304). Ann Surg. 2013;258(3):385–393. doi:10.1097/SLA.0b013e3182a1599b

[18] Lammert F, Gutt C. Prävention, Diagnostik und Behandlung von Gallensteinen [Prophylaxis, Diagnosis and Treatment of Gallstones - The Most Important Facts of the Updated S3-Guideline of the DGVS and DGAV]. Dtsch Med Wochenschr. 2019;144(3):194–200. doi:10.1055/a-0649-5391

[19] Bernardi et al. Gut. 2019.

[20] TheCurbSiders.com

[21] Rodrigues, S. G., Mendoza, Y., & Bosch, J. (2019). Beta-blockers in cirrhosis: evidence-based indications and limitations. JHEP Reports.

[22] ASGE. "The role of endoscopy in the management of variceal hemorrhage." Gastrointestinal Endoscopy. 80(2). 2014.

[23] Hepatitis C Online. Diagnosis and Management of Hepatic Encephalopathy. 2019.

[24] Runyon BA; AASLD Practice Guidelines Committee. Management of adult patients with ascites due to cirrhosis: an update. Hepatology. 2009;49(6):2087-2107.

[25] Rassi et al. JHep (2019).

[26] Schneiderhan et al. "Targeting gut flora to treat and prevent disease." J Fam Pract. 2016 January;65(1):34-38.

[27] Ford et al. "American College of Gastroenterology Monograph on the Management of Irritable Bowel Syndrome and Chronic Idiopathic Constipation." Am J Gastroenterol 2014; 109:S2 – S26.

[28] Ruepert L Quartero AO de Wit NJ van der Heijden GJ Rubin G Muris JW Bulking agents, antispasmodics and antidepressants for the treatment of irritable bowel syndrome. Cochrane Database Syst Rev 2011 CD003460.

[29] Jamshed N, Lee ZE, Olden KW. "Diagnostic approach to chronic constipation in adults." Am Fam Physician. 2011 Aug 1;84(3):299-306.

[30] Wald, Arnold. JAMA. 2019.

[31] Wilkins T, McMechan D, Talukder A. "Colorectal Cancer Screening and Prevention." Am Fam Physician. 2018 May 15;97(10):658-665.

[32] Diarrhea, Acute. In: Papadakis MA, McPhee SJ, Bernstein J. eds. Quick Medical Diagnosis & Treatment 2018 New York, NY: McGraw-Hill; . http://accessmedicine.mhmedical.com/content.aspx?bookid=2273&sectionid=178292926. Accessed March 13, 2018.

[33] MMWR. "Diagnosis and Management of Foodborne Illnesses." January 26, 2001 / 50(RR02);1-69.

[34] Diarrhea, Chronic. In: Papadakis MA, McPhee SJ, Bernstein J. eds. Quick Medical Diagnosis & Treatment 2018 New York, NY: McGraw-Hill; . http://accessmedicine.mhmedical.com/content.aspx?bookid=2273&sectionid=178292959. Accessed March 13, 2018.

[35] Jacobs, Danny. "Diverticulitis." N Engl J Med 2007;357:2057-66

[36] Savastano ME. The Role of Speech/Language Pathologists in Dysphagia Management. In: McKean SC, Ross JJ, Dressler DD, Scheurer DB. eds. *Principles and Practice of Hospital Medicine, 2e* New York, NY: McGraw-Hill

[37] Lembo A, Cremonini F. Chapter 35. Dysphagia. In: Henderson MC, Tierney LM, Jr., Smetana GW. eds. The Patient History: An Evidence-Based Approach to Differential Diagnosis New York, NY: McGraw-Hill

[38] Bono MJ. Esophageal Emergencies. In: Tintinalli JE, Ma O, Yealy DM, Meckler GD, Stapczynski J, Cline DM, Thomas SH. eds. *Tintinalli's Emergency Medicine: A Comprehensive Study Guide, 9e* New York, NY: McGraw-Hill

[39] McQuaid KR. Diseases of the Esophagus. In: Papadakis MA, McPhee SJ, Rabow MW. eds. Current Medical Diagnosis and Treatment 2020 New York, NY: McGraw-Hill

[40] Gralnek et al. "Acute Lower Gastrointestinal Bleeding." N Engl J Med 2017; 376:1054-1063.

[41] Stanley AJ, Laine L, Dalton HR, Ngu JH, Schultz M, Abazi R, et al; International Gastrointestinal Bleeding Consortium. Comparison of risk scoring systems for patients presenting with upper gastrointestinal bleeding: international multicentre prospective study. BMJ. 2017;356:i6432.

[42] Chey WD, Wong BC; Practice Parameters Committee of the American College of Gastroenterology. American College of Gastroenterology guideline on the management of Helicobacter pylori infection. Am J Gastroenterol. 2007;102(8):1808-1825.

[43] Barkun et al. "International Consensus Recommendations on the Management of Patients with Nonvariceal Upper Gastrointestinal Bleeding." Ann Intern Med. 2010;152:101-113

[44] Barkun AN, Almadi M, Kuipers EJ, et al. Management of Nonvariceal Upper Gastrointestinal Bleeding: Guideline Recommendations From the International Consensus Group. Ann Intern Med. 2019; [Epub ahead of print 22 October 2019]. doi: 10.7326/M19-1795

[45] Kilgore et al. "Bowel preparation with split-dose polyethylene glycol before colonoscopy: a meta-analysis of randomized controlled trials." Gastrointest Endosc. 2011 Jun;73(6):1240-5.

[46] Trikudanathan et al. "Current Controversies in Fluid Resuscitation in Acute Pancreatitis." Pancreas. 41(6). August 2012

[47] Clinical Practice and Economics Committee. "AGA Institute Medical Position Statement on Acute Pancreatitis." GASTROENTEROLOGY 2007;132:2019 –202162

[48] Baron, Todd. "Managing severe acute pancreatitis." CCJM. 80(6) June 2013

[49] Tenner at al. "American College of Gastroenterology Guideline: Management of Acute Pancreatitis." Am J Gastroenterol. July 2013.

[50] Conwell DL, Banks P, Greenberger NJ. Acute and Chronic Pancreatitis. In: Kasper D, Fauci A, Hauser S, Longo D, Jameson J, Loscalzo J. eds. *Harrison's Principles of Internal Medicine, 19e* New York, NY: McGraw-Hill; 2014. http://accessmedicine.mhmedical.com/content.aspx?bookid=1130&sectionid=79749276. Accessed February 08, 2018.

[51] Wu et al. "Lactated Ringer's Solution Reduces Systemic Inflammation Compared With Saline in Patients With Acute Pancreatitis." Clinical Gastroenterology And Hepatology 2011;9:710 –717

[52] De Waele et al. "Intra-abdominal Hypertension and Abdominal Compartment Syndrome." Am J Kidney Dis. 57(1):159-169.

[53] Tintinalli JE, Stapczynski JS, Cline DM, Ma OJ, Cydulka RK, Meckler GD. Chapter 86. Bowel Obstruction and Volvulus. In: Tintinalli JE, Stapczynski JS, Cline DM, Ma OJ, Cydulka RK, Meckler GD, eds. *Tintinalli's Emergency Medicine: A Comprehensive Study Guide.* 7th ed. New York: McGraw-Hill; 2011.

[54] AGA Institute. "American Gastroenterological Association Medical Position Statement on the Management of Gastroesophageal Reflux Disease." GASTROENTEROLOGY 2008;135:1383–1391.

[55] Katz et al. "Diagnosis and Management of Gastroesophageal Reflux Disease." Am J Gastroenterol 2013; 108:308–328.

[56] Keung C, Hebbard G. The management of gastro-oesophageal reflux disease. Aust Prescr. 2016;39(1):6–10. doi:10.18773/austprescr.2016.003

[57] Lanas, Angel et al. "Peptic ulcer disease." The Lancet , Volume 390 , Issue 10094 , 613 - 624

[58] Crowe et al. "*Treatment regimens for Helicobacter pylori.*" In: UpToDate, Basow, DS (Ed), UpToDate, Waltham, MA, 2012.

[59] Osama Siddique, Anais Ovalle, Ayesha S. Siddique, Steven F. Moss, Helicobacter Pylori Infection: an Update for the Internist in the Age of Increasing Global Antibiotic Resistance, The American Journal of Medicine (2018), https://doi.org/10.1016/j.amjmed.2017.12.024.

[60] Giannini et al. Liver enzyme alteration: a guide for clinicians. CMAJ. 2005 February 1; 172(3): 367–379.

[61] Oh, Robert C et al. "Mildly Elevated Liver Transaminase Levels: Causes and Evaluation." Am Fam Physician. 2017 Dec 1;96(11):709-715.

[62] Bénichou C. Criteria of drug-induced liver disorders. Report of an international consensus meeting. J Hepatol. 1990;11(2):272-6.

[63] Calderon et al. "Statins in the Treatment of Dyslipidemia in the Presence of Elevated Liver Aminotransferase Levels: A Therapeutic Dilemma." Mayo Clin Proc. 2010;85(4):349-356.

[64] Kopec, K. L., & Burns, D. (2011, October). Nonalcoholic fatty liver disease: A review of the spectrum of disease, diagnosis, and therapy. Retrieved from https://www.ncbi.nlm.nih.gov/pubmed/21947639

QUICK ACLS

Primary and Secondary ABCD Survey 80

Asystole 80

Bradycardia 80

Pulseless Electrical Activity 81

VFib/Pulseless VTach 82

Tachycardia 82

Code Cart / Common ICU Medications

Drug	Dose	Comments
Adenosine	Tachycardia Initial: 6mg IVP x1 Repeat @ 12mg prn after 1-2m May repeat 12mg once	Due to short half-life, must administer by rapid IV push (1-3 seconds) followed by 20 cc saline or sterile water flush.
Amiodarone	Pulseless VT/VF 300mg Stable VT 150mg	Pulseless VT/VF 300 mg IV push unfiltered/undiluted-may repeat with 150 mg if needed. Stable VT 150 mg diluted in 25-50 mL NS or D5W infused over 10 minutes. Max 2.2g/24h
Atropine	Bradycardia 0.5-1mg IV q3-5m	Maximum dose of 0.04 mg/kg Go directly to TC pacing or dopamine or epinephrine in pts likely to be unresponsive to atropine, incl. cardiac transplant pts, type II 2nd- or 3rd-degree block, or 3rd-degree AV block w/ new wide-QRS complex; caution if acute coronary ischemia or MI
Calcium Chloride	CCB overdose 1g/10cc over 10m q20m (1 amp = 10cc) Arrhythmia 500mg-1g IV q10m prn Hypocalcemia 500mg-1g IV over 5-10m	Given for known hyperkalemia, hypocalcemia, hypermagnesemia, or toxic effects of calcium channel blockers. May repeat as needed. Vesicant, use extreme caution when administering; incompatible with phosphate solutions. Central line preferred.
Calcium gluconate	CCB overdose 3-6g IV over 10m q20m Hypocalcemia 1-2g IV q6h prn Arrhythmia 1.5-3g IV q2-5m prn	Preferred over calcium chloride for non-emergent calcium supplementation. Dilute in 50 mL of NS or D5W and administer over 1 hour.
Dopamine	Bradycardia adjunct 2-10mcg/kg/m IV Post-resuscitation stabil. 5-10mcg/kg/min IV	For patients unresponsive to atropine for bradycardia
Epinephrine	PVT/VF/PEA/Asystole Dose: 1mg 1:10000 IVP IV/IO: q3-5m ETT: q3-5m Bradycardia Infusion 2-10mcg/min IV Anaphylaxis Auto-injector: 0.3mg SC/IM x1 (repeat p 5-15m) Cart: 0.2-0.5mg 1:1000 SC/IM q5-15m (max 1mg)	Use 1:10000 solution for cardiac arrest *If needing to use 1:1000 solution, then use 2-2.5mg of 1:1000 formulation)* For patients unresponsive to atropine for bradycardia
Magnesium Sulfate	1-2g	Dilute to 10 mL with D5W or NS; administer over 1-2 minutes. For general magnesium supplementation administer each 2 grams over 1 hr. Given for known hypomagnesemia and/or Torsade de Pointes
Naloxone	0.4-2mg q2-3m	Dilute in 10cc of NS or sterile water
Sodium Bicarbonate	1 mEq/kg (repeat ½ dose q10m)	Typical dose is 50 mEq
Vasopressin	40 U IVP (repeat in 10-20m)	Use is PVT or VF

PRIMARY AND SECONDARY ABCD SURVEY

Establish safety net: O2, tele, IV, help
- **Primary ABCD survey**
  - Focus: basic CPR and defibrillation
  - Airway: assess and manage the airway with noninvasive devices.
  - Breathing: assess and manage breathing (look, listen, and feel). If the patient is not breathing, give two slow breaths.
  - Circulation: assess and manage the circulation; if no pulse, start CPR.
  - Defibrillation: assess and manage rhythm/defibrillation; shock VF/VT up to 3 times (200 J, 300 J, 360 J, or equivalent biphasic) if necessary.
- **Secondary ABCD survey**
  - Focus: more advanced assessments and treatments
  - Airway: place airway device as soon as possible.
  - Breathing: assess adequacy of airway device placement and performance; secure airway device; confirm effective oxygenation and ventilation.
  - Circulation: establish IV access; administer drugs appropriate for rhythm and condition.
  - Differential Diagnosis: search for and treat identified reversible causes.
- Potentially reversible causes include: hypoxia, hypovolemia, hyperkalemia, hypokalemia and metabolic disorders, hypothermia, tension pneumothorax, tamponade, toxic/therapeutic disturbances, and thromboembolic/mechanical obstruction

ASYSTOLE

- CPR, obtain IV/IO access, prepare pt for intubation
- Epinephrine 1 mg Q 3-5 minutes up to 3 doses
- Atropine 1 mg Q 3-5 minutes up to 3 doses
- Consider high-dose Epinephrine or continue Epinephrine 1 mg IVP Q 3-5 minutes

BRADYCARDIA

- If possible, in any patient in whom you are worried about symptomatic bradycardia, try to have **atropine** at the bedside before the patient gets unstable. Always ask yourself the following two questions in the bradycardic patient:
  - Is the patient symptomatic or hemodynamically unstable? If so, place the patient in Trendelenburg and follow ACLS protocols (See ACLS: Bradycardia).
  - Does the ECG show either type II 2nd-degree or 3rd-degree AV block? If so, consider trans-cutaneously pacing the patient and prepare for possible transvenous pacer (consult Cardiology).
- If the patient is relatively stable hemodynamically and symptomatically and there is no sign of a dangerous form of AV block, you have some time to do a quick chart biopsy and look for clues from the patient's med list and admitting diagnoses.

Causes of Bradycardia	
Category Examples[65,66]	
Meds	ß blockers, calcium channel blockers, digoxin, amiodarone, clonidine (look at the MAR and remember to consider any eye drops—e.g. timolol)
Cardiac	Sick sinus, inferior MI, vasovagal, 2nd or 3rd degree heart block, junctional rhythm
Intrinsic Causes	Idiopathic degeneration (aging), infiltrative diseases (sarcoid, amyloid), collagen vascular disease, surgical trauma, endocarditis
Autonomically Mediated	Neuro cardiogenic syncope, carotid-sinus hypersensitivity, situational: coughing, micturition, defecation, vomiting
Other	Hypothyroidism, hypothermia, increased intracranial pressure (Cushing's reflex), hyperkalemia, hypokalemia, obstructive sleep apnea, normal variant

- In general, if the patient is not symptomatic and this is not a significant change from prior days/nights, then an exhaustive workup is unnecessary at night. However, have a low threshold to get an ECG in bradycardic patients and consider ischemia in any patient at risk.
- Take a focused H&P. Focus on signs and symptoms to distinguish the above (chest pain, prior MI, straining or other maneuvers prior to bradycardia, altered mental status, hypothermia, BP, etc.).
- If you believe the bradycardia is secondary to medications, be careful discontinuing them. Remember; treat the patient, not the numbers. Stopping rate control meds could cause a rebound tachycardia and precipitate myocardial ischemia
- Transcutaneous pacing can be quite uncomfortable. If there's time, short-acting analgesics and/or sedatives may be worthwhile considering.
- In asymptomatic patients with bradycardia, the class I indications for pacemakers are as follows:
  - 3rd-degree AV block with asystole lasting > 3 seconds or with escape rates < 40 while awake
  - 3rd-degree or 2nd-degree type II AV block in patients with chronic bifasicular or trifascicular block
- **ASx Bradycardia, AV Block 1 or AV Block Mobitz-type 1**
  - No specific therapy
  - *For AV block Mobitz type 1:* Stop B-blockers, CCBs, Digoxin
- **Symptomatic Bradycardia**
  - Call attending and transfer pt to ICU
  - Put pacer pads on just in case you might need them (bradycardia ACLS)
  - Give 0.5 mg Atropine IV Q 3-5 minutes up to 3mg
  - Transcutaneous pacemaker if no response to Atropine
  - Epinephrine and Dopamine may also be used if no response to Atropine
- **AV block Mobitz-type 2 and AV block 3rd degree**
  - Call attending and transfer pt to ICU
  - Put pacer pads on just in case you might need them (bradycardia ACLS)
  - Give 0.5 mg Atropine IV
  - Transcutaneous pacemaker must be placed (even if pt Asx), then arrange for permanent pacemaker

PULSELESS ELECTRICAL ACTIVITY

- Definition: ↓BP and absent pulse, but some type of electrical activity on ECG
- Find the cause and treat it
- <u>Treatment</u>: Epinephrine 1 mg Q 3-5 minutes up to 3 doses

QUICK ACLS

VFIB/PULSELESS VTACH

- Give 1 shock (or a precordial thump until a defibrillator is available) and resume CPR immediately
- Check for rhythm and pulse; give 1 shock and resume CPR immediately if no pulse present
- Epinephrine 1 mg IV/IO Q 3-5 minutes up to 3 doses
- Give drugs during active CPR
- Give 1 shock after drug administration and resume CPR immediately
- Consider Amiodarone 300mg (second dose is 150mg) or Magnesium (if evidence of Torsade's)

> Remember: Shock→CPR+drug→shock

TACHYCARDIA

1. **Tachycardia with Pulses**
   - ABCs; give O2
   - Identify reversible causes
   - Obtain IV access
   - Monitor ECG and identify rhythm
   - If pt unstable (altered mental status/signs of shock)→synchronized cardioversion
2. **Ventricular Tachycardia with Pulse**
   - Wide complex tachycardia (QRS >0.12 sec)
     - Use **Brugada Criteria** to differentiate VT from SVT
   - Uniform pattern on ECG; no P waves
   - Sustained vs. Nonsustained
     - *Nonsustained*: 3 beats to 29 seconds in duration → if structural heart disease consider ICD placement, otherwise if not then reassurance
     - *Sustained*: ≥30 seconds; often will require ICD placement
   - Amiodarone 150 mg IV over 10 minutes (**may repeat to max dose of 2.2 g/24 hours**)
   - May use Lidocaine or consider cardioversion if no initial response to Amiodarone
3. **Torsade's de Pointes**
   - Magnesium initial bolus 1-2 g, then continuous infusion
     - Check electrolytes
   - May try IV Lidocaine or Phenytoin. If no response to Mg and electricity, consider isoproterenol (beta agonist)
   - If hemodynamic instability→ immediate electrical cardioversion
4. **Pre-excitation / Wolff-Parkinson-White Syndrome**
   - Short PR intervals and wide QRS; Associated with SVT
   - Delta waves (slurred upstroke in QRS complex)
   - Synchronized cardioversion if unstable
   - Procainamide best alternative
   - **Avoid** CCBs, Beta blockers and Adenosine (will lead to uninterrupted action through accessory pathway)
5. **Narrow Complex Tachycardia**
   - STEP 1: Is the tachycardia regular or irregular?
     - If irregular, the differential is limited to:
       1. Atrial fibrillation
          - Rate vs rhythm control
            - Rate: metoprolol, diltiazem, digoxin

- Rhythm: chemical (amio) vs electrical (synchronized; 200J)
  Amiodarone
    - *Load*: 150mg bolus over 10 minutes with gtt 1mg/kg for 8h then 0.5mg/kg x16h (atrial source req 6-8g total; ventricular source req 10-12g total)
    - *Maintenance*: 200mg/d if atrial source; 400mg/d if ventricular source
  2. Atrial flutter with variable block
  3. Multifocal atrial tachycardia: defined as tachycardia with 3 or more different p wave morphologies
  - If regular, go to STEP 2
- STEP 2: Where is the p wave?
  - Look carefully for the presence of p waves- they are often embedded at the end of QRS complexes or within the T wave so always compare the tachycardia ECG to the NSR ECG to look for subtle changes in QRS/T wave morphology (e.g. in cases of atrial tachycardia with 2:1 block, undetected "hidden" p waves may lead to an incorrect diagnosis of sinus tachycardia)
  1. If the p wave is identified, measure the RP interval
     - If the RP interval is < ½ the RR interval, this is a SHORT RP tachycardia
       - Consider AVNRT, orthodromic AVRT, JT
     - If the RP interval is > ½ the RR interval, this is a LONG RP tachycardia
       - Consider atrial tachycardia, sinus tachycardia, etc.
  2. If the p wave is NOT found, one can probably assume that it is embedded within the QRS and is therefore a SHORT RP tachycardia, consider AVNRT

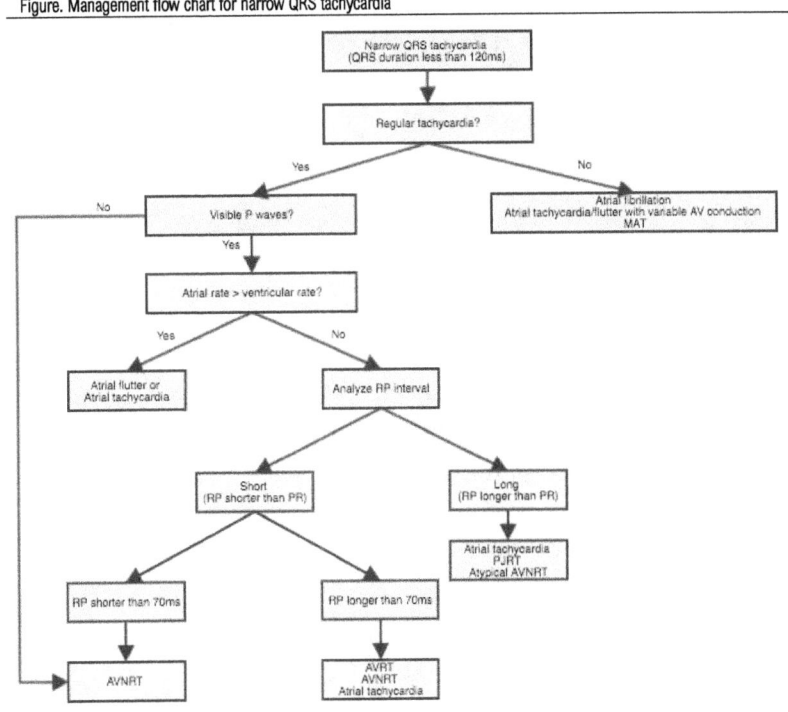

Figure. Management flow chart for narrow QRS tachycardia

- o **Treatment**
    - Adenosine (drug of choice) 6 mg IV **rapid** push initial dose; may give 2nd and 3rd dose of 12 mg IV **rapid** push
        1. Warn pts they may feel sense of impending doom or severe pain, which is self-limited and resolves quickly
        2. Therapeutic: if AVRT or AVNRT may terminate rhythm
            - AVRT – associated with WPW; look for delta wave
        3. Diagnostic: if not the above, will show fibrillation or flutter waves
    - Vagal Maneuvers
        1. Carotid sinus massage (R>L in effectiveness), Valsalva
    - Radiofrequency Ablation

Bibliography

[65] Montgomery Family Practice Residency Program, Intern Guide 2005-6
[66] Mangrum JM, DiMarco JP. The evaluation and management of bradycardia. N Engl J Med 2000; 342:703-9.

INFECTIOUS DISEASE

Reading Microbiology Report 86
Susceptibility Interpretation 88
Empiric Antibiotic Regimen 88
Fever of Unknown Origin 103
Cellulitis 105
Clostridium Difficile 107
Meningitis 112
Urinary Tract Infections 116
Pyelonephritis 120
Sepsis 121
Bacterial endocarditis 127
Pneumonia 129
Surgical Site Infections 137

INFECTIOUS DISEASE

READING MICROBIOLOGY REPORT

Figure. Distinguishing gram negatives and positives based on features

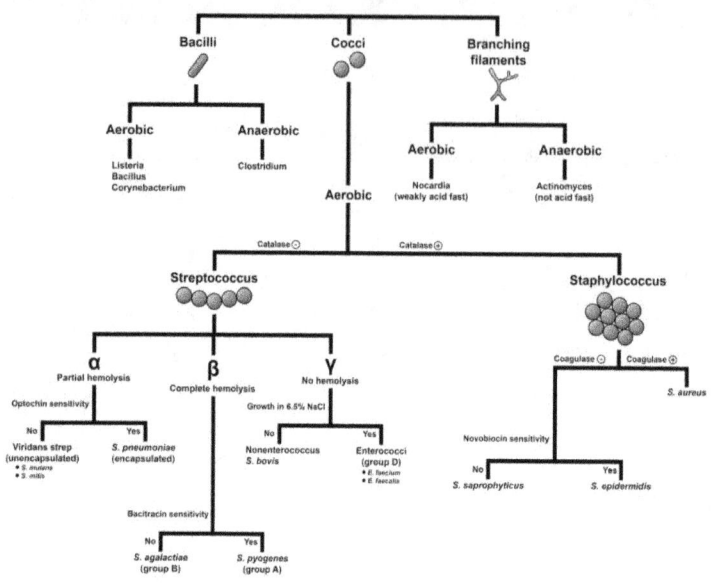

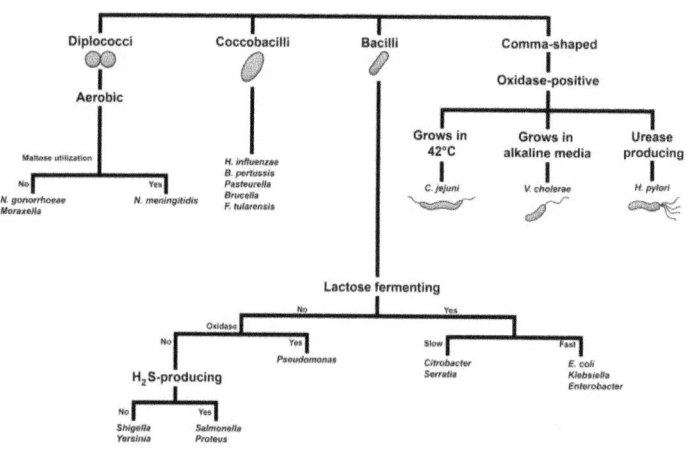

INFECTIOUS DISEASE

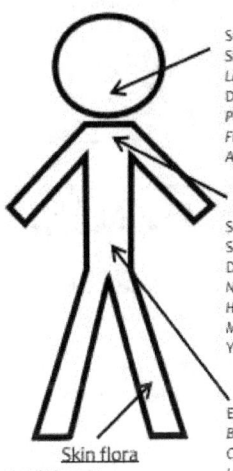

Oral flora
Streptococci
Staphylococci
Lactobacillus spp.
Diphtheroids
Porphyromonas spp.
Fusobacterium spp.
Actinomyces spp.

Respiratory flora
Streptococci
Staphylococci
Diphtheroids
Neisseria spp.
Haemophilus spp.
Moraxella spp.
Yeasts

Gut flora
Enterobacteriaceae
Bacteroides spp.
Clostridium spp.
Lactobacillus spp.
Candida spp.
Streptococci
Enterococci
Staphylococci

Skin flora
Staphylococci
Streptococci
Diphtheroids
Micrococci
Propionibacterium spp.
Peptostreptococci

Bacterial pathogens from different classes

Gram-positive cocci [67]
Aerobic
In clusters
- Coagulase (+): *Staphylococcus aureus*
- Coagulase (-): *Staphylococcus lugdunensis* and other coagulase-negative staphylococci

In pairs/chains
- Optochin sensitive: *Streptococcus pneumoniae*
- Alpha-hemolytic: Viridans group *Streptococcus*, *Enterococcus*
- Beta-hemolytic:
  o Group A Strep (*Streptococcus pyogenes*)
  o Group B Strep (*Streptococcus agalactiae*)
  o Group C, D, G Strep

Anaerobic: *Peptostreptococcus spp.* and many others

Gram-positive rods
Aerobic
- Large: *Bacillus spp*
- Cocco-bacillus: *Listeria monocytogenes*, *Lactobacillus spp*
- Small, pleomorphic: *Corynebacterium spp*
- Branching filaments: *Nocardia spp, Streptomyces spp*

Anaerobic
- Large: *Clostridium spp*
- Small: *P. acnes; Actinomyces spp*

Mycobacteria

Gram-negative cocci
Aerobic
- Diplococcus: *Neisseria meningitidis, N. gonorrhoeae, Moraxella catarrhalis*
- Cocco-bacillus: *Haemophilus influenzae, Acinetobacter*

Anaerobic: *Veillonella spp.*

Gram-negative rods
Aerobic
Lactose fermenting (Lactose positive):
- *Enterobacter spp, Escherichia coli, Klebsiella spp*
- *Citrobacter spp*, Serratia spp**

Non lactose-fermenting (Lactose negative):
- Oxidase (-): *Acinetobacter spp, Burkholderia spp, E. coli, Proteus spp, Salmonella spp, Shigella spp, Serratia spp*, Stenotrophomonas maltophilia*
- Oxidase (+): *P. aeruginosa, Aeromonas spp.*

Anaerobic: *Bacteroides spp, Fusobacterium spp, Prevotella spp.*

Spirochetes

M. tuberculosis	Treponema pallidum (syphilis)
M. leprae	Leptospira
M. bovis	Borrelia
M. abscess	
M. avium	
M. marinum	
M. kansasii	

SUSCEPTIBILITY INTERPRETATION

One of four interpretations:
- S (susceptible) - isolate is inhibited by the usually achievable concentrations of antimicrobial agent when the dosage recommended to treat the site of infection is used.
- I (intermediate) - isolate is not inhibited by these usually achievable concentrations, OR that the organisms might express a resistance mechanism.
- R (resistant) - the MIA is approaching the usually attainable concentration, but the response rates may be lower than for a susceptible isolate
- NS (non-susceptible) - A "NS" value does not necessarily mean that the isolate has a resistance mechanism, but rather that it has an unusually high MIA.

Specimen Gram Stains		
When You Know:	Gram Stain Results:	Think:
Meningitis (CSF)	Pleomorphic Gram negative bacilli	Haemophilus influenzae
	Gram negative diplococci	Neisseria meningitidis
	Gram positive cocci in pairs	Streptococcus pneumoniae
Wound infection	Gram positive cocci in clusters	Staphylococcus aureus
	Gram positive cocci in pairs	Streptococci
	Gram positive bacilli	Bacillus, Clostridium
	Gram negative bacilli	E coli, enterics, others
Bacteremia	Gram positive cocci in clusters	Staphylococcus aureus
	Gram positive cocci in chains	Streptococci
	Gram positive cocci in pairs	Streptococcus pneumoniae
	Gram positive bacilli	Bacillus, Corynebacterium, Clostridium
	Gram negative bacilli	E coli, enterics, Acinetobacter, Klebsiella
	Yeast	Candida albicans, Cryptococcus neoformans
Urinary tract infection	Gram positive cocci in clusters	Staphylococcus aureus
	Gram positive cocci in chains	Streptococci
	Gram positive cocci in pairs	Enterococci
	Gram negative bacilli	E coli, enterics, others
	Yeast	Candida albicans

EMPIRIC ANTIBIOTIC REGIMEN

- **Determining appropriate antibiotic selection**
    - Site of Infection: drug penetration, common organism
    - Host: immune status, past pathogens, drug-drug interactions, allergie
    - Susceptibility data

Common Antibiotic Classes and Uses					
	G+	G-	A	MRSA	PsA
PCN					
PCN	+				Not staph
Amp/Amox	+	?			
Oxacillin/Diclox	+				Sensitive staph
1st gen Cephalosporins	Less susceptible to B lactamases				

INFECTIOUS DISEASE

Common Antibiotic Classes and Uses

	G+	G-	A	MRSA	PsA	
Cefazolin/Cephalexin	+	+				Sensitive staph. Gram - ESBL are resistant
2nd gen Cephalosporins						
Cefuroxime	+	+	+			
3rd gen						
Ceftriaxone	+	+	+			
Cefotaxime	+	+	+			
Cefpodoxime PO	+	+				
Ceftazidime	+	+	?		+	
4th gen						
Cefepime	+	+			+	
5th gen						
Ceftaroline	+	+		+		SSSI CA-PNA Good against MRSA
Carbapenems	Highly resistant to B lactamases; Lowers seizure threshold					
Imipenem	+	++	+		+	
Ertapenem	+	++	+			No PsA!
Meropenem	+	++	+		+	
Doripenem	+	++	+		+	Complicated intraabdominal infection Complicated UTI Best to use against PsA
Combinations	Combo with B lactamase inhibitor					
Amox/Clavulanate (Augmentin)	+	+	+			
Amp/Sulbactam (Unasyn)	+	+	+			
Pip/Tazo (Zosyn)	+	+	+		+	
Aztreonam		+			+	Binds only Gram – penicillin binding proteins
Macrolides	Inhibits bacterial tRNA and ribosome translocation					
Azithromycin	+		+			atypical
Clarithromycin	+		+			
Erythromycin	+?		+			
Quinolones	Inhibit bacterial DNA gyrase and topoisomerase. Watch INR, CDif.					
Levofloxacin	+	++			+	And atypical
Ciprofloxacin	+	++			+	
Moxifloxacin	+	++	+			
Gatifloxacin	+	++	+			
Tetracyclines	Binds ribosome inhibits tRNA binding. Photosensitivity!					
Doxycycline	+	+	+	+		And most atypical (not Legionella)
Aminoglycosides	Binds ribosome inhibits protein synthesis. Nephrotoxic, ototoxic					
Gent		+			+	
Tobra		+			+	
Neomycin						Not absorbed
Other	G+	G-	A	MRSA	PsA	
Vancomycin	++		?	+		Inhibits cell wall synthesis. 15mg/kg bid (less if renal insuff); Redman
Clindamycin	+		+	?		Binds ribosome, inhibits tRNA and ribosomes (like macrolides).
Metronidazole			+			Taken up by anaerobes, forms toxic metabolites. Peripheral neuropathy
Linezolid	++		?	+		Prevents initiation complex of ribosomes. Marrow toxicity
Daptomycin	++			+		Alternative for MRSA SSTI (MRSA) Check CK weekly R side endocarditis No lung penetration

INFECTIOUS DISEASE

Common Antibiotic Classes and Uses

	G+	G-	A	MRSA	PsA	
Tigecycline	++	+	+	+		Complicated SSTI (MSSA, MRSA, VSE)
						Complicated intraabdominal infection (MSSA, VSE)
Nitrofurantoin	+	+				Toxic metabolites. e. coli only
Rifampin	+			+		Inhibits bacterial RNA polymerase. Neisseria
Trimethoprim/Sulfa	+	+		+		Inhibits successive steps in folate synthesis. Increases Cr but not nephrotoxic

Credit: UNC School of Medicine

Risk Factors for Select Organisms

Pseudomonas aeruginosa / GNRs
Community acquired:
- Prior IV antibiotics within 90 day
- Known colonization with MDROs

Hospital acquired:
- Prior IV antibiotics within 90 days
- 5 or more days of hospitalization prior to onset
- Acute renal replacement therapy prior to onset
- Septic shock
- Known colonization with MDROs

MRSA
Known colonization with MDROs
- Recent MRSA infection
- Known MRSA colonization
- Skin & Skin Structure and/or IV access site:
  - Purulence
  - Abscess
- Pneumonia
  - Severe, rapidly progressive necrotizing Pneumonia
  - Note: absence of nasal colonization is strong evidence against MRSA pneumonia

Invasive Candidiasis
Central venous catheter
- Broad-spectrum antibiotics
- + 1 of the following risk factors:
  - Parenteral nutrition
  - Dialysis
  - Recent abdominal surgery
  - Necrotizing Pancreatitis
  - Systemic steroids or other immunosuppressive agents

VRE
- Liver transplant
- Known colonization
- Prolonged broad antibacterial therapy
- Prolonged profound immunosuppression

Empiric Antibiotic Treatments

Neurological

Condition	Organisms	Treatments	Duration	Pearls
Meningitis	**Immunocompetent (<50)** S.pneumo N.meningitidis H.influenza **Immunocompetent (>50)** S.pneumo Listeria N.meningitidis GBS **Immunocompromised** S.pneumo N.meningitidis H.influenza Listeria GN **Post NS or Head Trauma** S.pneumo (if CSF leak) H.influenza Staphylococci GN **Shunt** S.aureus Coag neg staph GNs	**Immunocompetent (<50):** Vancomycin + CTX 2g IV BID **Immunocompetent (>50):** Vancomycin + CTX 2g IV BID + Ampicillin 2g IV Q4H **Immunocompromised** – Vancomycin + Cefepime + Ampicillin **Post NS or Head Trauma** – Vancomycin + Cefepime **Shunt** – Vancomycin + Cefepime **PCN Allergy:** Age<50: Vancomycin 15 mg/kg IV + Moxifloxacin 400 mg IV Q24H Age>50: Vancomycin IV + Moxifloxacin 400 mg IV Q24H + SMX/TMP 5 mg/kg IV Q6H	Stop tx if LP negative at 48h or no PMN on cell count S.pneumo: 10-14d N.mening: 7d Listeria: 21d H.flu: 7d GNB: 21d	Do not wait for CT or LP results to start Abx; if there is delay in LP obtain BCx and start Abx Dexamethasone advised in adult patients suspected of having pneumococcus dosed as 0.15mg/kg IV q6h for 4d and give it with Abx or 10-20min before Abx Indications for head CT prior or LP • History of CNS dz (lesion, CVA) • New seizure in last 7 d • Papilledema • Altered LOC • Focal neuro deficit LP Labs: -Viral culture - HSV PCR - Enteroviral PCR - Lyme Antibody (IgG index, requires simultaneous serum) - VDRL
Encephalitis	HSV, VZV	If HSV suspected: Acyclovir 10mg/kg IV Q8H If Lyme suspected: CTX 2g IV Q24H	14-21d	Have low threshold to treat

Oral

Thrush	Candida	Oropharyngeal Clotrimazole 10mg troch 5x/d Nystatin susp PO QID Fluconazole 100-200mg PO daily Itraconazole soln 200mg PO daily Voriconazole 200mg PO BID (for refractory disease) Esophageal Fluconazole 200-400mg PO daily Caspofungin 70mg load then 50mg daily	Oral: 7-14d Esophageal: 14-21d	Consider IV formulation if cannot tolerate PO
Respiratory				
CAP (non-ICU)	S.pneumo H.influenza M. Catarrhalis	Inpatient Ceftriaxone 1 gm iv q day + azithromycin 500 mg PO on day 1 then 250mg/d for 4 more days OR Moxifloxacin 400 mg IV/PO daily OR Ampicillin/Sulbactam 1.5g IV q6h + Azithromycin 500mg IV/PO daily OR Cefotaxime 1-2g/d + Azithromycin 500mg IV/PO daily OR Ceftaroline 600mg BID + Azithromycin 500mg IV/PO daily Outpatient (no comorbidities) Amoxicillin 1g TID Doxycycline 100mg BID Azithromycin 500mg day 1 then 250mg thereafter Clarithromycin ER 1g daily Clarithromycin 500mg BID Outpatient (with COPD, CHF, Cirrhosis, CRF, DM, EtOH) Augmentin 875/125 BID + Azithromycin/Doxy Cefpodoxime 200mg BID + Azithromycin/Doxy Cefuroxime 500mg BID + Azithromycin/Doxy Levofloxacin (Levaquin) 750 mg po QD Moxifloxacin 400mg/d	3-5 days if not immunocompromised and no structural lung disease 7 days if moderate immunocompromise and/or lung disease 10-14 days if they have a poor clinical response with significant immunocompromise	Consider addition of steroids in CAP for hospitalized patients

Condition	Treatment	Duration	Notes
CAP (ICU)	Gemifloxacin 320mg/d **Inpatient** *Not at risk for Pseudomonas* - Azithromycin 500 mg IV day 1 then 250mg thereafter + Ceftriaxone 2gm IV daily - Moxifloxacin 400mg IV P q24h *Risk for Pseudomonas/MDRO* - Cefepime 2 gm IV BID PLUS Azithromycin 500 mg IV daily - Zosyn 4.5mg IV PO q6h + Azithromycin 500 mg IV daily - Moxifloxacin 400mg IV P q24h + aztreonam 2g IV q8h IF anaphylactic Beta Lactam allergy: Levofloxacin 750 mg IV daily PLUS Aztreonam 1 gm every 8 hours **Outpatient** Levofloxacin 500 mg po QD Doxycycline 100 mg po BID	3-5 days if not immunocompromised and no structural lung disease 7 days if moderate immunocompromise and/or lung disease 10-14 days if they have a poor clinical response with significant immunocompromise	Consider addition of steroids in CAP for hospitalized patients
Aspiration	**Inpatient** Ceftriaxone 1g IV QD + Clindamycin 900mg IV Q8H OR Piperacillin/Tazobactam (Zosyn) 4.5 gm IV Q8H OR Ertapenem (Invanz) 1 gm IV daily **Outpatient** Augmentin 500 mg po TID		
HAP/VAP	Not at risk for MDR/MRSA/Pseudomonas (choose 1) Piperacillin-tazobactam, 4.5 g intravenously q6h Cefepime, 2 g intravenously q8h	5-7 days if PNA confirmed otherwise can stop after 3 days	Consdier covering with azithromycin 500mg IV/PO daily for patients coming from a nursing home or LTEC to cover Legionella
	Enterococci *Candida*		

Condition	Organisms	Treatment	Notes
COPD Exacerbation	H. flu, M. catarrhalis, S. pneumo. Consider pseudomonas and Enterobacter in severe COPD and extensive prior Abx	**Outpatient Uncomplicated** Doxycycline 100mg PO BID x 5d Amoxicillin 500mg PO Q8H Azithromycin 500mg PO/IV once then 250mg/d x 3d Bactrim 1 DS tablet BID Cefpodoxime 200mg PO BID x 5d Cefdinir 300mg PO BID x 5d **Outpatient Complicated/Failed Prior Abx Therapy** Augmentin 875mg PO BID x 5d Moxifloxacin 400mg/d x 5d **Inpatient** Augmentin 875mg PO BID x 5d Doxycycline 100mg PO BID x 5d Moxifloxacin 400mg/d x 5d Levofloxacin, 750 mg intravenously daily Imipenem, 500 mg intravenously q6h Meropenem, 1 g intravenously q8h **Risk for MRSA (add one of the following)** Vancomycin Linezolid 600mg IV BID **Risk for Pseudomonas (add one of the following)** Levofloxacin 750mg/d Ciprofloxacin 400mg IV q8h Aztreonam 2g IV q8h	Prophylactic azithro can reduce rates of exacerbations; dosed 250mg daily See left
Abdominal Tract			
Unspecified	GNR Anaerobes	**Inpatient** Ciprofloxacin 400 mg IV Q12H + Metronidazole 500mg IV Q8H OR Piperacillin/Tazobactam 3.375g IV Q6H MAY ADD IF PSEUDOMONAS SUSPECTED: Tobramycin 7 mg/kg IV x1 See page 107	
C. diff	N/A		

Condition	Organisms	Treatment	Duration / Notes
H.pylori	N/A	See page 70	
Biliary Tract (cholecystitis and cholangitis)	GNR (e.coli, kleb proteus) Anaerobes (bacteroides) Enterococcus Yeast	Community-acquired infections in patients without previous biliary procedures AND who are not severely ill • Ceftriaxone 1g IV q24h • Ertapenem 1g IV q24h • Ciprofloxacin 400mg IV q12h (PCN allergy) Hospital-acquired infections OR patients with multiple therapeutic biliary manipulations (e.g. stent placement/exchange, bilio-enteric anastomosis of any severity) OR patients who are severely ill • Zosyn 3.375 g iv q6h • Cefepime 1g IV q8h + Flagyl 500mg IV q8h • Aztreonam 1g IV q8h + Flagyl 500mg IV q8h +/- Vancomycin	*Uncomplicated treat until obstruction free, complicated requires 4 days and if septic then 7 days until source control*
Diverticulitis	Polymicrobial; Aerobic such as E.coli, K.pneumoniae, Enterobacter, Proteus, and Enterococcus. Anaerobes such as B.fragilis, Prevotella, and Peptostreptococci common	**Mild/Moderate** • Augmentin 875mg PO q12h • Ceftriaxone 1g IV q24h • Ertapenem 1g IV q24h • (Ciprofloxacin 400mg IV q12h or Ciprofloxacin 500mg Q12H) + Metronidazole 500mg IV/PO q8h (PCN allergy) **Severe** • Zosyn 3.375 g iv q6h • Cefepime 1g IV q8h + Flagyl 500mg IV q8h • Ciprofloxacin 400mg IV q12h or Aztreonam 1g IV q8h + Flagyl 500mg IV q8h (PCN allergy)	4 days unless source control not achieved Patients with uncomplicated diverticulitis (defined as CT Confirmed L sided dz w/o abscess, free air, or fistula ± fever and elevated inflammatory markers), can be treated conservatively without antibiotics based on a RCT.
Pancreatitis	GNs	• Zosyn 4.5 g iv q6h • Cefepime 1g IV q8h + Flagyl 500mg IV q8h	For infected pancreatic necrosis, continue abx for 14 days after source Only treat if suspected infection, prophylactic therapy not indicated

	Organisms	Treatment	Duration/Notes	Additional Notes
		• Ciprofloxacin 400mg IV q12h + Metronidazole 500mg IV/PO q8h	control is obtained. Continuation of antibiotics beyond this time places the patient at risk for colonization or infection with resistant organisms and drug toxicity.	
SBP	GNR, s.pneumoniae, enterococci. If polymicrobial, look for e/o perforation	**Treatment** • Ceftriaxone 1g IV q12h • Moxifloxacin 400mg IV/PO q24h **Prophylaxis (GIB)** • Ceftriaxone 1g IV q12h • Ciprofloxacin 500mg PO BID x 7 days **Prophylaxis (No bleed; used after treatment as outpatient)** • TMP/SMX 1 DS PO daily • Ciprofloxacin 500mg PO daily	All patients with cirrhosis + UGIB should be treated for 7 days First episode of SBP should prompt lifelong prophy treatment to prevent future exacerbations Treat for 5 days	Treat with 25% albumin 1.5g/kg if SCr>1, BUN>30, or TBILI >4 on day 1 and then decrease to 1g/kg on day 3 Diagnostic: 250 PMN per mm in ascitic fluid or Cx positive with <250 PMN (repeat tap advised) Repeat paracentesis 48h after tx and if PMN did not decrease by 25% consider changing Abx
Diarrhea	*Common CA* Salmonella, Shiga-E.coli, Campylobacter, C.diff *Immunocompromised* Giardia, crypto, cyclops, Isospora, Microsporidia, CMV	Campylobacter – Azithromycin 500mg PO daily for 1-3d E.coli – Ciprofloxacin 500mg PO BID for 1-3d Shiga E.coli – avoid treatment Salmonella – TMP-SMX 160/800mg PO BID x 3d Vibrio – Ciprofloxacin 500mg PO BID x 3d Yersinia – Ciprofloxacin 500mg PO BID x 3d E.histolitica – Metronidazole 750mg PO TID x5-10d Giardia – Metronidazole 250-500mg PO TID x 7-10d	See left	Avoid stool cx in pts hospitalized for >3d;

UTI

	Organisms	Treatment	Duration	Notes
Regular	Staphylococcus aureus Streptococci Enterococci E coli, enterics, others Candida albicans	**Inpatient** Trimethoprim/Sulfa DS (Septra DS) 1 tab po BID Ceftriaxone (Rocephin) 1 gm IV Q day Cefazolin 1g IV Q8H x 3d	3-5 days if uncomplicated 7-14 days if complicated (men, stones, urologic abnormality, pregnancy)	Pyuria = >10 WBC/hpf +UCx = ≥100k CFU/mL Nitrates = bacteria in urine LE = WBCs in urine Pyuria is more sensitive than LE

		Treatment	Duration	Notes
Nosocomial/CAUTI		**Outpatient** Trimethoprim/Sulfa DS 1 tab po BID x 3d Augmentin 500 mg po TID Nitrofurantoin 100mg PO BID x 5d Cephalexin 500mg PO Q6H x 5d Cefpodoxime 100mg PO BID x 5d **Candida** Fluconazole 200mg PO daily Remove catheter Ertapenem 1g IV daily Certriaxone 1g IV daily Ciprofloxacin 500mg PO BID or 400mg IV BID Cefepime 1g IV Q8H (severely ill pts) Aztreonam 1g IV Q8H (severely ill pts) Zosyn 3.375mg IV q6h (with nephrostomy tube)	14 days for candida 7 days if prompt improvement 10-14 days if delayed improvement 3 days if female and catheter removed and age ≤65	F/u ucx only if continued sx Positive culture is considered with only 1k CFU/mL Replace catheter prior to obtaining cx
Urosepsis		**Inpatient** Cefepime 1g IV q8h Aztreonam 1g IV q8h +/- Gentamycin **Outpatient** Levofloxacin (Levaquin) 500 mg po Q day Ciprofloxacin 400mg IV BID	7-10 days	Can transition to PO cipro or TMP/SMX as step down therapy Avoid PO beta-lactams in step down therapy
Pyelonephritis	GNR	Hospitalized <48h CTX 1g IV daily Ertapenem 1g IV daily (h/o ESBL) Aztreonam 1g IV q8h Gentamycin Hospitalized >48h	7-14 days	
	Candida		14 days for candida	

Cefepime 1g IV q8h
Aztreonam 1g IV q8h
Gentamycin

Step Down
Ciprofloxacin 500mg PO BID x 7d
TMP/SMX 1 DS tab PO BID x 7-10d
Cefpodoxime 400mg PO BID x 14d
Fosfomycin x1

Candida
Fluconazole 200-400mg PO daily

Soft Tissue

Cellulitis — MSSA

Inpatient
Cefazolin (Ancef) 1 gm IV Q8h
Nafcillin 2 gm IV Q4h
Clindamycin 300-450mg PO Q6H (or 600mg IV Q8H)

Outpatient
Cephalexin (Keflex) 500 mg po QID
OR
Dicloxacillin (Dynapen) 500 mg PO QID

MRSA

Inpatient
Vancomycin 1 gm Q12h per pharmacy protocol OR
Linezolid (Zyvox) 600 mg IV Q12h (for MRSA pneumonia)
Dalbavancin 1000mg once (or) 100mg once then 500mg 1w later
Oritavancin 1200mg single dose (over 3h)

Outpatient
Trimethoprim/Sulfamethoxazole DS BID
Doxycycline 100mg PO BID
Minocycline 100 mg Q12h
Clindamycin 300-450mg PO Q6H (or 600mg IV Q8H)

Severe

Inpatient
Ceftriaxone (Rocephin) 1 gm IV Q day + Clindamycin 900 mg 900 mg IV Q8H
Ertapenem (Invanz) 1 gm IV Q day
Ceftaroline 600mg IV BID

Condition	Organisms	Treatment	Duration	Notes
Orbital Cellulitis	S.aureus BH strep S.pneumo H.influenza M.catarrhalis	Daptomycin 4mg/kg/d IV daily Linezolid 600mg IV/PO BID Telavancin 10mg/kg/d IV daily MAY ADD TO ABOVE REGIMEN: Tobramycin 7 mg/kg IV once, then per pharmacy protocol Outpatient Augmentin 500 mg po TID OR Levofloxacin (Levaquin) 500 mg po Q day Empiric (choose one) – add Vanc if h/o MRSA colo Amp/Sulb 3g IV q6h CTX 2g IV daily Moxifloxacin 400mg IV daily Step-Down Augmentin 875 PO BID Cefpodoxime 400mg PO BID Moxifloxacin 400mg PO daily	7 days up to 6 weeks if bone involvement	Imaging is recommended for post-septal cellulitis (CT, MRI) Surgical intervention for abscess formation Antibiotic response should occur within 24-48h Poor response, worse visual acuity, or pupil changes are indications for surgery
Bacteremia / Sepsis				
Unclear	N/A	Urinary No MDR/ESBL -Zosyn 4.5g IV q8h -Aztreonam 2g IV q8h MDR/ESBL risk: Meropenam 1g q8h MRSA: Vancomycin VRE: Daptomycin 8-10mg/kg or Linezolid 600mg IV BID Pseudmonas: Tobramycin 5mg/kg IV daily	GN = can consider stopping after 7 days if responding and improved, otherwise 14 days advised	If suspect ESBL cover with meropenem 1g IV Q8H instead of zosyn/cefepime Repeat blood cultures 48h after are beneficial in G+ staph and candida infxn only, can consider for GNR RF for MRSA: -CV line

Category	Regimen	Notes
Respiratory	**Healthcare associated or immunocompromised** Zosyn 4.5g q8h MDR/ESBL risk: Meropenam 1g q8h MRSA: Vancomycin Cefepime 2g IV q8h Aztreonam 2g IV q8h Vancomycin 15mg/kg -OR- Linezolid 600mg IV daily PLUS Levofloxacin 750mg IV daily *(if FLQ allergy, use azithromycin 500mg daily plus tobramycin 7 mg/kg daily if at risk for pseudomonas)* **Community-Acquired** CTX 2g IV daily + Azithro 500mg IV daily CTX 2g IV daily + Doxy 100mg IV daily Levofloxacin 750mg IV daily	-Indwelling hardware -Known colonization -Prolonged hospitalization in last 90d for >14d -Nursing home or LTEC resident -IVDA Repeat BCx if +staph
GNR Bacteremia in febrile, neutropenic	Patients receiving chemotherapy - suspect S aureus, Pseudomonas, Klebsiella, E coli, and empirically administer ceftazidime, 2 g IV q8h or cefepime 2 g IV q8h	
Candidemia	N/A	Caspofungin IV 70mg then 50mg daily Fluconazole 800mg then 400mg daily Voriconazole IV/PO 400mg BID (2 doses) then 200mg Q12H	14 days after first negative culture Remove all IV catheters Consider eye exam Transition to fluconazole advised when stable Repeat bcx until negative
Vascular device	*Staph* *Strep*	Zosyn 4.5g IV Q8H Cefepime 2g IV Q8H Aztreonam 2g IV q8h Vancomycin 15mg/kg VRE risk: Linezolid 600mg IV BID ESBL risk: Meropenem 1g IV Q8H P.aeruginosa risk: Tobramycin 7mg/kg IV daily Fungal risk: Caspofungin 70mg IV once then 50mg IV daily	

Abdominal

Zosyn 4.5 IV q8h
MDR/ESBL risk: Meropenam 1g q8h
VRE risk: Linezolid 600mg IV BID
Cefepime 2g IV q8h + Flagyl 500mg IV q8h
Aztreonam 2g IV q8h + Flagyl 500mg IV q8h

OR FOR PCN ALLERGIC...

Aztreonam 2g IV q8h (or Ciprofloxacin 400mg IV Q8H
+
Gentamycin
+
Vancomycin

GN = can consider stopping after 7 days if responding and improved, otherwise 14 days advised

If suspect ESBL cover with meropenem 1g IV Q8H instead of zosyn/cefepime

Repeat blood cultures 48h after are beneficial in G+ staph and candida infxn only, can consider for GNR

RF for MRSA:
- CV line
- Indwelling hardware
- Known colonization
- Prolonged hospitalization in last 90d for >14d
- Nursing home or LTEC resident
- IVDA

Repeat BCx if +staph

INFECTIOUS DISEASE

Common pathologies and empiric treatments

Infection	Bugs	Drugs
Meningitis	S. pneumoniae N. Meningitidis, H. influenzae Listeria	Ceftriaxone + vancomycin ± ampicillin
If post-op	Staphylococcus sp. Gram negative rods (GNR)	Ceftazidime + vancomycin
Ventriculitis due to an infected VP shunt	S. epidermidis S. aureus Coliforms† Diphtheroids P. acnes	Vancomycin + Cefepime
Encephalitis (viral)	Herpes simplex virus Varicella zoster virus West Nile virus	Acyclovir
Sinusitis	S. pneumoniae	Amoxicillin or Augmentin (if prior antibiotic exposure)
Mastoiditis	M. catarrhalis Staphylococcus sp.	Ceftriaxone ± vancomycin
Pharyngitis	Group A, C, G streptococcus	Penicillin
	N. gonorrhea	Ceftriaxone (IM) + treat for Chlamydia with azithromycin OR doxycycline
Retropharyngeal/neck abscess	Streptococcus sp. Oral anaerobes	Clindamycin
Pneumonia		
Community-acquired	S. pneumoniae H. influenzae Chlamydia Mycoplasma Legionella	Levaquin OR Ceftriaxone + azithromycin
	Consider addition of steroids in severe CAP	
Hospital-acquired (48 hours)	S. pneumoniae S. aureus Enteric GNR (i.e. klebsiella)	Levaquin + Zosyn OR Ceftriaxone/ceftazidime + vancomycin ± gentamicin
Ventilator-associated (48-72 hours)	P. aeruginosa MRSA Acinetobacter Multidrug resistant GNR Stenotrophomonas	Imipenem + levofloxacin ± (vancomycin OR linezolid if suspect MRSA)
Pneumonitis	PCP Cytomegalovirus	High-dose Bactrim OR High-dose Ganciclovir
Endocarditis	S. aureus (MRSA) Viridans streptococcus Enterococcus Coagulase-negative staph Enteric GNR	Blood cultures first! Vancomycin + gentamicin + rifampin (if valve)

INFECTIOUS DISEASE

FEVER OF UNKNOWN ORIGIN

- **Defined** – 100.9F x 3 weeks with no obvious source despite investigation
- **HPI**[68,69]
    - Fevers + NS + chills → infection
    - NS + chills + anorexia + wt loss → neoplasm
    - Myalgias + joint pains → rheumatologic
- **Workup**
    - Travel history
    - Pet exposure
    - Work environment
    - Sick contacts
    - New Medications
- **Full Fever Workup**
    - CBC, ICU panel, CXR, blood cultures x2, UA, Urine culture x1, respiratory (if applicable)
    - Chest X-ray
    - UA
    - Consider cortisol if pt on steroids for ↑period of time
    - Consider lactate +/- procalcitonin (red misc. tube) if sepsis is a concern
    - If patient has an indwelling line, culture from that line
    - PE for skin evidence of infection
    - Re-address ABx therapy if applicable

Limited differential diagnosis list for FUO			
Infections	Malignancies	Autoimmune	Misc.
Endocarditis	Lymphoma	Temporal arteritis	Drug-induced fever
Abdominal abscesses	Renal cell carcinoma	Adult Still's disease	2/2 cirrhosis
TB (extrapulmonary)	Chronic leukemia	SLE	Factitious fever
Pelvic abscesses	Colon carcinoma	PAN	Hepatitis (alcoholic, granulomatous, or lupoid)
Dental abscesses	Metastatic cancers	PMR	
Osteomyelitis	Hepatoma	RA	
Sinusitis	Myelodysplastic syndromes	Rheumatoid fever	DVT
--------------------		IBD	Sarcoidosis
CMV	Pancreatic carcinoma	Reiter's syndrome	Medications
EBV	Sarcomas	Vasculitides	
HIV			
Lyme disease			
Prostatitis			
Sinusitis			

- **Preliminary Evaluation**
    - Labs
        - CBC
        - HFP
        - ESR/CRP
        - UA
        - Cultures
        - HIV
        - 1-step PPD +/- CXR
    - Imaging
        - CXR
        - Abdominal CT

INFECTIOUS DISEASE

- ▫ PET
- ▫ MRI brain
- ▫ Duplex US
- TTE

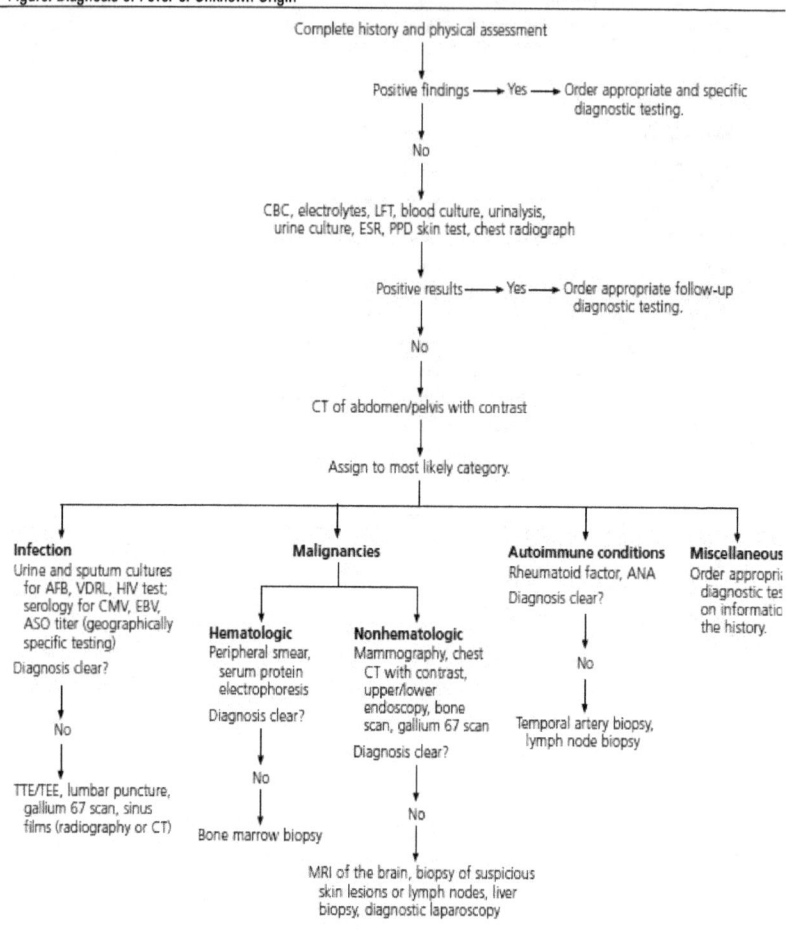

Figure. Diagnosis of Fever of Unknown Origin

INFECTIOUS DISEASE

CELLULITIS

- **Defined**
  - Mild - patients without systemic signs/symptoms of infection
  - Moderate - systemic signs of infection
  - Severe – system signs of infection, associated with penetrating trauma, failed Abx, immunocompromised, deep infection
- **Overview**[70,71,72]
  - Look for predisposing disease/condition that may cause recurrence:
    - PVD
    - T2DM
    - Onychomycosis
    - Tinea pedis (low involvement → tx with imidazole BID x 2-4w)
    - Lymphedema
    - S/P saphenous vein grafting d/t lymphatic vessel disruption
    - S/P mastectomy
- **Causes**
  - BHS, S. aureus, GN aerobic bacilli
- **Mimics**
  - Stasis Dermatitis
    - Long-standing, progressive
    - Ill-defined borders, bilateral, nontender, hyperpigmentation (bronzing, hemosiderin deposits), overlying superficial desquamation, serous drainage, no systemic symptoms
    - Due to chronic venous insufficiency → edema → RBA extravasation (↑pigmentation) → ↓O2
    - If chronic, can lead to lipodermatosalerosis
  - Lipodermatosalerosis
    - Sclerosing panniculitis 2/2 chronic venous insufficiency
    - "inverted champagne bottle" appearance to legs
    - Usually involves the lower 1/3 of the leg(s)
    - Known venous insufficiency, hyperpigmentation, lack of systemic symptoms, skin is "bound-down", no systemic symptoms
    - Chronic course may be associated with scattered ulcerations
  - Contact Dermatitis (ask about new medications, topicals, band aids, adhesives)
  - Lymphedema (high risk in patient's s/p lumpectomy, overweight). Thought to be secondary to compression of lymphatics → ↓O2 distribution → fibrosis. Often no warmth, tenderness, systemic symptoms.
- **Risk factors**
  - CaMRSA
    - Health care professional
    - Military
  - Necrotizing Fasciitis (calculate LRINEC score)
    - DM
    - EtOH
    - Trauma/Surgery
  - HaMRSA
    - DM
    - Dialysis
    - Long term IV access
    - Prolonged hospitalization
  - Others

- Puncture Wound
- Post-operative infection at incision site
- Skin Ulcer
- Neoplasms
- Lymphatic Cutaneous metastases from neoplasms
- Chronic Dependent edema (may progress rapidly)
- **Diagnosis**
  - Based on clinical manifestations
    - Fever
    - ↑WBC (check for ↑eosinophil count which may be s/o eosinophilic cellulitis)
    - Warmth
    - Erythema
    - Somewhat clear borders (if not clear; and not stasis dermatitis; consider erysipelas)
    - TTP
    - Often associated with puncture wound or ulcer
  - Cultures necessary for suspected systemic toxicity or extensive skin involvement or underlying comorbidities
- **Assessment**
  - Presence of crepitus should lead you to look for *Clostridium* or *Bacteroides*
  - Source
    - Skin – MRSA, GAS
    - Seawater – *Vibrio spp.*
    - Freshwater – *Aeromonas spp.*
- **Treatment**[73]
  - Elevated affected extremity
  - Antibiotics
    Coverage should include **GBS and MSSA** but if no improvement in 48 hours, include **MRSA** coverage. Total duration of treatment should be 7-10 days.

Pharmacologic management of purulent vs non-purulent treatment of SSTI	
Non-Purulent	Purulent
▫ Mild/Moderate Targeting streptococci, particularly Group A streptococci; other streptococcal species may also be present. Use IV therapy for moderate level infxn. • Augmentin 875mg PO BID • Cefazolin 1g IV/IM q8h • Cephalexin 500mg QID • Cefadroxil 500mg PO BID • PCN VK 200-500mg PO Q6H / Dicloxacillin 250mg PO q6h • Clindamycin 300mg PO TID if mild and PCN allergy; 600-900mg IV Q6H if moderate • Doxycycline 100mg BID • Ciprofloxacin 500mg BID • Mupirocin 1% BID x5d • Bactrim 1-2 DS BID • PCN 2-4mil U IV Q4-6H • Ceftriaxone 1g IV/d	▫ Mild (PO) • TMP-SMX 1-2ds tablets BID • Doxycycline/Minocycline 100mg BID • Clindamycin 300-450mg PO TID/QID only if resistance <10-15% • *If MSSA:* Dicloxacillin 500mg PO QID or Cephalexin 500mg PO QID ▫ Moderate to Severe (IV) *Failed I&D and PO antibiotics* • Vancomycin 15mg/kg IV +/- [zosyn 3.375mg IV Q6H or clindamycin 900mg IV Q8H) • Cefazoline 600mg IV Q12H • Delafloxacin 300mg IV Q12H for 5-14d • Linezolid 600mg IV/PO BID x 7-10 days • Tedizolid 200mg daily • Daptomycin 6mg/kg IV daily • *If MSSA:* Nafcillin 1-2g IV Q4H, Cefazolin 1g IV Q8H, or clindamycin 600mg IV Q8H
▫ Severe infections (requiring IV antibiotics) *MRSA infection elsewhere, IVDA, SIRS, oral antibiotic failure, etc., antimicrobials targeting both streptococci and MRSA are indicated* • Ampicillin/Sulbactam 1.5g IV Q6H	

INFECTIOUS DISEASE

- Penicillin G 2 million units IV every 6 hours or
- Cefazolin 1 gram IV every 8 hours or
- Clindamycin 600 mg IV every 8 hours or
- Vancomycin 15 mg/kg IV every 12 hours
- Metronidazole 600-900mg IV q8h
- Zosyn 3.375g IV q8h
- Telavancin 10mg/kg IV/d
- Delafloxacin 300mg IV Q12H for 5-14d or 450mg PO Q12H
- Ceftriaxone, 1.0 g intravenously every 24 hr
- Linezolid, 0.6 g intravenously every 12 hr.

- **Necrotizing Infections**
  - *Streptococcus pyogenes*: PCN 2-4M U IV q4-6h + clindamycin 600-900mg IV Q8H
  - *Vibrio vulnificus*: Ceftriaxone 1g IV daily + doxycycline 100mg PO BID
  - *Aeromonas hydrophila*: Doxycycline 100mg IV q12H + Ciprofloxacin 400mg IV BID
  - *Polymicrobial*: Vancomycin 15mg/kg IV + Zosyn 3.375g IV Q4H
- **Diabetic Foot Infection**
  - Mild (1-2 weeks treatment)
    - MSSA: Augmentin 875mg BID or Cephalexin 500mg PO Q6H or Dicloxacillin 250-500mg PO Q6H
    - MRSA: Doxycyclin 100mg PO BID or Bactrim DS 2 tablets PO BID
  - Moderate (deep or >2cm of erythema; 1-3 weeks treatment)
    - MSSA: Unasyn 1.5-3g IV Q6H/Ceftriaxone 1g IV daily
      - PCN allergy use combination Ciprofloxacin 500mg PO BID + Clindamycin 300mg PO Q6H
    - MRSA: Linezolid 600mg IV/PO BID or Daptomycin 6mg/kg IV/d or Vancomycin 15mg/kg IV
  - Severe (same as moderate with systemic signs; 2-4 weeks treatment)
    - Vancomycin 15mg/kg IV plus either the combination of Cefepime 2g IV Q8H/Flagyl 500mg IV Q6H or Zosyn 3.375g Q4H alone
- **Pseudomonal coverage**
  - Ceftazidime
  - Zosyn
- Erysipelas (Streptococcus coverage)
  - Mild-Moderate infections (oral, outpatient management)
    - Penicillin VK 500 mg orally four times per day for 7-10 days or
    - Amoxicillin 500 mg orally three times per day for 7-10 days or
    - Cephalexin 500 mg orally four times per day for 7-10 days
  - Penicillin Allergy
    - Azithromycin 500 mg orally on day 1, then 250 mg orally on days 2-5
    - Clindamycin 300 mg orally four times per day for 7-10 days
- **Recurrence**
  - Seen in 17% of patients
  - Consider prophylactic therapy if 2 episodes in 3 years with PAN 250mg/d x 1 year[74]

CLOSTRIDIUM DIFFICILE

- **Overview**[75,76]
  - G+ obligate anaerobic bacillus that can exist in both vegetative and spore forms
- **Diagnosis**

- o Only consider in patients with ≥3 loose stools in 24h (watery) not on laxatives
- o Lab options: toxin A+B via EIA (cannot determine if toxigenic), NAAT (can confirm toxigenic species), PCR, toxigenic culture, glutamate dehydrogenase, cell culture cytotoxicity
  - In general, perform EIA/NAAT first and if positive, confirm with toxin A/B EIA
  - Nucleic acid amplification tests (NAAT) for *C. difficile* toxin genes such as PCR are superior to toxins A+B EIA testing as a standard diagnostic test for CDI; do not solely perform NAAT for diagnosis.
  - Insufficient data to support testing for fecal lactoferrin or any other biologic markers
- **Risk Factors**
  - o Recent ABx use
  - o PPI
  - o Older age likely due to change in gut microbiota
  - o Severity of underlying illness
  - o Long-term care facility
  - o Recent abdominal surgery
- **Treatment**
  - o See table on prior page
  - o Testing for cure should not be done.
  - o If a patient has strong a pre-test suspicion for CDI, empiric therapy for CDI should be considered regardless of the laboratory testing result, as the negative predictive values for CDI are insufficiently high to exclude disease in these patients.
  - o Contact precautions should be continued for 48 hours after last occurrence of diarrhea
  - o In patients in whom oral antibiotics cannot reach a segment of the colon, such as with Hartman's pouch, ileostomy, or colon diversion, vancomycin therapy delivered via enema should be added to treatments above until the patient improves.
  - o Probiotics[77]
    - No sufficient evidence to support concomitant treatment with probiotics
- **Patients Requiring Antibiotics**[78]
  - o In patients who have a history of CDAD or cannot safely stop the antibiotics that precipitated their condition, IDSA recommends concomitant treatment for CDAD.
    - **Already on Abx and present with CDAD**
      - Extend CDAD treatment by providing a "tail" coverage with an agent effective against CDAD for 7-10 days following the completion of the inciting antibiotic.
    - **Prior history of CDAD and require Abx for another condition**
      - Concomitant prophylactic doses of oral vancomycin have been found to be effective in preventing recurrence.[9] The IDSA/SHEA recommend using low doses of vancomycin or fidaxomicin (e.g., 125 mg or 200 mg, respectively, once daily) while systemic antibiotics are administered.
- **Recurrent CDI**
  - o RCDI is a therapeutic challenge because there is no uniformly effective therapy.
  - o After treatment of an initial episode of *C. difficile*, the chance of RCDI within 8 weeks is 10-20%.
  - o Recurrence can be due to the same strain or to a different strain.
  - o First Reoccurrence
  The first recurrence of CDI can be treated with the same regimen that was used for the initial episode. If severe, however vancomycin should be used
    - 14d of Oral Vancomycin 125mg QID OR Metronidazole 500mg TID
    - Probiotics (lactobacillus and Saccharomyces bouldardii)
  - o Second Recurrence
  The second recurrence should be treated with a pulsed vancomycin regimen
    - Tapered dose regiment of oral vancomycin
    - 125mg QID x 7 days THEN
    - 125mg BID x 7 days THEN

INFECTIOUS DISEASE

- 125mg DAILY x 7 days THEN
- 125mg QOD x 7 days THEN
- 125mg qTHIRDday x 14 days WITH probiotics for 30 days beginning on first day
  - Third/Subsequent Recurrences
    - Tapered dose oral vancomycin with probiotics
    - Followed by:
      - 14d course of rifaximin (400-800mg daily)
      - Consider IVIG (200-500 mg/kg/day)
      - Consider fecal transport through colonoscopy (first degree relative, collect 1L, instill 200-400cc total during operation)
      - Consider chronic low dose vancomycin (not metronidazole d/t s/e) in elderly
    - Consider fecal transplantation (capsule vs. colonoscopy)
- **Prevention**
  - Common probiotics include Lactobacillus, Bifidobacterium, and Saccharomyces bouldardii.
  - Growing evidence supports the benefits of probiotics in preventing CDI in patients requiring hospitalization, who are at the highest risk of CDI infection.
  - Probiotics are most effective when given within 2 days of antibiotic initiation compared with later administration.

Treatment regimen based on severity/occurrences

Severity	Clinical Manifestations	Treatment
Carrier	No discernible clinical symptoms or signs	No treatment is indicated
Initial Episode/Non-severe WBC≤15k -and- SCr<1.5 mg/dL	• Mild diarrhea < 12 stools/day • Afebrile • Mild to Moderate discomfort or tenderness • Nausea With rare or absent vomiting • With or without hospitalization • Not in ICU • Dehydration • WBC < 15k • SCr<1.5 mg/dL	• Discontinuation of predisposing antibiotics, hydration, monitor clinical status, isolation • Oral vancomycin 125 mg QID x10-14d -or- • Fidaxomicin 200mg BID x 10d • *Alternative: Metronidazole 500mg TID x10d* • *No ↑ in morbidity or mortality seen with Metronidazole in mild/moderate C. diff* • Consider extending to 14d of therapy if improvement in symptoms or worsening*
Initial Episode / Severe WBC≥15k -or- SCr >1.5 mg/dL	• Severe or bloody diarrhea >12 stools/day • Pseudomembranous colitis • N/V • Ileus • Temp > 38.9 C • Age > 60 YO • In ICU • Renal failure Criteria: • WBC ≥ 15k or SCr>1.5	**No Distention** • Oral Vancomycin 125mg QID x10-14d* or • Fidaxomicin 200mg BID x10d *consider extending to 14d of therapy if improvement in symptoms or worsening*
Initial Episode / Complicated / Fulminant	• Hypotension / Shock • Toxic megacolon • Peritonitis • Ileus	• Surgical consultation • Vancomycin 500 mg QID PO or by NG tube x 14d -and- • Metronidazole 500mg IV TID (if perforation suspected) x 14d

Treatment regimen based on severity/occurrences

Severity	Clinical Manifestations	Treatment
Severe criteria above PLUS 1 of the following: ↓BP/shock, Ileus, Perforation, Megacolon		• If ileus, add rectal instillation of Vancomycin (500mg PR in 100cc saline as enema) QID x 14d
First Recurrence / Fulminant	As above	• Vancomycin 125 mg QID PO for 10-14 days if metronidazole was used for the initial episode OR • Use a prolonged tapered and pulsed VAN regimen if a standard regimen was used for the initial episode (e.g., 125 mg 4 times per day for 10–14 days, 2 times per day for a week, once per day for a week, and then every 2 or 3 days for 2–8 weeks) OR • Fidaxomicin 200 mg BID for 10 days if Vancomycin was used for the initial episode
Subsequent Recurrence / Fulminant	As above	• Vancomycin in a tapered and pulsed regimen >125mg PO Q6H x 14d >125mg PO Q12H x 7d >125mg PO daily x 7d >125mg PO QOD x 8d >125mg PO Q3D x 15d OR • Vancomycin 125 mg QID PO for 10 days followed by rifaximin 400 mg TID for 20 days OR • Fidaxomicin 200 mg BID for 10 days (if severe) OR • Fecal microbiota transplantation

INFECTIOUS DISEASE

MENINGITIS

- **Overall**[79]
  - Encephalitis (most commonly of viral origin 2/2 HSV esp. in older population >70) will present with AMS and focal neurological deficits. These patients require treatment with Acyclovir
  - 95% of patients with meningitis will present with headache, fever, AMS, and neck stiffness
- **Etiology**
  - Bacterial:
    - S. pneumoniae (+latex agglutination) most common cause of bacterial meningitis
    - N. meningitides
    - GNR
    - Listeria monocytogenes
    - H. influenza
    - E. coli K1
    - S. agalactiae
  - Fungal: cryptococcus
  - Arboviruses: West Nile, St. Louis, La Crosse, eastern and western equine
  - Viral: HSV, CMV, enterovirus, human parechovirus, varicella zoster
- **Labs/Diagnostic Testing**
  - CT prior to LP
  - Lumbar puncture may be performed without computed tomography of the brain if there are no risk factors for an occult intracranial abnormality. Signs that should warrant CT first prior to LP:
    - Immunocompromised (+HIV, AIDS, s/p chemotherapy)
    - Hx of CNS disease (mass, lesion, stroke, infection)
    - New seizure (within 1 week of presentation or in post ictal state)
    - Papilledema
    - Abnormal LOC/AMS
    - Focal neurological deficit
  - Performing lumbar puncture
    - Measure opening pressure (normal 10-20 cm if average wait, up to 25cm if obese)
      - Measured in the left lateral decubitus position

Labs obtained in lumbar puncture			
Tube #	Amount (cc)	Studies:	
#1	3cc	Cell count	
		Differential	
#2	3cc	Glucose	
		Protein	
#3	5-10cc	HIV-	HIV+
		- Gram stain	Gram stain
		- Culture	Culture
		- Cytology	India Ink
			VDRL (and serum RPR)
		Optional	Cocci serology
		- India Ink	Crypto antigen
		- VDRL (and serum RPR)	Fungal Culture
		- Cocci serology	Viral culture
		- Crypto antigen	AFB smear/Culture

INFECTIOUS DISEASE

			- Fungal Culture - AFB smear/Culture - Viral culture - TB PAR - Bacterial Antigen Panel	Toxo serology Cytology to eval for ANS lymphoma Consider JA Virus PAR
#4	3cc	Cell count Differential		

- o **Remember however, still give the ABx, then get CT, then LP!**
- o Serum: PCT, CRP
- Treatment
  - o ABx **should not** be delayed in patients suspected of having bacterial meningitis if lumbar puncture cannot be performed in a timely manner
  - o A large prospective, randomized, double-blind trial that established the use of adjuvant dexamethasone in adults found that patients who received dexamethasone had a significantly lower risk of an unfavorable outcome than patients who received placebo
    - Most often used in patients with diplococci on GS or culture + *S.pneumoniae* in blood or CSF
    - Dexamethasone 10mg x1 before or w/ first dose of ABx then 10mg q6h x4d
  - o Vaccination for Streptococcus pneumoniae, Haemophilus influenzae type B, and Neisseria meningitidis is recommended for patients in appropriate risk groups and significantly decreases the incidence of bacterial meningitis.
  - o Below are treatment regiments, those that are starred (*) are preferred overall

CSF findings and associated etiologies					
	Glucose	Protein	WBC	Opening Pressure	Cell differential
Normal	>40	<60	<5 cells	6-20cm	Lymphocytes
Bacterial	<40	100-500	1000-10,000	15-50cm	PMNs
Viral	Normal (30-70)	Normal (30-150)	<1000 ↓PMN ↑Lymph	60-30cm	Lymphocytes
TB	<40	High	<1000	15-50cm	Lymphocytes
Fungal	<40	High	<1000	15-50cm	Lymphocytes

CSF Findings in Meningitis by Etiology

Agent	Opening Pressure (mm H₂O)	WBC count (cells/μL)	Glucose (mg/dL)	Protein (mg/dL)	Microbiology
Bacterial meningitis	200-300	100-5000; >80% PMNs	< 40	>100	Specific pathogen demonstrated in 60% of Gram stains and 80% of cultures
Viral meningitis	90-200	10-300; lymphocytes with PMN in first 48h	Normal, reduced in LCM and mumps	Normal but may be slightly elevated	Viral isolation, PCR assays
Tuberculous meningitis	180-300	100-500; lymphocytes	Reduced, < 40	Elevated, >100	Acid-fast bacillus stain, culture, PCR
Cryptococcal meningitis	180-300	10-200; lymphocytes	Reduced	50-200	India ink, cryptococcal antigen, culture
Aseptic meningitis	90-200	10-300; lymphocytes	Normal	Normal but may be slightly elevated	Negative findings on workup
Normal values	80-200	0-5; lymphocytes	50-75	15-40	Negative findings on workup

LCM = lymphocytic choriomeningitis; PCR = polymerase chain reaction; PMN = polymorphonuclear leukocyte; WBC = white blood cell.

Common causes of meningitis and treatments

Bacteria	Susceptibility	Antibiotic(s)	Duration (days)
Streptococcus pneumoniae	Penicillin MIC ≤0.06 µg/mL	Recommended: Penicillin G or ampicillin Alternatives: Cefotaxime, ceftriaxone, chloramphenicol	10-14
	Penicillin MIC ≥0.12 µg/mL	Recommended: Cefotaxime or ceftriaxone Alternatives: Cefepime, meropenem	
	Cefotaxime or ceftriaxone MIC ≥0.12 µg/mL Cefotaxime or ceftriaxone MIC ≥1.0 µg/mL	Recommended: Vancomycin plus cefotaxime or ceftriaxone** Alternatives: Vancomycin plus moxifloxacin	
Haemophilus influenzae	Beta-lactamase–negative	Recommended: Ampicillin Alternatives: Cefotaxime, ceftriaxone, cefepime, chloramphenicol, aztreonam, a fluoroquinolone	7
	Beta-lactamase-positive	Recommended: Cefotaxime or ceftriaxone** Alternatives: Cefepime, chloramphenicol, aztreonam, a fluoroquinolone	
	Beta-lactamase–negative, ampicillin-resistant	Recommended: Meropenem Alternatives: Cefepime, chloramphenicol, aztreonam, a fluoroquinolone	
Neisseria meningitidis	Penicillin MIC < 0.1 µg/mL	Recommended: Penicillin G or ampicillin** Alternatives: Cefotaxime, ceftriaxone, chloramphenicol	7
	Penicillin MIC ≥0.1 µg/mL	Recommended: Cefotaxime or ceftriaxone Alternatives: Cefepime, chloramphenicol, a fluoroquinolone, meropenem	
Listeria monocytogenes	...	Recommended: Ampicillin or penicillin G** Alternative: TMP-SMX	14-21
Streptococcus agalactiae	...	Recommended: Ampicillin or penicillin G** Alternatives: Cefotaxime, ceftriaxone, vancomycin	14-21
Enterobacteriaceae	...	Recommended: Cefotaxime or ceftriaxone Alternatives: Aztreonam, a fluoroquinolone, TMP-SMX, meropenem, ampicillin	21
Pseudomonas aeruginosa	...	Recommended: Ceftazidime or cefepime Alternatives: Aztreonam, meropenem, ciprofloxacin	21
Staphylococcus epidermidis		Recommended: Vancomycin Alternative: Linezolid Consider addition of rifampin	

INFECTIOUS DISEASE

Organisms to consider based on population demographic

Population	Organism	Treatment
Adults 16-50 YO	N. meningitidis	Dexamethasone
	S. pneumoniae	Ceftriaxone
	H. influenzae	Vancomycin
Adults >50 YO	N. meningitidis	Dexamethasone
	S. pneumoniae	Ceftriaxone
	L. monocytogenes	Vancomycin
	GNR	Ampicillin (cover for L. Monocytogenes)
Post-NSurg/Shunt	S. aureus	Vancomycin
	S. pneumoniae	Cefepime
	GNR	
Immunocompromised	N. meningitidis	Vancomycin
	S. pneumoniae	Ampicillin
	H. influenzae	Cefepime
	GNR	
Penetrating trauma		Vancomycin
		Cefepime
HSV Encephalitis	HSV	Acyclovir

URINARY TRACT INFECTIONS

- **Definition**: LUTS with concurrent growth of significant pathological organisms
- **General Considerations**[80]
    - Although a urine Gram stain may be useful in guiding therapy, all antibiotics recommended as empiric therapy are effective against Gram-negative bacilli (pyelonephritis is not treated empirically with ampicillin or sulfonamides alone due to E. coli resistance to these antibiotics).
    - In patients with nosocomial pyelonephritis, a history of recurrent UTI, or prior infection with a resistant organism, *initial antimicrobial therapy should cover Pseudomonas aeruginosa* (I.e. cefepime, tobramycin, imipenem, ciprofloxacin, or piperacillin/tazobactam).
    - In all cases, antibiotic therapy should be revised once susceptibility data are available.
    - If bacteriuria persists > 24-48 hours, switch the antibiotic based on susceptibility data.
    - If fever or toxicity persists despite adequate antibiotics, consider perinephric or renal cortical abscess and evaluate with imaging of kidneys.
    - Signs of pyelonephritis (i.e. fever, leukocytosis) may not be present in the elderly.
- **Etiologies**: E coli (80% of outpatient UTIs), Staphylococcus saprophyticus (5–15% of outpatient UTIs), Klebsiella Proteus, Pseudomonas, Enterobacter, Enterococcus, Candida, Adenovirus type 11
- **Symptoms**
    - Urethral discharge (consider STD)
    - Dysuria
    - Urinary frequency
    - Malodorous urine does not correlate well with likelihood of infection
    - Systemic sx (fever, chills, n/v, flank pain) → consider pyelonephritis

Complicated vs. Uncomplicated UTI

Uncomplicated	Complicated
Lack of any identified risk factors that would otherwise predispose the patient to a UTI	*Infection associated with a condition such as structural or functional abnormality of the GU*

INFECTIOUS DISEASE

• Non-pregnant, premenopausal females • Healthy men • Acute pyelonephritis in an otherwise healthy patient • Recurrent UTI risk factors (i.e. controlled T2DM, sexual behavior)	tract or the presence of an underlying disease that increases the patient's risk of having a UTI • Pregnant females • Renal insufficiency (relevant, not well defined) • Asx bacteriuria if pregnant or undergoing urology procedure • Immunosuppression • Urinary obstruction (congenital, enlarged prostate, urinary stones) • Incomplete bladder emptying due to anatomic or neurogenic causes (e.g., spinal cord injury) • MDR bacteria • Foreign bodies (e.g., catheters, drainage tubes, instruments) • Systemic condition (e.g., diabetes, pregnancy) • Male participating in anal intercourse

- **Types**
  - Uncomplicated
  - Complicated
  - Asymptomatic – growth in asymptomatic pt
  - Recurrent - ≥2 infections in 6 months or ≥3 culture proven in one year
  - CAUTI - Indwelling urethral or suprapubic catheter or intermittent catheterization with 10^3 CFU/mL of one bacterial species cultured
- **Risk Factors**: sex, spermicide use, family h/o UTI, new sexual partner, h/o UTI during childhood, urinary incontinence, cystocele, atrophic vaginitis, high PVR
- **Diagnostics**
  - UA
    - ↑WBC (pyuria is >10 WBCs/mm^3; 95% sens)
    - +LE
    - +Nitrite
    - Contamination considered if more than 15-20 squamous cells/HPF
  - UCx (considered significant if > 100k CFU; less can be considered significant if obtained via sterile manner such as cath or suprapubic aspiration)
  - In appropriate population, consider gonorrhea/chlamydia testing
- **Organisms**
  - E.coli, enterococcus, klebsiella, Enterobacter, and proteus
- **Empiric Treatment**
  - Pain: Phenazopyridine 200mg PO TID after meals x48h
  - Antibiotics:
    - Acute, uncomplicated cystitis in women
      - First Line Therapy
        1. Nitrofurantoin 100 mg BID x5d (with meals; avoid if G6PD, pregnant, or has renal failure)
        2. TMP-SMX 160/800 mg twice daily for 3 days
        3. Fosfomycin 3g once
           - DM, >7 days of symptoms, recent UTI, age > 65, or diaphragm use: treat for 7 days with above
      - Second Line Therapy (must prove that above options either did not work or are contraindicated)
        1. Ciprofloxacin 250mg BID x3d or 500mg BID x7d
        2. Levofloxacin 250 mg daily x5d

INFECTIOUS DISEASE

3. Amoxicillin-Clavulanate 500mg PO BID x5-7d
4. Cefdinir 300mg BID x5-7d
5. Cefadroxil 500mg PO BID x5-7d
6. Cephalexin 500mg PO BID x5-7d
- **Pregnant**: PO amoxicillin, nitrofurantoin, cefpodoxime, OR TMP/SMX (do not use near term) for 3-7 days.
- Acute, uncomplicated cystitis in men *(recommended duration ≤7d assuming no sx of pyelonephritis or prostatitis)*
  - Nitrofurantoin 100mg BID
  - TMP-SMX DS BID
  - Fosfomycin 3g x1
- Acute, uncomplicated pyelonephritis in women
  - Mild/moderate symptoms without nausea/vomiting
    1. FQ x7 days OR amoxicillin/clavulanate or cephalexin or TMP/SMX (DS) x14 days
  - Severe/urosepsis requiring hospitalization
    1. IV FQ OR (ampicillin + gentamicin)
    2. 3rd generation cephalosporin
    3. piperacillin/tazobactam until afebrile then oral TMP/SMX (DS) or FQ x14 days
  - Pregnancy: IV ceftizoxime OR gentamicin ± ampicillin OR aztreonam OR TMP/SMX until afebrile then oral amoxicillin OR cephalosporin OR TMP/SMX (DS) x14 days
  - If fever persists beyond 5 days with continued symptoms, US should be obtained to r/o perinephric abscess
- Pain
  - Phenazopyridine 200mg PO TID x2d after meals
- Asymptomatic
  - 15-50% of patients in long term care facilities harbor bacteria
  - Treat in pregnant women and any patient undergoing urological manipulation
- Complicated UTI
  - Mild/moderate symptoms without nausea/vomiting: oral FQ x10-14 days
  - Severe/urosepsis requiring hospitalization: IV ciprofloxacin OR (ampicillin + gentamicin) OR ceftizoxime OR aztreonam OR piperacillin/tazobactam OR imipenem until afebrile then oral TMP/SMX (DS) or FQ x14-21 days
- ESBL UTI
  - Risk factors: hospitalization, catheter placement, CV catheter, feeding tube, prior ABx, ventilator usage, residence in nursing home
  - Treatment: carbapenems (ertapenem, meropenem, and imipenem) cefepime, ceftarolene, ceftazidime
- Recurrent UTI (women)
  - Postcoital or daily prophylactic ABx are recommended
    1. Options include TMP-SMX, Nitrofurantoin, Cephalexin, and Ciprofloxacin

INFECTIOUS DISEASE

Treatment of Urinary Tract Infection

Population	Organism	Treatment
Uncomplicated	E. coli (75% to 95%) P. mirabilis K. pneumoniae S. saprophyticus E. faecalis E. faecium	• Trimethoprim 100 mg or TMP/SMX 160/800 mg BID 3d • Nitrofurantoin 100 mg BID x 5d • Amoxicillin-clavulanate 875/125 mg BID • Cephalexin 500 mg BID – QID • Fosfomycin 3 gm single dose • Ciprofloxacin 250 mg BID x3d • Levofloxacin 250 mg daily x3d
Acute self-treatment	As above	TMP/SMX 160/800 mg BID for three days
Complicated	E. coli Citrobacter, Enterobacter, M. Morgani S. marcescens, P. aeruginosa K. pneumoniae P. mirabilis	Duration: 7d if only LUTS; extend to 10-14d for more severe infections (and in men per AUA) unless otherwise noted below. • PO: ciprofloxacin 500 mg BID x7d, levofloxacin 750 mg daily x5d, ciprofloxacin 1g ER x7d • TMP-SMX BID x14d (except enterococcus and pseudomonas) • IV: ceftriaxone 1 to 2 gms daily, ciprofloxacin 400 mg q12h, levofloxacin 750 mg daily, ertapenem 1 gm daily
CAUTI	P. mirabilis M. morganii K. pneumonia P. aeruginosa P. stuartii	Duration: 7d in most patients, 10-14d in those with delayed response • Remove and replace the catheter PRIOR to treatment. Collect the urine specimen for C&S from the newly placed catheter • Ampicillin 2 gm q6h + gentamicin 5 mg/kg, then adjusted based on kinetics. • Piperacillin-tazobactam 3.375 gm q6h • Ciprofloxacin 400 mg IV BID or levofloxacin 750/d • ESBL: Imipenem 0.5 gm IV q12h, meropenem 2 gm IV q8h

Pyelonephritis	E. coli (>80%)
	Other gram negatives
	Enterococci
	Pseudomonas spp.
	Staph
		• Outpatient
		  o Ciprofloxacin, 500 mg given orally twice daily x7d (preg cat C)
		  o TMP-SMX 160/800mg BID x14d
		  o Levofloxacin, 750 mg given orally once daily for 5 days
		  o Cefixime 400mg/d x10-14d (active against many FLQ-res and Bactrim-res GNB
		• Inpatient
		  o Ciprofloxacin 400mg Q12H
		  o Levaquin 750mg daily
		  o Ceftriaxone 1-2g/d
		  o Cefotaxme 1g q8-12h up to 2g q4h
		  o Ertapenem 1g q24h x7-10d
		  o Meropenam 500mg q12h x7-10d
		  o Ticarcillin-clavulanate: 3.1g q4-6h
		  o Imipenem 500mg IV q6h (covers ESBL but not CRE)
		  o Amikacin 15-20 mg/kg q24h x7-10d

PYELONEPHRITIS

- **Pearls**[81]
  - Fever can last (on average) 3 days in patients
  - After 3 days, consider complications such as abscess
  - Absence of fever is common in the geriatric population
  - Has potential to cause sepsis, shock, and death
- **Symptoms**
  - Flank Pain
  - Fever>103F common
  - Anorexia
  - N/V
  - Myalgias
  - Dysuria, ↑frequency, urgency
- **Diagnosis**
  - CT abd/pelv if suspected sepsis+/-shock, known urolithiasis, pH>7, or ↓GFR to 40 or if symptoms not improving after 24-48h
  - Labs
    - UA: WBC casts, +LE, pyuria (>5 WBCs), +nitrites, WBC cast (renal origin)
    - CBC, BUN/SCr, hCG, GFR
    - UCx: $\geq 10^5$ CFU **cardinal confirmatory diagnostic test
    - CRP
    - Albumin (<3.3 ↑ risk for need to hospitalize)
- **Etiology**
  - E. coli (>80%)
  - Other gram negatives
  - Enterococci
  - Pseudomonas spp.
  - Staph
- **Commonly Associated Conditions**
  - Indwelling catheters
  - Renal calculi
  - BPH
- **Rule out**
  - Complications such as hydronephrosis, concomitant nephrolithiasis, abscess (persistent fevers after 3 days of treatment, hx of DM, flank pain/abdominal pain, bacteremia). Consider re-imaging (or initial imaging) with CT, US, or cystoscopy.
  - Most common causes of failure are ABx resistance and nephrolithiasis
- **Treatment**

Triaging patients with pyelonephritis			
Triage	Home	Observation	Admission
Symptoms/Hx	Mild; no vomiting	Moderate; +/-vomit	Sepsis
	No other PMHx	None or stable	Potential PMHx
Fluids	None/minor	Moderate +/- maintenance fluids	Vigorous
Imaging	None	Only if risk for obstruction, abscess, or emphysematous pyelo	
ABx	IV/Oral/Both	Start on IV in ER and	No PO therapy until
	Can give single IV dose then continue PO	continue on floor then switch to PO	stabilized

  - Antibiotics:

INFECTIOUS DISEASE

In general, start broad then tailor therapy to culture and sensitivities. PO transition from IV can occur after patient has been afebrile for 24-48 hours. Most Abx require 14 days duration except ciprofloxacin which only requires 7 days.

- Outpatient
  1. Ciprofloxacin, 500 mg given orally twice daily x7d (preg cat C)
  2. TMP-SMX 160/800mg BID x14d
  3. Levofloxacin, 750 mg given orally once daily for 5 days
  4. Cefixime 400mg/d x10-14d (active against many FLQ-res and Bactrim-res GNB
- Inpatient
  1. Ampicillin 2g IV q6h + Tobramycin 6mg/kg IV daily x14d
  2. Ampicillin 2g IV q6h + gentamicin 1mg/kg IV q8h x14d
  3. Ciprofloxacin 400mg Q12H
  4. Levaquin 750mg daily
  5. Ceftriaxone 1-2g/d
  6. Cefotaxime 1g q8-12h up to 2g q4h
  7. Ertapenem 1g q24h x7-10d
  8. Meropenem 500mg q12h x7-10d
  9. Ticarcillin-clavulanate: 3.1g q4-6h
  10. Imipenem 500mg IV q6h (covers ESBL but not CRE)
  11. Amikacin 15-20 mg/kg q24h x7-10d
- o <u>Anesthetic</u>: Phenazopyridine 200mg PO TID x2d after meals unless CKD or ↑LFT
- o <u>Analgesic</u>: Tylenol, Opiate
- o <u>Anti-emetic</u>: prochlorperazine, Zofran
- o <u>Referral Indications</u>
  - UT obstruction and/or high urinary post void residual volumes
  - Nephrolithiasis
  - Intrarenal abscess
  - Perinephric abscess
  - Urology/IR for percutaneous nephrostomy tube if there is concern for pyelonephritis or ureteral obstruction with proximal infection

SEPSIS

- **Definition**[82]
  - o <u>Sepsis</u> is defined as the presence (probable or documented) of infection together with systemic manifestations of infection (SIRS).
    - Systemic Inflammatory Response Syndrome (SIRS) ≥ 2 of
      - T > 100.4F or < 96.8F
      - HR > 90
      - RR > 20 or PaCO2 < 32 mmHg
      - WBC > 12,000/mm^3 or WBC < 4,000/mm^3 or > 10% immature neutrophils (bands)
  - o <u>Severe Sepsis</u> – sepsis with evidence of acute organ dysfunction or tissue hypoperfusion
    - Tissue hypoperfusion:
      - Vitals: SBP<90, MAP<70, ↓SBP by 40
      - Labs: lactate > 2, SCr > 2, BILI > 2, PLT < 100k, INR > 1.5
      - UOP <0.5cc/kg/h x 2h despite fluids
    - End organ dysfunction (AMS, hypoxemia, oliguria, ileus, thrombocytopenia)
    - Organ dysfunction can be also predicted with change in qSOFA score of ≥2
  - o <u>Septic Shock</u> - subset of sepsis; defined by vasodilatory hypotension (MAP<65 mmHg and lactate > 2) despite <u>adequate</u> fluid resuscitation requiring vasopressors to maintain MAP>65
- **Screening**
  - o <u>qSOFA</u>; helps predict pts who may benefit from ICU transfer (mortality of appx 10%)
  - o Nonspecific symptoms: weakness, falls

INFECTIOUS DISEASE

- **Diagnostics**
    - CBC
    - CMP with amylase and lipase
    - Coag panel
    - Lactate
    - Cx if not already done (BCx, UCx) x2 sets
    - UA
    - ABG

Interpretation of elevated lactate

Type A – due to poor tissue perfusion or hypoxia		
Shock	Trauma	Limb/mesenteric ischemia
Profound hypotension	Burns	Compartment syndrome
Severe anemia	Carbon Monoxide	Seizure
Cardiac arrest	Cyanide	Increased work of breathing
Type B - accumulation in absence of tissue hypoperfusion or hypoxia		
Underlying disease process	Drug/Toxin	Congenital Errors in Metabolism
Malignancy	Metformin	G6PD
Sepsis	Tylenol	Mitochondriopathies (MELAS)
Thiamine deficiency	SABA	
Cirrhosis	EtOH	
AKI	CO	
DKA/AKA		

Severe sepsis

Sepsis + sepsis-induced organ dysfunction or tissue hypoperfusion
Sepsis-induced ↓BP
Lactate above upper limits laboratory normal
Urine output < 0.5 mL/kg/hr for more than 2 hrs despite adequate fluid resuscitation
Acute lung injury with Pao2/Fio2 < 250 in the absence of pneumonia as infection source
Acute lung injury with Pao2/Fio2 < 200 in the presence of pneumonia as infection source
Creatinine > 2.0 mg/dL (176.8 μmol/L)
Bilirubin > 2 mg/dL (34.2 μmol/L)
Platelet count < 100,000 μL
Coagulopathy (international normalized ratio > 1.5)

- **Treatment**[83]
    - Hour-1 Bundle
        - Initiated within the **first hour** of presentation; this is highly debated as many feel it is unrealistic to meet such a time marker.
            - **Bundle consists of**:
                - Measurement of the lactate level; remeasure if >2 mmol/L
                - Obtaining blood cultures before giving antibiotics
                - Maintain MAP≥65
                - Administering antibiotics
                - Giving 30 mg/kg crystalloid (LR) for ↓BP or lactate ≥4 mmol/L.
                    - Some will extend this to within the first 3 hours
                    - Consider albumin in cirrhosis with hypoalbuminemia
                    - Worse outcomes (↑death) were noted in patients who received >5L total in the first day
                - Giving vasopressors if patient remains hypotensive despite fluid resuscitation.
    - Rapid fluid infusions
        - *Fluid Choice*
            - Balanced crystalloids (LR, plasma-lyte) are more like plasma and associated with ↓30-day in-hospital mortality compared to NS (*SMART*)

INFECTIOUS DISEASE

- Normal saline (0.9%) causes ↑Cl, metabolic acidosis, renal vasoconstriction
- Trials have found no benefit comparing crystalloid to colloid (*SAFE, 6S*)
- Initial fluid challenge should be 1L or more of crystalloid, and a minimum of **30 mL/kg** of crystalloid (2.1 L in a 70 kg or 154-pound person) in the first 4-6 hours.
  - Grade 2B recommendation for adding albumin as necessary (in patients who require "substantial amount" of fluid)
  - Monitor lactate every 2 hours for 8 hours, aiming for reduction in 20% every 2 hours (*LACTATE trial*)

Hemodynamic management of early septic shock

Intervention	Recommendation	Considerations
MAP Target	≥65 mmHg	Permissive ↓BP may be considered in cases of trauma
Fluid resuscitation	30 cc/kg at least within 1 hour	Consideration that large amounts may increase fluid overload and worsen outcomes
What fluids to give and for how long	Crystalloids for at least 1 hour, then re-assess clinically	Consider adding albumin with "substantial" fluid requirements
Pharmacologic vasopressor support	NE remains #1 choice with vasopressin as #2 to support NE. Add dobutamine only after #1 and #2 given to reach MAP goal	Should fluids always be given first then vasopressors?

- o Vasopressors are next choice when fluids are not adequate
  1. First start should be norepinephrine (levophed) at 0.03U/minute (grade 2A)
  2. When additional pressors required: options should be **epinephrine or vasopressin** (0.03U/min) (grade 2B)
     - Patients at low risk for arrhythmias with low HR/CO can use dopamine otherwise avoided (grade 2C)
  3. **Dobutamine** should be added to above vasopressor if:
     - Signs of cardiac dysfunction (grade 1C) as evidenced by low CO or continued hypoperfusion with above pressors
     - Concern for cardiogenic shock (combine with dopamine, avoid PE, NE); add balloon pump if BP does not respond (acts to ↓ afterload); ↑survival if used after PCI
- o Antibiotics
  - Administration of effective intravenous antimicrobials **within the first hour** of recognition of septic shock
  - Obtain PCT level to assist in determining if a pt needs ABx but have no evidence of infection
  - Empiric combination therapy should not be administered for more than 3–5 days. De-escalation to the most appropriate single therapy should be performed as soon as the susceptibility profile is known (grade 2B).
  - Duration of therapy typically 7–10 days; longer courses may be appropriate in patients who have a slow clinical response, undrainable foci of infection, bacteremia with S. aureus; some fungal and viral infections or immunologic deficiencies, including neutropenia
- o Stress Ulcer Prophylaxis *(PEPTIC)*
  - H2-blockers are non-inferior for stress ulcer prophylaxis in ICU
  - PPI therapy remains appropriate for patients with evidence of UGIB
- o Neuromuscular blockers
  - The ACURASYS trial showed benefit of 48 hours of NM blockade in patients with ARDS

- ▫ Studies have shown early severe ARDS may benefit from NMBA especially if elevated pressures are noted
- ▫ 48-hour infusion of cisatracurium (Nimbex) with 15mg bolus f/b 37.5 mg/hr had lower 90-day mortality, morbidity, and quicker discharge from ICU than placebo
- o Glucose
  - Upper limit should be 180 mg/dL *(NICE-SUGAR)*
  - Initiate feeds 48 hours after dx of sepsis
- o Steroids
  - If patient does not adequately respond (↓BP) to vasopressors, should add IV hydrocortisone gtt at 200mg/day (grade 2C)
  - Also add if patient has adrenal insufficiency
- o Ventilation
  - ARDS patients should be kept at TV 0.6cc/IBW

> IBW Males = 0.91 × (height [cm] − 152.4) + 50
> IBW Females = 0.91 × (height [cm] − 152.4) + 45.5

- o Transfusion
  - Target HGB 7-9 g/dL in absence of sx (tissue hypoperfusion, ischemic CAD, acute bleeding) (Grade 1B)

Vasopressors

α_1 – vasoconstrictor effects, increases SVR
α_2 – inhibits pre-sympathetic release of NE thus no action on alpha1 receptors!
β_1 – think 1 heart, positive inotropic effects (↑Ca release at SR) from FS mech and ↑HR
β_2 – think 2 lungs, increases dilation of smooth muscle in arteries and bronchioles

Name	Recep/Eff	Dose	Action	Use
Phenylephrine	α_1 ↑MAP ↑SVR ↔HR	Continuous infusion for ↓BP: Start at 0.1-0.5 mcg/kg/min, titrate to effect, range: 0.5-1 mcg/kg/min	Potent α vasoconstriction can cause significant distal tissue hypoxia; ensure appropriate volume resuscitation	↓BP from low peripheral vascular tone. Pressor of choice for septic patients with cardiovascular disease, though patients likely have significant intrinsic sympathetic (and consequent) β1 stimulation anyway
Epinephrine (third)	$\alpha_1\alpha_2\beta_1\beta_2$ ↑↑MAP ↑↑SVR ↑↑HR	0.01-0.05 mcg/kg/min (upper range 0.5-1 mcg/kg/min) titrated every 1-2 minutes Anaphylaxis: 0.1-0.5 mg SC/IM (usual dose is 0.3 mg, 1:1,000)	Highly arrhythmogenic, can cause myocardial ischemia/infarct; not for prolonged use, watch for unopposed α stimulation in patients on β-blockers	Cardiac arrest, refractory ↓BP, status asthmaticus, anaphylaxis
Norepinephrine (first)	$\alpha_1\alpha_2\beta_1$ ↑↑MAP ↑↑SVR ↑↑HR	Continuous infusion for hypotension: Start 0.1-0.5 mcg/kg/min, titrate to effect (~SBP>90, MAP>60), range: 0.5-3 mcg/min	Potent α vasoconstriction can cause significant distal tissue hypoxia; ensure appropriate volume resuscitation	↓BP from low peripheral vascular tone, myocardial depression, or both **Convenient initial pressor choice** as it causes peripheral vasoconstriction, via α effect, and increased inotropy/chronotropy, via β1 effect
Dopamine	δ ↔MAP ↔SVR ↑HR	Continuous infusion for hypotension: Start 5-10 mcg/kg/min, titrate to effect: (0-2 mcg/kg/min "renal dose", 2-5 mcg/kg/min β1 dose, >5 mcg/kg/min α1 dose)	Less potent α _vasoconstriction, but increased risk of tachyarrhythmias 2°/2 β activity vs. norepinephrine	At lower doses, hypotension from decreased myocardial contractility and at higher doses, from low peripheral vascular tone.
	β_1	2-10 mcg/kg/min	Positive inotropy, causes arrhythmias	
	↑MAP			

Drug	Receptors	Effects	Dose	Comments
	α₁	↑SVR, ↑↑HR ↑MAP, ↑SVR, ↑↑↑HR	10-20 mcg/kg/min	Vasoconstriction, causes arrhythmias
Dobutamine	β₁,β₂		Continuous infusion: Start at 2 mcg/kg/min, titrate to effect (usually Cardiac Index > 2), range: 2-20 mcg/kg/min	Low cardiac output states; produces significant inotropy/chronotropy, and "afterload" reduction with peripheral vasodilation. Expect hypotension, if needed support BP with dopamine first, and then start dobutamine - Risk of tachyarrhythmias, though less then epinephrine, dopamine, and isoproterenol; increased myocardial oxygen consumption, with resultant risk of ischemia
Vasopressin (second)	V₁	↑↑↑MAP, ↑↑↑SVR, ↔HR	Start at 0.03U/min with upper limit of 0.06U/min	Antidiuretic hormone that causes vasoconstriction and works to supplement catecholamine therapy (NE) particularly (see *VASST Trial*) Combine with NE to increase its effectiveness (can be secondary medication for septic shock)
Angiotensin II	AT₁, AT₂	↑↑MAP, ↑↑HR	Start: 20 ng/kg/minute IV by continuous infusion Maintenance: do not exceed 40 ng/kg/min; doses as low as 1.25 ng/kg/min may be used	↑BP by vasoconstriction and ↑ aldosterone release; direct action of angiotensin II on the vessel wall, stimulates smooth muscle contraction Approved for use in septic, anaphylactic or neurogenic shock; be aware of s/e which include thrombosis, tachycardia which warrants concurrent systemic anticoagulation *(ATHOS-3)*

INFECTIOUS DISEASE

Physiologic effects of hemodynamic medications			
Drug	Effect on HR	Effect on contractility	Arterial constriction effects
Dobutamine	+	+++	↔ (dilates)
Dopamine	++	++	++
Epinephrine	+++	+++	++
Norepinephrine	++	++	+++
Phenylephrine	↔	↔	+++
Amrinone	+	+++	↔ (dilates)

BACTERIAL ENDOCARDITIS

- **Clinical Manifestations**[84]
    - Signs/Symptoms
    - Fever, chills, sweats, anorexia, weight loss, malaise, myalgias, arthralgias, heart murmur, arterial emboli, splenomegaly, petechiae, peripheral manifestations (Osler's nodes, subungual hemorrhages, Janeway lesions, Roth's spots) and signs of CHF.
- **Risk Factors**
    - Structural heart disease, IVDU, indwelling vasc devices, bacteremia with other infection, prior history of infective endocarditis
- **Laboratory manifestations**
    - Anemia, leukocytosis, microscopic hematuria, elevated ESR, CRP, RF, circulating immune complexes, decreased serum complement
- **Microbiology**
    - S. aureus (30-40%), viridians group strep, enterococci (1%), coagulase-staph, culture negative (2-20%)
- **Work-Up**
    - Blood Cultures
        - If not critically ill: 3 blood cultures over 12-24 hours (can delay treatment)
        - If critically ill: 3 blood cultures over 1 hour (treat)
    - Echo (TTE or TEE)
    - ECG: evaluate for conduction abnormalities, ischemia, infarction
    - CXR: evaluate for septic emboli, valvular calcification, CHF
- **Diagnosis**
    - Modified Duke Criteria (2 major OR 1 major and 3 minor OR 5 minor criteria)
        - Major Criteria
            - Positive blood cultures
                - Typical microorganisms from two separate blood cultures: viridians strep, Strep bovis, HACEK, or community acquired Staph aureus or enterococci in absence of primary focus
                - Persistently positive blood culture: recovery of organism from blood cultures drawn > 12hrs apart OR all of 3 or majority of 4 or more separate blood cultures with first and last > 1hr apart
            - Evidence of endocardial involvement
            - Positive echo: oscillating intracardiac mass or abscess or new partial dehiscence of prosthetic valve
                - TEE recommended as first test in the following patients prosthetic valve endocarditis; or those with at least "possible" endocarditis by clinical criteria; or those with suspected complicated endocarditis, such as perivalvular abscess.
                - TTE recommended as first test in all other patients
                - Definition of positive findings: oscillating intracardiac mass, on valve or supporting structures, or in the path of regurgitant jets, or on implanted

material, in the absence of an alternative anatomic explanation or myocardial abscess or new partial dehiscence of prosthetic valve
- New valvular regurgitation
- Minor Criteria
  - Predisposing heart condition or injection drug use
  - Fever ≥ 38.0°C
  - Vascular phenomena: major arterial emboli, septic pulmonary infarcts, mycotic aneurysm, intracranial hemorrhage, conjunctival hemorrhages, Janeway lesions
  - Immunologic phenomena: glomerulonephritis, Osler's nodes, Roth's spots, RF
  - Microbiologic evidence: positive blood culture but not meeting above major criteria or serologic evidence of active infection with organism consistent with infective endocarditis
- **Treatment**
  - Empiric
    - For culture-positive endocarditis, use Sanford Guide to determine regimen
      - Unless the pt has a toxic appearance or clinical or echo evidence of progressive valvular regurgitation or CHF, empiric antibiotics should be delayed until blood cultures are drawn. Administration of antibiotics before blood cultures are obtained reduces recovery rate of bacteria by 30-45%.
    - Native valve without IVDU
      - [Penicillin G 20 million units q24h continuous or divided q4h OR ampicillin 12gm IV q24h continuous or divided q4h] AND oxacillin 2 gm IV q4h AND gentamicin 1mg/kg IV q8h
      - Alternative regimen is vancomycin + gentamicin
    - Native valve with IVDU (S. aureus)
      - Vancomycin 1gm IV q12h OR daptomycin 6mg/kg q24h
    - Prosthetic valve
      - Vancomycin 15mg/kg IV q12h + rifampin 600mg PO q24h + gentamicin 1mg/kg IV q8h
      - Prophylaxis (indirect evidence, no randomized trials)
  - Cardiac lesions for which endocarditis prophylaxis is advised:
    - High risk: prosthetic valves, prior bacterial endocarditis, complex cyanotic heart disease (except isolated secundum ASD and completely corrected PDA, VSD or pulmonary stenosis), PDA, coarctation of the aorta, surgically constructed systemic-pulmonary shunts
    - Moderate risk: congenital cardiac malformations, VSD, bicuspid AV, acquired AV and MV, hypertrophic CMY, MVP with valvular regurgitation and/or thickened leaflets
  - Procedures for which endocarditis prophylaxis is advised (moderate and high risk patients):
    - Dental procedures: extractions, periodontal procedures, implant placement, root canal, surgery beyond apex, subgingival placement of antibiotic fibers/strips, placement of orthodontic bands but not brackets, intraligamentary injections
  - Respiratory procedures: operations involving mucosa, rigid bronchoscopy
  - GI procedures: Esophageal variceal sclerotherapy, stricture dilatation, ERCP, biliary tract surgery, bowel surgery involving the mucosa
  - Oral cavity, respiratory tract, or esophageal procedures
    - Amoxicillin 2gm orally 1 hour before procedure
    - Unable to take oral medications: ampicillin 2gm IV or IM within 30mins of procedures
  - PCN allergy options:
    - Clarithromycin 500mg PO 1h before procedure

- Cephalexin 2gm PO 1h before procedure
- Clindamycin 600mg PO 1h before procedure or IV 30mins before procedure
- Cefazolin 1gm IV/IM 30mins before procedure
  - GU/GI procedures
    - *High risk:* ampicillin 2gm IM/IV and (gentamicin 1.5mg/kg within 30min of procedure); repeat ampicillin 1gm IM/IV or amoxicillin 1g PO 6h later
    - *High risk with PCN allergy:* vancomycin 1gm IV over 1-2h AND gentamicin 1.5mg/kg IV/IM completed within 30 minutes of procedure
    - *Moderate risk:* amoxicillin 2g PO 1h before procedure or ampicillin 2g IV/IM within 30min before procedure
    - *Moderate risk with PCN allergy:* vancomycin 1g IV over 1-2h completed within 30 min of procedure

PNEUMONIA

- **Types**
  - Community Acquired (CAP)
  - Hospital Acquired (HAP) – pneumonia acquired after 48h in the hospital
  - Ventilator Associated (VAP) – HAP subset; acquired after 48h of being intubated
  - Aspiration
- **Diagnostic Workup**
  - Serum: CBC, LFTs, ICU panel (↓Na may be indicative of legionella), ABG
  - Respiratory viral panel
  - Influenza testing advised during flu season (molecular assay > antigen)
  - Urinary antigens for legionella and pneumococcal if high risk locally, known outbreak, or recent travel.
  - CRP *can* be used to guide ABx therapy
    - No ABx if CRP <20
    - Delay ABx if CRP 20-100
    - Use ABx if CRP >100
  - Urine: UA, Urinary antigens for pneumococcal only in severe CPA; legionella indicated if travel history, local outbreak, or severe disease
  - CXR (repeat 7-12 weeks after therapy in patients with high risk characteristics such as age>50, and smoking history or with persistent symptoms despite therapy)
    - Consider repeating 24-72h after event if aspiration to r/o bacterial cause
    - Any effusions should be diagnostically tapped
  - Cultures (blood, sputum, endotracheal aspirate, viral) only in severe cases and those suspected of having MRSA or *Pseudomonas*.
    - Good quality sputum culture
      - <10 epithelial cells
      - >25 PMN
  - QuantiFERON if suspecting TB
  - HIV (if age<55yo, homeless or other risk factors)
  - AFB stain and culture (if cough>1mo, homeless, other risk factors)
  - PCT (may help delineate viral vs bacterial; shortens length of ABx in the ED and wards)[86]
    - No specific cut-off can sufficiently distinguish between viral and bacterial CAP
    - Do not get if CXR positive and clinical suspicion present
    - Likely if >0.25, very likely if >0.5
    - If abx started, repeat PCT on days 3, 5, and 7
    - If abx not started, can repeat if high suspicion remains
- **Severity/Disposition (Admission vs. Outpatient therapy for CAP)**

INFECTIOUS DISEASE

Criteria for Severe CAP (1 major or 3 minor)			
Minor	RR ≥ 30	Confusion	PLT<100k
	PaO2/FIO2 < 250	Uremia (≥20)	Temp<36c
	Multilobular infiltrates	WBC<2000	↓BP
Major	Mechanical ventilation		
	Vasopressor support		

- o PSI to determine severity (preferred by ATS)
  - Low risk: ≤90 (outpatient)
  - Moderate risk: 91-130 (wards)
  - High risk: >130 (wards vs ICU)
- **Risk factors associated with increased morbidity and mortality:**
  - o Age > 65
  - o Coexisting illnesses: DM, renal failure, CHF, chronic lung disease, EtOH, aspiration, recent hospitalization, altered mental status
  - o PE: RR>30, BP<90/60, T≥38.3°c, confusion or lethargy
  - o Labs: WBC <4,000 or >30,000, PaO2<60, PCO2>50, SCr>1.2, BUN>20, HCT<30, coagulopathy; multilobar disease or effusions on CXR
- **Risk factors for MDR pathogens causing HAP, HCAP, and VAP**
  - o ABx in preceding 90 d
  - o Current hospitalization of 5d or more
  - o High frequency of antibiotic resistance in the community or in the specific hospital unit
  - o Presence of risk factors for HCAP:
    - Hospitalization for 2 d or more in the preceding 90 d
    - Residence in a nursing home or extended care facility
    - Home infusion therapy (including antibiotics)
    - Chronic dialysis within 30 d
    - Home wound care
    - Family member with multidrug-resistant pathogen
  - o Immunosuppressive disease and/or therapy
- **Treatment**
  - o Overall management based on severity determination (CURB-65, PSI)
  - o See table on next page for ABx coverage
  - o Corticosteroids only for those with refractory septic shock (weak evidence)
  - o Speech path c/s for aspiration PNA
  - o F/u CXR not advised
- **Failure to Improve**
  - o May take up to 72h on ABx to improve
  - o Insufficient coverage of ABx
  - o Resistant organisms (consider RF for expanded coverage)
  - o Para pneumonic effusions (need to be tapped for both diagnostic and tx purposes)
  - o Insufficient drug levels (i.e. vanc trough should be 15-20)
- **Discharge Criteria**
  - o Do not discharge if any of the following have occurred in the past 24h:
    - Temp >100.4F
    - RR>24
    - HR>100
    - SBP<90
    - SaO2<90
    - Confusion
    - Cannot tolerate PO intake

INFECTIOUS DISEASE

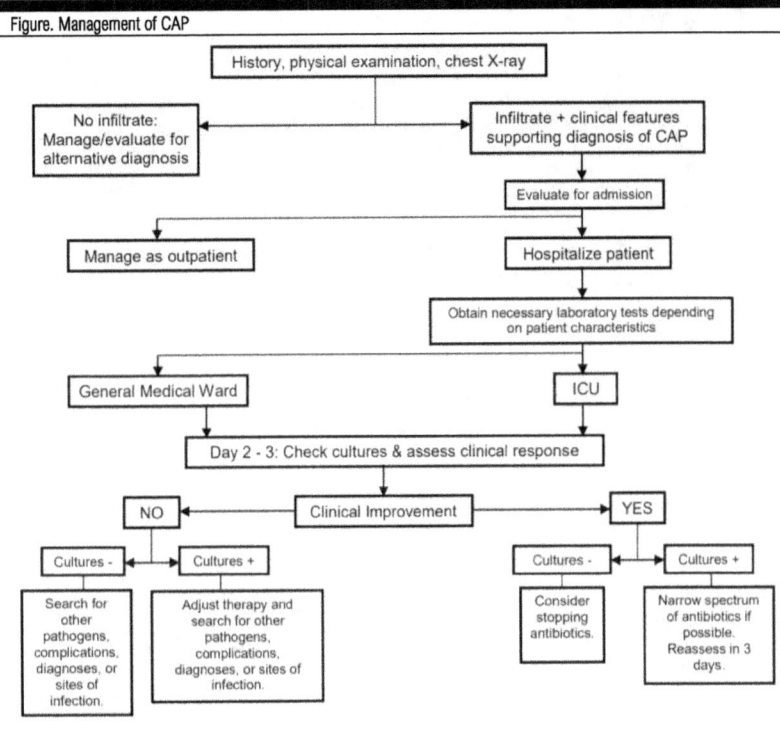

Figure. Management of CAP

Review of pneumonias by type

CAP

Pathogens: viruses (RSV, rhino, parainfluenza, influ, corona), bacteria (S.pneumo, S.auerus, mycoplasma, chlamydia, H.influ, Legionella, Kleb in EtOH and aspiration)

Outpatient
CURB-65: 0-1
PSI: <90

Previously Healthy and No Antibiotics in Past 3 Months (low risk for MRSA)

Treat for total of 5 days unless otherwise noted; ABx should be extended if patients are not improving by day 3

- Amoxicillin 1g TID
- Doxycycline 100 mg po BID
- Clarithromycin 500 mg po BID
- Clarithromycin ER 1g daily
- Azithromycin (500 mg po once, then 250 mg daily) x 3 days

Comorbidities (CHF, CRF, COPD, DM, EtOH, Asplenia, Malignancy) or Antibiotics in Past 3 Months: Select an Alternative from A Different Class

Treat for total of 5 days; ABx should be extended if patients are not improving by day 3

- Moxifloxacin (400 mg po qd) or Levofloxacin (750 mg po qd) or Gemifloxacin 320mg daily

or

Combination of group 1 and group 2

GROUP 1
- Amoxicillin/clavulanate 500 mg/125 mg TID
- Amoxicillin/clavulanate 875 mg/125 mg BID
- Cefpodoxime 200 mg BID
- Cefuroxime 500 mg BID

GROUP 2
- Azithromycin 500 mg on first day then 250 mg daily
- Clarithromycin 500 mg twice daily
- Clarithromycin ER 1,000 mg daily
- Doxycycline 100 mg twice daily

Hospitalized
PSI: 91-130
CURB-65: 2-3

Medical Ward / Nonsevere

Treat for total of 7-10 days (longer if extrapulm involvement). IDSA suggests 5 days minimum, pt should be afebrile for >48-72h. Re-evaluate diagnosis if no response in 72 hours

- Moxifloxacin (400 mg po or iv daily) or levofloxacin (750 mg PO or IV daily)

or

An antipseudomonal β-lactam [cefotaxime (1–2 g iv q8h), ceftriaxone (1–2 g IV QD), ampicillin-sulbactam (1.5-3g iv q6h), Ceftaroline (600mg BID)]
plus
Macrolide [azithromycin (500mg/d), clarithromycin 500mg BID])

ICU (PSI>130; CURB-65 >3) / SEVERE CAP / See table above

In patients with refractory septic shock, consider addition of steroids

- An antipseudomonal β-lactam [cefotaxime (1–2 g iv q8h), ceftriaxone (2 g iv daily), ampicillin-sulbactam (2 g iv q8h)]
plus
Azithromycin/Doxycycline/FLQ

or

β-lactam + Fluoroquinolone

- If PCN allergy, use FLQ+aztreonam

Special Considerations

- If pseudomonas is a consideration, multiple regimens possible:

  Regimen Option 1   An antipneumococcal, antipseudomonal β-lactam [piperacillin/tazobactam (4.5 g iv q6h), cefepime (1–2 g iv q12h), imipenem (500 mg iv q6h), meropenem (1 g iv q8h)]
  +
  Either ciprofloxacin (400 mg iv q12h) or levofloxacin (750 mg iv qd)

  Regimen Option 2   Beta lactam + aminoglycoside + azithromycin
  Regimen Option 3   Beta lactam + aminoglycoside + cipro/levo
  Regimen Option 4   Aztreonam + aminoglycoside + azithro/cipro/levo
  for PCN allergy

- If CA-MRSA is a consideration

- Add linezolid (600 mg iv q12h) or vancomycin (1 g iv q12h) NOT tigecycline

HAP

Defined: pneumonia that occurs 48 hours or more after admission and did not appear to be incubating at the time of admission.
RF: hosp or ABx in past 3 mo, nursing home dwelling, receiving home infusions or wound care, dialysis, immunosuppressed
Pathogens: Staph aureus, strep pneumoniae MRSA, enteric gram negative rods (enterobacter species, e. Coli, klebsiella, proteus species, Serratia marcescens), Hemophilus influenzae, anaerobes, pseudomonas aeruginosa, Acinetobacter, fungi (candida, aspergillus) in neutropenic patients
Duration: 7 days (IDSA/ATS) or 5-10 days (NICE) of Abx (except GNR which require 15d), 14 days (if pseudomonas), 14-21 days (if MRSA)

No MDR Risk Factors
- Cefepime 2g IV q8h
- Ceftazidime 2g q8h
- Pip-Tazo 4.5g IV q6h
- Imipenem 500mg IV q6h
- Meropenem 1g IV q8h
- Aztreonam 2g q8h

If risk factors for MRSA present, then add
Vancomycin 15 mg/kg IV q12h (goal trough 15-20 mg/mL) -or- Linezolid 600mg IV q12h

MDR Risk Factors (Treat For 7 Days)

For patients at high risk of mortality or who have received IV antibiotics in the past 3 mo or who have other risk factors for pseudomonas infection or MDR pathogens, use a 3 drug regimen from the tables below (use 2 agents (from different classes) that target Pseudomonas aeruginosa and other gram-negative bacteria (IDSA/ATS Weak recommendation, Low-quality evidence) as well as one agent effective against MRSA

Anti-Pseudomonal / MSSA Coverage				MRSA Coverage
Beta-lactam/beta-lactam-like		Non-beta-lactams		
piperacillin-tazobactam 4.5 g IV q6h cefepime or ceftazidime 2 g IV q8h imipenem 500 mg IV q6h meropenem 1 g IV q8h aztreonam 2 g IV q8h	+	Levofloxacin 750 mg IV daily Ciprofloxacin 400 mg IV q8h Amikacin 15–20 mg/kg IV daily Tobramycin 5–7 mg/kg IV daily	+	Vancomycin 15 mg/kg IV q8-12h (target trough levels of 15-20 mg/mL) Linezolid 600 mg IV q12h

Legionella
Add macrolide (iv erythromycin or azithromycin)
MSSA

Nafcillin 2 g iv q4h or oxacillin 2 g iv q4h

Fungal Component/Neutropenic
- Add amphotericin b (traditional 1st line agent)
  - Consider alternatives such as itraconazole, voriconazole, caspofungin as less side effects (similar efficacy per RCT)

ESBL
imipenem-cilastatin, ertapenem, meropenem, or doripenem

HIV Positive Patient
- Organisms:

S. Pneumoniae, h. Influenzae, PCP, m. Tuberculosis, aerobic GNRs (e. coli, klebsiella), MAI, fungi (cryptococcus, histoplasmosis), CMV, toxoplasmosis

Use therapy for cap and high-dose trimethoprim/sulfamethoxazole to cover PCP (add prednisone for PaO2<70) and high-dose ganciclovir to cover CMV

Aspiration

<u>Types</u>: chemical (aspiration of only gastric material causing pneumonitis) and bacterial (leads to sx 24-72h after event)
<u>Risks</u>: impaired swallowing, stroke, cardiac arrest, EtOH, GERD, tube feeds, impaired cough reflex, poor dentition
<u>Pathogens</u>: outpatient (strep, s.aureus, anaerobes), inpatient (GNR such as pseudomonas) and s. aureus
<u>Diagnosis</u>: If no infiltrates are present on CXR after 72 hours can stop ABx if they were started empirically; Look for foul smelling sputum suggestive of anaerobic disease

Community-acquired
- If CXR abnormal (RLL apical segment, RUL inferior segment; look for cavitation's and abscesses):
  - Poor dentition: Amoxicillin-clavulanate 875mg po bid x 7-10 days, Ampicillin-Sulbactam 1.5-3g q6h IV, Moxifloxacin 400mg qd, Levofloxacin 500mg qd, Ertapenem 1g qd
  - Normal dentition: same as above as well as Ceftriaxone 1-2g IV qd
- If CXR clear
  - If patient is stable, consider withholding ABx and observing
  - If intubated or septic, treat based on dentition above and MDR with re-assessment in 48-72h

Hospital-acquired
- If CXR abnormal (RLL apical segment, RUL inferior segment; look for cavitation's and abscesses):
  - No risk of MDR: Amoxicillin-clavulanate 875mg po bid x 7-10 days, Ampicillin-Sulbactam 1.5-3g q6h IV, Moxifloxacin 400mg qd, Levofloxacin 500mg qd, Ertapenem 1g qd, Ceftriaxone 1-2g IV qd
  - Risk of MDR: Zosyn 4.5g q8h or 3.37g q8h, cefepime 2g q8-12h, Levaquin 750mg PO qd, Meropenem 1g q8h, Imipenem 500mg q6h or 1g q8h
    PLUS
    Aminoglycoside (Gentamycin 5-7mg/kg qd) or Colistin 9mil IU/d in 2-3 doses
- If CXR clear

- If patient is stable, consider withholding ABx and observing
- If intubated or septic, treat based on dentition above and MDR with re-assessment in **48-72h**

SURGICAL SITE INFECTIONS

- **Antibiotic Administration**[86]
  - Best to give within 1 hour prior to incision (except FLQ and VANC which require 2)
    - 2gm cefazolin for pts <120kg; use 3gm if >120kg
    - Re-dose if surgery >4h
    - D/c within 24 hours (except cardiac, extend for 48h)
  - The CDC recommend that ABx prophylaxis be used for all clean-contaminated procedures and certain clean procedures.
- **Screening for MRSA**[87]
  - Patients undergoing cardiac or orthopedic surgery should be screened for S. aureus carriage 2 weeks prior to surgery, and carriers should undergo decolonization with intranasal mupirocin and chlorhexidine bathing for 5 days.
  - For patients at highest risk of carrying CA-MRSA (e.g., those with a history of MRSA infection, history of dialysis, recent healthcare exposure, or history of recurrent furunculosis), it would be reasonable to include vancomycin in the perioperative antibiotic prophylaxis regimen.
  - In high-risk patients, decolonize with topical mupirocin nasal ointment and daily chlorhexidine bathing before surgery.
- **Selecting Abx prophylaxis**

Typical microbiologic flora at surgical sites	
Grafts	S.aureus, Coag negative Staph species
Cardiac	S.aureus, Coag negative Staph species
NS	S.aureus, Coag negative Staph species
Breast	S.aureus, Coag negative Staph species, streptococci
Ophthalmic	S.aureus, Coag negative Staph species, streptococci, GNR
Orthopedic	S.aureus, Coag negative Staph species, streptococci, GNR
Thoracic	S.aureus, Coag negative Staph species, strep pneumo, GNR
Vascular	S.aureus, Coag negative Staph species
Appdendicitis	GNR, anaerobes
Biliary tract	GNR, anaerobes
Colorectal	GNR, anaerobes
GI	GNR, streptococci, oropharyngeal anaerobes
ENT	S.aureus, streptococci, oropharyngeal anaerobes
OB GYN	GNR, enterococci, GBS, anaerobes
Urologic	GNR

- **Post-operative fever/infection**
  - <48 hrs of surgery: only treat if systemic sx exist
  - >48 hrs of surgery: treat with ABx if >5cm of erythema beyond incision exists and consider I&D

Bibliography

[67] The Antimicrobial Stewardship Program. UCLA Health System.
[68] Roth et al. "Approach to the Adult Patientwith Fever of Unknown Origin." Am Fam Physician 2003;68:2223-8.
[69] Berthold, Jessica. "It's all about the history: Diagnosing fever of unknown origin." ACP Hospitalist. May. 2014.
[70] Baddour et al. "Cellulitis and Erysipelas." UpToDate.com
[71] Swartz, Morton N. Cellulitis. N Engl J Med 2004;350:904-12.
[72] Keller et al. "Distinguishing cellulitis from its mimics." CCJM. Vol 79 (8). 547-552.
[73] Johns Hopkins Antibiotic Guide, 2019.
[74] Thomas KS, Crook AM, Nunn AJ, et al; U.K. Dermatology Clinical Trials Network's PATCH I Trial Team. Penicillin to prevent recurrent leg cellulitis. N Engl J Med. 2013 May 2;368(18):1695-703. PMID: 23635049

[75] Surawicz, Christina M. "Guidelines for Diagnosis, Treatment, and Prevention of Clostridium difficile Infections." Am J Gastroenterol 2013; 108:478–498; doi:10.1038/ajg.2013.4; published online 26 February 2013.

[76] McDonald et al. "Clinical Practice Guidelines for Clostridium difficile Infection in Adults and Children: 2017 Update by the Infectious Diseases Society of America (IDSA) and Society for Healthcare Epidemiology of America (SHEA)." Clinical Infectious Diseases: An Official Publication of the Infectious Diseases Society of America 2018 February 15.

[77] Shen NT et al. Timely use of probiotics in hospitalized adults prevents clostridium difficile infection: A systematic review with meta-regression analysis. Gastroenterology 2017 Feb 10; [e-pub].

[78] Roberts, M. A., Md, W. H., & Manian, F. A. (2018, November 02). How do you evaluate and treat a patient with C. difficile–associated disease? Retrieved from https://www.the-hospitalist.org/hospitalist/article/178718/gastroenterology/how-do-you-evaluate-and-treat-patient-c-difficile

[79] Lin et al. "The Evaluation and Management of Bacterial Meningitis Current Practice and Emerging Developments." The Neurologist 2010;16: 143–151.

[80] AUA Medical Student Curriculum: Adult UTI.

[81] Johnson JR, Russo TA. "Acute Pyelonephritis in Adults." N Engl J Med. 2018 Jan 4;378(1):48-59.

[82] Dellinger et al. "Surviving Sepsis Campaign: International Guidelines for Management of Severe Sepsis and Septic Shock: 2012." Critical Care Medcine. February 2013 • Volume 41 • Number 2

[83] 2012 Society of Critical Care Meeting

[84] Baddour LM, Wilson WR, et. al. "Infective endocarditis: diagnosis, antimicrobial therapy, and management of complications: a statement for healthcare professionals from the Committee on Rheumatic Fever, Endocarditis, and Kawasaki Disease, Council on Cardiovascular Disease in the Young, and the Councils on Clinical Cardiology, Stroke, and Cardiovascular Surgery and Anesthesia, American Heart Association: endorsed by the Infectious Diseases Society of America." Circulation. 2005;111:e394.

[85] Sager et al. BMC Medicine (2017).

[86] "Prevention And Treatment Of Surgical Site Infections." Society of Hospital Medicine Learning Portal.

[87] Schweizer ML, Chiang HY, Septimus E, Moody J, Braun B, Hafner J, et al. Association of a bundled intervention with surgical site infections among patients undergoing cardiac, hip, or knee surgery. JAMA. 2015;313:2162-71. PMID: 26034956 doi:10.1001/jama.2015.5387

CARDIOLOGY

How to Read an ECG	140
Heart Failure	150
Coronary Artery Disease	167
Stress Testing	172
Chest Pain & ACS	176
UA/NSTEMI	188
STEMI	194
Murmurs	203
Cardiomyopathy	205
Hypotension	205
Hypertension	207
Resistent Hypertension	219
Aortic Stenosis	219
Atrial Fibrillation	221
Pacemakers	229

HOW TO READ AN ECG

Figure. Placement of ECG leads and associated cardiac anatomy

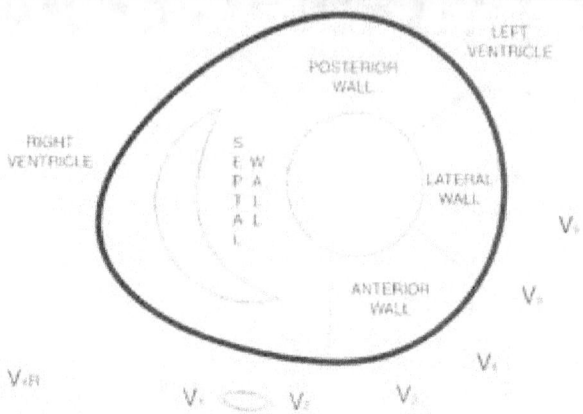

Waveform Measurements	
Baselines	
One large box	0.20s
One small box	0.04s
Normal measurements ECG	
P wave	<.11s
PR interval	0.12-0.20s
QRS interval	<0.10s
QTc interval	0.33-0.47s

1. **Background**
   - Paper
     - Each small box represents 1mm, and is 0.04 seconds
     - This means that one large box, which is comprised of 5 small boxes, represents 5mm, or 0.2 seconds
     - Each small box is 1mm / 1mV tall
   - Normal ECG Complex
     - *P Wave* - Caused by depolarization of the atria. With normal sinus rhythm, the P wave is upright in leads I, II, aVF, V4, V5, and V6 and inverted in aVR.
       1. Best read in leads II, III → ensure normal morphology
       2. AVR should have inverted p wave
       3. *Above 3 together = NSR*
     - *QRS Complex* - Represents ventricular depolarization
     - *Q Wave* - The first negative deflection of the QRS complex (not always present and, if present, may be pathologic)
     - *R Wave* - The first positive deflection (R) is the positive deflection that sometimes occurs after the S wave)
     - *S Wave* - The negative deflection following the R wave

- *T Wave* - Caused by repolarization of the ventricles and follows the QRS complex.
- Normally upright in leads I, II, V3, V4, V5, and V6 and inverted in aVR
    o Axis Deviation
    - The QRS axis is midway between two leads that have QRS complexes of equal amplitude, or the axis is 90 degrees to the lead in which the QRS is isoelectric, that is, the amplitude of the R wave equals the amplitude of the S wave.
    - Normal Axis. QRS positive in I and aVF (0–90 degrees). Normal axis is actually –30 to 105 degrees
    - LAD. QRS positive in I and negative in aVF, –30 to –90 degrees. Seen with LVH, LAHB (–45 to –90 degrees), LBBB, and in some healthy individuals
    - RAD. QRS negative in I and positive in aVF, +105 to +180 degrees. Seen with RVH, RBBB, COPD, LPFB, WPW, and acute PE (a sudden change in axis toward the right), as well as in healthy individuals (occasionally)
    - Extreme Right Axis Deviation. QRS negative in I and negative in aVF, +180 to +270 or –90 to –180 degrees
    o Bipolar Leads
    - Lead I: Left arm to right arm
    - Lead II: Left leg to right arm
    - Lead III: Left leg to left arm
    o Precordial Leads: V1 to V6 across the chest
    o ECG Paper: With the ECG machine set at 25 mm/s, each small box represents 0.04 s and each large box 0.2s. Most ECG machines automatically print a standardization mark.
2. Introduction
    o Standardization. With the ECG machine set on 1 mV, a 10-mm standardization mark (0.1 mV/mm) is evident
3. Axis. If the QRS is upright (more positive than negative) in leads I and aVF, the axis is normal. The normal axis range is –30 degrees to +105 degrees.
4. Intervals. Determine the PR, QRS, and QT intervals (Figure 19–2). Intervals are measured in the limb leads.
    o The PR should be 0.12–0.20 s
    o The QRS, <0.12 s.
    o The QT interval increases with decreasing heart rate, usually <0.44 s. The QT interval usually does not exceed one half of the RR interval (the distance between two R waves).
5. Rate. Count the number of QRS cycles in a 6-s strip and multiply it by 10 to roughly estimate the rate. If the rhythm is regular, you can be more exact in determining the rate by dividing 300 by the number of 0.20-s intervals (usually depicted by darker shading) and then extrapolating for any fraction of a 0.20-s segment.
    - *Bradycardia*: Heart rate <60 bpm
    - *Tachycardia*: Heart rate >100 bpm
6. Rhythm. Determine whether each QRS is preceded by a P wave, look for variation in the PR interval and RR interval (the duration between two QRS cycles), and look for ectopic beats.
    o **Sinus Rhythms**
    - *Normal*: P waves (which are positive in II and negative in aVR) with a regular PR and RR interval and a rate between 60 and 100 bpm. There should be one P wave for every QRS wave. Understand that truly "regular" rhythm is ultimately under the influence of the autonomic nervous system therefore variations may exist on the paper due to this, and or the patient's respiratory cycle.
    - *Sinus Tachycardia*: Normal sinus rhythm with a heart rate >100 bpm and <180 bpm Clinical Correlations. Anxiety, exertion, pain, fever, hypoxia, ↓BP, increased

sympathetic tone (secondary to drugs with adrenergic effects [e.g., epinephrine]), anticholinergic effect (e.g., atropine), PE, COPD, AMI, CHF, hyperthyroidism, and others
- *Sinus Bradycardia*: Normal sinus rhythm with a heart rate <60 bpm. Clinical Correlations. Well-trained athlete, normal variant, secondary to medications (e.g., beta-blockers, digitalis, clonidine), hypothyroidism, hypothermia, sick sinus syndrome (tachy–brady syndrome), and others
- *Sinus Arrhythmia*: Normal sinus rhythm with a somewhat irregular heart rate. Inspiration causes a slight increase in rate; expiration decreases the rate. Normal variation between inspiration and expiration is 10% or less.
1. **Atrial Arrhythmias**
    - PAC: Ectopic atrial focus firing prematurely followed by a normal QRS. The compensatory pause following the PAC is partial; the RR interval between beats 4 and 6 is less than between beats 1 and 3 or 6 and 8.
        - Clinical Correlations. Usually not of clinical significance, can be caused by stress, caffeine, and myocardial disease
    - PAT: A run of three or more consecutive PACs. The heart rate is usually between 140 and 250 bpm. The P wave may not be visible, but the RR interval is very regular.
        - Clinical Correlations. Can be seen in healthy individuals but also occurs with a variety of heart diseases. Symptoms include palpitations, light-headedness, and syncope.
        - Treatment: Increase Vagal Tone. Valsalva maneuver or carotid massage.
            - Medical Treatment. Can include adenosine, verapamil, digoxin, edrophonium, or beta-blockers (propranolol, metoprolol, and esmolol). Verapamil and beta-blockers should be used cautiously at the same time because asystole can occur.
            - Cardioversion with Synchronized DC Shock. Particularly in the hemodynamically unstable patient
    - MAT: An atrial arrhythmia that originates from ectopic atrial foci. It is characterized by varying P-wave morphology and PR interval and is irregular.
        - Clinical Correlations. Most commonly associated with COPD, also seen in elderly patients, CHF, diabetes, or use of theophylline. Antiarrhythmics are often ineffective. Treat the underlying disease.
    - AFib: Irregularly irregular rhythm with no discernible P waves. The ventricular rate usually varies between 100 and 180 bpm. The ventricular response is slower with digoxin, verapamil, or beta-blocker therapy and with AV nodal disease.
        - Clinical Correlations. Seen in some healthy individuals but commonly associated with organic heart disease (CAD, hypertensive heart disease, or rheumatic mitral valve disease), thyrotoxicosis, alcohol abuse, pericarditis, PE, and postoperatively.
        - Treatment
            - Pharmacologic Therapy. Intravenous adenosine, verapamil, digoxin, and betablockers (propranolol, metoprolol, and esmolol) can be used to slow down the ventricular response, and quinidine, procainamide, propafenone, ibutilide, and amiodarone can be used to maintain or convert to sinus rhythm.
            - DC-Synchronized Cardioversion. Indicated if associated with increased myocardial ischemia, ↓BP, or pulmonary edema
    - Atrial Flutter: Characterized by sawtooth flutter waves with an atrial rate between 250 and 350 bpm; the rate may be regular or irregular depending

on whether the atrial impulses are conducted through the AV node at a regular interval or at a variable interval.
- **Example**: One ventricular contraction (QRS) for every two flutter waves = 2:1 flutter.
- **Clinical Correlations**. Seen with valvular heart disease, pericarditis, ischemic heart disease, pulmonary disease including PE, and alcohol abuse
- **Treatment**.
  - Diltiazem is considered drug of choice for rate control (↑AV node refractoriness)
    - Diltiazem drip (*Diltiazem Atrial Fibrillation/Atrial Flutter Study Group*):
      - IV bolus 0.25 mg/kg over 2 minutes
      - Wait 15 minutes
      - Second bolus of 0.35mg/kg over 2 minutes if first dose tolerated, but inadequate response
      - Continuous infusion @ 10-15 mg/h
      - Expect response in 4-5 minutes
    - Monotherapy with PO: 30mg q6h ↑ to max 360 mg/day
      - Calculate monotherapy from drip dose by totaling drip dose over 24 hours then providing that dose through long acting daily Diltiazem (Tiazac)
  - Rate control with BB or CCB.
  - Amiodarone used to slow AV node conduction.
  - Digoxin used to enhance vagal tone.
- **Nodal Rhythm**
  - AV Junctional or Nodal Rhythm: Rhythm originates in the AV node. Often associated with retrograde P waves that may precede or follow the QRS. If the P wave is present, it is negative in lead II and positive in aVR (just the opposite of normal sinus rhythm). Three or more premature junctional beats in a row constitute a junctional tachycardia, which has the same clinical significance as PAT
  - AVNRT – pseudo R' in V1 or pseudo S in II/III/AVF; commonly presents as SVT with short RP interval.
  - AVRT – ST elevation in AVR; commonly presents as SVT with short RP interval.
- **Ventricular Arrhythmias**
  - PVC: As implied by the name, a premature beat arising in the ventricle that is caused by **presence of a re-entrant circuit at the level of the Purkinje fibers**. P waves may be present but have no relation to the QRS of the PVC. The QRS is usually >0.12 s with a left bundle branch pattern. A compensatory pause follows a PVC that is usually longer than after a PAC. The RR interval between beats 1 and 3 is equal to that between beats 3 and 5. Thus, the pause following the PVC (the fourth beat) is fully compensatory. The following patterns are recognized:
    1. *Bigeminy*. One normal sinus beat followed by one PVC in an alternating fashion
    2. *Trigeminy*. Sequence of two normal beats followed by one PVC
    3. *Unifocal PVCs*. Arise from one site in the ventricle. Each has the same configuration in a single lead.
    4. *Multifocal PVCs*. Arise from different sites; therefore, have different shapes
    5. *Clinical Correlations*. PVCs occur in healthy persons and with excessive caffeine ingestion, anemia, anxiety, organic heart disease (ischemic, valvular, or hypertensive), secondary to medications (epinephrine and isoproterenol; from toxic level of digitalis and theophylline), or predisposing metabolic abnormalities (hypoxia, hypokalemia, acidosis, alkalosis, or hypomagnesemia)

CARDIOLOGY

6. *Criteria for Treatment.* In the setting of an AMI:
   - >5 PVCs in 1 min (many clinicians would treat any PVC associated with an MI or injury pattern on ECG)
   - PVCs in couplets (two in a row)
   - Numerous multifocal PVCs
   - PVC that falls on the preceding T wave (R on T)
7. *Treatment*
   - Lidocaine. Most commonly used; other antiarrhythmics include procainamide, and amiodarone.
   - Treatment of aggravating cause often sufficient (e.g., treat hypoxia, hypokalemia, or acidosis

- <u>Ventricular Tachycardia</u>:
  1. By definition, **three or more beats with QRS>0.12sec at rate of >100 bpm.**
     - <u>Sustained</u>: >30 seconds
  2. Types
     - <u>Monomorphic</u> – due to circuit through region of old myocardial infarction
     - <u>Polymorphic</u> – active ischemia vs. electrolyte disturbance vs. drugs that prolong QT (torsade's)
     - <u>AIVR</u> – wide complex @ 40-100bpm; occur after reperfusion in acute MI or ↑symp tone; no tx necessary
  3. Work up
     - M/c caused by structural heart dz → TTE
     - Check for channelopathies → ECG
     - Review medication list
     - Check patient's magnesium and potassium levels
     - Hypoxia, hypoventilation
     - Ischemia → ECG +/- TROP
  4. Treatment
     - *Stable*
       o EF<40%
         ▪ Amiodarone 150mg load x1 order (IVPB); Amio gtt AMOUNT: 900; comment: 1.8mg/ml (33.3ml/hr.) x 6 hours then decrease to 0.5mg/min (16.6ml/hr.)
         ▪ Lidocaine 1-1.5mg/kg IVP then 1-4mg/min maintenance, or cardioversion
       o EF>40%: Procainamide 20-30mg/min IVP then 1-4mg/min maintenance, Amiodarone
     - *Unstable*
       o Rapid defibrillation (up to 3 shocks)
       o If persists, use Epinephrine (1mg IVP q3min) with alternations with vasopressin 40U IVP as single bolus
       o If persists, use Amiodarone, Procainamide, Lidocaine
       o Consider AICD placement in patient that survives for long-term protection from sudden death if repeat TTE in 40 days confirms low EF

- AIVR
  1. Benign
  2. Not treated successfully with antiarrhythmics
  3. Wide-complex, usually has a rate of 60-110bpm vs. 120-250bpm seen with VT
  4. *Caused by presence of a ventricular focus that assumes control over the SA node because it is shooting faster; can be sign of early AV block; marker of spontaneous/induced reperfusion of the myocardium*

- Ventricular Fibrillation: Erratic electrical activity from the ventricles, which fibrillate or twitch asynchronously. No cardiac output occurs with this rhythm.
    1. *Clinical Correlations.* One of two patterns seen with cardiac arrest (the other would be asystole or flat line)
- Supraventricular Tachycardia[88]
    1. Defined as HR≥100 with short QRS (<120ms)
    2. Multiple causes: Atrial fibrillation, Atrial flutter, Multifocal Atrial Tachycardia (MAT), Atrial Tachycardia (AT), AVNRT (AV nodal re-entrant tachycardia), AVRT (AV re-entrant tachycardia), Sinus tachycardia (ST)
        - AVNRT – most common cause; two different pathways exist to the AV node (fast and slow)
        - AVRT – accessory pathway exists which is faster than normal pathway to ventricle (not limited by AV node; thus, it bypasses the AV node which would normally slow down and regulate the electrical signal)
            o Two types: orthodromic and antidromic
                - Orthodromic – travels to AV node normally but then returns back to atria via fast path
                - Antidromic – travels to ventricle via fast path and returns to atria via the slow normal path
        - AT and ST – abnormal cells in the atria automatically fire independent of the SA node; this is what differs it from ST where the original source of stimulation is from the SA node.
        - MAT – common in patients with chronic lung conditions causing RA enlargement causing a classic ECG appearance with 3 different P wave morphologies.
        - AFib/Aflutter – defined elsewhere in book

    Steps to Identification
    Recommended step by step approach to identification of SVT is to (1) first determine if you have a narrow complex tachycardia (NCT) which is suggestive of SVT or a wide complex tachycardia (WCT) which can be SVT with aberrancy due to a BBB or VT/paced/artifact. Next, (2) determine if you have a regular or irregular rhythm and then (3) identify if P waves exist and if they do (4) see if their morphology is the same or if it changes between beats.
    - NCT with regular rhythm
        o First determine the RP interval
        o Short RP: AVNRT vs Orthodromic Tachycardia (ORT; may have delta wave)
        o Long RP: AT, ST
    - NCT with irregular rhythm
        o No P waves → AFib
        o P waves present
            - Sawtooth: Aflutter
            - 3 Different P waves: MAT
    3. Management
        - Stable and regular → vagal and consider adenosine 6mg IVP; avoid CCB if WPW
        - Stable and irregular WCT → avoid BB/CCB if AF with pre-excited tachy → instead consider ibutilide
        - Unstable → synchronized cardioversion
        - AVNRT → BB or cardio ablation
        - AVRT/ORT → cardio ablation; avoid AV nodal blockers

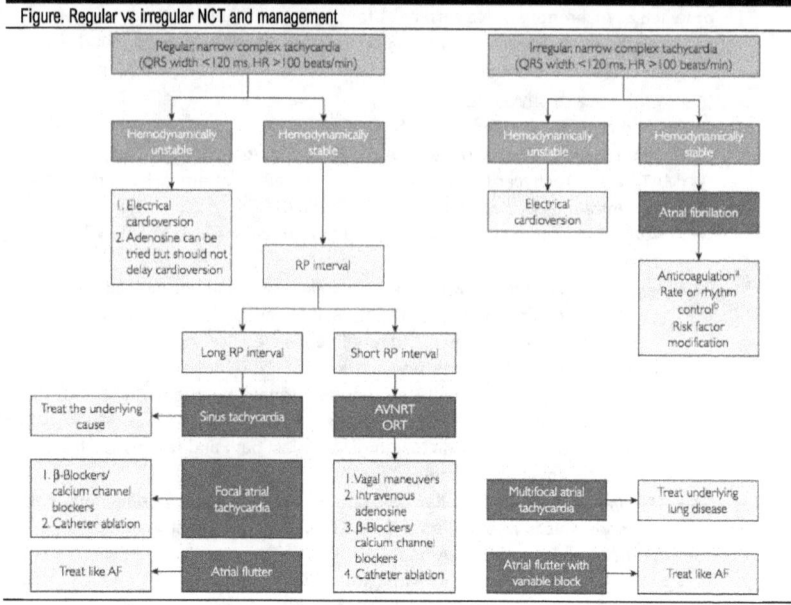

Figure. Regular vs irregular NCT and management

7. Hypertrophy
   - **Atrial hypertrophy:**
     - Right = biphasic P in precordium or > 3 mm in II, III.
     - Left = P duration > 0.12 sec, biphasic in V1 or notched in II, III.
   - **Ventricular hypertrophy**

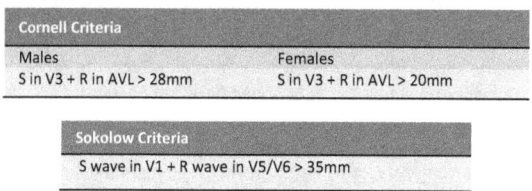

Cornell Criteria	
Males	Females
S in V3 + R in AVL > 28mm	S in V3 + R in AVL > 20mm

Sokolow Criteria
S wave in V1 + R wave in V5/V6 > 35mm

8. Blocks
   - Fascicular Blocks
     - *LAFB* – LAD in conjunction with negative overall deflection in lead II and III (rS)
     - *LPFB* – RAD in conjunction with positive overall deflection in lead II and III (qR)
   - Bundle Branch Blocks[89]
     - If the electrical impulse traveling down the bundle of his (BIH) is unable to travel down the right bundle due to a RBBB, then it will go down the intact left bundle.
       1. The impulse travels fast down the intact left bundle and then moves slowly up towards the right. This slow depolarization to the right ventricle causes it to contract, but now takes slightly longer than the left and leads to a prolonged QRS. This slow swing of electricity to the right may cause a right axis deviation.
     - If the electrical impulse traveling down the bundle of his (BIH) is unable to travel down the left bundle due to a LBBB, then it will go down the intact right bundle.

1. The impulse travels fast down the intact right bundle and then moves slowly up towards the left. This slow depolarization to the left ventricle causes it to contract, but now takes slightly longer than the right and leads to a prolonged QRS. This slow swing of electricity to the right may cause a left axis deviation.
2. May cause poor R-wave progression

LBBB	RBBB
QRS > 0.12	QRS > 0.12
V1: Q wave or QRS mostly negative	V1: QRS with a RSR pattern or mostly positive
T wave inversion in all or some of the leads over the left : V5, V6, I, and aVL	T wave inversion in all or some of the leads over the right V1, V2, and V3

Determining location of infarct based on ECG pattern				
Leads	Wall affected	ECG Δ	Artery	Reciprocal Δ
II, III, AVF	Inferior	Q, ST-T, T	RCA (90%) CIRC (10%)	I, aVL
	With any inferior MI, always consider the following complications: 1) AV node dysfunction 2) Posterior MI 3) RV infarction			
I, aVL	High lateral	Q, ST-T, T	Early diagnosis Circ branch	V1, V3
I, aVL, V5-6	Lateral	Q, S-T, T	Diagonal branch- LAD Circ Early marginal	I, III, aVF
V1-4, I, aVL	Anterior	Q, S-T, T Loss of RWP	LAD	
V1-2 (more than inferior leads)	Posterior	R>S S-T depression T-wave depression	RCA Circ	
V3-6	Apical	Q, S-T, T Loss of septal R in V1	LAD RCA	
I, aVL, V5-6	Anterolateral	Q, S-T, T	LAD Circ	I, III, AVF
V1-4	Anteroseptal	Q, S-T, T Loss of septal R in V1	LAD	

9. **Infarction or Ischemia**. Check for the presence of ST-segment elevation or depression, Q waves, inverted T waves, and poor R-wave progression in the precordial leads.
    o Requires ≥1mm of ST↑ in 2 contiguous leads except:
        - Anterior STEMI: 2mm of ST↑ in V2 and V3 (men >40) and 2.5mm (men <40) and 1.5mm in women
        - Posterior STEMI: ST↑ in V7-9
    o **Inferior infarctions** must be further analyzed to r/o posterior or RV infarction[90, 91]
        - RV Infarction – d/t complication of RCA pts present with ↓BP and ↑JVP but **clear lung fields**
            1. Indications for RV wall infarction include:
                - ST elevation in inferior leads
                - ST elevation in V1
                - RBBB
                - 2 or 3rd degree AVB
                - ↓BP, clear lung fields
            2. ECG Lead Placement:
                1) V1R: 4th ICS at left sternal border

2) V2R: 4th ICS at right sternal border
3) V3R: halfway between V2R and V4R on a diagonal line
4) V4R: 5th ICS, right midclavicular line
5) V5R: right anterior axillary line, same horizontal line as V4R and V6R
6) V6R: right mid-axillary line; same horizonal line as V5R and V6R

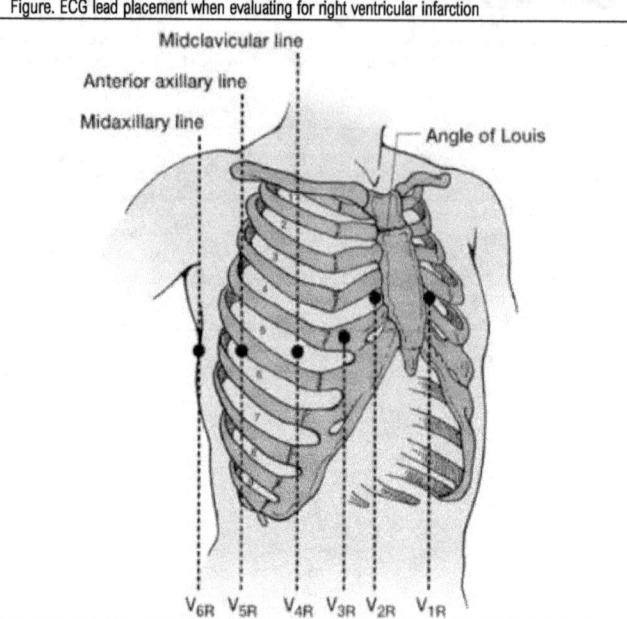

Figure. ECG lead placement when evaluating for right ventricular infarction

- The ST-segment elevation in **V4R** is a strong independent predictor of major complications and in-hospital mortality.
3. Treatment:
    - The initial therapy of a patient with RVI, who has ↓BP and no pulmonary congestion, should start with **volume expansion**, often by infusion of isotonic saline to increase the filling of the right ventricle which in turn will increase the filling of the underfilled left ventricle and increase cardiac output. Avoid nitroglycerin!
    - For patients who are unresponsive to initial trial of fluids, hemodynamic monitoring may be necessary, and subsequent volume challenge may be appropriate if the estimated central venous pressure is < 15 mmHg.
- Posterior Infarction[92]
1. In patients presenting with ischemic symptoms, horizontal ST depression in the anteroseptal leads (V1-3) with tall R waves should raise the suspicion of posterior MI or ST↑.
    - Horizontal ST depression
    - Tall, broad R waves (>30ms)
    - Upright T waves
    - Dominant R wave (R/S ratio > 1) in V2

2. **Posterior infarction is confirmed by the presence of ST elevation and Q waves in the posterior leads (V7-9).**
    - Leads V7-9 are placed on the posterior chest wall in the following positions:
        o V7 – Left posterior axillary line, in the same horizontal plane as V6.
        o V8 – Tip of the left scapula, in the same horizontal plane as V6.
        o V9 – Left paraspinal region, in the same horizontal plane as V6.

Figure. Placement of posterior thoracic ECG leads in suspected posterior infarction

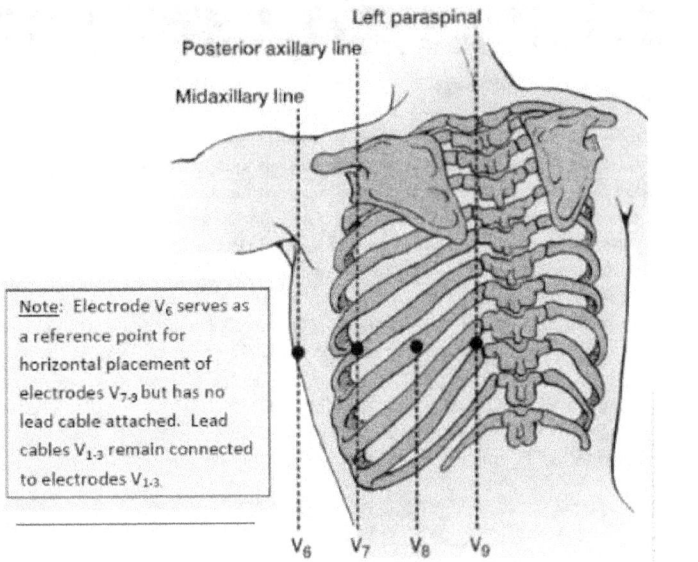

Note: Electrode V_6 serves as a reference point for horizontal placement of electrodes V_{7-9} but has no lead cable attached. Lead cables V_{1-3} remain connected to electrodes V_{1-3}.

Figure. Various signs of early-repolarization

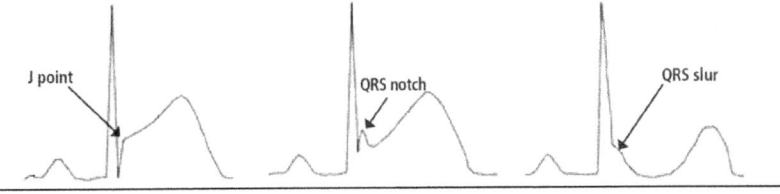

J point · QRS notch · QRS slur

- o **Early Repolarization**
    - Seen in 5-15% of general population, m/c in AA and young, healthy individuals
    - Presents as J-point elevation, QRS slur, or terminal QRS notch (see above)
    - Defined as $\geq$0.1mV of J point in 2+ contiguous leads (not including V1-3) with QRS<120ms
    - Pattern is almost always benign, high risk features include h/o syncope, FHx of SCD, J point noted in inferior leads or globally, a J point amplitude of $\geq$0.2 mV, horizontal or down sloping ST segment

10. **Poor R-wave progression**[93]
    - o Physiology
        - Electrical depolarization from the AV node often moves down through the ventricles in a L→R direction

CARDIOLOGY

- As a result, the initial vector seen is a small R wave in V1-3
- At V3-4, known as transition zone, the QRS complex changes from a predominantly negative to predominantly positive pattern
    1. The R/S ratio becomes >1
    2. The R wave should be >2mm by V3, if not 2-4mm tall by V3-4, this is known as **poor r-wave progression**
- Cause
    - Commonly due to anterior MI, LBBB, or LVH

HEART FAILURE

Contributors: Robert Pangilinan, MD, Jone Flanders, DO, Irena Crook, MD[94,147,95,96,97,98,99,100]

- **Definition**
    - HF is a <u>clinical syndrome</u> characterized by typical symptoms (e.g. breathlessness, ankle swelling and fatigue) that may be accompanied by signs (e.g. elevated jugular venous pressure, pulmonary crackles and peripheral edema) caused by a structural and/or functional cardiac abnormality, resulting in either preserved (EF>50%), reduced (EF<40%) or mixed range (EF 40-50%) cardiac output and/or elevated intracardiac pressures at rest or during stress.
        - Some suggest that reduced should be considered a level below 50% as the mixed range responds the same to those with <40% *(TOPCAT, CHARM)*[101]
- **Types**
    - <u>Reduced</u> (HFrEF) - reduced ejection fraction (<40%)
    - <u>Midrange</u> (HFmrEF) - any percentage between 40-50%
    - <u>Preserved</u> (HFpEF) - preserved ejection fraction, (≥50%)

Characteristics of HFpEF as Compared with HFrEF		
Characteristic	HFpEF	HFrEF
Symptoms (dyspnea)	Yes	Yes
Congestive State (LE edema)	Yes	Yes
EF	Normal	↓
LV Mass	↑	↑
Relative Wall Thickness	↑	↓
EDV	Normal	↑
EDP	↑	↑
LA size	↑	↑
Exercise capacity	↓	↓
CO	↓	↓

AHA Stages of Heart Failure[102]	
Stage	Definition
	Emphasize development and progression of the disease
Stage A	At risk (HTN, DM, cardiotoxic rx) for heart failure but without structural heart disease or symptoms
Stage B	Asymptomatic but has structural heart disease (prior MI, valvular dz, LV enlargement, low EF)
Stage C	Structural heart disease is present, AND symptoms have occurred
Stage D	Presence of advanced heart disease (EF <30%) with continued heart failure symptoms at rest (inability to exercise, <300m on 6 min walk) requiring aggressive medical therapy (refractory) often with ≥ 1 hospitalization in past 6 months

NYHA Functional Classification of Heart Failure		
Focuses on exercise capacity and symptomatic status		
Class I:	None	Patients with cardiac disease but asymptomatic
Class II:	Mild	Patients with cardiac disease that causes symptoms with normal physical activity
Class III:	Moderate	Patients with cardiac disease resulting in symptoms with ADLs; symptoms with moderate activity
Class IV:	Severe	Patients with cardiac disease resulting in symptoms at rest

- **Symptoms**
  No significant difference in physical exam findings between HFpEF and HFrEF
  - SOB
  - LE edema
  - Cough
  - Orthopnea
  - ↓exercise tolerance
  - ↑JVP
  - PND
  - Ankle swelling
- **Diagnosis** - made based on clinical symptoms (along with radiographic as needed) along with echocardiographic findings. S3 associated with HFrEF.
- **Exacerbation Factors**
  - Non-adherence to medical regimen with ↑Na and without fluid restriction
  - ACS
  - HTN (↑140/90)
  - AF and other arrhythmias (commonly lead to HFpEF)
  - Obesity (BMI >35, commonly leads to HFpEF)
  - Recent initiation of negative inotrope (CCB, BB)
  - Diuretic resistance[103] (consider addition of thiazide to patient already on loop diuretic)
  - PE
  - Pacemaker (commonly leads to HFpEF)
  - Initiation of steroids, NSAIDs
  - Illicit drugs (i.e. cocaine), EtOH
  - DM, ↑thyroid, ↓thyroid
  - Infections
- **Assessment**
  - Baseline GFR is a better predictor of mortality than NYHA class or EF
    - Renal disease patients with concomitant LVH have accelerated rates of coronary events and uremia
  - Rapid history, vital signs, exam of neck, lungs, heart, extremities.
  - Determine if left-sided, right-sided, or both

Symptoms in infarction based on infarct location	
Left Sided	Right Sided
Tachypnea	Elevated JVP
Rales	Hepatojugular reflex, RUQ tenderness, congestive hepatopathy
Left-sided S3	Ascites, peripheral edema

  - Sit patient up with legs off bed.
  - IV access
- **Evaluation/Work-up**
  - Inpatient Setting

- Interventions
  - STAT pulse ox (ABG)
  - ECG (if arrhythmia/ MI suspected)
- Imaging
  - CXR
    - Radiologic Findings
      - Cardiomegaly
      - Bilateral cephalization
      - Blunting of the CPA
      - ↑lung markings
  - TTE to assess valve status and for hypertrophy along with LV cavity size
    - Can help distinguish systolic from diastolic heart failure
  - Can order CCTA if low risk (see page 169)
  - Patients with new HFpEF or HFrEF should have coronary w/u performed which may include CCTA vs. heart cath vs MPS.
  - PFTs (presence of COPD or PHTN)
- Labs
  - CMP
    - BUN/SCr (r/o anemia 2/2 renal failure as ↑BUN/SCr may be seen with advanced disease due to cardio-renal syndrome)
    - K
    - Mg
  - CBC
    - leukocytosis → consider cultures as well
    - Iron deficiency anemia may be present and exacerbate symptoms
  - TSH
  - LFTs
  - Lipid panel
  - Urinalysis
  - Iron panel
    - In patients with NYHA class II and III HF and iron deficiency (ferritin <100 ng/mL or 100 to 300 ng/mL if transferrin saturation is <20%), intravenous iron replacement might be reasonable to improve functional status and QoL.
  - cTnI (and trended if initial is positive)
  - If high suspicion for drug use, obtain UDS (r/o cocaine) and EtOH (holiday heart)
  - Lactate - assess for ↓ end organ perfusion
  - BNP vs. NT-proBNP (prohormone)
    - <100 excludes cardiac source
    - >400 likely CHF with BNP
    - >900 likely CHF with NT-proBNP
    - Falsely low in patients with elevated BMI
- Outpatient Setting
  - Interventions
    - ECG (if arrhythmia/ MI suspected).
  - Imaging
    - PA/LAT CXR (see above for expected findings in fluid overload)
    - TTE to assess valve status and for hypertrophy along with LV cavity size
      - Can help distinguish systolic from diastolic heart failure
    - Can order CCTA if low risk (see page 169)
    - Patients with new HFpEF or HFrEF should have coronary w/u performed which may include CCTA vs. heart cath vs. MPS
    - Cardiac MRI to distinguish ischemic vs nonischemic
    - Coronary Angiography – advised for new dx of CHF

- Labs
  - CMP – obtain **at least** daily if not BID depending on aggressiveness of diuretic therapy (if adding thiazide to loop, consider TID labs to monitor K)
    - BUN/SCr (r/o anemia 2/2 renal failure as ↑BUN/SCr may be seen with advanced disease due to cardiorenal syndrome)
    - K
    - Mg
  - CBC (leukocytosis → consider cultures as well, anemia)
    - Iron panel
      - In patients with NYHA class II and III HF and iron deficiency (ferritin <100 ng/mL or 100 to 300 ng/mL if transferrin saturation is <20%), intravenous iron replacement might be reasonable to improve functional status and QoL. (*IRONOUT-HF*)
  - TSH
  - LFTs
  - Lipid panel
  - Urinalysis
  - BNP vs. NT-proBNP (prohormone)
    - <100 excludes cardiac source
    - >400 likely CHF with BNP
    - >900 likely CHF with NT-proBNP
    - Falsely low in patients with elevated BMI
- **Admission Criteria**
  - Critically ill (hypoxia, shock, anuria, respiratory distress)
  - No prior history of HF
  - Marked degree of congestion on examination
    - Orthopnea
    - DOE
    - PND
    - Nocturnal cough
    - Abdominal swelling
    - Anorexia
    - Peripheral edema
  - Medium to High complexity of medical risk
- **Discharge from ER Criteria**
  - Documented history of CHF and mild exacerbation
  - Return to baseline function s/p treatment
  - No evidence of dysrhythmia or infarction
  - Known cause: i.e. medication noncompliance
  - Not requiring supplemental oxygen
- **Inpatient nursing interventions**
  - Maintain strict I/O's
  - Daily weights (for more accurate fluid management, weight loss may be seen with cardiac cachexia) → goal -1kg/d during diuresis
  - Heart healthy 2g Na diet
    - NPO if doing stress test
  - 2L fluid restriction
  - Frequent electrolyte checks
    - K due to Lasix
    - ↑Na seen with advanced disease
  - VS q4h (SBP <90 is seen with advanced disease)

Figure. Treatment for patients with HFrEF and stage C symptoms

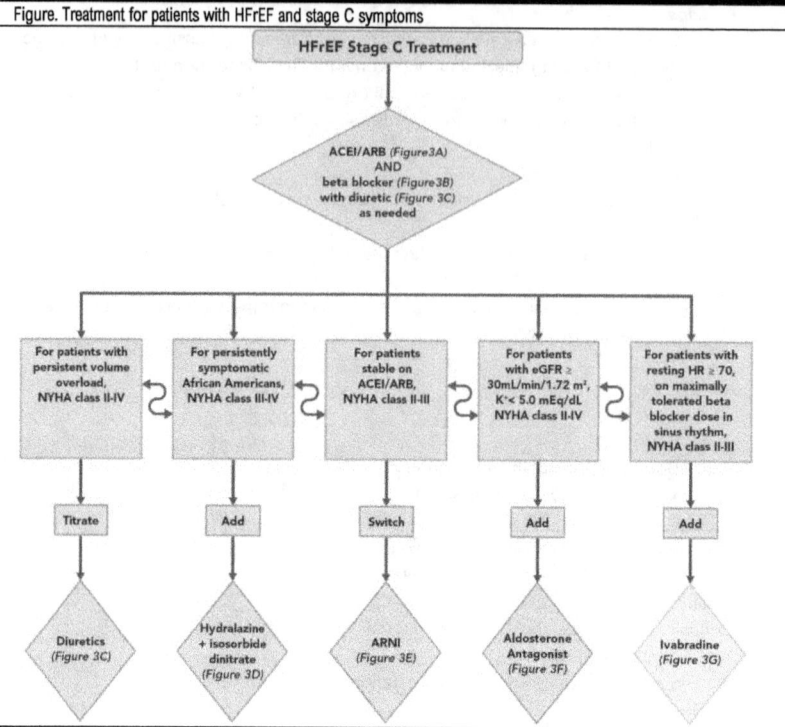

- **Treatment**[104]
  - Acute Decompensated Heart Failure (both HFpEF and HFrEF)
    - Diuresis
      - Goals of treatment are daily urine volume of 3-5L.
        - For Lasix, IV to PO dosing represents a bioavailability of 2.0, thus if a patient is taking 80mg of PO Lasix, then the IV dosing would be 40mg in IV form. Boluses should not exceed 80mg/d.
          - Initial dose usually 1-2.5 times total daily oral loop diuretic in Lasix equivalents given q8h or q12h; if naïve, may want to start lower.
            - Intermittent dosing is not inferior to continuous/drip *(DOSE trial)*
            - High-dose bolus loop diuretics are associated with better symptom improvement than low-dose *(DOSE trial)*
              - Threshold dose for loop diuretic varies by patient; 10mg if nml renal fx, up to 160mg with chronic kidney disease (with minimum given often at 80mg), and up to 80mg in CHF.[105]
        - Monitor Trajectory of Diuretic Therapy
          - Improving – continue dosing until relief of congestion, consider PO conversion
          - Initial improvement then stalled –
            - Escalate diuretic dose by 50-100% until total dose exceeds 500mg of the equivalent **oral** dose
            - Increase frequency of dosing to TID-QID
            - Consider metolazone 2.5-5mg 1-2x/d (see *diuretic resistance* below).
            - Consider acetazolamide 250-500mg/d[106]

- Typically initiated if HCO3 reaches 32
    - Not improved or worsening – escalate diuretics, consider inotropes, resistance as below. Can consider acetazolamide 250-500mg/d.
- If diuretic resistance suspected (U_{Na}<20, see figure below), consider addition of a thiazide diuretic (chlorthalidone, metolazone) to loop diuretic but beware ↓K, ↓Mg, and metabolic alkalosis. This is based on the concept of "sequential nephron blockade."[107]
    - If using metolazone 2.5mg, its long duration of action limits use to 2-3x/week. Has also been studied given as 10mg daily x 3 days.[108]
    - Consider cutting loop diuretic dose in half when adding a thiazide to limit adverse effects
    - Concurrent NSAID can limit loop diuretic effectiveness
    - Consider adding aldosterone antagonist to not only limit effects on K but may reduce mortality in those with advanced HF.

> SCr x 20 = ### mg of IV Lasix
> *Avoid more than 80mg for initial dosing*

- Blood Pressure Control
    - IV NTG or paste (SBP 160-220 and no severe AS) with gtt if >220
    - Pressors (dobutamine 2 mcg/kg/min or milrinone) if ↑SCr and hypotensive
- Avoid Antiarrhythmics
    - Amiodarone okay
- Medications
    - *See following table on next few pages*
    - Avoid rate controlling CCB such as Diltiazem/verapamil unless AF with RVR and preserved EF
    - ACEi
    - Sacubitril/ARB should **not be** initiated in the acute setting in patients with acute decompensated heart failure as it was only studied in stable patients. Can start if they have not received IV diuretics in the past 6 hours (or inotropes in past 24 hours)
        - Do not start unless you know the patient can continue uninterrupted therapy as an outpatient
        - Consider transitioning from ACEi to ARB prior to starting if concern about pre-authorization, etc. to prepare patient for eventual tx.
    - BB
        - Do not start if low blood pressure or cold/dry profile
        - ½ dose if poor response to diuresis and more aggressive diuresis required
        - When administering test doses, consider carvedilol 3.125mg or metoprolol succinate 6.25mg
    - CAD management drugs
    - Aldactone/Eplerenone (beneficial in patients with ↑pro-BNP)
    - Hydralazine+Isordil (African American population)
- Others
    - Oxygen
    - Rx: Morphine, ACEi/ARB (see choices below),
    - Daily imaging may be considered
    - Diet: low sodium diet imperative, less sodium ingested means less available to reabsorb to cause HTN
- Chronic
    - Treatment depends on HFrEF vs HFpEF

- HFrEF has guideline-based treatment regimens (see page *159*)
    - IV diuretics if evidence of fluid overload
    - Beta-blockers (continue during decompensated HF, but do not start) ACE-I or ARB
    - Aldosterone antagonist (NYHA class II-IV) if LVEF≤35%
- HFpEF does not have clear guideline-based evidence
- Consults: Referral to cardiac rehab, heart failure clinic
- **Iron Deficiency**[109]
    - Common in patients with HFrEF (≤45%) and NYHA II-III symptoms
    - Look for ferritin <100 -or- (combination of ferritin 100-300 and saturation <20%) in the setting of HGB<10
    - Treatment
        - IV iron 1g on week 0 with additional 500mg (if wt. 35-70kg on week 6) or 1000mg (if wt. >70kg)
- **HFrEF (previously termed 'systolic')**
    - ACEi/ARB
    - Consider sacubitril/valsartan as long as their symptoms are **stable** and tolerating max dose ACEi (i.e. enalapril 10mg BID)
    - Start at lowest dose and increase dose every 2 weeks until maximum tolerated dose achieved.
    - If ACE-I not tolerated, can try ARB (angiotensin II receptor blocker) e.g. Losartan.
        - For patients with elevated blood pressure despite maximum ACE inhibitor and β-blocker dosing, consider adding an ARB in non-AA or the **combination of hydralazine and long acting nitrates in AA**[110]

Figure. When to consider addition of CRT or ICD in patients with HFrEF

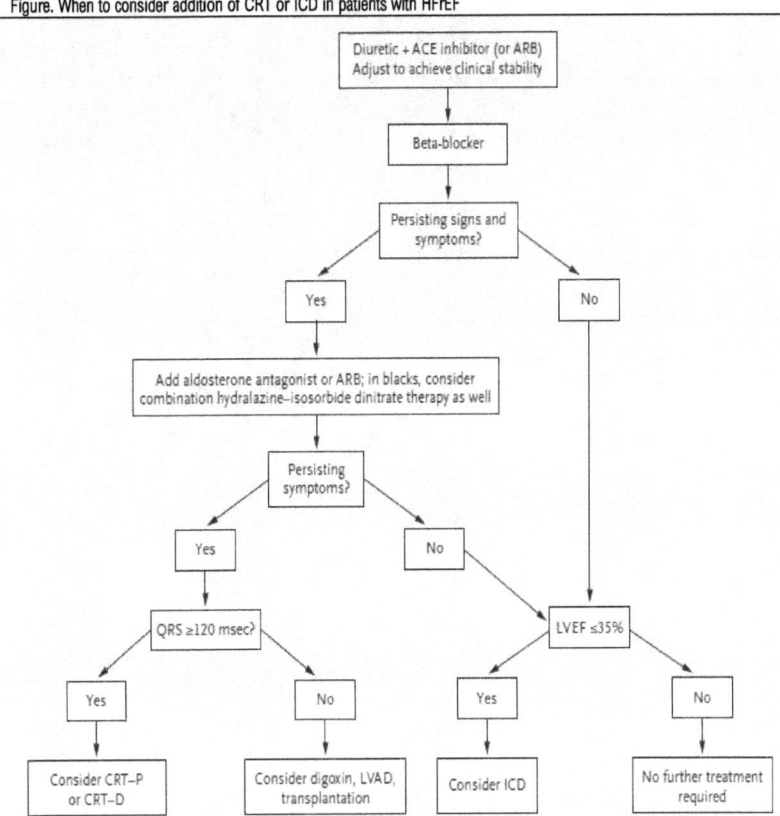

Heart Failure

At Risk for Heart Failure

STAGE A
At high risk for HF but without structural heart disease or symptoms of HF

e.g., Patients with:
- HTN
- Atherosclerotic disease
- DM
- Obesity
- Metabolic syndrome

or

Patients:
- Using cardiotoxins
- With family history of cardiomyopathy

THERAPY

Goals:
- Heart healthy lifestyle
- Prevent vascular, coronary disease
- Prevent LV structural abnormalities

Drugs:
- ACEI or ARB in appropriate patients for vascular disease or DM
- Statins as appropriate

↓ Structural heart disease

STAGE B
Structural heart disease but without signs or symptoms of HF

e.g., Patients with:
- Previous MI
- LV remodeling including LVH and low EF
- Asymptomatic valvular disease

THERAPY

Goals:
- Prevent HF symptoms
- Prevent further cardiac remodeling

Drugs:
- ACEI or ARB as appropriate
- Beta blockers as appropriate

In selected patients:
- ICD
- Revascularization or valvular surgery as appropriate

↓ Development of symptoms of HF

STAGE C
Structural heart disease with prior or current symptoms of HF

e.g., Patients with:
- Known structural heart disease and
- HF signs and symptoms

HFpEF

THERAPY

Goals:
- Control symptoms
- Improve HRQOL
- Prevent hospitalization
- Prevent mortality

Strategies:
- Identification of comorbidities

Treatment:
- Diuresis to relieve symptoms of congestion
- Follow guideline driven indications for comorbidities, e.g., HTN, AF, CAD, DM

HFrEF

THERAPY

Goals:
- Control symptoms
- Patient education
- Prevent hospitalization
- Prevent mortality

Drugs for routine use:
- Diuretics for fluid retention
- ACEI or ARB
- Beta blockers
- Aldosterone antagonists

Drugs for use in selected patients:
- Hydralazine/isosorbide dinitrate
- ACEI and ARB
- Digitalis

In selected patients:
- CRT
- ICD
- Revascularization or valvular surgery as appropriate

↓ Refractory symptoms of HF at rest, despite GDMT

STAGE D
Refractory HF

e.g., Patients with:
- Marked HF symptoms at rest
- Recurrent hospitalizations despite GDMT

THERAPY

Goals:
- Control symptoms
- Improve HRQOL
- Reduce hospital readmissions
- Establish patient's end-of-life goals

Options:
- Advanced care measures
- Heart transplant
- Chronic inotropes
- Temporary or permanent MCS
- Experimental surgery or drugs
- Palliative care and hospice
- ICD deactivation

Pharmacologic therapy in Heart Failure with Reduced Ejection Fraction

Type	Trials	Class Restriction	Starting Dose	Target Dose
ACEi	CONSENSUS SOLVD SAVE TRACE	I, II, III, IV	Captopril∞ 6.25mg TID Enalapril 2.5mg BID Lisinopril 2.5-5mg/d Ramipril 1.25mg-2.50mg daily or BID	50mg TID 10-20mg BID 20-40mg/d 10mg/d

First line therapy for afterload reduction in all pts with reduced EF (because heart failure is characterized by systemic vasoconstriction). If cannot be used d/t ↑SCr → use isosorbide denitrate-hydralazine instead. Start lowest dose and increase every 2 weeks until maximum tolerated dose achieved. ↓mortality, HF hospitalization, symptoms.
∞ Captopril superior in patients with CKD (SAVE) however questionable whether improved outcomes noted in other ACEi

| Beta Blocker** | CIBIS-II%
MERIT-HF#
COPERNICUS$
CAPRICORN
SAVE
REVERT
COMET → carvedilol>Lopressor | I, II, III, IV | Carvedilol[111]✝
1.25mg daily (10mg daily)
Bisoprolol
1.25mg daily (10mg)
Metoprolol succinate[112]
12.5mg-25mg/d (200mg/d) | 10mg
10mg
200mg |

Only initiate when patient stable; Help decrease remodeling, ↓ all-cause mortality, hospitalization, and prevent further adrenergic mediated dysfunction. Offer to patients with LVEF < 40% and no contraindications (dyspneic, signs of congestion, hemodynamically unstable). Target HR<64; titrate up every 2-4 weeks. Carvedilol specifically is good in patients with nonischemic cardiomyopathy. Avoid sotalol, nadolol, and atenolol in patients with CKD
✝Carvedilol advised in CKD patients.

| Mineralocorticoid Receptor Antagonists | RALES
EPHESUS
EMPHASIS-HF | II-IV and with EF<35%
-or-
Post-STEMI+EF<40%
-and- | Eplerenone
25 mg daily
Aldactone
25 mg
Spironolactone | 50 mg
25-50 mg
25-50mg |

Pharmacologic therapy in Heart Failure with Reduced Ejection Fraction

Type	Trials	Class Restriction	Starting Dose	Target Dose
		Symptomatic CHF or DM -or- Class IIb recommendation for HFpEF	12.5-25mg daily (goal K≤5) (↓dose if GFR<50) Amiloride 5mg	5-20mg

Indicated for patients with continued symptomatic HF and LVSD (≤35%) and those who develop LVSD after MI on maximum therapy of ACEi/ARB and BB. Beware ↑K. Spironolactone is 2x as powerful as eplerenone. Often used in combination with loops to increase diuresis. Eplerenone is used for Class II, Spironolactone used for III, or IV.

Type	Trials	Class Restriction	Starting Dose	Target Dose
Combination ARB+Neprilysin Inhibitor	PARADIGM-HF	II-IV with EF<40% and can tolerate max ACEi/ARB	Valsartan-sacubitril 24/26mg BID or 49/51mg BID if SBP≥120 mmHg	After 2-4 weeks double the dose to maintenance of 97/103mg PO BID

Indicated to reduce the risk of cardiovascular death and hospitalization for heart failure (HF) in patients with NYHA class II-IV HF and reduced ejection fraction ≤40% as initial therapy (not prev. on ACEi) or on target dose ACEi already (replacement). Avoid in patients with ↓BP or orthostatic symptoms. Can be used in patients not previously on ACE/ARB. To convert from patient previously on enalapril (≤10mg) and/or valsartan (≤160mg daily) you can start 24/26mg BID of sacubitril/valsartan (otherwise use 49mg/51mg if enalapril/valsartan dosing was >10/>160mg. Do not use with ACEi – instead, stop ACEi and after 36 hours start on combo arb/neprilysin inhibitor.

Type	Trials	Class Restriction	Starting Dose	Target Dose
ARBs	CHARM* ELITE* Val-HeFT®		Candesartan* 4-8mg/d Valsartan® 40 mg BID Losartan* 25-50 mg/d	32 mg daily 160 mg BID 150 mg/d
Isosorbide denitrate/hydralazine Symptomatic African Americans, NYHA III-IV, HFrEF only	A-HeFT	Selected patients who do not respond to ACEi and BB; beneficial in African Americans	Hydralazine 37.5 mg TID Isosorbide denitrate 20 mg TID	75 mg TID 40mg TID

Pharmacologic therapy in Heart Failure with Reduced Ejection Fraction

Type	Trials	Class Restriction	Starting Dose	Target Dose
Milrinone *Phosphodiesterase-3 Inhibitor; Inotrope that functions by ↑CO, ↓preload + afterload (both inotrope and vasodilator)*	OPTIME-CHF	III, IV (with EF <25%); short term therapy; best if combined with B-blocker	**Milrinone** LD 50 mcg/kg over 10 minutes then gtt based off hemodynamics **often used in patients on maximum therapy with continued symptoms of dyspnea, advanced CHF (stage IV), marginal SBP. Use is associated with ↓BP, ↑arrhythmias, ↑mortality	
Ivabradine *I_f inhibitor*	SHIFT	Indicated for patients with symptomatic heart failure, II or III, and LVEF ≤ 35% in NSR with heart rate that persists at 70+ despite maximal beta blocker therapy	Ivabradine 5mg BID for 14 days then increase to 7.5mg/BID	2.5-7.5mg/tablet with a daily dose range of 5-15mg/d
Drugs for Symptomatic Therapy				
Diuretic *NYHA II-IV with volume overload*		Used to manage fluid overload (symptoms), beware ↓K and ↓Mg. High effectiveness when combined with thiazide (30 min prior). Better to ↑dose prior to adding a second dose (need to reach threshold concentration for it to be effective)		
		Loop *Function by binding to NKCC at the ascending loop of henle and macula densa resulting in inhibition of JG feedback but stimulating renin (bad; increases aldosterone and thus Na reabsorption). Vasodilation also will occur which may decrease end organ perfusion to the kidney.* *Highly dependent on proteins (thus affected by low albumin level)*	**Furosemide*** (DOA 6-8h) PO: 20-80mg daily/BID IV: 40-160mg IV once-TID Infusion: 5-20mg/h **Bumetanide*** (DOA 4-6h) bumex 2mg = lasix 80mg PO: 0.5-2mg daily or BID Infusion: 0.5-2mg/h IV: 0.5-4mg once-TID	600mg daily-TID *Increase 20-40 q6h* Max gtt: 40mg/h Max: 1500mg/d 1-2mg daily-BID (10mg/d) High dose considered >2.5mg/d Max: 10mg/d

Pharmacologic therapy in Heart Failure with Reduced Ejection Fraction

Type	Trials	Class Restriction	Starting Dose	Target Dose
			Torsemide** *(TORIC)* (DOA 12-16h) torsemide 40mg = lasix 80mg 10-40mg/d	20-100mg daily-TID Max: 200mg/d (TID preferred given DOA 4hrs but up to 6 hrs in CHF patients)
		Thiazide-type	HCTZ (DOA: 6-12h) PO: 25-50mg daily (or BID if inpatient)	100mg/d
			Metolazone (DOA: 12-24h) 2.5-5mg daily (or BID if inpatient)	20mg daily/BID/weekly
			Chlorothiazide (DOA: 6-12h) IV: 0.5-1g IV daily-BID	2g/d
			Chlorthalidone (DOA 24-72h) 12.5-25mg daily (or BID if inpatient)	100mg/d

-A dose of Lasix 40mg is equivalent to 1mg of bumex and 20mg of torsemide
*Lasix has inconsistent bioavailability (10-90%) therefore in patients who do not respond over time to increasing doses of Lasix, bumetanide or torsemide should be considered. Given natruretic threshold, must have high enough dose with low Na intake before it will have an effect.
**Torsemide and Bumetanide are used for patients not responding adequately to furosemide; torsemide is 2x more effective than Lasix and not affected by gut edema
-In patients nonresponsive to loop diuretics (160-320mg/d), initial dose of thiazide 30-60m prior to loop may help improve diuresis at the expensive electrolyte abnormalities. If using metolazone, 2-3x/week dosing max due to long DOA
-Diuretics should be given prior to meals, as food disrupts absorption
-Repeat or follow K level at least 2 weeks after medication initiation or change
-The kidney will learn from subsequent diuretic administration ☆ retains more Na when the diuretic wears off. Diurese enough to cause mild ↑SCr but then don't continue past this

Inotrope	DIG		Digoxin 0.125mg QHS	0.125-0.375mg nightly (check levels in AM)
			Often utilized in patients with concurrent arrythmia (i.e. AF); prn (no mortality benefit); use when low output or ↓organ perfusion.	

Pharmacologic therapy in Heart Failure with Reduced Ejection Fraction

Type	Trials	Class Restriction	Starting Dose	Target Dose
AICD	DINAMIT REVERSE MADIT-CRT SCD HeFT	Only if EF<30%, SE gallop Keep serum levels <0.8 II-III if EF≤ 35% -or- EF≤30% at least 40 days post MI (or 3 months post CABG/PCI) on optimal therapy	Not to be placed <40 days after MI, <3 months after CABG, survival expected of >1 year	
CRT/Bi-V	CARE-HF	III-IV if EF≤ 35, QRS≥120ms -or- I-II, EF≤30%, QRS≥130	Best for those with <35% EF and QRS>150ms due to mechanical desynchrony and ↓CO that results. Greatest benefit seen in those with LBBB	

- Avoid NSAIDS as it can worsen acute exacerbation (↓prostaglandin production which aids in vasodilation) leading to ↓ renal perfusion leading to fluid retention and worsening symptoms.[113]
  - Diuretics: acutely used to reduce **clinical** symptoms of pulmonary edema and **weight loss**
    - Choices include furosemide, bumetanide, and torsemide
      - Start with furosemide, and if patient does not respond (no change in weight/symptoms) and are adhering to restricted diet, try doubling, then tripling the dose.
        - Outpatient starting dose of 20-40mg is adequate
        - Goal is 1 kg/day **weight loss**
        - Consider twice daily dosing if diuresis is occurring but not adequate
          - BID = upon awakening and then at 1300
        - If inadequate diuresis with furosemide alone, try **adding** thiazide (Metolazone, HCTZ 25 mg)
        - If this does not work, consider switching from Lasix to bumetanide or torsemide
    - Monitor BUN/SCr for hypoperfusion
    - Watch serum electrolytes (especially K+) carefully and replete as necessary
    - *Drip:* Furosemide 0.5-1.0 mg/kg IV. If inadequate response, double the dose. Remember half-life is 90min.
      - When transitioning to PO, it is 2.5x the IV dose
  - Digoxin
    - Recommended to be used in patients with LVSDF who have **symptomatic** HF despite the use of triple therapy (BB, ACEi, and diuretic) and have multiple hospitalizations over the past year
    - No survival benefits
    - Best given at night, levels checked in AM (normal 0.5-0.9ng/dL)
    - Optimal level is 0.5-0.8; higher levels are associated with toxicity
  - Nitrates: also useful in acute setting to reduce pulmonary edema by decreasing preload.
    - Sublingual, nitro paste, or IV nitroglycerin (start at 10-20 mcg/min and titrate as BP allows). When stable, can convert to PO nitrate (e.g. start with Isordil 10 mg PO TID).
  - Vasodilators: Add hydralazine up to 100mg p.o. QID, Isordil up to 80mg TID if patient's BP remains high despite maximum dose of ACE-I. Also, if pt is intolerant to ACEI/ARB due rise in Cr, regimen provides good afterload reduction.
    - Both hydralazine and isosorbide denitrate are **particularly effective in AA** when combined with ACEi and BB → should be considered standard therapy in patients with **symptomatic HF**[114]
  - Spironolactone[115]
    - Demonstrated mortality benefit in Class II-IV CHF
    - Best when used concurrently with ACEi or ARB
    - Start at 12.5-25mg PO daily
      1. Consider switching to Eplerenone 25mg x 4 weeks then 50mg/day if pt has side effects as it is associated with less s/e such as **gynecomastia**
    - Must check potassium **after 7 days and every week** until stabile; closely monitor K, BUN, Cr. Goal is ≤5.
    - *Contraindications:* Male Cr > 2.5, Female Cr > 2.0. Only benefit patients with Class III-IV HF (EF <40%), ischemic etiology
  - Intravenous Inotropes

- Patients presenting with predominantly low output syndrome or combined congestion and low output may be considered for intravenous inotropes (e.g., dopamine, dobutamine, milrinone)
- May help relieve symptoms caused by poor perfusion and preserve end-organ function in those with severe systolic dysfunction and dilated cardiomyopathy.
- **HFpEF (previously termed 'diastolic')**
  - No proven treatment exists, currently empiric
    - Treat based on causes: treat hypertension, control HR using BB or CCB, ↓sx via diuretics
  - May benefit from cardiac catheterization (Yusef, Lancet 362: 777-281)
  - Goals of treatment are to "keep 'em dry, keep 'em slow":
    - Reduce congestion
      - Angiotensin II–receptor blockers (Candesartan, 4–**32 mg**, Losartan, 25–100 mg)
        - Candesartan is the only agent studied in a randomized, controlled trial involving patients with diastolic heart failure.
      - Salt restriction (<2g/day)
      - Diuretics (Furosemide, 10–120 mg; Hydrochlorothiazide, 12.5–25 mg)
        - Torsemide 10-40 mg IV or PO daily
        - Furosemide 20-80 mg IV or PO daily
      - ACE Inhibitors (Enalapril, 2.5–40 mg, Lisinopril, 10–40 mg)
    - Decrease incidence of tachycardia, maintain LA contraction
      - Prevent atrial fibrillation, cardioversion if it does occur
      - Beta blockers (Atenolol, 12.5–100 mg, Metoprolol, 25–100 mg)
      - CCB (Verapamil, 120–360 mg, Diltiazem, 120–540 mg)
    - Prevent myocardial ischemia
      - Nitrates (Isosorbide dinitrate, 30–180 mg, Isosorbide mononitrate, 30–90 mg)
      - BB (see above)
      - CCB (see above)
      - CABG vs. PCI
    - Control high blood pressure (<130/80)
      - Chlorthalidone, 12.5–25 mg
      - Hydrochlorothiazide, 12.5–50 mg
      - Atenolol, 12.5–100 mg
      - Metoprolol, 12.5–200 mg
      - Amlodipine, 2.5–10 mg
      - Felodipine, 2.5–20 mg
      - Enalapril, 2.5–40 mg
      - Lisinopril, 10–40 mg
      - Candesartan, 4–32 mg
      - Losartan, 50–100 mg
  - **Other things to consider**
    - Alternating leg tourniquets, phlebotomy if truly desperate.
    - Check electrolytes and replace K+ early, especially if heavy diuresis.
    - New diagnosis of heart failure warrants MPS or cardiac catheterization
    - Swan-Ganz line may be helpful if hemodynamically unstable. Remember: CHF and bilateral pneumonia can be hard to differentiate. PCWP helps.
    - Intra-aortic balloon pump for cardiogenic shock from acute MI.
- **Consequences**
  - Cardiorenal Syndrome (CRS)[116]
    - Acute or long-term dysfunction in one organ induces acute or long-term dysfunction in the other. CRS is characterized by the **triad** of concomitant

decreased kidney function, diuretic-resistant heart failure with congestion, and worsening kidney function during heart failure therapy.
- *Pathophysiology*
  - Not due to impaired renal flow from depressed EF but instead a multitude of factors interacting to include: CV congestion, anemia, oxidative stress (HGB is an antioxidant), renal sympathetic activity
  - Low-Flow-State: old hypothesis was that depressed EF (CO) resulted in inadequate renal perfusion prompting RAS to ↑renin release. This is true however is not the sole mechanism at play
  - Another hypothesis is based off that patients with HF have ↑CV congestion which leads to ↑gradient across the glomerular capillary network → ↑renal venous pressure
- *Types*
  - Type 1: worsening kidney function in patients with acute worsening of cardiac function (decompensated HF, ACS, cardiogenic shock)
  - Type 2: chronic cardiac dysfunction leads to kidney dysfunction
  - Types 3-5: beyond scope of this book
- *Treatment*
  - Fluid removal – no diuretic superior over another; limited by ↑SCr, azotemia, contraction alkalosis
  - Inotropes – mixed reviews on efficacy
- *Discharge* - Do not hold ACEi on discharge

- **Primary Prevention**
  - HF clinic for frequent monitoring
    - 6-minute walk test – document distance each time to look for worsening function
      - Formal exercise or pharmacologic stress testing
  - Hyperlipidemia[117]
  - Hypertension
  - Hyperglycemia
  - Check of OSA
  - Tobacco Cessation
  - Sodium restriction
  - Daily Weights
- **Secondary Prevention**
  - Implantable cardioverter-defibrillator (AIAD)[118]
    - Placement of an IAD is recommended in patients with:
    Assuming patients are on optimal medical therapy with an expected life span of >1 year
    - With LVEF ≤ 35% due to prior MI who are at least 40 days post-MI and are in NYHA Functional Class II or III
    - With LV dysfunction due to prior MI who are at least 40 days post-MI, have an LVEF ≤ 30%, and are in NYHA Functional Class I
    - As secondary prevention to prolong survival in patients with current or prior symptoms of HF and reduced LVEF who have a history of cardiac arrest, ventricular fibrillation, or hemodynamically destabilizing ventricular tachycardia (Level of evidence A).
  - Cardiac Resynchronization Therapy
    - *Indications*
      - QRS>150
      - NYHA Class II, III, or IV with LBBB with QRS>150
      - EF<35%
  - Heart Transplant

- Refractory NYHA Class IV, 65% 5-year survival and 55% 10 year survival

CORONARY ARTERY DISEASE

- **General**[119]
  - Synonymous with **Ischemic Heart Disease**
  - **Types**: obstructive and non-obstructive
  - ASCVD is any of the following: CAD such as MI, angina, or known stenosis >50%, CVD, TIA, ischemic stroke, and carotid stenosis >50%, PAD, Aortic disease
  - Cardiovascular disease is the leading cause of death among **women**.
- **Definitions**
  - Typical angina is defined as having **all three** of the following: substernal chest pain or discomfort, provocation by exertion or emotional stress, and relief with rest or nitroglycerin.
  - Atypical angina has two of the three characteristics.
  - Non anginal chest pain may have one or none.
- **Pathophysiology**
  - Atherosclerosis with superimposed thrombosis is the main cause of myocardial infarction, coronary death, heart failure, and large-artery stroke
  - The plaques that have overlying thrombus are at risk for thrombosis and are thus called "high-risk" plaques when they are present in the coronary or carotid vessels
  - It is important to find patients at risk for ASCVD because the first indicator of its presence often is an MI leading to unexpected death and thus, we can do our best to ↓ their risks for further progression of the disease if present
- **Patient with Known CAD/IHD**
  - Stable – see page 177
  - Unstable – see page 176
    - Further classified as high, moderate, or low risk
- **MINOCA (MI with Non-Obstructive Coronary Arteries)**
  - Defined as AMI with non-obstructive CAD (<50%) with no e/o cardiac trauma
  - Nonischemic etiologies thought to be d/t:
    - Coronary artery spasm
    - Microvascular dysfunction
    - Thrombophilic states (Factor V Leiden, Protein C & S deficiency)
    - ↓troponin clearance (d/t renal impairment)
    - ↑RH pressure (d/t PE)
- **Assessing risk in patients without known CAD between ages 45-70**

ASCVD Risk Levels based on pooled cohort calculation	
Low	<5%
Borderline	5-7.4%
Intermediate	7.5-19.9%
High	>20%

  - Screening Tools (for those 40-75)
    No single calculator is superior to others
    - **Pooled Cohort Equation Calculator**
    - **ACC ASCVD Calculator**
      http://tools.acc.org/ASCVD-Risk-Estimator-Plus/
    - MESA (combines ASCVD risk with CAC score)
    - QRISK2
    - Framingham/ATP III Risk Score

CARDIOLOGY

- SCORE

Figure. How to asses recommended interventions based on atherosclerosis test results

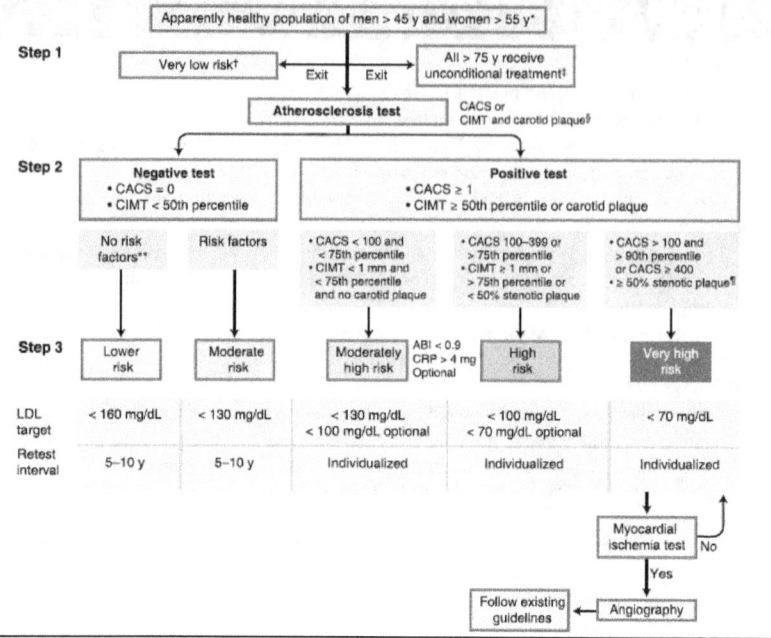

- **Risk Factors**
  - HLD (LDL>100 and CHOL>240)
    - Goal is LDL<100 or 50% reduction; high risk patients should have LDL<70
    - Non-HDL-C is better predictor of morbidity than LDL alone
    - HDL<40
  - HTN (SBP>140, DBP>90), see page 207
  - Smoking, see page *722* for cessation options
  - DM (FS>126x2, random>200, HbA1c>6.5)
  - Age (45/55 for male/female)
  - Family Age of MI (55/65 for male/female)
- **Labs/Diagnostics**
  - Screening tool as above
  - Cholesterol panel (start at 40 unless major CV risk factor present such as DM, HTN, smoking, or +fam hx)
  - hsCRP (if at moderate risk)
  - A1c
  - Coronary CTA
  - LFTs
  - TSH
  - SCr/GFR
- **Imaging/Diagnostics**
  - Stress Testing (see page 172 for full discussion)
    - ECG/Treadmill
    - Nuclear
    - TTE

- Coronary CTA[120,121]
  - Risk stratification tool used in **asymptomatic** patients at **intermediate** risk of CAD based on ACC ASCVD risk calculator to look for subclinical CAD. In this population, found to be noninferior to functional stress testing (*PROMISE*). It has a high negative predictive value for detection of CAD
  - *Who to test*
    - Can use for **low** risk patients if they have a family history of premature CAD.
    - *2016 ACC/AHA guidelines recommend:*
      - **Asymptomatic** patients at **intermediate** risk
      - Known family history of premature CAD (male <55; female <65) and 10 year risk < 5%
    - ER patients (low or intermediate risk) with chest pain suggestive of possible ACS (TIMI<=2) *(CT-STAT, ACRIN-PA, ROMICATT-II)*
      - Safe and effective means to discharge low to intermediate-risk patients from the ED
      - The significance/appropriate management of a positive CCTA study is less clear (angiography vs stress testing). See figure above for flow chart management options.
  - *Who not to test*
    - Patients at high risk for CAD (consider proceeding straight to cath) or known CAD
  - *Coronary Artery Calcium Score (CACS)*
    - The imaging allows for one to calculate a coronary calcium score (CAC) by measuring density and extent of calcifications in coronary artery walls.
      - High negative predictive value
      - The amount of calcium deposits correlates to the risk of future cardiac events, it does NOT tell you about the severity of luminal obstruction
        - Provides information on coronary plaque morphology and stenosis
      - With the CAC score, you can then use the **MeSA calculator** to determine the 10 year CAD risk score which determines statin eligibility
        - Consider starting a statin in patients with a score >0
        - Consider starting ASA in patients with a score >100

CACS Interpretation	
0	No CAD
1-99	Mild CAD
100-399	Moderate CAD
≥400	Severe CAD

- Coronary Cath

Algorithm for Treatment Approach to CAD		
	No History of CAD	Known History of CAD
1	Assess Pretest Probability of CAD using risk calculators	Assess Risk in patients with stable IHD using imaging
	-Obtain lipid, HgA1c, LFTs, TSH	-Standard exercise ECG if able to exercise, add radionuclide MPI or TTE to the standard exercise ECG if the resting ECG is uninterpretable -Only perform MPI/TTE/CMI or CCTA if unable to exercise -If patient is presenting with new CHF, consider going straight to angiography

CARDIOLOGY

	-Calculate ASCVD risk based on one of the calculators above (pooled cohort, Diamond/Forrester, ACC, etc.) if patient not presenting with acute symptoms (**asymptomatic**)
	  -Based on low/mod/high risk, obtain imaging (low/mod do CCTA; high then consider straight to cath)
	  -Use flow chart above to determine how to manage based on CACS
	-If patient presenting with acute symptoms (**symptomatic**) then calculate CAD Consortium Clinical Score (see below) if in clinic or HEART score if in ER to determine admission criteria.
		Assess Risk in patients with unstable IHD by evaluating for specific features
		-High: prolonged (>20m) chest pain at rest, pulmonary edema, dynamic ST$\Delta \geq$ 1mm, new or worsening MR, ↓BP
		-Intermediate: prolonged (>20m) chest pain at rest that has resolved spontaneously or with NTG, nocturnal angina, dynamic T-wave Δs, pathologic Q waves, ST seg ↓ $\leq$1mm, age>65
		-Low: no high or intermediate risk features, normal or unchanged ECG, ↑ angina frequency, severity or duration

2	**Determine treatment of primary or secondary prevention based on treatment above** See treatment below based on imaging results above	**Determine treatment of primary or secondary prevention based on intervention above** -Unstable: see NSTEMI on page 183 -Stable: see treatment below

- **Pretest Probability of Obstructive Coronary Artery Disease**
  - Estimate pretest probability of CAD in patients **with chest pain** on the basis of age, sex, pain characteristics, and cardiovascular risk factors (Bayes theorem)
    - Use the CAD Consortium clinical score, or HEART score (only validated in ER population)

Interpretation based on CAD Consortium Clinical Score		
<5%	5-80%	>80%
Evaluate for non-cardiac causes of CP	If patient has no prior PCI, CABG, or MI then: ↓GFR? IV contrast allergy? CCTA in past 5 years? If none of above.	Refer to cardiology
	Stress echo or MPS if cannot walk or abnormal EKG If Yes, then perform non-cardiac w/u Perform CCTA	

HEART Score (for use in ER; total possible score 10)[122]		
Variable		Score
Hx	2	History highly suspicious for coronary syndrome
	1	History moderately suspicious for coronary syndrome
	0	History slightly suspicious for coronary syndrome
ECG	2	ECG with Significant ST Depression
	1	ECG with Non-specific repolarization disturbance
	0	ECG Normal
Age	2	65+
	1	45-64
	0	<45
RF	2	Three or more risk factors for or history of atherosclerotic disease
	1	One to 2 risk factors for atherosclerotic disease
	0	No risk factors for atherosclerotic disease
Troponin	2	More than twice the normal Troponin upper limit
	1	One to 2 times the normal Troponin upper limit
	0	Within normal limits for Troponin levels
Scoring		
0-3		Adverse outcome risk: 2.5% (very low) Supports early discharge with appropriate f/u

	Adverse outcome risk: 20.3% (moderate risk)
4-6	Supports admission with standard rule-out management (serial TROP) and stress testing
	Score of 4 has SENS of 96% and SPEC of 45% for MAC
	Adverse outcome risk: 72.7% (high to very high)
7-10	Risk in first 30 days >50%
	Supports early aggressive management and typically with cardiac cath

- **Treatment**
  - Primary Prevention - the prevention of cardiac events and mortality in patients **without** a history of previous major adverse cardiac events (MACE).
    - Assess 10-year ASCVD risk for patients 40-75 via pooled cohort equations
    - Maximum dose high-intensity statin in those at high risk (see page 669 for medication dosing) aiming for LDL<55 mg/dL *(2019 ESC/EAS guidelines)*. Very-high risk patients should target even lower LDL at <40 mg/dL.
      1. Atorvastatin 40-80mg
      2. Rosuvastatin 20-40mg
      3. Add ezetimibe (*IMPROVE-IT*) if LDL is not at goal of ≥50% reduction (remains ≥70) despite high dose statin in those at very high risk
         - Very high risk defined as multiple ASCVD events (ischemic CVA, ACS, PAD, h/o revascularization, s/p amputation) or 1 major ASCVD+multiple high risk conditions
           - High risk conditions defined as age ≥65 years, heterozygous familial hypercholesterolemia, prior coronary revascularization outside of the major ASCVD events, diabetes, hypertension, chronic kidney disease with estimated glomerular filtration rate 15-59, current smoker, and LDL-C ≥100 mg/dl despite maximally tolerated statin therapy and ezetimibe
      4. Add PCSK9 inhibitors (alirocumab 75mg SQ q2w and evolocumab) in those who are not at an "LDL goal" (*ODYSSEY LONG TERM*) defined as patients **with ASCVD with LDL 70-189mg/dl on maximum statin+ezetimibe**[123]
         - Other indication for starting therapy include stable ASCVD, HDL>190, and statin intolerance (*GLAGOV, FOURIER*)
    - ASA not indicated in primary prevention due to ↑ bleed risk.
  - Secondary Prevention – prevention of recurrent cardiac events or mortality in patients **with** a previous history of MACE.
    - Complete smoking cessation (see page 720)
    - Blood pressure control (see page 207)
    - Appropriate lipid management (see page 667)
    - Physical activity goal of at least 30 minutes, 7 days per week
    - Prevention of metabolic syndrome and weight control
    - Antiplatelet agents
      1. ASA 81mg/d indicated in secondary prevention of CAD (Plavix is an alternative in patients with ASA allergy)
         - ASA should be started within 6 hours post CABG started at 100-325mg/d for 1 year then 81mg/d thereafter
      2. Concurrent ASA+P2Y12 indicated in patients with stent placed for maximum of 12 months (minimum 12mo if ACS; otherwise dependent on type of stent)
         - Prasugrel only indicated after PCI
         - Ticagrelor, Plavix can be used if medical intervention only; neither is superior to the other[124]
      3. In those with Atrial Fibrillation, consider DAPT with NOAC+Plavix for 12 months after any intervention (PCI or CABG) f/b NOAC alone (*AFIRE*)
    - Diabetes mellitus management (see page 244)

CARDIOLOGY

1. Focus on agents that have known benefits in patients with CVD (i.e. SGLT-2 inhibitors and GLP-1 agonists, see page 247)
- ACEi/ARB (see page 212)
  1. Should be implemented in patients with known ↓EF, DM, CKD, and HTN (unless AA)
  2. Lisinopril 5-40mg/d and Enalapril 2.5-20mg BID
  3. ARB (Candesartan 4-32mg/d) should be considered in patients intolerant to ACEi
- β-Blockers
  1. Similar to ACEi/ARB, indicated in patients with ↓EF or prior ACS limited to metoprolol succinate 25-400mg/d or divided BID (tartrate), carvedilol 3.125mg-25mg BID. See page 188 for more information.
  2. If patients have normal EF, then only use for 3 years and re-assess thereafter if continued use is indicated
- Calcium Channel Blockers
  1. Similar effectiveness as beta blockers
  2. Nifedipine 30-90mg/d, amlodipine 5-10mg/d, or felodipine 2.5-10mg/d
  3. Avoid diltiazem or verapamil in those with EF>40% as they may precipitate HF
- Nitrates
  1. Dilate systemic veins, arteries decreasing preload
  2. SBL NTG 0.4mg q5m x3 for acute anginal episodes
  3. Long acting: isosorbide mononitrate 30-240mg/d for anginal prophylaxis
- Ranolazine
  1. Dosed 500-1000mg BID
  2. Anti-anginal and anti-ischemic agent
  3. Use as adjunctive therapy when symptoms persist despite optimal doses of other antianginals
- Keep patients up to date on all vaccines
- Consider cardiac rehab consultation

STRESS TESTING

- **Purpose**[125,126,127,187,128]
  o Most helpful when pre-test probability between 10-90%
  o Detect inducible cardiac ischemia in symptomatic **intermediate-risk** patients
    - Low pre-test – don't test
    - High pre-test – do cath
  o Detection of CAD in patients with anginal chest pain
  o Evaluation of anatomic and functional severity of CAD (TTE/MRI)
  o Assessment of response to medical interventions
  o Atypical symptoms but risk factors for CAD
  o Coronary Calcium score >100 in patients with ↑RF but **asymptomatic**
  o Evaluation post PCTA @ 2 years or CABG @ 5 years
- **Choosing Between Stress Tests**
  o First, there are 3 major choices for stressing: exercise, inotropes, and vasodilators
    - Exercise- for patients with intermediate probability of ischemic heart disease who have at least moderate physical functioning or no disabling comorbidity and only *intermediate* pre-test risk.
    - Exercise Stress with Nuclear MPI or TTE – for patients with *intermediate to high* pretest probability of IHD with at least moderate physical functioning or no disabling comorbidity

- Next, you determine how to measure response to the stressor (EKG, TTE, Nuclear-SPECT, MRI)
  - Overall, decision should be determined off your pre-test probability (10-90%)
    - ECG: must have normal baseline ECG and intermediate pre-test probability at most of IHD
    - Others: abnormal baseline ECG (LVH with strain, digoxin, LBBB, ST/T changes) with intermediate to moderate pre-test probability of IHD

Figure. How to determine which type of stress test to order

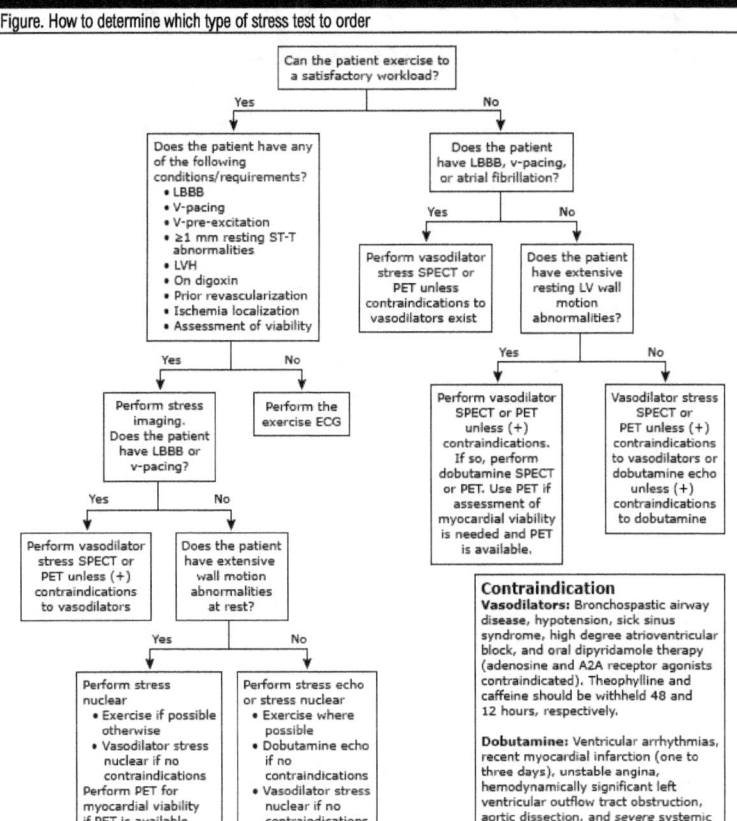

What type of stress test to get

Type of stress	Cons	Mechanism	Best for	Not for
Exercise Exercise ECG	Lowest SN/SP (45-67%/72-90%) Cannot localize ischemia Many C/I	↑HR, ↑BP	Patients able to reach target HR of (85% x 220-age), men, patients who desire no radiation exposure, least $$$	LBBB Pacer Cannot reach HR ST elevations/deviations at baseline WPW
Exercise Echo	SN of 85% <u>TTE</u> Subjective interpretation of results <u>SPECT</u> Cannot differentiate if balanced ischemia present, also subjective interpretation of results			
Vasodilator Regadenoson, adenosine, dipyridamole (RAD)		Dilates coronary arteries without ↑HR or BP	LBBB Pacer Cannot reach HR H/O PCI or CABG Obesity SENS: 87-90% SPEC: 73-89% *most sens/spec*	Reactive airway dz Taking theophylline Adenosine and Dipyridamole c/i if pmhx of asthma, 2-3" HB or severe COPD (FEV1<30%), ↓BP Avoid adenosine in pts with HA
Inotrope Dobutamine stress echo		↑HR + BP	Cannot reach HR Reactive airway dz (asthma/COPD) SENS: 68-98% SPEC: 44-100% *no radiation but quicker results	Tachyarrhythmias Significant obesity LBBB (↑ false +)
<u>MRI/CT</u> Not always available, high $$$				

- **Contraindications to stress testing**
  - Absolute Contraindications
    - Severe/Symptomatic AS
    - Acute MI (within 2 days)
    - Unstable Angina
    - Decompensated HF
    - Unstable Arrhythmias
    - Acute PE
    - Suspected Aortic Dissection
  - Relative Contraindications
    - Left Main CAD
    - Moderate AS
    - HOCM
    - Electrolyte Abnormalities
    - AFib with RVR
    - 3rd degree AV block
    - Resting BP > 200/110
- **When to including imaging (SPECT/TTE/MRI)**
  - Imaging is often added to exercise testing if there is one of the following:
    - Baseline abnormality on ECG that may make interpretation difficult
    - Symptoms at rest or poor exercise tolerance that may limit their ability to achieve full BRUCE protocol
    - Anatomic abnormalities expected
    - High pretest probability for CAD
    - Abnormal baseline ECG (BBB)
    - Previous myocardial damage or revascularization procedure
    - If you want to analyze wall motion function and to determine the physiologic significance of a lesion that is presence and the probable success of an intervention
- **Preoperative Use**
  - Preoperative exercise stress testing is not indicated for risk stratification before non-cardiac surgery in patients who are able to achieve a minimum of 4 METs (e.g., walking up one flight of stairs) without cardiac symptoms, even if they have a history of CAD.
  - Exercise stress testing is helpful for risk stratification in patients undergoing vascular surgery and in those who have active cardiac symptoms before undergoing non emergent non cardiac surgery.
  - Patients with poor functional capacity (unable to achieve 4 METs) should undergo stress echocardiography or exercise single-photon emission computed tomography (SPECT) before undergoing vascular surgery or a kidney or liver transplant.
- **Results**
  - If your patient had a positive or negative exercise treadmill test, consider calculating his **Duke Treadmill Score (DTS)**, which is predictive of 5-year survival and significant severe CAD for patients who are younger than 75 years
    - DTS helps you to exclude low-risk patients from further invasive testing and ensure high-risk patients receive further evaluation and appropriate treatment. DTS appears to be more useful in women with an intermediate pretest score but not with a low pretest score.

Interpretation of DUKE treadmill score			
Score (Duke)	Risk Group	1 year mortality	Management
≥ 5	Low	0.25%	medical management with ASA, BB, CCB, statin, and long acting nitrate
-10 to 4	Intermediate	1.25%	Cardiology referral
≤ -11	High	5.25%	

- **Findings associated with poor outcomes**
  - Poor exercise capacity (<5 METS)
  - Exercise-induced angina during minimal exercise

- Inability to achieve 85% of age-predicted maximum HR
- Fall in SBP during exercise from baseline
- ST elevation
- ≥2mm ST depression during minimal expenditure
- Early onset or prolonged duration of ST depression during exercise test
- ST depression in multiple leads
- Ventricular couplets or tachycardia during recovery

CHEST PAIN & ACS

Immediate Approach
- <u>Do first</u>: IV access, O2, cardiac monitoring, ECG (compare to prior; repeat q15m if ACS concern), CXR
- <u>History</u>: Obtain HPI of pain (position, quality, radiation, severity, timing, associated sx, alleviating & exacerbating factors), cardiac risk factors (ie: CAD, aortic dz, PE), prior cardiac testing (timing & results of last stress test, catheterization, TTE) & prior cardiac events/procedures (i.e. myocardial infarction [MI], CABG, valve repair, etc.)
- Empiric tx: ASA 325 mg (if considering ACS & low suspicion for AD), NTG for pain (unless R-sided ischemia, hypotension, PDEinh)
- Risk stratify for dxs being considered: ACS (TIMI, GRACE, or PURSUIT), PE (Well's), AoD (Aortic Dissection Detection risk score)

- **Define** –any type of pain in the central chest region, this is **not** the same as angina.
  - There are five important causes of chest pain, which should be diagnosed/treated at night; the other causes can wait until morning.
    1. **Cardiac**[129]
        - <u>Determine risk categorization</u>: if concerned for ACS/AMI; calculate TIMI, HEART, or COMPASS-MI score
        - Typical angina (definite):
            - All 3 of the following: Substernal chest discomfort with (1) a characteristic quality and duration (typically 20-30 minutes) that is (2) provoked by exertion or emotional stress and (3) relieved by rest or nitroglycerin
                - Most common cause and takes many forms: chest, arm, back, jaw pains, sometimes dizziness, nausea and vomiting. Diagnosis of acute myocardial infarction occurs in the setting of appropriate symptoms with an elevated hs-cTn with characteristic rise and fall.
                    - <u>Unstable</u> (*defined as* rest angina lasting **>20min**, new-onset angina within 2 months of initial presentation, or increasing angina with crescendo pattern)
                        - Rx with sublingual NTG q 2-4 minutes. Keep checking BPs to be sure SBP > 90 before the next dose!
                        - Use dilaudid 0.5 to 1 mg IV if NTG unsuccessful. (Can also try Maalox 30 cc p.o.) Be aware that Procardia can cause a reflex tachycardia. Unrelieved angina or recurrent/prolonged angina in a post-MI patient should go to the PCU. Don't wait. Call the upper year resident.
                        - Acute ST elevations require IV nitro, heparin, TPA or streptokinase, Lopressor if no contraindications (low BP, HR, CHF, RAD hx). For IV nitro, use Tridil 50/250 D5W, titrate to pain free and SBP > 100.
                        - Heparin 5000 u bolus, then run at 18 unit/kg/hour and check PTT in 6 hours. You should call the attending (cardiology) to

start TPA/strepto, notify ICU/PCU for transfers to the respective unit.
- Stable (*defined as* chest pain or discomfort that reliably/predictably occurs with activity or stress lasting a short time of **5 min or less**, and resolves with rest or NTG)
  - Stress testing and outpatient management (ASA, BB, statin, CCB, long acting nitrate, prn NTG)
- Atypical angina (probable): *Meets 1-2 of the above criteria.*
  - Determine risk factors present (see AAS criteria on page 184) and do stress test if necessary (see page 167)
- Non-cardiac chest pain: *Meets none of the above criteria.* MSK, GI, psychogenic, continued below

2. **Pericarditis** -- sharp or dull ache, patient wants to sit up, friction rub, pulsus paradoxus. Only two of the symptoms are required for diagnosis (typical chest pain, rub, ECG changes with diffuse ST elevation and PR depression in AVR, effusion). Consider myocarditis if the previous symptoms are present along with ↑CK-MB/TROP, ↓EF on TTE, or MRI showing myocarditis. Treatment first with NSAIDs (i.e. indomethacin, ibuprofen) + colchicine. Only use steroids if refractory symptoms or allergies to former as they can actually ↑ relapse rates otherwise. ASA should be used if post-MI pericarditis is the diagnosis.

3. **Aortic aneurysm** -- "tearing pain," asymmetric pulses suspicious especially with pain to back or right side
   - Stat ECG and CXR; if still suspicious, CT of chest. Try to lower the BP (nitro or Lopressor).

4. **Pulmonary embolus** -- sudden onset, often pain more peripheral, suspect especially with tachypnea and tachycardia, pO2<80
   - Risk factors: inactivity, venous stasis, post-op (esp. ortho and urology), hx of DVT, cancer, pre or post-partum, OCP's, HRT, CHF, COPD.
   - Signs/symptoms: tachypnea, dyspnea, pleuritic chest pain, sinus tachycardia (or bradycardia, esp. w/ β-Blocker), anxiety, S1/Q3T3, new RBBB, RAD.
   - Tests
     - Stat ABG – resp. alkalosis with normal/↓ pO2 (and poor response to O2) (90% with PE have low pO2; therefore, 10% of PE presents with nml O2).
     - CXR (need to r/o pneumothorax, CHF, pneumonia).
     - TTE
     - U/S for DVT
   - Treatment
     - Hemodynamically stable: UFH
     - Hemodynamically unstable: alteplase
     - Contraindication to AC or thrombolytics: IVC filter

5. **Esophageal reflux/PUD/pancreatitis** -- can masquerade as substernal chest pain; need to belch, burning sensation in throat

6. **Others** – see table below

CARDIOLOGY

Brief Differential of Chest Pain

Cardiac Related	GI Related
o ACS/Myocardial infarction must always be ruled, see below	o GERD
o Aortic dissection	o Esophageal spasm
o Pericarditis	o Mallory-Weiss
	o Peptic ulcer disease
Pulmonary Related	**Others**
o Pneumothorax (PTX)	o MSK (costochondritis)
o Pneumonia	o Anxiety
o Pleuritis	o Zoster
o PE	

- **Approach**
  - History
    - Characterize the pain (site, severity, time/duration, stabbing/gripping, radiation, precipitating and relieving factors, previous history of similar sx
      - Symptoms not suggestive of ACS: lasting seconds, or lasting >24h
    - Associated symptoms (SOB, n/v, palpitations, dizziness)
    - Drug history, ECGs
    - Cardiac history in self or family
  - Exam
    - VS, cardiac exam, reproducible, lung exam, edema
  - Diagnostics
    - CXR
    - ECG (w/i 10 minutes of symptoms; serially thereafter)
      - Remember to get posterior ECG if ST↓ noted in V1-V3
    - Pulse ox
    - Labs: CBC, d-dimer if indicated, CMP, BNP if indicated[130]
      - High sensitivity troponin (cTnI): 2 sets separated by 1-2h unless the onset of sx was >8-12 hours ago, then a single cTnI is appropriate
        - more sensitive for early cardiac injury; elevations should be repeated to determine the likely cause:

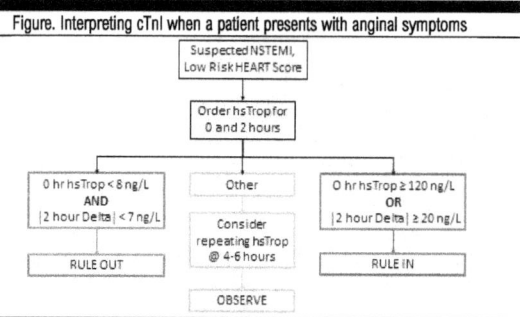

Figure. Interpreting cTnI when a patient presents with anginal symptoms

Thrombotic and Nonthrombotic Causes of Elevated Troponin

- Thrombotic
  - *Atherosclerotic plaque disruption with thrombosis (AMI)*
    - Acute Myocardial Infarction (AMI) defined as anginal symptoms with ECG changes (STΔ, LBBB, and pathologic Q waves), loss of viable myocardium on imaging, and/or new wall motion abnormality on TTE.

- Nonthrombotic
  - *Supply/demand mismatch*
    - ↓Supply: coronary spasm, embolism, resp failure, ↓HGB, ↓BP, shock, sustained bradyarrhythmia, coronary dissection, burns, sepsis
    - ↑Demand: tachyarrhythmia, ↑BP w/wo LVH
  - *Myocardial Ischemia*: coronary vasospasm, acute stroke, sympathomimetics, aortic dissection, AV dz
  - *Myocardial strain* – CHF, pulmonary embolism, extreme exertion, AV dz
  - *Direct myocardial damage* – infiltrative dz, inflammatory dz 2/2 myocarditis, drug toxicity, rhabdomyolisis, defibrillation

- Follow angina pathway on following pages if necessary, otherwise for other specific conditions see their respective sections in this book.
- Risk Score - after performing your exam, obtaining biomarkers, and getting an ECG, now determine the risk score (TIMI and HEART) which will predict the risk of adverse short-term outcomes in 30 days.
- Based on the risk score, then go down appropriate management (early invasive, delayed, stress testing).

CARDIOLOGY

Figure. Interpreting myocardial injury as seen with ↑cTnI

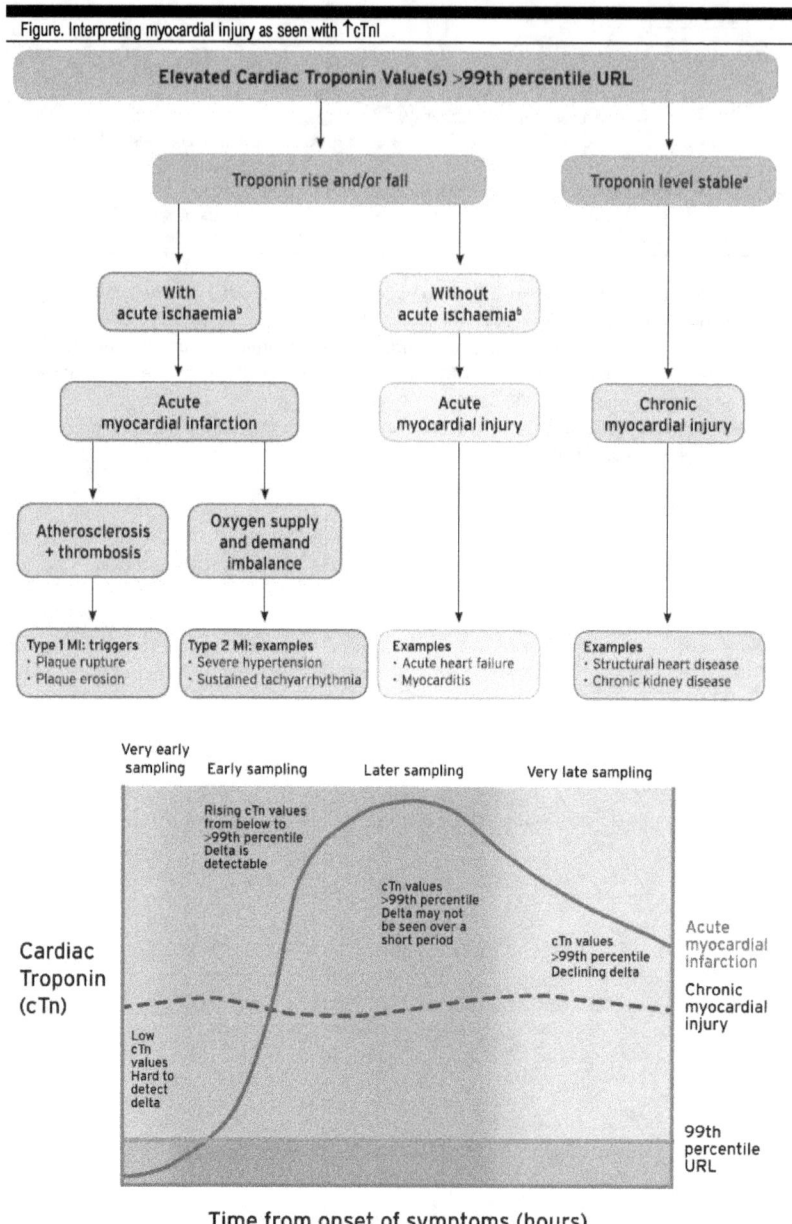

CARDIOLOGY

Figure. Approach to patients presenting with anginal symptoms suspicious for acute myocardial ischemia[131]

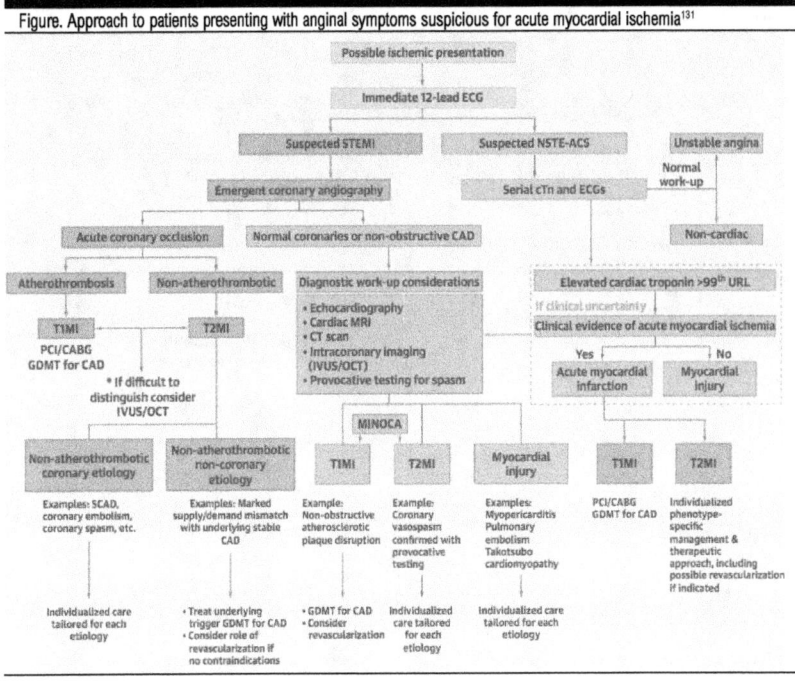

CARDIOLOGY

Figure. Algorithm if suspecting NSTEMI

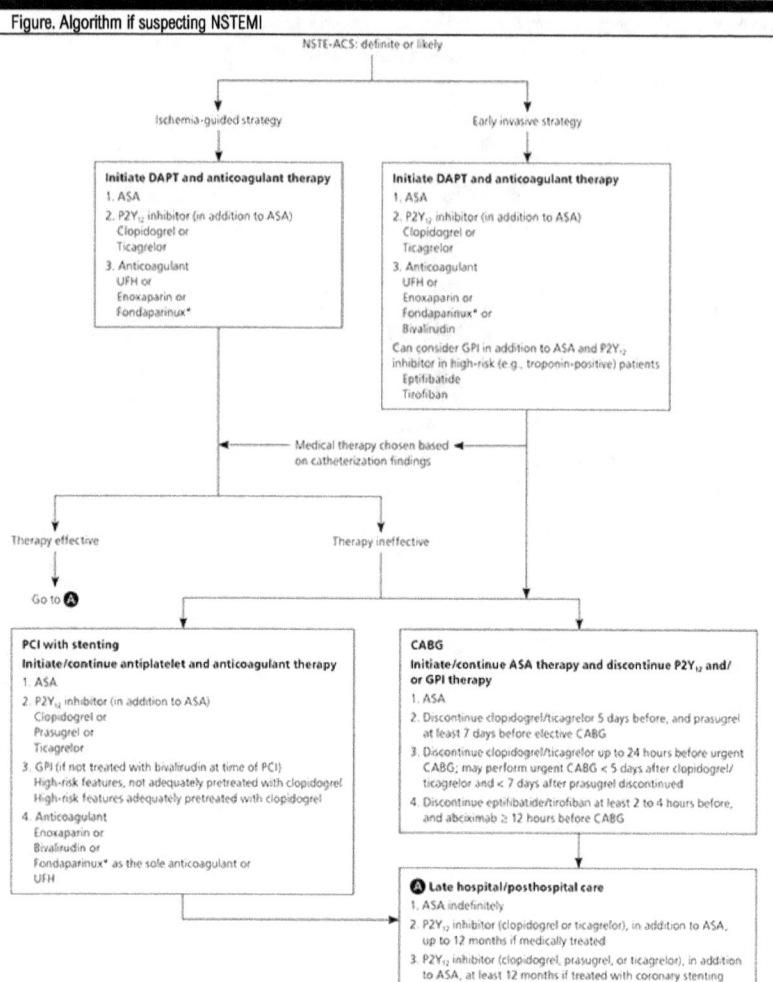

CHEST PAIN EVALUATION

	STEMI	NSTEMI	UA	Atypical Chest pain

MYOCARDIAL INFARCTION: typical rise and fall in troponin in the setting of either: (1) anginal symptoms (2) ECG changes (ST or T wave; new LBBB) or (3) Echo changes

IS THIS ACUTE CORONARY SYNDROME?

	STEP 1	STEP 2	STEP 3	
	Ask 3 questions: • Is chest pain substernal? • Is chest pain brought on by exertion? • Is chest pain relieved within 10 minutes by rest or nitroglycerin?	Total the number of "yes" answers to identify symptom pattern: 0 of 3=Asymptomatic 1 of 3=Non anginal chest pain 2 of 3=Atypical angina 3 of 3=Typical angina	Find the cell in the matrix (below) where age, gender, and symptom pattern converge: High probability — >90% Intermediate — 10%–90% Low — <10% Very low — <5%	
Symptoms	Chest pressure (often lasts 10 sec – 30 min) +/- with NTG Dyspnea Diaphoresis Nausea, Vomiting Dizziness Fatigue Symptoms at rest/↑frequency/Δ from normal pattern			Atypical
ECG	ST elevation	ST depression TWI	Normal or ST depression/TWI	Normal
Cardiac Enzymes	+	+	Normal	Normal
Universal Classification of MI	1) **Type 1 MI** – ischemia due to primary ACS (plaque rupture, erosion); detection of a rise/or fall of cTnI with at least one value above the 99th percentile and at least one of the following:			

i. Symptoms of acute MI
ii. New ischemic ECG Δs
iii. Development of pathological Q waves
iv. Imaging s/o new loss of viable myocardium or new WMA
v. Imaging showing coronary thrombus
2) Type 2 MI[132] – Rise and/or fall of cTnI (one should be >99th percentile) with e/o supply/demand mismatch. This likely unmasks underlying CAD; examples include anemia, vasospasm, ↓BP, arrythmia, fixed coronary atherosclerosis, or ↑BP. Ultimate management is based on having rising/falling cTnI with at least 1 ≥99th percentile and clinical evidence of myocardial ischemia (less commonly have angina, m/c have dyspnea and atypical sx). If unclear, obtain cardiac imaging, coded as "myocardial injury."
3) Type 3 MI – sudden unexpected cardiac death
4) Type 4A MI – ACS secondary to PCI
5) Type 4B MI – documented stent thrombosis
6) Type 5 MI – related to CABG

Classification

Canadian Cardiovascular Society Grading System

Grade I – Angina with strenuous, rapid, or prolonged exertion; ordinary physical activity, such as climbing stairs, does not provoke angina
Grade II – Slight limitation of ordinary activity; angina occurs with postprandial, uphill, or rapid walking; when walking more than 2 blocks of level ground or climbing more than 1 flight of stairs; during emotional stress; or in the early hours after awakening
Grade III – Marked limitation of ordinary activity; angina occurs with walking 1-2 blocks or climbing a flight of stairs at a normal pace
Grade IV – Inability to carry on any physical activity without discomfort; rest pain occurs

AAS Risk Assessment

High	Intermediate	Low
Prev MI	Age>70	Atypical AP

Risk Assessment

- HEART Score, T-MACS, EDACS (in ER)

		Reproducibility
Hx AAD	Male	TWI <1mm
ECG Δ w/ sx	DM	ØECG
Sym TWIs	PVD	
EF<40	ST↓ <1mm	
↑cTnI	TWI >1mm w/ ↑R	
VT or VF		
Prior CABG		

Management | See STEMI on page 194 | Calculate TIMI to determine invasive vs conservative. See NSTEMI management on page 188 | ACS rule out to include either stress test or coronary CTA

- CAD Consortium: https://qxmd.com/calculate/calculator_287/pre-test-probability-of-cad-cad-consortium

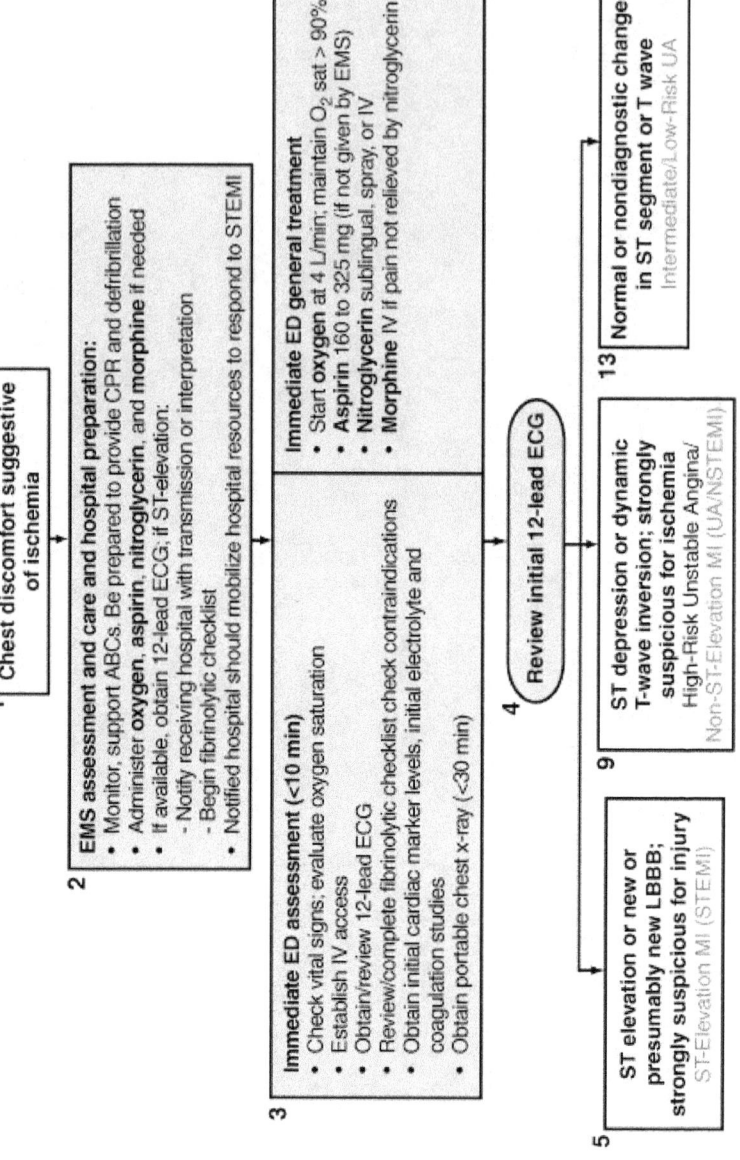

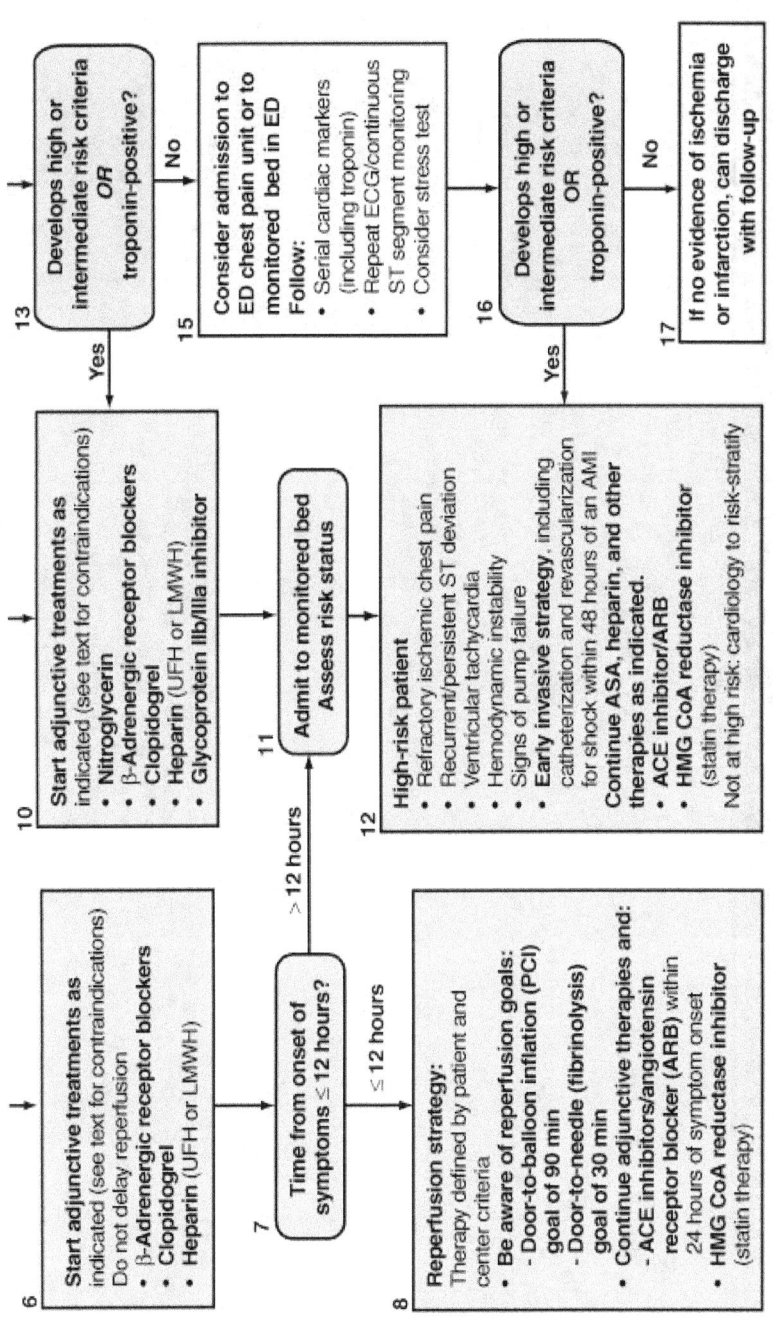

UA/NSTEMI

	IMMEDIATE INVASIVE	DELAYED INVASIVE	EARLY INVASIVE (TIMACS trial)	ISCHEMIA-GUIDED / CONSERVATIVE
TIME	Within 2 hours	24-72 hours	<24 hours	N/A
SCORE	TIMI ≥ 3 GRACE > 140 ACCF/AHA: intermediate/high HEARTS3: 35.3%	TIMI ≥ 2 GRACE 109-140 ACCF/AHA: intermediate/high HEARTS3: 35.3%	GRACE > 140 ACCF/AHA: intermediate/high HEARTS3: 4.6%	TIMI 0-1 GRACE < 109 ACCF/AHA: low HEARTS3: 0%
SYMPTOMS /INDICATIONS	• Refractory angina • Sustained VT/VF • Hemodynamic instability • Electrical instability • New signs of heart failure	• PMHx of DM, CHF, Hx PCI<6mo ago, prior CABG • +MPS • EF<40% • Hx of PCI in last 6 months or prior CABG • Not at high/intermediate risk • GRACE 109-140. TIMI ≥ 2	• Temporal change in Troponin • New or presumably new ST depression • GRACE > 140 • High risk for clinical events	• Patient or clinician preference in the absence of high-risk features • Low TIMI (0 or 1) or GRACE (<109) • Patient/Physician preference
ORDERS	• Admit directly to cath unit or "step-down" unit			• Admit to telemetry (call MD for > 6 PVC/min, A-fib, V-fib, > 3 beat run of VT, R on T). • Bed rest until ruled out
MEDS	1. ASA 325mg chewed 2. Beta Blocker - only if no active HF, PR prolongation, or RAD - Metoprolol 5mg IVP q5min x 3 OR Metoprolol 25-50mg PO to target HR<60 (other options include carvedilol or bisoprolol) 3. P2Y12 Inhibitor see below	1. ASA 325mg chewed and continued daily until discharge then 81mg/d 2. Beta Blocker - only if no active HF, PR prolongation, or RAD - Metoprolol 5mg IVP q5min x 3 OR Metoprolol 25-50mg PO to target HR<60 (other options include carvedilol or bisoprolol) 3. P2Y12 Inhibitor with Ticagrelor 180mg loading f/b 90mg BID or Plavix (300-600mg loading f/b 75mg daily)		1. ASA 325mg then ASA 81mg/d indefinitely (coronary CTA score of >100 suggests initiation of ASA; primary prevention recommended only if 10-year risk score ≥ 10%) 2. Morphine 3. Oxygen via NC at 2 L/min if SpO2 <90% 4. Metoprolol 25 mg **PO** BID

4. **Statin** (atorvastatin 80mg/day) even if LDL is known to be <70
5. **ACEi** (Captopril 6.25mg PO TID) for HF; EF<40%, or STEMI in anterior location
6. **Supplemental Oxygen**[133] – only if SaO2 is <90%

4. **Statin** (simvastatin 80mg/day) even if LDL is known to be <70. Can also be considered if coronary CTA is >0.
5. **ACEi** (Lisinopril 5mg/d titrated to 10mg/d; Captopril 6.25mg → 12.5mg after 2 hrs. → 25mg 12 hours later → 50mg BID; Ramipril 1.25mg BID titrated to 5mg BID)
6. **Supplemental Oxygen** – only if SaO2 is <90%

- If this IV dose is tolerated, you can usually start 25 mg PO bid but be sure to write hold parameters.
- Can consider statin however can also use coronary CTA results to guide initiation (score > 0 should have statin initiated)
- If C/I (active wheezing, allergy) then give Diltiazem
  - NTG
  - Lipitor 80mg/day or Crestor 20mg/d
  - ACEi indicated if patient has evidence of LVD/CHF

P2Y12

- In patients going to the cath lab, give one of the following **before** cath:
  - Clopidogrel 300/600mg load then 75mg/d (if fibrinolysis then use 75mg/d dose)
  - Ticagrelor 180mg load (recommended over Plavix if early invasive strategy used) then 90mg BID
- If giving Prasugrel 60mg load then 10mg/d, give **after** cath if NSTEMI, and **before** cath if STEMI *(ISAR-REACT 5)*
  - Prasugrel outperformed Ticagrelor in patients presenting with ACS[134]

ANTICOAG

- Enoxaparin 30mg IV load then 1mg/kg SC q12h (reduce to 1mg/kg SC daily if CrCl < 30cc/min) and continue until PCI or for duration of hospitalization (max 8 days)
- Heparin (UFH) 60 IU/kg (maximum 4000 IU) loading dose with initial infusion of 12 IU/kg per hour (maximum 1000 IU/h) adjusted per APTT to maintain therapeutic anticoagulation according to the specific hospital protocol, continued for 48 hours or until PCI is performed

Alternatives
- Bivalirudin 0.1mg/kg loading dose followed by 0.25mg/kg per hour (**only if early invasive strategy**)

RADS/PROC

Angiography

Stress testing should be done within 72 hours of presentation.

MPS (if no ischemia sx in 24 hours)
- ECG with ischemic change (ST depression >1mm) → exercise echo test

- Uninterpretable ECG (LBBB, paced, LVH) – stress echo
- ECG without changes → exercise ECG
- Patients with COPD, obesity, chest wall deformities → MPS
- Patients unable to exercise → MPS
- For more detailed information, see page 172

TTE (look at LV function)
ECG – avoid in women (high false +)
CORONARY CTA (see page 169)
- Troponin q6-12h x 2
- PT/PTT
- Cholesterol panel if no previous workup
- HgA1C if diabetic.

If patient classified as low risk after stress test, then:
- No angiography is indicated
- ASA 81mg, BB, statin, CCB, nitrate indefinitely
- Ticagrelor 90mg BID x 12 month (PLATO)
- Stop GP2B3A if already started
- Continue heparin x 48 hours or Lovenox x 8 days
- Cardiac rehab referral

LABS
- Troponin q3-6h x 2 (or further if sx develop)
- PT/PTT
- Cholesterol panel if no previous workup
- HgA1C if diabetic

OUTCOME

1. CABG
   - Continue ASA 81mg/d
   - Discontinue clopidogrel 5 to 7 d prior to elective CABG or 24 hours before urgent CABG
   - Discontinue IV GP IIb/IIIa 2-4 h prior to CABG
   - Continue UFH; discontinue enoxaparin 12 to 24 h prior to CABG;
   - Treat exacerbations of chest pain with NTG prn → Nitro paste (1" removed daily) → nitro gtt
   - Cardiac rehab referral
   - Avoid concurrent NSAIDs
   - Beta blocker for 3 years duration if nml LV function

2. PCI
   - DAPT required (ASA+P2y12) for minimum 12 months then calculate DAPT score and if ≥ 2 then continue dual therapy for 30 months.
     o Continue ASA 81mg/d
     o Loading dose of clopidogrel (600mg) if not given pre angio, maintained at 75mg after
     o After 3 months of DAPT, ticagrelor for 12 mo vs continued DAPT noninferior[135]
     o Consider GPI if not treated with bivalirudin at time of PCI
     o If concurrent Afib:

- Consider DAPT only (stop ASA after 14 days of DAPT+anti-coagulation) with:
  - Apixiban+plavix (*AUGUSTUS*)
  - Edoxaban+Plavix (*ENTRUST-AF*)
  - Dabigatran+Plavix (*RE-DUAL PCI*)
  - Rivaroxiban+Plavix (*PIONEER AF-PCI*)
- Short period of triple therapy (ASA+Plavix+OAC) f/b DAPT (OAC+ASA/Plavix) per ESC guidelines
- Discontinue anticoagulant after PCI for uncomplicated cases
- Cardiac rehab referral
- Beta blocker for 3 years duration if nml LV function
- Avoid concomitant NSAIDs

3. Medical Therapy
   - No significant obstruction → ASA and Plavix
   - CAD → continue ASA, continue UFH x 48 hours or Lovenox for hospitalization
   - P2y12 inhibitor (clopidogrel 75mg/d or ticagrelor 90mg BID) for 12 months
   - Consider PPI if patient on triple therapy (+warfarin) or h/o GIB
   - If Warfarin required, consider lower INR goal of 2.0-2.5. Calculate HAS-BLED score
   - Cardiac rehab referral
   - Beta blocker for 3 years duration if nml LV function
   - Avoid concomitant NSAIDs

DECISION: SELECT MANAGEMENT STRATEGY

Favors Invasive Strategy:
Recurrent chest pain despite maximal medical therapy
Elevated cardiac biomarkers
New ST-segment depression
Signs of heart failure
New or worsening mitral regurgitation
Hemodynamic instability
Sustained ventricular tachycardia
Prior CABG
High risk score (e.g., TIMI 5–7)
PCI within 6 months
Reduced LV ejection fraction

Favors Conservative Strategy:
Low risk score (e.g., TIMI 0–2)
Patient or physician preference
Risk of revascularization outweighs benefits

Calculated TIMI Score	14-day Risk of MACE
0 or 1	5%
2	8%
3	13%
4	20%
5	28%
6 or 7	41%

INVASIVE STRATEGY
(i.e., Diagnostic catheterization with intent to perform PCI)

Early invasive strategy (i.e., requiring immediate catheterization) should be considered in patients with:
- Refractory chest discomfort despite vigorous medical therapy
- Hemodynamic or rhythm instability

CONSERVATIVE STRATEGY

DRUGS—Unless contraindicated, all patients should receive the following regardless of the strategy:
- Anticoagulant therapy:
  Unfractionated heparin: 60 U/kg IV bolus, max 4000 U; then 12 U/kg/hr, max 1000 U/hr
  OR,
  Enoxaparin (Lovenox): If <75 years, then 30 mg IV bolus followed 15 min later with 1 mg/kg SQ q12h (or q24h if CrCl < 30). If >75 years, then omit IV bolus and inject 0.75 mg/kg SQ avoid if Cr > 2.0
  OR,
  Fondaparinux (Arixtra): 2.5 mg SQ daily (avoid if CrCl < 30)
  OR,
  Bivalirudin (Angiomax): 0.1 mg/kg IV bolus; then 0.25 mg/kg/h
- Dual antiplatelet therapy:
  For the invasive strategy, If there is a high suspicion for CAD that may require CABG (i.e., diabetes or known multi-vessel CAD) then consider withholding therapy and starting a GP IIb/IIIa inhibitor until the anatomy is defined:
  Clopidogrel (Plavix): 300–600 mg PO loading dose then 75 mg daily
  For patients undergo PCI, you may consider Prasugrel (Effient) 60 mg PO loading dose at the time of PCI then 10 mg daily (see Algorithm 19.1 for contraindications)

Continued on next page

Continued on next page

CARDIOLOGY

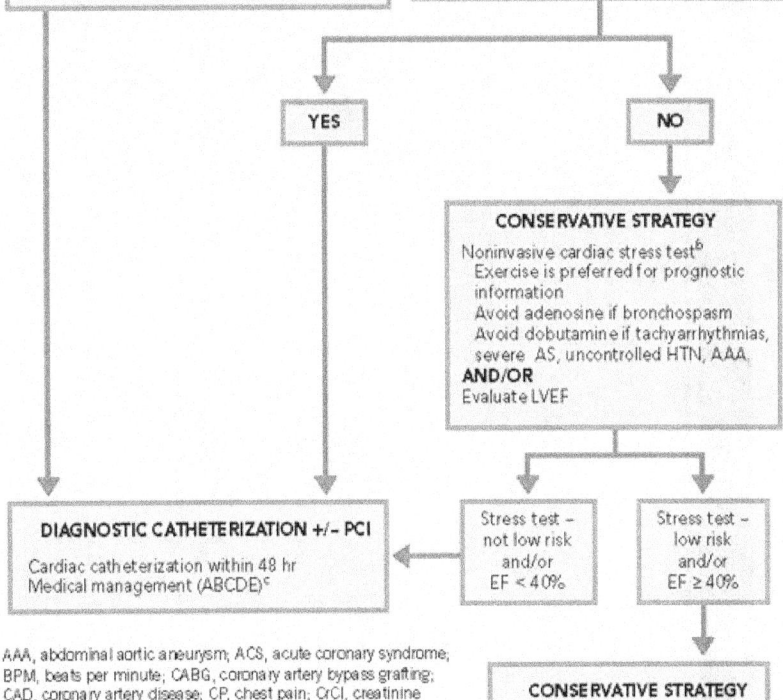

AAA, abdominal aortic aneurysm; ACS, acute coronary syndrome; BPM, beats per minute; CABG, coronary artery bypass grafting; CAD, coronary artery disease; CP, chest pain; CrCl, creatinine clearance; CVA, cerebrovascular accident; DM, diabetes mellitus; ECG, electrocardiogram; GP, glycoprotein; HR, heart rate; HTN, hypertension; IV, intravenous; LVEF, left ventricular ejection fraction; MACE, major adverse cardiac events; MI, myocardial infarction; PAD, peripheral arterial disease; PCI, percutaneous coronary intervention; PO, by mouth; SBP, systolic blood pressure; SQ, subcutaneous; TIMI, thrombolysis in myocardial infarction. [a]Coronary risk factors include diabetes mellitus, cigarette smoking, hypertension (>140/90 mm Hg or on antihypertensive medication), low HDL cholesterol (<40 mg/dL), family history of premature CAD (male first-degree relative ≤55 years old or female first-degree relative ≤65 years old), and age (men ≥45 years old; women ≥55 years old). [b]Diagnostic accuracy of various stress tests are exercise treadmill: men—68% sensitive, 77% specific, women—61% sensitive, 70% specific; exercise, adenosine thallium—88% sensitive, 77% specific; exercise or dobutamine echo—76% sensitive, 88% specific. [c]See Table 19.2

STEMI

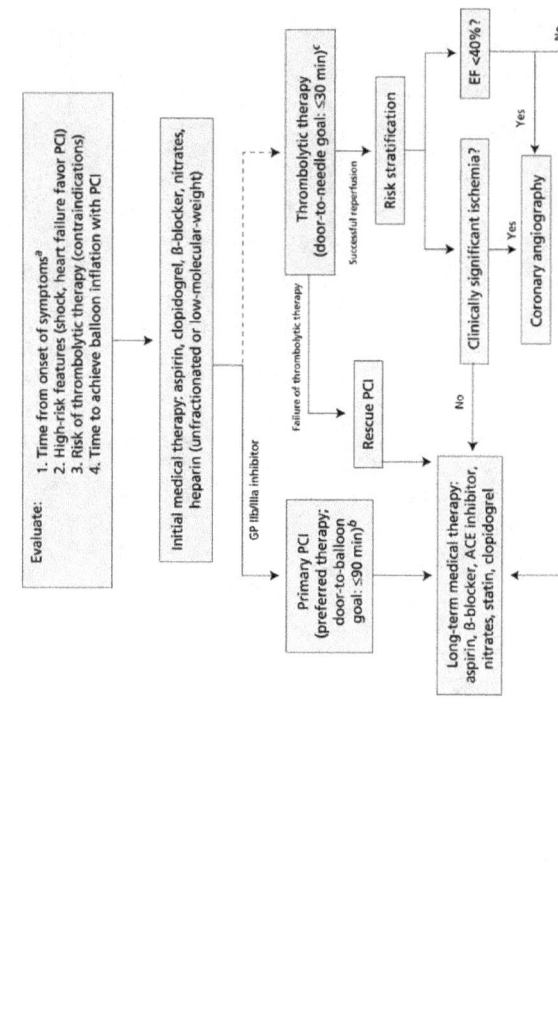

- Definition[136,147,137,138,139,140]
  - **Acute ST elevation MI requires two of the following:**
    1. Chest pain or chest pain-equivalent (indigestion, SOB, dizziness, etc.)

2. ECG with ≥ 1mm ST elevation in ≥ 2 contiguous leads
   - Inverted T waves
   - Consider posterior infarction if ST↓ in V1-4 with posterior ECG showing ST↑ in V7-9
   - Elevated ST segment (area of injury)
     o Leads V1-V4 → anterior wall → LAD
     o Leads V1-V2 → anteroseptal → Proximal LAD
     o Leads V2-V3 → anteroapical → LAD or branches
     o Leads I and aVL → lateral → CFX
     o Leads II, III, or aVF → inferior wall → RCA
     o Leads V1 R>S, Q in V6 → posterior wall → PDA
     o **Asymmetric ST depression is associated with strain not ischemia**
     - Q waves (area of infarction, usually develop during 12-36 hr)
3. Left bundle branch block, not known to be old (*Scarbossa criteria*)
   - ST-segment elevation at least 1mm concordant with a predominantly positive QRS complex in at least one lead
   - ST depression at least 1mm in leads V1, V2 or V3
   - ST elevation at least 5mm discordant (in the opposite direction) from a predominantly negative QRS complex
     ▪ Patients with sustained symptoms in absence of diagnostic ECG should have repeat ECG in 30mins
     ▪ Patients who have symptoms associated with an ECG showing ST depression unrelieved within 30 minutes of initiating medical therapy should be considered to have refractory unstable angina.
     ▪ As the resident, call cardiology immediately if suspected AMI patient (meeting above criteria); perform a brief evaluation of all chest pain/rule out MI patients and review ECG within 10 minutes of being informed of admission; call MOD if any question on ECG.
   o **Assessment**
     ▪ **Rapid** assessment is key → should receive an ECG within 10 minutes of symptoms:
     ▪ **Focused H&P:**
       1. Current symptoms: onset, duration, and quality; exacerbating/alleviating factors; associated symptoms.
       2. Prior ischemic disease? CHF? Arrhythmia? Other cardiac disease?
       3. Cardiac risk factors: Age, HTN, DM, PVD, CVD, hyperlipidemia, family history of premature CAD, smoking
       4. Other medical problems: renal failure, bleeding disorders, GI bleeds
       5. Assess vital signs—look for signs of cardiogenic shock or CHF; BP in both arms, JVP, murmurs (MR, VSD, etc.)
     ▪ **Diagnostic tests:**

1. ECG: (with rapid interpretation) call resident with any questions; repeat ECG in 6 hrs., or if any recurrent symptoms, then QD x 2d and on day prior to discharge; in reperfusion patients, check an end of therapy and repeat in 4-6hrs, then as above
2. Labs: CBC with platelets, Chem 7, PT/PTT, non-fasting lipid panel; others as indicated (ABG for respiratory insufficiency, hypoxia, etc.).
   - Cardiac enzymes:
     - Measure troponin I or T at presentation and 3—6 h after symptom onset in all patients with suspected ACS to identify pattern of values
     - Obtain additional troponin levels beyond 6 h in patients with initial normal serial troponins with electrocardiographic changes and/or intermediate/high risk clinical features
3. CXR to r/o mediastinal widening (c/f aortic dissection)
4. Echocardiography: indicated acutely if you suspect pericarditis, aortic dissection (TEE), tamponade, acute MR; also, useful to assess LV dysfunction, size, location and severity of regional wall motion abnormalities, valvular abnormalities. Otherwise, obtained after thrombolytics provided for risk stratification.
5. Acute coronary angiography: for urgent reperfusion by angioplasty or CABG, or localization of lesions for further management. Obstructive CAD defined as ≥50% obstruction noted on cath.
6. Right heart catheterization: for complicated MI—↓BP, oliguria, CHF, cardiogenic shock. Considered if you have inferior wall infarction (II, III, aVF) with V3R and V4R ST elevation.
   o Initial Therapy for planned PCI[136]
     - Access: IV: 2 lines, large bore; Foley catheterization
     - Oxygen: >90%
     - ASA: 325mg chewed immediately → 81mg afterwards if received Ticagrelor otherwise continue 325mg/d
       1. If ASA allergy, use Plavix
     - Thienopyridine
       1. Prasugrel: 60mg loading dose then 10mg daily *(ISAR-REACT 5)* showed superiority over Ticagrelor
       2. Ticagrelor: 180mg loading dose then 90mg BID
       3. Plavix: 600mg loading dose then 75mg for one year (with ASA 81mg)
     - GP2B3A
       1. *Only ordered by cardiology!*
       2. *For expected PCI intervention*
       3. Eptifibatide dosing 180mcg/kg IV bolus over 1-2min then cont. infusion 2mcg/kg/min as long as SCr <2 6 hours before PCI and for 18-24 hours after
         - If SCr 2-4 then cont. infusion ↓ to 1 mcg/kg/min.
         - If SCr >4 then use abciximab instead
         - After first bolus, give second bolus after 10 minutes.
     - Metoprolol[141]
       1. Oral β-Blockers should be initiated in the first 24 hours in patients with STEMI who do not have any of the following: signs of HF, evidence of a low output state, AVB, increased risk for cardiogenic shock (age>70, BP<120, ST at 110bpm)
         - Newer research is suggesting that if patients do not have evidence of depressed EF (nml TTE) beta blockers may not be as beneficial after 3 years duration.[142]
       2. *Contraindicated if in HF, bradycardic, or SBP<90*
       3. *Generally, only given if HR>90*
       4. *If allergy, then use CCB such as verapamil or diltiazem*

5. Reduce oxygen demand via contractility, HR, and pressure
6. Metoprolol 5mg x 3 IV then 50mg q6h PO x 24 hours → 100mg BID thereafter with target HR <60
7. Other options include carvedilol and bisoprolol
- ACEi
  1. To all patients with STEMI with anterior location, HF, or ejection fraction (EF) less than or equal to 0.40, unless contraindicated
     - Contraindicated: CKD (SCr > 2.5), RAS, ↓BP
  2. ↓workload and post-MI remodeling
  3. Start within 24 hours of symptoms
  4. Lisinopril 5mg daily titrated to 10mg/day[143]
  5. Captopril 6.25mg → 12.5mg after 2 hrs. → 25mg 12 hours later → 50mg BID
  6. Ramipril 1.25mg BID titrated to 5mg BID
- Heparin/Lovenox
  1. Patients with STEMI undergoing reperfusion with fibrinolytic therapy should receive anticoagulant therapy for a minimum of 48 hours, and preferably for the duration of the index hospitalization, up to 8 days or until revascularization if performed
  2. Depending on renal function (heparin preferred if SCr elevated)
     - UFH: Bolus of 60 units/kg (maximum, 5000 units) followed by infusion of 12 units/kg/h (maximum, 1000 units/h) *titrated to an APTT time 50-70 sec (1.5-2x control) for 48 hours.*
       - Check PT/PTT every 6 hours
       - Stop when patient about to go to cath lab
       - Continue **48 hours after PCI** if *large thrombus found, AFib, or EF<30%*
     - Enoxaparin: 1mg/kg milligrams IV bolus followed by 1 milligram/kg SC every 12 h until discharge
       - Hold 6 hours prior to PCI
     - Fondaparinux: <50kg: 5mg SC once daily; 50-100kg: 7.5mg SC once daily; >100kg: 10mg SC once daily
  3. If history of HIT, recommend bivalirudin
- NTG
  1. Contraindications: R heart failure, dehydration, ↓BP (SBP>90)
  2. Sublingual
  3. Consider drip if recurrent unresolved CP
- Statin:
  1. Check lipid profile
  2. Goal LDL <70 mg/dL

3. Start atorvastatin 80mg

FIBRINOLYSIS / NON-PCI

- Invasive strategy is not an option (e.g., lack of access to skilled PCI facility or difficult vascular access) or would be delayed
- **Goal fibrinolysis initiated within 30 minutes** if patient cannot be transported to PCI capable hospital within **120 minutes**
- No contraindications to fibrinolysis (*see table below*)
- For patients with STEMI, fibrinolytic therapy should be simultaneously accompanied by antithrombotic (e.g., heparin 4-5k IU and then titrated to reach aPTT 1.5-2x normal values i.e. 75-80s) and antiplatelet (aspirin plus clopidogrel 300mg load if <75yo or 75mg if >75 and then 75mg/d thereafter) therapies.
- Urgent angiography with a view toward "rescue PCI" should be pursued if there is less than 50% resolution of ST-segment elevation 90 minutes after administration.
- Resolution of chest pain and the presence or absence of reperfusion arrhythmias (i.e. AIVR) are also useful markers of successful reperfusion. Importantly, patients should be given a full 90 minutes after fibrinolytic therapy before being taken to the catheterization laboratory because percutaneous intervention immediately after fibrinolysis (i.e, so-called facilitated PCI) has been shown to worsen outcomes. Moreover, patients who receive fibrinolytic should be routinely transferred to a PCI-capable hospital for planned angiography (3-16 hours after receiving fibrinolytic) regardless of clinical status as part of the delayed-invasive strategy of care (class IIa recommendation).
- **Door-to-needle goal (initiation of therapy): ≤ 30 min**

Fibrinolytic Agents

Tenecteplase

Weight	Dose
<60 kg	30 milligrams
>60 but <70 kg	35 milligrams
>70 but <80 kg	40 milligrams
>80 but <90	45 milligrams
>90	50 milligrams

Streptokinase 1.5 million units over 60 min.

PCI

- Late presentation (sx onset >3 hr ago)
- **Medical contact-to-balloon / door-balloon ≤90 min**
- Outside transfer from non-PCI center to PCI center time <120 min
- Contraindications to fibrinolysis, including ↑ risk of bleeding and ICH
- High risk from STEMI (CHF, Killip class is ≥3)
- Dx in doubt

Glycoprotein IIb/IIIa Inhibitors

Abciximab	0.25 milligram/kg bolus followed by infusion of 0.125 microgram/kg/min (maximum, 10 micrograms/min) for 12–24 h.
Eptifibatide	180 micrograms/kg bolus followed by infusion of 2.0 micrograms/kg/min for 72–96 h.
Tirofiban	0.4 micrograms/kg/min for 30 min followed by infusion of 0.1 microgram/kg/min for 48–96 h.

P2Y$_{12}$ Inhibitors

Clopidogrel	Load: 600mg Daily: 75mg Onset: 2-6h depending on loading dose Duration: 3-10d
Prasugrel	Load: 60mg Daily: 10mg Onset: 30min Duration: 7-10d W/d before surgery: 7d
Ticagrelor	Load: 180mg Twice a Day: 90mg Onset: 60min Duration: 3-5d W/d before surgery: 5d

Anistreplase	30 units IV over 2–5 min.
Alteplase	Body weight >67 kg: 15 milligrams initial IV bolus; 50 milligrams infused over next 30 min; 35 milligrams infused over next 60 min. Body weight <67 kg: 15 milligrams initial IV bolus; 0.75 milligrams/kg infused over next 30 min; 0.5 milligram/kg infused over next 60 min.
Reteplase	10 units IV over 2 min followed by 10 unit's IV bolus 30 min later.

Contraindications to fibrinolytic therapy

Absolute	Relative
Active internal bleeding	BP > 180/110
History of CNS hemorrhage	Recent internal bleeding
Ischemic stroke within 3 mo.	Prolonged CPR (<10m)
Head trauma within 3 mo.	Pregnancy
CNS neoplasm	Surgery in past 3 weeks
Known AVM	
Suspected AD	

- **Post Catheterization/PCI**
  - Immediate Care
    - Check groin for oozing, bleeding, hematoma, or bruit.
      - Oozing: direct pressure for at least 10 minutes, pressure bandage.
      - Bleeding: manual compression ASAP and contact cath team. Consider FemoStop®.
      - Hematoma: check HCT, platelets, type and cross. Outline borders in ink, document lower limb neuro exam, follow size, and ensure blood bank sample and IV access.
      - Treat as medically indicated. For groin bleeding, apply direct pressure
      - CBC, platelets, and type and cross STAT to monitor HCT and to rule-out immune mediated thrombocytopenia
      - Transfuse PRBC, FFP, and platelets as indicated. For abciximab (ReoPro) consider platelet transfusions even if platelet count is normal; for eptifibatide (Integrilin) consider platelets only if patient thrombocytopenic
  - Procedures
    - TTE or stress testing not typically required unless patient has new chest pain and question if its cardiac in etiology
  - Consults
    - Cardiac Rehab[144]
  - Counseling
    - *Smoking*: all ACS patients who smoke should be counseled to quit smoking. Document this in the medical record.
    - *Diet*: all ACS patients should be counseled on a diet low in saturated fat and cholesterol.
      - Provide the patient with educational materials if available.
  - Medications
    - **ASA** 325mg for 1 month then 81mg/d indefinitely
      - In patients with concurrent AF, consider only P2Y12+apixiban[145] or NOAC (Rivaroxaban) alone without ASA, 12 months after intervention in those with atrial fibrillation *(AFIRE)*
    - **ACEi** (*GISSI-3; ISIS-4*)
      - Indicated if CHF or LV dysfunction present
      - Titrate to maximal dose
      - Zofenopril+ASA combination was found to be superior than Ramipril+ASA combination in patients post MI with LVEF<40% (*SMILE-4*)
    - **β-Blocker**
      - Expert opinion is to continue **for 1-3 years if normal EF**, no clear benefit after (*REACH registry and ISIS-1*)
      - In patients with LV dysfunction, long term treatment recommended
      - Most evidence supports use of propranolol, timolol, and metoprolol.
    - **Aldosterone Antagonists**
      - *Eplerenone* (if concomitant HF with EF<40% that is symptomatic or concomitant DM)[146]
    - **Heparin/Lovenox**
      - Continued for DVT prophylaxis
      - Lovenox 40mg SQ daily
      - Heparin 5000U TID
    - **Statin**
      - Atorvastatin 80mg daily or Rosuvastatin 40mg/d regardless of LDL level however in patients with an LDL on admission of <50, may consider starting on low dose. Add ezetimibe if further reduction in LDL desired (LDL remains above 70) in very-high risk patients.

- **GB2B3A**
  - Decided by cardiology
  - Abciximab: 0.25-mg/kg IV bolus, then 0.125 mcg/kg/min (maximum 10 mcg/min)
  - Tirofiban: (high-bolus dose): 25-mcg/kg IV bolus, then 0.15 mcg/kg/min
  - Eptifibatide: 180-mcg/kg IV bolus, then 2 mcg/kg/min; a second 180-mcg/kg bolus is administered 10 min after the first bolus
- **P2Y12 Inhibitors**
  - Plavix is the only P2Y12 inhibitor approved for triple therapy use (when treating for AFib) by combining with warfarin (INR goal 2.0-2.5)
  - P2Y12 Inhibitor (12 months minimum for DES; 1 month for BMS)
    - Plavix 75mg daily or Ticagrelor 90mg BID if ischemia driven NSTEMI or ACS for 12 months
    - Plavix 75mg/d, Prasugrel 10mg daily or Ticagrelor 90mg BID x12m in those receiving BMS or DES
- **Anticoagulation for Stents**
  - Overview[147] - The risk of coronary stent thrombosis is approximately 0.7% and is increased with early discontinuation of dual antiplatelet therapy (aspirin and clopidogrel).
  - Choosing
    - *DES* has a lower rate of repeat target vessel revascularization but requires longer-term platelet blocker therapy to prevent stent thrombosis. As a result, the risk of major bleeding on long term dual antiplatelet therapy is higher
    - *BMS* should be used when:
      - Patients are not a candidate for DES for technical reasons.
      - Patient is not likely to comply with recommended 12 months of dual antiplatelet therapy
      - Patient will require surgery (requiring cessation of dual antiplatelet therapy) in the coming year.
      - Patient is a high risk of bleeding

Anticoagulation Management in ACS[148]		
Indication	Recommended loading and maintenance dose	Recommended duration of therapy
Medical Management	Plavix 75mg/day Prasugrel 10mg daily Ticagrelor 90mg BID Cangrelor 4 mcg/kg/m	Depends on type of intervention 12 months 12 months 2h or duration of PCI
BMS	Plavix 600 mg load / 75 mg po daily Prasugrel 60mg load / 10mg daily Ticagrelor 180mg load / 90mg BID Cangrelor 30 mcg/kg load	ACS: minimum 1 year; may extend to 30 months if tolerated 12 months Non-ACS: Preferably 1 year; minimum 1 month in any case but push for 6 weeks; extend to 30 months if DAPT score ≥ 2
DES	Plavix 600 mg load / 75 mg po daily	ACS: minimum 1 year; extend to 30 months if DAPT score ≥ 2 Non-ACS: Preferably 1 year; minimum 6 months; ↓ to 3 months if surgical delay outweighs risk of thrombosis (urgent surgery)

- **PCSK9 Inhibitor**
  - Patients with angiographic evidence of nonobstructive coronary artery disease (20% to 50% stenosis in a target vessel) treated with statin and evolocumab after 76 weeks of treatment had significantly greater reduction in percent atheroma volume, as measured by serial intravascular ultrasound (*GLAGOV* trial)

CARDIOLOGY

- See *Hyperlipidemia* section for more details
- **Post Fibrinolysis**
  - ASA 81mg indefinitely
  - Plavix 75mg (at least 14 days, ideal 1 year)

MURMURS

Differential of Murmurs

Cause[147]	Characteristics	Location	Radiation	Findings	Serial Evaluation
Systolic					
AS	Crescendo-Decrescendo midsystolic	Base	Carotids	Accentuation Valsalva release Sudden squatting Passive leg raising Decrease Handgrip Valsalva Standing	Mild (Vmax <3 m/s, AVA >1.5 cm2) → yearly clinical exam Mod (Vmax 3-4 m/s, AVA 1-1.5 cm^2) → echo 1-2 year Severe (Vmax >4 m/s, AVA <1.0 cm^2) → echo every year
Pulmonic stenosis	Crescendo-decrescendo, midsystolic	Base	None	Valve opening click, right-sided S4	
HOCM	Crescendo, mid-or late systolic	Base	Carotids	Accentuation Valsalva strain Standing Decrease **Handgrip** Squatting Leg elevation	
Mitral Regurgitation	Holo- or late Systolic	Apex	Axilla or Back	Accentuation Sudden squatting **Isometric handgrip** Decrease Valsalva Standing	Mild (VC <0.3 cm, ROA <0.10 cm2, RV <30 mL/beat); normal EF mL/beat); EF normal; LV size normal → echo if sx Severe (VC_0.7 cm, ROA_0.4 cm2, RV_60 mL/beat, RF >50%) → echo q6-12mo
Tricuspid Regurgitation	Holosystolic	LLSB	LRSB	Accentuation Inspiration	

Diastolic				
Aortic Regurgitation	Decrescendo	LLSB	None	Passive leg raising _Decrease_ Expiration	Mild (VC <0.3 cm, ROA <0.10 cm2, RV <30 mL/beat) → echo q2-3y
				Increase Sudden squatting Isometric handgrip	Severe (VC >0.6 cm, ROA ≥0.3 cm2, RV ≥60 mL/beat, RF >50%) EF >50%; LV size normal → echo yearly
					EF >50%; LV size increased → echo q6-12mo
Mitral stenosis	Low-pitched Rumble	Apex	None	_Increase_ Exercise Left lateral position Isometric handgrip Coughing	
Tricuspid Regurgitation	Mid-diastolic Loud S2	LLSB	None	_Increase_ Inspiration Passive leg raising _Decrease_ Expiration	

CARDIOLOGY

CARDIOMYOPATHY

- **Definition**: disease of the myocardium resulting in ventricular dysfunction and clinical heart failure
- **Types**[149]
    - Ischemic – due to myocardial ischemia and infarction related CAD
    - Non-ischemic –
        - *Genetic* – HOCM, ARVD
        - *Mixed* – idiopathic dilated, restrictive
        - *Acquired* – inflammatory (myocarditis), peripartum, 2/2 ↑HR
        - *Secondary* – infiltrative (amyloid, hemochromatosis), toxin (EtOH, chemo), endocrine (↓thyroid), inflammatory (sarcoid), autoimmune (SLE, RA)
- **Evaluation**

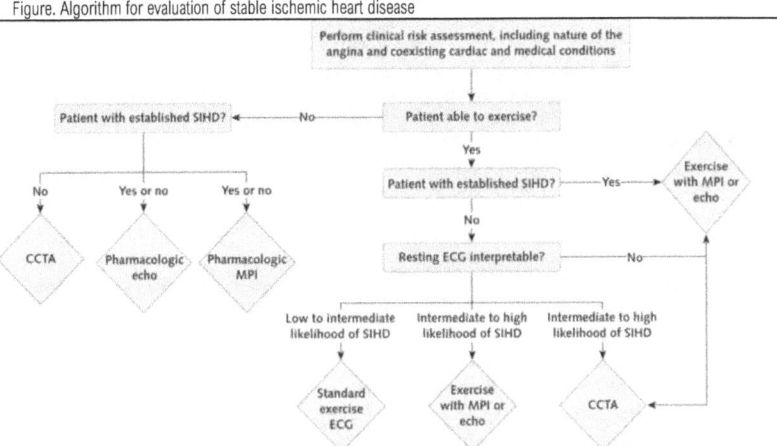

Figure. Algorithm for evaluation of stable ischemic heart disease

- TTE - Ejection fraction and functional capacity are frequently used markers of disease severity
- **Management**
    - The same as that for heart failure
    - Stable IHD should be managed medically *(ISCHEMIA)*
    - RX:
        - BB – carvedilol>metoprolol (*COMET trial*)
        - ACEi/ARB
            - Hydralazine+nitrate for those unable to take ACEi/ARB +/- AA descent (*A-HeFT trial*)
        - Aldosterone antagonist if NYHA>3
    - ICD (ventricular arrythmia, HF<35%+QRS prolonged, cardiac arrest)

HYPOTENSION

- **Causes**[150]
    - Hypovolemia: hemorrhage (internal or external), vascular dissection, GI losses, over-diuresis, post-dialysis, third spacing

- o Cardiogenic: MI, valvular dysfunction, arrhythmia
- o Obstructive: PE, tamponade, tension pneumothorax, atrial myxoma
- o Distributive: sepsis, anaphylaxis, medications, neurogenic, adrenal insufficiency
- **Evaluation**
  - o Any signs or symptoms of hypoperfusion or shock? (i.e. altered mental status, cool, clammy skin, diaphoresis, chest pain, ↓ urine output, ↓peripheral pulses) If so, call for back up and begin initial management listed below.
  - o Hypovolemia: volume status (mucous membranes, low JVP, skin turgor), post cath bleed, GI bleed, aortic dissection, LV free wall rupture s/p MI.
  - o Cardiac ischemia: chest pain, SOB, history of CAD, ECG
  - o Arrhythmia: pulse rate & rhythm, rhythm strip
  - o Tamponade: pulsus paradoxus, distant heart sounds, JVD, electrical alternans on ECG
  - o Pneumothorax: tracheal deviation, JVD, unequal breath sounds, hyperresonance
  - o Pulmonary Embolism: dyspnea, hypoxia, JVD, loud P2, RV strain/S1Q3T3 pattern on ECG (sinus tachycardia occurs in 80% of the time), see page 340
  - o Hemorrhage: GI, retroperitoneum, thigh, abdomen, pancreas, adrenal, hip or pelvic fracture
  - o Anaphylaxis: stridor, wheezing, urticaria, flushed skin, pruritus, angioedema
  - o Sepsis: fever or hypothermia, leukocytosis or leukopenia
  - o Adrenal insufficiency: history of steroid use, hypopituitarism, adrenal hemorrhage/infection/trauma
- **Specific Management**
  - o Cardiac ischemia: see acute MI protocol.
  - o Tamponade: call resident/cardiology fellow for emergent echo and pericardiocentesis
  - o Pneumothorax
    - SOB and or rim of air >2cm on CXR?
      1. If yes then place 14 or 16 gauge needle into second intercostal space at midclavicular line ASAP. Call pulmonary fellow for chest tube placement/drain if aspiration does not relieve symptoms.
      2. If not, then discharge and outpatient review in 2-4 weeks
  - o Pulmonary Embolism: see page 340
  - o Bleeding: large bore IV, NS, blood product repletion, reverse any coagulopathy,
  - o Anaphylaxis: (see page 461)
  - o Sepsis: start broad spectrum ABx emergently (always double gram negative, and don't be afraid to give aminoglycosides) and pressors (Levophed > dopamine > vasopressin > Neo-Synephrine) as needed
  - o Adrenal insufficiency[151]: suspect in patients with ↑K, ↓Na, NAGMA who do not respond to multiple fluid boluses, AM cortisol <3 mcg/dL is **diagnostic**; hydrocortisone 100mg IV bolus then 200mg over 24 hours (50mg q6h), after attaining ACTH and AM cortisol (levels higher than 15-18 mcg/dL helps rule out condition). If need to later do adrenal testing, must withhold hydrocortisone for 24 hours. After patient is stable, obtain abdominal CT to evaluate for adrenal hemorrhage. Formal diagnosis requires ACTH stimulation test (determine primary cortisol deficiency, secondary low ACTH, or tertiary low CRH).
    - *ACTH stim test*: Starting at any time of the day, provide IM or IV injection of high dose 250 µg cosyntropin and measuring total serum cortisol at baseline, 30 minutes, and 60 minutes to assess the response of the adrenal glands.
      1. If the cosyntropin is IV, any value > than 18 to 20 µg/dL indicates normal adrenal function and excludes adrenal insufficiency.
      2. If IM is used, any value > than 16 to 18 µg/dL at 30 minutes post-cosyntropin excludes adrenal insufficiency.
      3. The ACTH stimulation test may not exclude acute secondary or tertiary adrenal insufficiency.

- Patients who have the diagnosis require chronic treatment with oral hydrocortisone and fludrocortisone.

HYPERTENSION

- **Diagnosis** – high measurements on two or more occasions separated by time (1-2 min apart). Confirm stage 1 within 1-4 weeks but can start prescription medication immediately if patient presents in stage 2. Masked hypertension can be evaluated with ambulatory blood pressure testing.
  - Pregnancy: dx of HTN prior to pregnancy or in the undx, a BP >140/90 before 20w gestation.

Classifying BP		
Category	SBP	DBP
Normal	<120	<80
Elevated	120-129	<80
Stage 1 HTN	130-139	80-89
Stage 2 HTN	≥140	≥90
Ambulatory BP Monitor (ABPM)		
Daytime (awake)	140	90
Nighttime (sleep)	125	75
24 hour average	135	85
Non-dipper	Does not fall >10% at night	

*based on average of ≥2 careful readings obtained on ≥2 occasions

Etiologies
  - Essential: 30% of adults; only ½ may achieve target BP
  - Secondary: should consider in patients <30 (that are non-obese, nonblack, without family history) or sudden onset HTN or refractory (see page 219)[152]
  - Pregnancy: pre-eclampsia (high risk in first pregnancy, concurrent DM, twins). Look for concurrent HA, scotomas, renal disease (proteinuria), edema (face, hands), abdominal pain.

Conditions to consider in secondary hypertension			
	Conditions	Examination	Workup
Renal	Parenchymal (2-3%)	DM history	UA
	Renovascular (1-2%)	PCKD	SCr
	-Atherosclerosis	GN	UCx
	-Fibromuscular dysplasia		Urine albumin/protein
	-Polyarteritis nodosa		Evaluate for RAS only if ↓GFR
	-Scleroderma		also noted
Endocrine	Hyperaldosteronism (1-5%)	ARF secondary to ACEi/ARB	MRA w/ gad
	Crushing's (1-5%)	Flash pulm edema	CT angio
	Pheochromocytoma (<1%)	Renal bruit	TSH
	Myxedema (<1%)	↓K	Renal artery duplex US
	Hypercalcemia (<1%)		24-hr urinary free cortisol
	Thyroid dysfunction		24-hr urinary frx metneph
			Angio
			Aldosterone:renin ratio

CARDIOLOGY

Other	Pre-eclampsia
	Anxiety
	Pain
	Medication non-adherence
	Obstructive sleep apnea
	Alcohol
	Supplements (ginseng, ephedra, ma huang)
	Medications (OCP, steroids, NSAIDs, BuSpar, lithium, SNRI, decongestants)
	Psych (SSRI, clozapine)
	Aortic coarctation
	PCV

- **Labs** – lipids, sodium, potassium, calcium, TSH, uric acid, SCr, H/H, UA, ECG
- **High Risk Patients**
    - AA ethnicity
    - Pregnancy
    - LVH by electrocardiography (without critical coronary stenosis)
    - DM without orthostatic ↓BP
    - Prior stroke or TIA
    - Prior heart failure admissions
- **Goals**[153]

Hypertension Goals Based on Demographics		
Past Medical History Based Guidelines		
CHF, LVSD	<120/80	
CAD, AAA, PAD	<130/80	
CVA	<140/90 (previously dx/tx HTN)	
	<130/80 (lacunar, no h/o HTN)	
DM	<130/80 (ACC) <140/90 (ADA, JNC8)	
<60 CKD	<140/90	
>60	<150/90 (<140/90 if comorbid dz)	
Age		
<50	<120 (130 if high risk)	*SPRINT*
50-74	<130 (140 if DM)	>50 with h/o or high risk of CVD
≥75	<140	but no DM or TIA → restrictive to <120 goal
Patient Characteristics		
Nonblack	Thiazide CCB ACEi ARB	Level B
Black	Thiazide CCB	Level B
CKD	ACEi ARB	
Pregnancy		
SBP>160, DBP>105 mmHg		

- **Treatment**
    - Goal: <130/80
    - Taking antihypertensive medication at bedtime almost halves cardiovascular events (*Hygia Chronotropy Trial*)
    - Initial treatment should be based on 10 year risk assessment (www.cvriskcalculator.com) → if 130/80 and ≥10% -or- known CVD then treat with medication

- If less than 10% and no h/o CVD can trial lifestyle modifications for 3-6 months assuming no CKD, DM, and <65 YO

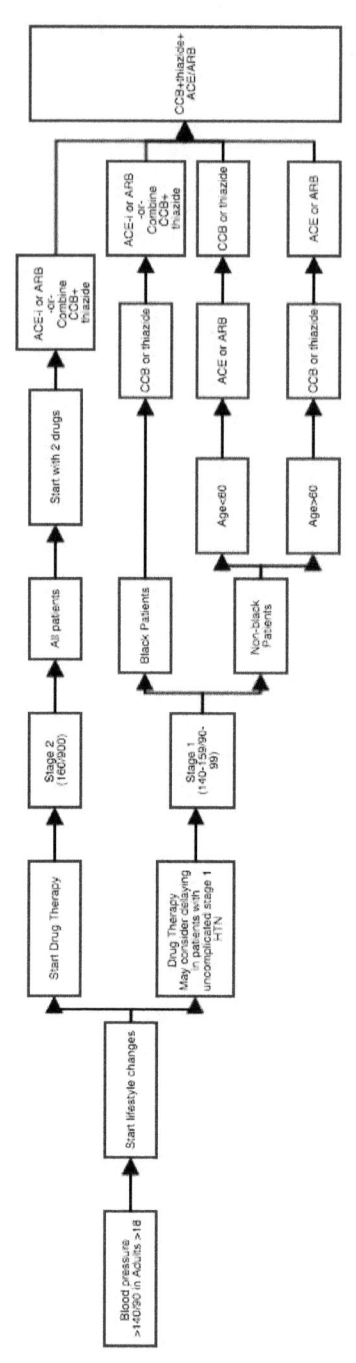

Treatment Decision				
Category	SBP	DBP	CVD Risk	Treatment
Normal	<120	<80	N/A	Healthy Lifestyle
Elevated BP	120-129	<80	N/A	Nonpharm Tx
Stage 1 HTN	130-139	80-89	ASCVD <10%	Nonpharm Tx
	130-139	80-89	ASCVD ≥10% -or- h/o CVD	Anti-HTN Tx
	130-139	80-89	DM, CKD, Age≥65	
Stage 2 HTN	≥140	≥90	N/A	(two medications recommended if Stage ≥2)

- o Treatment on Wards (IV Therapy)
  - ↑BP ↑HR
    - □ Labetalol 10 mg IV prn Q4hours
    - □ Lopressor (Metoprolol) 2.5-5 mg IV Q 6 hours OR 25 mg PO x1
    - □ IV Lasix
  - ↑BP ↓HR: Hydralazine 10 mg IV Q6H prn
  - Other Options
    - □ Furosemide 20mg PO daily
    - □ Clonidine 0.2mg/week
    - □ Captopril 6.25 mg PO TID (if normal K+ and Creatinine)
- o Diet Changes
  - Encourage healthy lifestyles for all individuals.
  - Prescribe lifestyle modifications for all patients with prehypertension and hypertension.
  - Components of lifestyle modifications include weight reduction, DASH eating plan, dietary sodium reduction, aerobic physical activity, and moderation of alcohol consumption
    - □ DASH can reduce BP by 11 mmHg
    - □ Active lifestyle can reduce BP by 2-5/1-4 mmHg
    - □ Moderate weight loss (>5%) can reduce BP by 5 mmHg
- o Essential/Benign[154]
  - See table on next page
  - Dose HS rather than AM leads to better CV outcomes
- o Pregnancy
  - *Chronic Hypertension*
    - □ See above for BP targets to initiate tx
    - □ *First choice:* Methyldopa
    - □ *Second choice:* Labetalol, hydralazine, CCB
    - □ *Avoid:* Atenolol (intrauterine growth retardation reported), diuretics, nitroprusside, ACEi, ARB
  - *Eclampsia*
    - □ Treatment options the same as those for chronic HTN above
    - □ Consider seizure prophy with Mg Sulfate IV
- o Combination hypertension treatments
  - *Preferred combinations*
    - □ ACEI + thiazide (likely more effective than combination with CCB; *LEGEND-HTN)*
    - □ ACEI + dihydropyridine CCB
    - □ ARB + thiazide
    - □ ARB + dihydropyridine CCB
  - *Acceptable combinations*
    - □ CCB + thiazide
    - □ Thiazide + K+-sparing diuretic
    - □ Aliskiren + thiazide or CCB
    - □ β-blocker + diuretic or dihydropyridine CCB

Pharmacologic Treatment of Essential Hypertension

Drug Class	Usual Dose	Indications	Side Effects
Thiazide			
Chlorthalidone	12.5-25mg/d	First-line or add-on	Hyponatremia, hypokalemia, orthostasis; not effective if GFR<30
HCTZ	12.5-50mg/d	Better BP reduction than ACEi *(LEGEND-HTN)*	
Indapamide	1.25-2.5mg/d	High quality evidence showed ↓mortality, cardiac events, stroke, and CAD	
Metolazone	2.5-5 mg once daily		
ACE Inhibitors			
Benazepril	5-80mg/d in one or two doses	First line or add on; CKD with albuminuria, CHF, post MI	Hyperkalemia
Enalapril	10-15mg/d		Angioedema
Fosinopril	10-80mg/d in one or two doses	ACEi specific: Low to moderate quality evidence showed ↓mortality, stroke, CAD	
Lisinopril	5-40mg/d		
Moexipril	7.5-30mg/d in one or two doses	ARB specific: good choice for gout patients and those intolerant to ACE inhibitors	
Perindopril	4-16mg/d in one or two doses		
Ramipril	2.5-20mg/d in one or two doses		
ARBs			
Candesartan	8-32mg/d in one or two doses		
Irbesartan	150-300mg/d		
Losartan	50-100mg/d in one or two doses		
Telmisartan	20-80mg/d		
Valsartan	80-320mg/d		
Loop			
Bumetanide	0.5-2 mg/day in 2 divided doses		
Furosemide	20-80 mg/day in 2 divided doses		
Torsemide	2.5-10 mg once daily		

Pharmacologic Treatment of Essential Hypertension

Drug Class	Usual Dose	Indications	Side Effects
Combination medications			
ACE+thiazide			
Captopril/HCTZ	25/15 25/25 50/15 50/25	Take 1hr before meals. Adjust at 6wk intervals. Usual max 150mg captopril, 50mg HCTZ daily.	
Benazepril/HCTZ	10/12.5 20/12.5 20/25	Switching from monotherapy with either component: initially 10/12.5mg once daily; may increase after 2–3wks as needed up to max 20/25mg daily.	
Lisinopril/HCTZ	10/12.5 20/12.5	Not for initial therapy. Initially 10mg/12.5mg or 20mg/12.5mg; increase HCTZ dose 2–3wks after. Max 80mg/50mg daily. CrCl <30mL/min: not recommended.	
ARB+thiazide			
Losartan/HCTZ *(Hyzaar)*	50/12.5 100/12.5 100/25	May increase after 3wks as needed to max 100/25mg daily	
Telmisartan/HCTZ *(Micardis HCT)*	40/12.5 80/12.5 80/25	Not for initial therapy. May titrate up to 160mg/25mg after 2–4wks. Severe renal or hepatic impairment: not recommended.	
Valsartan/HCTZ	80/12.5 160/12.5 160/25 320/12.5 320/25	Add-on or initial therapy and not volume-depleted: initially 160mg/12.5mg once daily; may increase after 1–2wks up to max 320mg/25mg daily.	
CCB+ACEi			

Pharmacologic Treatment of Essential Hypertension

Drug Class	Usual Dose	Indications	Side Effects
Amlodipine/benazepril	2.5/10 5/10 5/20 5/40 10/20 10/40	Unable to achieve BP control with amlodipine without developing edema: Initially 2.5mg/10mg once daily; may titrate up to 10mg/40mg once daily if BP remains uncontrolled. CrCl ≤30mL/min: not recommended.	
CCB			
Dihydropyridine			
Amlodipine	5-10mg/d	First line or add on therapy; minimal effect on CO	Edema of the legs, may worsen proteinuria
Felodipine	2.5-10mg/d		
Nicardipine ER	5-20mg/d		
Nifedipine ER	30-120mg/d in one or two doses		
Non dihydropyridine			
Diltiazem SR	180-360mg/d in one or two doses	Tachycardia; LVOT obstruction, migraine prophylaxis	Constipation, heart block if used with BB
Verapamil SR	120-480mg/d in one or two doses		
BB with sympathomimetic activity			
Acebutolol	200-1200mg 1-2 doses	Indications - myocardial infarction, angina	Contraindications - asthma, chronic obstructive pulmonary disease (COPD) however cardioselective are okay such as atenolol, bisoprolol, metoprolol, heart block
Penbutolol	10-80mg/d		
Pindolol	10-60mg/d		
BB without intrinsic sympathomimetic activity			
Atenolol	50-100mg/d		
Betaxolol	5-20mg/d		
Bisoprolol	5-20mg/d		
Toprol XL	25-400mg/d	Cardioselective	
Lopressor	25-200mg in 1-2 doses		
Nadolol	20-320mg/d	Not cardioselective	
Propranolol	40-240mg/d in 2 doses	Not cardioselective	

Pharmacologic Treatment of Essential Hypertension

Drug Class	Usual Dose	Indications	Side Effects
Potassium-sparing diuretics			
Amiloride	5-10mg/d in 1-2 doses		
Triamterene	50-100mg in 1-2 doses		
Aldosterone antagonists			
Eplerenone	50-100mg/d	May increase to 50 mg twice daily if needed after 4 weeks; initial dose 25 mg once daily if concomitant weak CYP3A4 inhibitors (erythromycin, verapamil, saquinavir, fluconazole)	
Spironolactone	25-50mg/d		
Others			
Clonidine	PO: 0.1mg BID-0.2mg BID Patch: 0.1mg applied for 24h qweek		
Minoxidil	5-10mg/d		
Hydralazine	25-100mg BID		

CARDIOLOGY

- Hypertensive Crises (3/4 are urgency, ¼ are emergency)[155]
  - Understand that oscillometric devices (and manual) are likely underestimating blood pressure by up to 50/30 mmHg in comparison to intraarterial when BP levels exceed 180/100
  - **Hypertensive Urgency**
    - Defined
      1. BP≥180/110 without evidence of end-organ damage
    - General
      1. No evidence to support treatment of patients with asymptomatic hypertensive urgency; can f/u in 1-7 days after adjusting long-acting medications as needed
         - If they have nonspecific symptoms, can give rapid acting oral rx while also adjusting long acting medications as needed
         - Safe to discharge when BP <180/110 mmHg
         - Follow up in 1-7 days
      2. No indication to treat with IV medications; review home medications (if applicable) and slowly start PO medications over 24-72 hours
    - Causes – pain, EtOH w/d, volume overload, missed rx, increased Na, NSAID use, high-dose steroids, anxiety, CHF
    - Goal: If no other conditions exist, then reduce mean blood pressure by 25% in first hour then reduce to goal SBP 160-180 in next 2-6 hours.
      1. Reach goal BP within 48 hours
    - Management (usually treated with short acting oral medications; *no inpatient admission required):*
      1. *Clonidine*: 0.2mg orally, followed by 0.1mg q hour to total of 0.8mg. Watch for sedation, bradycardia with AV nodal blockers. Onset in 30-60 minutes. Rebound hypertension if abruptly stopped.
      2. *Captopril* 12.5-25mg orally works in 15-30 minutes with variable episodes of excessive response. May increase to 50-100mg q90-120min
      3. *Metoprolol* 12.5-100mg PO BID (ok to start titrating 25 mg p.o. q6hrs x 48 hrs. -> then convert to BID). Try to avoid IV MTP as it lasts a short time. (2.5 mg PO MTP = 1 mg IV MTP)
      4. *Labetalol* PO 200-400mg
      5. *Topical Nitropaste* 1-2 inches to chest wall q6hr; wipe off for BP < (your parameter)
  - **Hypertensive Emergency**
    - Defined: BP≥180/110 *with end-organ damage*
    - End-Organ Injury (AKI, T2MI, ICH)
    - Signs/Symptoms
      1. *CNS*: AMS, seizure, stroke, irritability, ICH, PRES
         - *Preferred agents: labetalol, nicardipine, nitroprusside, clevidipine; avoid hydralazine*
      2. *Pregnancy*: eclampsia, or preeclampsia
      3. *Eyes*: blurred vision, papilledema, exudates, flame hemorrhages
      4. *Cardiac*: ACS, ECG strain or ischemic changes, pulmonary edema, SOB
         - *Preferred agents: NTG, labetalol, esmolol, metoprolol; avoid hydralazine*
         - *Preferred agents for CHF: NTG, nitroprusside, loop diuretics, hydralazine; avoid BB*
      5. *Vascular*: aortic dissection
         - *Preferred agents: esmolol, labetalol + nicardipine/Clevidipine/nitroprusside/or NTG; consider BB unless bradycardic*
      6. *Renal*: low urine output, edema, hematuria, azotemia

- Management
    1. Hypertensive emergencies require admission to ICU
    2. Start arterial line
    3. Initiate reduction of BP with IV medications, to reduce permanent organ dysfunction and death
    4. Per ACC/AHA 2017 guidelines, if above conditions present then reduce SBP to <140 in the first hour.
    5. Resume home meds within 6-12 hours of treatment
- Hypertensive Crisis
    - **Do not** reduce MAP > 20–25% over 30–60 min.
        1. Sodium Nitroprusside 0.5 mcg/kg/min to max (10 mcg/kg/min)

CARDIOLOGY

Pharmacologic management of hypertensive emergency

Drug	Dose	Onset	Information
IV Nicardipine	5-15mg/hr increased by 2.5mg/hr q5-15min up to max 30 mg/hr	≤5m	Good first choice agent Great for SAH, CVA (ischemic) Avoid in HF and known coronary ischemia Causes reflex tachycardia ↑ICP DOA 1-4h
IV Clevidipine	1-16mg/hour doubled q90s	≤1m	Good for most hypertensive emergency Avoid in Atrial fibrillation Avoid in soy allergy ↑CO DOA 5-15m
IV Labetalol	10-20mg bolus f/b 0.5-10mg/m IV infusion (can repeat bolus 10m after first dose before gtt) -or- 10-80mg q10min prn	5-10m	• First choice agent for patients with myocardial ischemia, acute aortic dissection, pregnancy, CVA • Most potent adrenergic blocker. • Favorable response in hypertension associated with pregnancy. • Do not lower BP too abruptly as sudden drop in BP may lead to cerebral and other organ hypoperfusion; goal is 25% reduction in mean arterial pressure or to reduce DBP to no lower than 100-110mmHg in first 12-24 hrs. • DOA 3-6h
IV Nitroprusside	0.25-10 mcg/kg/min IV titrated to 8-10mcg/min and adjusted by 0.5 mcg/kg/m q5m	1-2min	• Not often first line due to tendency to overshoot BP goal, risk of cyanide toxicity, and ↑ICP • C/I in pregnancy • Arteriolar and venous dilation • Toxicity with thiocyanate and cyanide metabolite must be considered with several days of therapy and with renal and hepatic insufficiency
IV Esmolol	500-1000mcg/kg loading (80mg) over 1 minute, then continue infusion at 100-300 mcg/kg/min adjusting by 50mcg/kg/m q5m	2-10m	• Short acting • Titratable • Good for aortic dissection • DOA 10-30m
IV Hydralazine	5-20mg q15-20m then q3-4h	10-20m	• Good for pregnancy/eclampsia • Avoid in ischemia pts (coronary steal) • DOA 3-6h
IV Nitroglycerin	5mcg/min titrated up to 100mcg/min	1-5m	• First choice agent for patients with myocardial ischemia • May cause Venous dilation
NTG	10-400 mcg/m adjusted by 10-20mcg/m q5-15m	5-10m	• C/I in RV infarction • Prolonged use may lead to diminishing effect

CARDIOLOGY

RESISTENT HYPERTENSION

- **Define**
  - JNC 7 and AHA define resistant hypertension as the failure to reach target BP despite treatment with 3 concurrent antihypertensive medications.
  - Both JNC 7 and AHA require that each medication should be from a different class of antihypertensive medications, with 1 medication from the diuretic class, and that all medications should have been optimally dosed.
    - Data from large clinical trials of antihypertensive therapy place the prevalence at 13% to 54%
- **Population** - Patients have higher risk for stroke, MI, CHF, and CKD
- **Causes**
  - Nonadherence to prescribed medications and the white coat syndrome are the 2 main reasons for failure to control BP.
    - White coat syndrome can be ruled out by performing 24-hour ambulatory BP monitoring (ABPM) or home BP monitoring.
    - Officially diagnosed if office blood pressure is $\geq$ 140/90 and 24 hour average of ABPM is $\leq$ 130/80
  - Excessive dietary salt and alcohol consumption as well as nonsteroidal anti-inflammatory drugs (NSAIDs), sympathomimetic agents (e.g., decongestants, diet pills, and cocaine), and stimulants (e.g., methylphenidate, dexmethylphenidate, dextroamphetamine, amphetamine, methamphetamine, and modafinil) can all elevate BP.
  - Some forms of secondary hypertension, are more common in individuals with resistant hypertension, including **obstructive sleep apnea, chronic kidney disease, primary aldosteronism, and renal artery stenosis.**
- **Treatment**
  - The first 3 agents recommended by treatment guidelines for the management of hypertension include a diuretic, a CCB, and an ACE inhibitor or an ARB, either as monotherapy or as combination therapy.
  - At equivalent doses, chlorthalidone is a more effective BP-reducing agent than hydrochlorothiazide.
    - It also has a longer duration of action.
  - **Beta-blockers or alpha blockers** may be used as fourth agents after inadequate BP control on CCB + ACE inhibitor + diuretic combination therapy. **Mineralocorticoid receptor antagonists (MRAs), spironolactone** or eplerenone, are also often recommended as the fourth agent in individuals with resistant hypertension. They are especially helpful in patients with concomitant **OSA**. Eplerenone may be a better option as it **does not** have the gynecomastia effects like spironolactone.

AORTIC STENOSIS

- **Define** – left ventricular outflow obstruction across the aortic valve due to pathologic narrowing from calcification. It is usually progressive in nature.[156]
- **Risk factors**
  - Age>60
  - Genetic
  - Anatomical (bicuspid valve accounts for 60% of cases)
  - Clinical (h/o rheumatic dz, CAD, HLD, tobacco, T2DM, h/o mediastinal irradiation, CRF)
- **Symptoms**
  - Classic triad of symptoms are: CHF, angina, and syncope

- patients may be asymptomatic but can progress to decreased exercise capacity, exertional chest pain (angina), heart failure, fatigue, weakness, and syncope.
- **Examination**
    - Crescendo-decrescendo SEM at the RUSB radiating to the carotid arteries and delayed diminished carotid pulse
        - Time to peak intensity correlates with severity (later peak = more severe)
    - Displaced PMI
    - Evidence of heart failure
- **Severity** – determined by different measurements on echocardiography:
    - Maximum transvalvular velocity: (≥4m/s in severe cases)
    - Mean transaortic pressure gradient

Stages of Progression in Aortic Stenosis				
Stage	Degree	Description	Defined	Management
A	Normal	Asymptomatic, at risk	Aortic-valve sclerosis or bicuspid valve; Vmax of <2 m/sec	Primary prevention, patients have 50% increased risk of MI
B	Mild/Moderate	Progressive	Mild/moderate calcification; -Vmax of 2-3.9 m/sec -MTAPG 20 to 39 mm Hg	Primary prevention TTE q1-2y if moderate AS (Vm 3-3.9m/s) TTE q3-5y if mild AS (Vm 2-2.9m/s)
C	Severe	C 1 Remains asymptomatic but severe AS noted but normal LVEF C 2 As above but now with LVEF<50%	Severe valve calcification; -Vmax ≥4m/s -MTAPG≥40mmHg -EF varies depending on stage	Monitor q6m clinically with TTE done yearly. If patients have severe AS but remain asymptomatic, can consider treadmill exercise testing. In patients with Stage C(2), AV replacement recommended to preserve what LV function is left
D	Very Severe	D 1 Symptomatic, severe, high-gradient stenosis D 2 Symptomatic, severe, low-gradient stenosis with reduced EF D 3 Symptomatic, severe, low-flow and low-gradient stenosis with nml EF	Severe calcification with reduced leaflet motion -Vmax ≥ 4m/s (type 1; less if type 2 or 3) -MTAPG ≥ 40 mmHg	Prompt AVR is only therapy advised in Type 1, if type 2 and 3, AVR is reasonable in symptomatic patients

MTAPG = mean transaortic pressure gradient

- **Management**
    - Always control underlying risk factors (diabetes, hypertension, dyslipidemia)
    - Those who are asymptomatic (no chest pain, exertional dyspnea, syncope, dizziness) with normal EF often are followed clinically despite severity of valve disease
    - ECG – can obtain at any point, evaluate for e/o LVH (seen in 90% of patients), atrial fibrillation, LAE

- o CXR – cardiomegaly, calcification of the aorta/valve
- o Cardiac Catheterization
  - In symptomatic patients with SEM and inconclusive AS on TTE or the severity of symptoms does not correlate with non-severe AS findings on TTE
- o Exercise Stress Testing
  - Can help risk stratify in those with symptom-limited stress testing in otherwise asymptomatic patients with severe AS based on Vm (≥4m/s or MTAPG≥40mmHg)
  - → look to provoke symptoms or look for a drop in BP/poor exercise capacity
- o Echocardiograms
  - Look for valvular abnormality (tricuspid vs bicuspid), can calculate valve area, peak gradients, transvalvular mean
  - Stage A: follow clinically
  - Stage B: TTE q1-2y if moderate AS (Vm 3-3.9m/s); extend to q3-5y if mild AS (Vm 2-2.9m/s)
  - Stage C: Q6-12mo in asymptomatic patients
- o Aortic Valve Replacement
  - Presence or absence of symptoms related to AS is key
  - AVR has shown to prolong life in those with symptomatic severe AS (Vmax≥4m/s)

ATRIAL FIBRILLATION

Section Editor: Kourtney Aylor, DO

- **Definition** - Irregular ventricular rate in the absence of P waves or well-defined flutter waves in all leads
- **Classifications**
  - o Paroxysmal AF - recurrent AF (≥2 episodes) that terminates spontaneously within 7 days
  - o Persistent AF - sustained beyond 7 days
  - o Long-standing persistent AF - continuous AF >1 year.
  - o Permanent AF - AF in which cardioversion either has failed or has not been attempted because the patient has decided not to pursue restoration of sinus rhythm by any means.
- **Etiology/Risk Factors**
  - o Idiopathic: Age, >BMI
  - o Pulmonary: COPD, PNA, OSA
  - o Cardiac: HTN (#1 cause), CAD, valvular disease, rheumatic heart disease, CHF, myocarditis, pericarditis, WPW (consider if HR>200)
  - o Idiopathic (common cause)/Ischemia (rarely causes Afib acutely)
  - o Metabolic: Ethanol, cocaine, amphetamines, stress, infection, post-operative state pheochromocytoma), thyrotoxicosis, DM
- **Symptoms**[157]
  - o Many patients are asymptomatic at diagnosis
  - o Most common symptom otherwise is palpitations
    - Others include fatigue, chest pain, tachycardia, syncope, presyncope
- **Work-up**
  - o History: EtOH, caffeine, stimulants, supplements, family history, recent surgery, medications
  - o Lab: TSH, Mg, K, CMP, cardiac enzymes
  - o Diagnostics: TTE, ECG, CXR
- **Screening**
  - o Currently, screening for AF not advised
- **Monitoring**
  - o Event, implantable, loop, Holter

- Short term (<30 days) monitoring is not enough time for detection of new dx of silent AF (*REACH AF*)
- **Immediate Treatment (summarized on next table)**
  1. *First determine stability*
     - Unstable: DCCV + anticoagulation
     - Stable: see table
  2. *Determine duration of AF if unstable*
     - if new AF for <48h then consider DCCV + anticoagulation
     - if new AF>48h then one of two options (1) anticoagulation x 4w →DCCV→ anticoagulation or (2) TEE to r/o LA thrombus then DCCV.
     - Otherwise if this is chronic, then treat per next section

Immediate treatment of Atrial fibrillation with RVR in the inpatient setting	
Scenario	Treatment
Unstable (i.e. ↓BP, ↓mentation, angina)	Direct Current Cardioversion • Synchronized DC (100J, 200J, 300J, 360J) • Requires 1 month of anticoagulation no matter the CHA2DS2-VASc score

Stable (goal HR<110)	No active COPD, asthma or CHF
	Rate Control Method
	Metoprolol/Lopressor 5mg IV over 2 min q5min x3 (contraindicated in COPD and acute decompensated HFrEF) with IV magnesium 4.5mg[158]
	• If initial stabilization is achieved with this, consider starting Metoprolol Tartrate PO (dosed as below) or succinate (daily dose)
	    o Total 5mg IV given → start 12.5mg PO Q6H
	    o Total 10mg IV given → start 25mg PO Q6H
	    o Total 15mg IV given → start 37.5mg PO Q6H
	    If further doses needed, can increase to 50mg PO Q6H
	• IV maintenance dose: 60-200 mcg/kg/min
	• Addition of Mg 4.5g may be useful addition for rate control
	
	Esmolol 50 mcg/kg/m infusion for 4 minutes then continue at 50 mcg/kg/m or if response subpar then increase every 4 minutes in 50mcg/kg incriments to max 200 mcg/kg/m
	
	Cardioversion
	• Consider elective electrical synchronized cardioversion 100 joules, then 200 then 360
	• Pretreatment with amiodarone, flecainide, ibutilide, propafenone, or sotalol can be useful to enhance direct current cardioversion and prevent recurrent AF
	• For patients with AF of 48-h duration or longer, or when the duration of AF is unknown, anti-coagulation (INR 2.0 to 3.0) is recommended for at least 3 wks. prior to and 4 wks. after cardioversion
	• Heparin should be administered concurrently by an initial intravenous injection followed by a continuous infusion (aPTT 1.5 to 2x control). Thereafter, oral anticoagulation (INR 2.0 to 3.0) should be provided for at least 4 wks., as for elective cardioversion.
	• For patients with AF of less than 48-h duration associated with hemodynamic instability, cardioversion should be performed immediately without anticoagulation.
	• Contraindicated if patient is hypokalemic!
	Active COPD
	Calcium Channel Blocker
	• Can pretreat with calcium chloride 200mg if worried about ↓BP
	• **Diltiazem** 0.25 mg/kg IV bolus (over 2 min) with IV magnesium 4.5mg.

- If no response after 15 minutes → either (1) give 2nd bolus at 0.35mg/kg IV, (2) start 5-10mg/h infusion, or (3) try giving 30mg PO IR q6h to see if you can avoid the need of a drip.
  - If response to 2nd bolus → convert to PO dosing 3 hours after 2nd bolus was given
  - If response to drip → convert to PO dosing at least 1 hour after infusion started
- Convert from drip to oral (give first dose 1 hr prior to decreasing gtt by 2.5mg/hr until off[159]
  - Oral dose (in mg per day) IR = [rate (mg/hr) x 3 + 3] x 10
    Divide above by 4 to dose q6h then can transition to ER dose
  - Standard conversion table:
    3 mg/hr IV = 120 mg daily (divided q6h)
    5 mg/hr IV = 180 mg daily (divided q6h)
    7 mg/hr IV = 240 mg daily (divided q6h)
    11 mg/hr IV = 360 mg daily (divided q6h)
    15 mg/hr IV = 480 mg daily (divided q6h)
- **Verapamil** 5-10mg IV over 2 min (can repeat in 30m)
  - PO: 120-360 mg/d in divided doses

Low blood pressure or Acute Decompensated Heart Failure (EF<40%)
Digoxin
- Can combine with Lopressor
- Load 0.25 mg IV q2h up to 1.5mg/24h, then 0.125mg-0.375mg PO/IV daily; check level after 3-4d in AM; slow onset of action; adjust dose in renal failure, with amiodarone, etc.
- Should be added to CCB or BB, NEVER used alone!
- Not considered effective rate control with atrial fibrillation (only provides control at rest)

Amiodarone *(CHF-STAT)*
- <u>IV</u>: 150mg bolus (IVPB); then 1mg/minute x 6 hours and 0.5mg/minute x 18 hours. If the HR remains >110 about 1 hour after bolus then can give 2nd bolus of 150mg IV while continuing drip
- PO (if conversion to NSR or after 24 hours)
  - Day 1: start 400mg PO BID
  - Day 2: continue at 200mg for 1-3 months (can decrease dose by 50% if HR<50)

- **Chronic Treatment**
  - *Rate Control*
    Goal is to achieve resting HR 60-80 and max HR 110; rate vs rhythm not important (AFFIRM trial)
    - <u>Beta-blocker</u> - Lopressor PO 12.5-25mg PO q6h
    - <u>Ca-channel blockers</u> (good option if pt has pre-existing pulm dz)
      - Diltiazem IR 60-90mg PO q4-6h *high doses can ↑ HF risk
      - Verapamil PO: 80-120mg q6-8h
    - <u>Digoxin</u> (good for patients that are hypotensive, can combine with Lopressor)
      - Daily dose is 0.125-0.25mg
      - Should be **added** to CCB or BB, NEVER used alone!
    - <u>Magnesium</u> - Addition of Mg 4.5g may be useful addition for rate control[160]

Antiarrhythmics for Atrial Fibrillation

Factors	Medication	Conversion Dose	Maintenance Dose	Pearls
HTN with LVH Known CAD Known CHF Paroxysmal AF Persistent AF	Amiodarone	5-7 mg/kg IV over 30-60m → 1 mg/min, 10g load	200-400 mg daily	↑QT, can lead to pulm, liver, and thyroid dz. ↑INR if taking warfarin
Known CAD Avoid in NYHA IV or NYHA II-III with recent decomp Avoid in perm AF	Dronedarone	N/A	400mg BID	↓s/e compared to amio; ↑liver tox, avoid in AECHF
Known CAD	Ibutilide	1 mg IV over 10 min; may repeat once	N/A	C/I if ↓K or ↑QT interval Pretreatment before cardioversion
	Sotalol	N/A	80-160 mg BID	May ↓HR, ↑QT interval
Known CAD Known CHF Struct nml heart	Dofetilide	500mcg PO BID	500 mcg BID	↑QT interval
No HTN, LVH, or ischemic heart dz	Flecainide Propafenone Procainamide	300mg PO once 600mg PO once 10-15 mg/kg IV over 1 h	100-150 mg BID 150-300mg TID N/A	May ↓BP, ↑QT interval

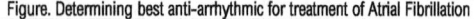

Figure. Determining best anti-arrhythmic for treatment of Atrial Fibrillation

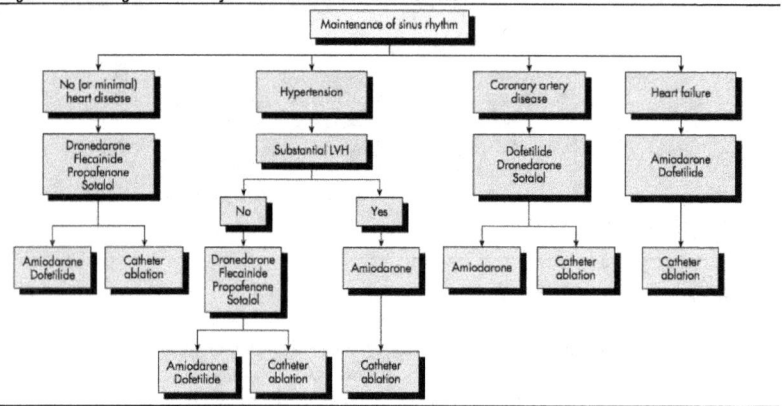

- Rhythm control (see table above also)
  - *Pharmacologic Options*
    1. **Known structural heart disease +/- CAD**
       - Amiodarone
         - Inpatient pharmacologic conversion: 150mg load x1 order (IVPB); Amio gtt AMOUNT: 900; comment: 1.8mg/ml (33.3ml/hr) x 6 hours then decrease to 0.5mg/min (16.6ml/hr) for 18 hours
           - <1 week – 800 – 1600mg PO/day
           - 1-3 weeks – 600-800mg PO/day
           - >3 weeks – 400mg PO/day
         - Outpatient pharmacologic conversion: 600-800mg daily for total load up to 10g then maintenance dose of 400-600 mg/d for 2-4 weeks f/b 100-200mg/d

- o S/e include ↓BP, bradycardia, QT prolongation, torsade's de pointes (rare), GI upset, constipation, phlebitis (IV)
- Ibutilide—risk of torsade's; use with guidance of Cardiology
- Can pursue catheter ablation as discussed below

2. *No structural heart disease or CAD*
   - Flecainide[161]: pill in the pocket approach (300mg if wt. >70kg and 200mg if <70kg); studied in patients who suffer from infrequent paroxysms, few symptoms, without known structural dz, arrhythmias, and hemodynamically stable when in AF
     - o IV dosing: 1.5-3.0 mg/kg over 10-20 min
   - Procainamide: 1gm IV over 1 hour, then Procan SR 750mg PO QID (daily dose 1g-4g); check for QT prolongation, QRS prolongation, ↓BP; follow procainamide and NAPA (toxic metabolite) levels (total level of 10-20 is therapeutic); be sure to give AV nodal blocking agent (e.g. Digoxin) first
   - Dofetilide: Must renal dose but can start at 500mcg BID (contraindicated if GFR<20). S/e include QT prolongation.
   - Dronedarone (used if paroxysmal or persistent, not permanent): 400-800mg PO BID WF
   - Sotalol 240-320mg

- Non-Pharmacologic Options

1. *Cardioversion*
   Indications: hemodynamic instability, angina, decompensated heart failure, ACS with new onset AFib
   - Can also be considered in patients nonresponsive to pharmacotherapy
   - AF onset within 48 hours (+ low risk for stroke):
     - o Cardioversion with anticoagulation x 4 weeks
       - Synchronized DC (100J, 200J, 300J, 360J)
     - o Anticoagulation can be withheld if CHA2DS2-VASc score (0 in men; 1 in women) both before and after cardioversion (IIb evidence)
   - AF onset after 48 hours (+/- high risk for stroke) or unknown duration:
     - o Can perform TEE and if no thrombus then cardiovert with 4 weeks of anticoagulation. If thrombus noted, then perform below:
       -or-
     - o Empiric oral anticoagulation for 3 weeks then perform cardioversion with 4 weeks of post cardioversion anticoagulation as well.

2. *Ablation*
   - Catheter radiofrequency ablation or balloon cryoablation (targeting pulmonary vein) is superior over AADs in paroxysmal and persistent AF.
   - Balloon cryoablation noninferior to radiofrequency ablation *(FIRE AND ICE)*
     - o Consider in patients with:
       - Individuals seeking to maintain sinus rhythm and who have an AF breakthrough while on AAD
       - Concomitant CHF and unable to tolerate antiarrhythmic therapy
       - Young adults thought to have AF d/t cardiac remodeling
       - Those who have persistent symptomatic AF despite treatment *(AATAC)*
   - Biventricular pacemaker implantation post AV node ablation is recommended in patients with medically refractory AF, symptomatic CHF, and low LVEF. *(PAVE)*

- **Anticoagulation**
  - o Primary vs. Secondary stroke prevention
  - o If not candidate for anticoagulation, can consider left atrial appendage closure device *(PROTECT AF)*
  - o When to initiate anticoagulation is based on stroke risk (CHA_2DS_2VASc score) and risk factors of major bleeding on anticoagulation (HASBLED, ABC, mOBRI, ORBIT, ATRIA)

- Balanced assessment tool: HAS-BLED
- High Sensitivity: ABC, mOBRI
- High Specificity: ORBIT, ARIA, Shireman, GARFIELD-AF
- **HAS-BLED**[162]

    Low:0; Moderate:1-2; High≥3
    - Hypertension
    - Abnormal Liver/Renal Function
    - Stroke History
    - Bleeding Predisposition
    - Labile INRs
    - "Elderly" (Age >65)
    - Drugs/Alcohol Usage
- **CHA2DS2VASc** (score ≥2 in men and ≥3 in women requires anticoagulation. See table below to calculate.

Scoring Risk of Stroke in AFib	
CHA_2DS_2-VASc Risk Criteria	Score
Congestive Heart Failure	1
Hypertension	1
Age > 75	2
DM	1
Prior stroke or TIA	2
Vascular Disease (prior MI, PAD, aortic plaque)	1
Age > 65-74	1
Gender (F)	1
MAX SCORE	**9**

- o Any pt with AF>48hours (or unknown) duration should be anticoagulated if no definitive contraindication (active hemorrhage, recent neurosurgery, recent hemorrhagic CVA, etc.) to prevent risk of thrombo embolization
    - Start with Heparin drip (see protocol under Hematology), then Coumadin
    - Pt must be therapeutic (INR 2-3) for 3 weeks prior to attempt at cardioversion and must remain on anticoagulation for 1 month subsequent to successful cardioversion
    - Patients requiring DAPT in combination with anticoagulation should be started on low dose ASA (100mg) and Plavix (75mg)
    - Alternatively get TEE to r/o atrial appendage clot and proceed with earlier cardioversion, still need to anticoagulate for **4 or more weeks post cardioversion**
- o Interrupting anticoagulation/DOAC for procedure: see table below
- o Choosing VKA vs DOAC
    - VKA
        1. Warfarin remains the standard of care for the management of patients with valvular AF or mechanical heart valves[163,164]
            - **Valvular AF** defined as:
                - o moderate or severe AS
                - o mechanical/bioprosthetic heart valve
                - o rheumatic heart disease with mitral stenosis
            - Patients with hepatic dysfunction or associated coagulopathies or impaired renal function (CrCl <30 mL/min per 1.73 m2) are not good candidates for NOACs owing to their hepatic metabolism and renal excretion.
    - NOAC (contraindicated in valvular AF)
        1. Obtain RFP and HFP prior to initiation
        2. If compliance is an issue, rivaroxaban, with its once-daily administration, might be a better choice than dabigatran or apixaban.

3. Dabigatran is best avoided in patients with ulcer/non ulcer dyspepsia given its tartaric acid core and described associations with GI adverse effects.
4. In patients with a recent history of GI bleeding, apixaban may be a better choice as it has a lower incidence of GI bleeding than dabigatran and rivaroxaban.
5. Given the recent association of dabigatran with a trend toward an increase in the incidence of myocardial infarction, rivaroxaban or apixaban should possibly be considered when selecting an NOAC in this subset of patients.
    - On the other hand, in patients with a history of ischemic strokes while taking warfarin, dabigatran and apixaban may be suitable alternatives as they are the only NOACs with a lower rate of ischemic stroke than warfarin.
- **Reversal Agents**
  - Dabigatran - Idarucizumab (*REVERSE AD*)
  - Rivaroxiban or Apixaban – Andexant alfa
  - Warfarin – Vitamin K

DOAC options approved by ACA/AHA

	MOA	Nonvalvular Afib	VTE/PE	VTE prophy	Convert from VKA	Best population	Side Effects	Preoperative Interruption
Dabigatran *Pradaxa*	Direct thrombin inhibitor	RE-LY SCr<30: 75mg BID SCr>30: 150mg BID	RE-COVER 150mg BID	RE-MODEL RE-NOVATE I Hip surgery prophylaxis: 110mg day 1 then 220mg daily for 28-35 days	When INR<2	Hx of TIA or CVA (superior to warfarin) For stroke while on Warfarin: 150mg BID	Dyspepsia Abdominal pain Diarrhea	High Risk Procedure: stop 3 days prior (4 if SCr≤50cc and 6 days if <30) Low Risk Procedure: stop 2 days prior (3 if SCr≤50cc and 4 days if <30)
Apixaban *Eliquis*	Factor XA inhibitor	AVERROES ARISTOTLE 5mg BID (or 2.5mg BID if any of the 2: age≥80, BW≤60kg or SCr≥1.5	10mg BID x 7d then 5mg BID	ADVANCE 2.5mg BID -Knee: x12 days -Hip: x35 days	When INR<2	Hx of MI ESRD Hx of TIA or CVA (superior to warfarin; also ↓ systemic embolization) Hx of PUD or GI bleed Fewer strokes and major bleeding than rivaroxaban[165]	Bleeding complications Nausea	High Risk Procedure: stop 3 days prior (4 if SCr≤30cc) Low Risk Procedure: stop 2 days prior
Rivaroxaban *Xarelto*	Factor XA inhibitor	ROCKET-AF SCr>50: 20mg/d SCr 30-50: 15mg/d	EINSTEIN EINSTEIN-PE 15mg BID x 3w then 20mg/d for 3-6m	10 mg daily -Knee: x12 days -Hip: x35 days	When INR<3	Hx of MI Hx of PUD Wants a once-daily dosing option	Itch HA	High Risk Procedure: stop 3 days prior (4 if SCr≤30cc) Low Risk Procedure: stop 2 days prior (3 if SCr≤30cc)
Edoxaban *Savaysa*	Factor XA inhibitor	60mg daily	10 days IV Lovenox then 60mg daily	Not FDA indicated	When INR<2.5	High overall bleed risk Dyspepsia Wants a once-daily dosing option	Dizziness HA Pain Nausea Itch	High Risk Procedure: stop 3 days prior (4 if SCr≤30cc) Low Risk Procedure: stop 2 days prior (3 if SCr≤30cc)

Low Risk Procedure: Colonoscopy, breast bx, minor orthopedic, cardiac cath | High Risk Procedure: Abdominal, Cardiac, Kidney, Neuro, Prostate, Spinal, and Vascular surgery

PACEMAKERS

- **Indications for Permanent Pacemaker**[166]
  - Guidelines for implantation of cardiac pacemakers have been established by a task force formed jointly by the American College of Cardiology, the American Heart Association, and the Heart Rhythm Society (ACC/AHA/HRS).
  - Symptoms
    - Dizziness, lightheadedness, syncope, fatigue, poor exercise tolerance all which may be due to bradyarrhythmias (SA node dysfunction)
    - AV node dysfunction may lead to PR prolongation, AV blocks
  - Sinus Node Dysfunction Indications
    - *Class I* — The following conditions are considered class I indications for pacemaker placement:
      - Sinus bradycardia in which symptoms are clearly related to the bradycardia (usually in patients with a heart rate below 40 beats/min or frequent sinus pauses).
      - Symptomatic chronotropic incompetence.
    - *Class II* — The following are considered to be class II, or possible, indications for pacemaker placement in patients with sinus node dysfunction:
      - Sinus bradycardia (heart rate <40 beats/min) in a patient with symptoms suggestive of bradycardia, but without a clearly demonstrated association between bradycardia and symptoms.
      - Sinus node dysfunction in a patient with unexplained syncope.
      - Chronic heart rates <40 beats/min while awake in a minimally symptomatic patient.
      - A less distinct group of patients with sinus bradycardia of lesser severity (heart rate >40 beats/min) who complain of dizziness or confusion that correlates with the slower rates.
  - AV Node Block Indications
    - AV block is the second most common indication for permanent pacemaker placement. Causes include the following: fibrosis and sclerosis of the conduction system, ischemic heart disease, digitalis, calcium channel blockers, beta blockers, amiodarone, increased vagal tone, valvular disease, congenital heart disease, cardiomyopathies, myocarditis, hyperkalemia, and infiltrating malignancies
    - *Class I Indications* — The following conditions represent severe conduction disease and are generally considered to be class I indications for pacing, regardless of associated symptoms:
      - Complete (third-degree) AV block*
      - Advanced second-degree AV block (block of two or more consecutive P-waves)
      - Symptomatic Mobitz I or Mobitz II second-degree AV block
      - Mobitz II second-degree AV block with a widened QRS or chronic bifasicular block, regardless of symptoms
      - Exercise-induced second or third degree AV block (in the absence of myocardial ischemia)
    - Current ACC/AHA/HRS guidelines classify asymptomatic third-degree AV block with average awake ventricular rates ≥ 40 beats/min, in a patient with normal left ventricular size and function, as a class IIA indication for permanent pacemaker implantation. Yet many cardiologists consider this condition a definite indication for pacemaker placement. The ACC/AHA/HRS guidelines consider asymptomatic complete AV block in the setting of cardiomegaly or left ventricular dysfunction to be a class I indication

- *Class II Indications* — Patients with less severe forms of acquired AV block may still benefit from pacemaker placement. In such patients, determinations are often based upon correlation of bradycardia with symptoms, exclusion of other causes of symptoms, and/or results of electrophysiology (EP) testing.
  - Other indications for possible pacemaker implantation:
    - Asymptomatic Mobitz II second-degree AV block with a narrow QRS interval; patients with associated symptoms or a widened QRS interval have a class I indication for pacemaker placement.
    - First-degree AV block when there is hemodynamic compromise because of effective AV dissociation secondary to a very long PR interval.
    - Bifasicular or trifascicular block associated with syncope that can be attributed to transient complete heart block, based upon the exclusion of other plausible causes of syncope (specifically ventricular tachycardia)
    - Patients that meet Class I indications for pacing after myocardial infarction, regardless of symptoms:
      - Third-degree AV block within or below the His-Purkinje system.
      - Persistent second-degree AV block in the His-Purkinje system, with bilateral bundle branch block.
      - Transient advanced infranodal AV block with associated bundle branch block.
    - Patients that meet class I indications in patients with neurocardiogenic syncope:
      - Significant carotid sinus hypersensitivity, defined by syncope and >3 seconds of asystole following minimal carotid sinus massage

Pacemaker Modes				
1st letter	2nd Letter	3rd letter	4th letter	
Chamber Paced	Chamber Sensed	Response to sensed beat	Program features	
Antitachycardia Function				
A	A	T	P	P (pacing)
V	V	I	M	S (shock)
D	D	D	C	D (dual shock+pace)
O	O	O	R	
			O	

A = atrium
V = ventricle
D = dual (both chambers)
O = none
T = triggered I = inhibited
R = rate adaptable available

Mode	Description
AAI	Demand atrial pacing: output inhibited by sensed atrial signals
AAIR	Demand atrial pacing: output inhibited by sensed atrial signals
	Atrial pacing rates ↓ and ↑ in response to sensor input up to the programmed sensor-based upper rate
VVI	Demand ventricular pacing: output inhibited by sensed ventricular signals
VVIR	Demand ventricular pacing: output inhibited by sensed ventricular signals.
	Ventricular paced rates ↓ and ↑ in response to sensor input up to the programmed sensor-based upper rate
VDD	Paces ventricle, senses in both atrium and ventricle
	Synchronizes w/atrial activity and paces ventricle after a preset AV interval up to the programmed upper rate
VDDR	Paces ventricle, senses in both atrium and ventricle
	Synchronizes w/atrial activity and paces ventricle after a preset AV interval up to the programmed upper rate; in absence of spontaneous atrial activity, functions as VVIR
DDD	Paces and sense in both atrium and ventricle
	Paces ventricle in response to sensed atrial activity up to the programmed upper rate
DDDR	Atrial and ventricular paced rates can both ↑ and ↓ in response to sensor input up to the programmed sensor-based upper rate

- o The first 3 letters are used most commonly. More modern pacemakers have multiple functions. A pacemaker in VVI mode denotes that it paces and senses the ventricle and is inhibited by a sensed ventricular event.
- o Alternatively, AAT mode represents pacing and sensing in the atrium, and each sensed event triggers the generator to fire within the P wave.
- o The DDD mode denotes that both chambers are capable of being sensed and paced. This requires two functioning leads, one in the atrium and the other in the ventricle. In the ECG, each QRS is preceded by two spikes. One indicating the atrial depolarization and the other indicating the initiation of the QRS complex. Given that one of the leads is in the right ventricle, a left bundle branch pattern may also be evident upon the ECG. Note that a two-wired system need not necessarily be in DDD mode, since the atrial or ventricular leads can be programmed off. Additionally, single tripolar lead systems are available that can sense atrial impulses and either sense or pace the ventricle.
- o Thus, this system provides for atrial tracking without the capability for atrial pacing and can be used in patients with atrioventricular block and normal sinus node function.
- **Early Pacemaker Complications**
  - o Pneumothorax (check CXR)
  - o Hematoma formation (especially if patient on anticoagulation)
  - o Lead perforation of RA or RV (suspect if hemodynamically unstable)
  - o Lead dislodgment or pacemaker failure (suspect if failure to sense or capture)

Bibliography

[88] DeSimone et al. Mayo Clin Pro. 2018.
[89] EKGS Made Simple: Bundle Branch Blocks" < https://sites.google.com/site/ekgsmadesimple/h-bundle-branch-blocks>
[90] Haji, Showkat. Right Ventricular Infarction—Diagnosis and Treatment. Clin. Cardiol. 23, 473–482 (2000)
[91] Emergency Nurses Association (ENA). "Translation into Practice: Right-sided and Posterior ECGs." December 2012.
[92] Edhouse J, Brady WJ, Morris F. ABC of clinical electrocardiography: Acute myocardial infarction-Part II. BMJ. 2002; 324: 963-6.
[93] MacKenzie, Ross M.D. "Poor R-Wave Progression" J Insur Med 2005;37:58–62
[94] American College of Physicians "In the Clinic: Heart Failure." Annals of Internal Medicine 1 June 2010
[95] Aurigemma, Gerard P. Diastolic Heart Failure. N Engl J Med 2004; 351:1097-1105 September 9, 2004
[96] Nicklas et al. Heart Failure: Clinical Problem and Management Issues. Prim Care Clin Office Pract 40 (2013) 17–42
[97] Brown, Jennifer. "Acute Decompensated Heart Failure." Cardiol Clin 30 (2012) 665–671

[98] Cullington D, Goode KM, Clark AL, Cleland JG. Heart rate achieved or beta-blocker dose in patients with chronic heart failure: which is the better target? Eur J Heart Fail. 2012 May 22

[99] American College of Physicians "In the Clinic: Heart Failure." Annals of Internal Medicine 1 June 2010

[100] Hollenberg et al. 2019 ACC Expert Consensus Decision Pathway on Risk Assessment, Management, and Clinical Trajectory of Patients Hospitalized With Heart Failure: A Report of the American College of Cardiology Solution Set Oversight Committee. Journal of the American College of Cardiology 2019 September 10.

[101] Butler et al. JAMA (2019).

[102] The American College of Cardiology and the American Heart Association Stages of Heart Failure

[103] Ellison DH. The Physiologic Basis of Diuretic Synergism: Its Role in Treating Diuretic Resistance. Ann Intern Med. ;114:886–894.

[104] Epocrates Online

[105] Oh SW, Han SY. Loop Diuretics in Clinical Practice. Electrolyte Blood Press. 2015;13(1):17–21. doi:10.5049/EBP.2015.13.1.17

[106] Imiela T, Budaj A. Acetazolamide as add-on diuretic therapy in exacerbations of chronic heart failure: a pilot study. Clin Drug Investig. 2017;37:1175–81.

[107] Jentzer et al. Combination of Loop Diuretics With Thiazide-Type Diuretics in Heart Failure. JACC. 56(19). 2010: 1527-1534.

[108] Channer KS, McLean KA, Lawson-Matthews P, Richardson M.Combination diuretic treatment in severe heart failure: a randomisedcontrolled trial. Br Heart J 1994;71:146 –50.

[109] Zhou X, Xu W, Xu Y, Qian Z. Iron supplementation improves cardiovascular outcomes in patients with heart failure. Am J Med. 2019.

[110] Evidence from the randomized, placebo- controlled CHARM (Candesartan Cilexitil [Atacand] in Heart Failure Assessment of Reduction in Mortality and Morbidity)- Alternative trial showed that the ARB candesartan decreased a combined end point of death from cardiovascular causes or hospitalization due to heart failure when compared with placebo in patients with left ventricular dysfunction who could not tolerate ACE inhibitors

[111] The CAPRICORN (Carvedilol Post-Infarct Survival Control in Left Ventricular Dysfunction) trial showed that the B-blocker carvedilol significantly reduced mortality in patients with left ventricular dysfunction with or without heart failure after MI and who also received ACE inhibitors, revascularization, and aspirin

[112] The MERIT-HF (Metoprolol CR/XL Randomized Intervention Trial-Heart Failure) randomly assigned 3991 patients with NYHA class II to IV heart failure to metoprolol CR/XL, up to 200 mg/d, versus placebo. All-cause mortality was reduced 34% (P < 0.001), and sudden death was reduced 59% (P < 0.001) for patients receiving metoprolol versus placebo

[113] Feenstra J et al. Association of nonsteroidal anti-inflammatory drugs with first occurrence of heart failure and with relapsing heart failure: The Rotterdam Study. Arch Intern Med 2002 Feb 11; 162:265-70.

[114] A-HeFT (African American Heart Failure Tri- al), which compared isosorbide plus hydralazine with placebo in African Americans with heart failure, showed that adding this therapy increased survival in those who were already taking other neurohormonal blockers, including ACE inhibitors and B-blockers

[115] ALES (Randomized Aldosterone Evaluation Study), a large, randomized, placebo- controlled trial involving 1663 patients with NYHA class III to IV heart failure on appropriate therapy with or without spironolactone, was halted 18 months early by the Data Safety Monitoring Board because there were significantly fewer deaths in the spironolactone group than in the placebo group (284 vs. 386 deaths; 35% reduction; P < 0.001)

[116] Verbrugge FH, Grieten L, Mullens W. Management of the cardiorenal syndrome in decompensated heart failure. Cardiorenal Med. 2014;4:176-88. PMID: 25737682

[117] The CARE (Cholesterol and Recurrent Events) trial found that pravastatin significantly reduced the incidence of heart failure, subsequent cardiovascular events, and mortality.

[118] ACC/AHA/HRS 2008 Guidelines for Device-Based Therapy of Cardiac Rhythm Abnormalities: Executive Summary

[119] Fihn SD, Gardin JM, Abrams J, et al. 2012 ACCF/AHA/ACP/AATS/PCNA/SCAI/STS guideline for the diagnosis and management of patients with stable ischemic heart disease: a report of the American College of Cardiology Foundation/American Heart Association Task Force on Practice Guidelines, and the American College of Physicians, American Association for Thoracic Surgery, Preventive Cardiovascular Nurses Association, Society for Cardiovascular Angiography and Interventions, and Society of Thoracic Surgeons. J Am Coll Cardiol. 2012;60(24):e44-e164.

[120] Raff et al. "SCCT guidelines on the use of coronary computed tomographic angiography for patients presenting with acute chest pain to the emergency department: A Report of the Society of Cardiovascular Computed Tomography Guidelines Committee." Journal of Cardiovascular CT. (2014). 254-271.

[121] Parikh et al. "Coronary artery calcium scoring: Its practicality and clinical utility in primary care." Cleveland Clinic Journal of Medicine. 2018 September;85(9):707-716.

[122] Six (2008) Neth Heart J 16(6):191-6 [PubMed]

[123] Lloyd-Jones DM, et al. J Am Coll Cardiol. 2017;70(14)1785-1822.

[124] Turgeon et al. JAMA. 2020.

[125] Diamond GA. A clinically relevant classification of chest discomfort. J Am Coll Cardiol 1983;1:574–575.

[126] Gibbons RJ, Balady GJ, Bricker JT, et al. ACC/AHA 2002 guideline update for exercise testing: A report of the American College of Cardiology/American Heart Association Task Force on practice guidelines (Committee on Exercise Testing). 2002. Available at: www.acc.org/qualityandscience/clinical/guidelines/exercise/exercise_clean.pdf. Accessed on March 6, 2007.

[127] Askew et al. Selecting the optimal cardiac stress test. UpToDate. Last update: 15FEB2013

[128] Garner et al. "Exercise Stress Testing: Indications and Common Questions." Am Fam Physician. 2017 Sep 1;96(5):293-299A.

[129] Snow V, Barry P, Fihn SD, et al. Primary care management of chronic stable angina and asymptomatic suspected or known coronary artery disease: A clinical practice guideline from the American College of Physicians. Ann Intern Med. 2004;141(7):562-767.

[130] Petrilli CM, Giacherio DA. Annals for Hospitalists Inpatient Notes - Clinical Pearls—A Middle-Aged Man With Pneumonia and Elevated High-Sensitivity Troponin Levels. Ann Intern Med. ;169:HO2–HO3. doi: 10.7326/M18-2296

[131] Sandoval, Y. et al. J Am Coll Cardiol. 2019;73(14):1846–60.

[132] Sandoval et al. JACC: 73(14). 2019.

[133] Stub D et al. Air versus oxygen in ST-segment–elevation myocardial infarction. Circulation 2015 Jun 16; 131:2143.

[134] Schupke et al. Ticagrelor or Prasugrel in Patients with Acute Coronary Syndromes. New England Journal of Medicine 2019 September 1

[135] Mehran R, Baber U, Sharma SK, et al. Ticagrelor with or without aspirin in high-risk patients after PCI. N Engl J Med. 2019;381:2032-42. 31556978

[136] O'Gara et al. "2013 ACCF/AHA Guideline for the Management of ST-Elevation Myocardial Infarction: Executive Summary: A Report of the American College of Cardiology Foundation/American Heart Association Task Force on Practice Guidelines." Circulation. 2013;127:529-555

[137] Spaulding CM, Joly LM, Rosenberg A, et al. Immediate coronary angiography in survivors of out-of-hospital cardiac arrest. N Engl J Med 1997; 336:1629-33.

[138] The ESPRIT Investigators. Novel dosing regimen of eptifibatide in planned coronary stent implantation (ESPRIT): a randomized, placebo-controlled trial. Lancet 2000;356:2037-44.

The PURSUIT trial investigators. Inhibition of platelet glycoprotein IIb/IIIa with eptifibatide in patients with acute coronary syndromes. N Engl J Med 1998;339:436-43.

Cohen M, Demers C, Gurfinkel E et al for the ESSENCE Trial. A comparison of lowmolecular-weight heparin with unfractionated heparin for unstable coronary artery disease. N Engl J Med. 1997;337:447-52.

Grines CL, Browne KF, Marco J et al. A comparison of immediate angioplasty with thrombolytic therapy for acute myocardial infarction. (PAMI-1). N Engl J Med 1993;328:673-9.

Antman EM, Cohen M, Bernink PJ, McCabe CH, Horacek T, Papuchis G, Mautner B, Corbalan R, Radley D, Braunwald E. The TIMI risk score for unstable angina/non-ST elevation MI: A method for prognostication and therapeutic decision making. JAMA. 2000;284:835-842.).

Braunwald E, Antman EM, Beasley JW, Califf RM, Cheitlin MD, Hochman JS, Jones RH, Kereiakes D, Kupersmith J, Levin TN, Pepine CJ, Schaeffer JW, Smith EE III, Steward DE, Theroux P. ACC/AHA guideline update for the management of patients with unstable angina and non-ST-segment elevation myocardial infarction: a report of the American College of Cardiology/American Heart Association Task Force on Practice Guidelines (Committee on the Management of Patients with Unstable Angina). 2002. Available at: http://www.acc.org/clinical/guidelines/unstable/unstable.pdf.).

Tcheng JE. Clinical challenge of platelet glycoprotein IIb/IIIa receptor inhibitor therapy: Bleeding, reversal, thrombocytopenia, and retreatment. Am Heart J 2000;139:S38-S45.

Yusuf S, Zhao F, Mehta SR, Chrolavicius S, Tognoni G, Fox KK; The Clopidogrel in Unstable Angina to Prevent Recurrent Events Trial Investigators. Effects of clopidogrel in addition to aspirin in patients with acute coronary syndromes without ST-segment elevation. N Engl J Med 2001 Aug 16;345(7):494-502.

Packer M, Poole-Wilson PA, Armstrong PW, Cleland JG, Horowitz JD, Massie BM, Ryden L, Thygesen K, Uretsky BF. Comparative effects of low and high doses of the angiotensinconverting enzyme inhibitor, lisinopril, on morbidity and mortality in chronic heart failure. ATLAS Study Group. Circulation 1999 Dec 7;100(23):2312-8.

[139] 2011 ACCF/AHA Focused Update of the Guidelines for the Management of Patients With Unstable Angina/Non-ST-Elevation Myocardial Infarction.

[140] Widmer et al. "The Evolving Face of Myocardial Reperfusion in Acute Coronary Syndromes: A Primer for the Internist." Mayo Clinic Proceedings, Volume 93, Issue 2, 199 – 216.

[141] MIAMI trial research group

[142] Mandrola John. "Beta-Blockade After MI: No Practice Should Be Set in Stone ." Medscape. September, 13, 2018.

[143] GISSI-3. Lancet. 1994, 343: 1115-1122

[144] Consensus Panel statement on Cardiac Rehabilitation of the AHA, the U.S. Department of Health and Human Services, and the Agency for Health Care Policy and Research.

[145] Lopes RD et al. N Engl J Med 2019 Mar 17 Mehta SR. N Engl J Med 2019 Mar 17

[146] Hunt SA, Abraham WT, Chin MH, et al. 2009 Focused update incorporated into the ACC/AHA 2005 guidelines for the diagnosis and management of heart fail- ure in adults: a report of the American College of Cardiology Foundation/Ameri- can Heart Association Task Force on Prac- tice Guidelines developed in collabora- tion with the International Society for Heart and Lung Transplantation. J Am Coll Cardiol 2009;53(15):e1-e90. [Erra- tum, J Am Coll Cardiol 2009;54:2464.]

[147] MKSAP 15

[148] Levine GN, Bates ER, Bittl JA, Brindis RG, Fihn SD, Fleisher LA, et al. 2016 ACC/AHA guideline focused update on duration of dual antiplatelet therapy in patients with coronary artery disease: a report of the American College of Cardiology/American Heart Association Task Force on Clinical Practice Guidelines. J Am Coll Cardiol. 2016;68:1082-115. PMID: 27036918

[149] Wu, Audrey. "Management of Patients with Non-ischaemic Cardiomyopathy." Heart. 2007; 93. 403-408.

[150] UCLA Inpatient Handbook 2010-2011

[151] Zaghlol RY et al. "A 71-year-old woman with shock and a high INR." Cleveland Clinic Journal of Medicine. 2018 April;85(4):303-312.

[152] Charles et al. "Secondary Hypertension: Discovering the Underlying Cause." Am Fam Physician. 2017 Oct 1;96(7):453-461.

[153] Reference card from the Seventh Report of the Joint National Committee on Prevention, Detection, Evaluation, and Treatment of High Blood Pressure (JNC 7)

[154] DynaMed

[155] Peixoto, Aldo. NEJM. 2019.

[156] DynaMed [Internet]. Ipswich (MA): EBSCO Information Services. 1995 - . Record No. T114195, Aortic Stenosis; [updated 2018 Nov 30].

[157] Reiffel et al. JAMA Cardiol. 2017.

[158] Bouida W et al. LOw dose MAGnesium sulfate versus HIgh dose in the early management of rapid atrial fibrillation: Randomized controlled double blind study. Acad Emerg Med 2018 Jul 19

[159] https://www.ebmconsult.com/articles/diltiazem-iv-to-oral-dose-conversion

[160] Acad Emerg Med. 2018 Jul 19.

[161] Alboni et al. "Outpatient Treatment of Recent-Onset Atrial Fibrillation with the "Pill-in-the-Pocket" Approach." N Engl J Med 2004;351:2384-91.

[162] Pisters R, Lane DA, Nieuwlaat R, de Vos CB, Crijns HJ, Lip GY. A novel user-friendly score (HAS-BLED) to assess 1-year risk of major bleeding in patients with atrial fibrillation: the Euro Heart Survey. Chest. 2010 Nov;138(5):1093-100. Epub 2010 Mar 18. PubMed PMID: 20299623. Lip GY, Frison L, Halperin JL, Lane DA. Comparative validation of a novel risk score for predicting bleeding risk in anticoagulated patients with atrial fibrillation: the HAS-BLED (Hypertension, Abnormal Renal/Liver Function, Stroke, Bleeding History or Predisposition, Labile INR, Elderly, Drugs/Alcohol Concomitantly) score. J Am Coll Cardiol. 2011 Jan 11;57(2):173-80. Epub 2010 Nov 24. PubMed PMID: 21111555.

[163] Gonsalves et al. "The New Oral Anticoagulants in Clinical Practice." Mayo Clinic Proceedings. May 2013; 88(5): 495-511.

[164] Mandell et al. "Selecting antithrombotic therapy for patients with atrial fibrillation." CCJM. 2015: 82(1)

[165] Fralick et al. Ann Intern Med. 2020.

[166] UCLA CCU Resident Housebook Version 3

ENDOCRINOLOGY

Adrenal Incidentaloma 235
Osteoporosis 236
Sexual Dysfunction 241
Diabetes Mellitus 244
Insulin Management 260
Diabetic Ketoacidosis (DKA) 267
Hyperosmolar Nonketotic Coma 275
Hypoglycemia 277
Hyperthyroidism 277
Hypothyroidism 281
Pituitary Incidentaloma 284
Steroids 285
Thyroid Nodule 286
Vitamin D Deficiency 288

ADRENAL INCIDENTALOMA

- The objective in devaluating an adrenal incidentaloma is to determine the risk of malignancy and assess for subclinical endocrine activity.
  - Must first determine if it is secreting hormones!
- Imaging
  - Imaging cannot distinguish functioning from nonfunctioning (need for hormonal evaluation)
  - After initial diagnosis on CT, follow up with triphasic scan (10-15min delay)
    - Benign lesions enhance up to 80-90HU with wash out up to 50% on delay
    - Metastatic/CA/Pheo will show enhancement to >100HU
- Differential Diagnosis[167]
  - Benign
    - If surgical resection is not recommended, then follow-up every 3-6 months and then every 1-2 years
    - Hormonal evaluation at time of diagnosis and every annually for 5 years
    - If during this time, it grows > 1cm consider surgical resection
  - Malignant Characteristics
    - Adenoma > 4 cm
    - Irregular borders
    - >50% contrast retention after 10 minutes
    - Unilateral
    - Calcifications/heterogenous
    - HU>10
    - ↑ growth over short time period
  - Pheochromocytoma
    - *Labs*: plasma/24-hour urine fractionated metanephrine and normetanephrine with fractionated catecholamines (urine or plasma), aldosterone:renin ratio (+ if >20:1), dexamethasone suppression test
    - Prescribe alpha-adrenergic blocker prior to surgery
    - Should have surgical resection with long term follow-up afterwards due to ↑ rate of reoccurrence
  - Cushing's Disease
    - Look for elevated 24 hr urine cortisol (normal < 90 mcg/day) in setting of patient with obesity, diabetes, osteoporosis, and HTN
    - If elevated, follow up with either:
      - Midnight salivary cortisol
      - 1mg-dexamethasone suppression test which will show serum cortisol level > 5 (lack of suppression). Performed by:
        - 1mg given at 11-pm to midnight
        - 0800 cortisol checked the following AM, should be low (<5mcg/dl)
          - A value >10 mcg/dl suggests Cushing's Syndrome
    - If (+) and surgical resection done, f/u with exogenous glucocorticoids until HPA axis recovers
  - Aldosterone secreting tumor
    - Look for Aldosterone:Renin ratio > 20 with absolute aldosterone level > 15
    - If above are positive, follow up with 24 hour urine study to look for **lack of** suppression after salt load (saline infusion or oral sodium) which confirms diagnosis if persistent aldosterone production exists despite this load.
- Workup
  - Labs

ENDOCRINOLOGY

- 24 Hour Urine Metanephrine
- 24 Hour Urine Catecholamines
- Serum aldosterone (if hypertensive)
- Serum renin activity factor (if hypertensive)
- Urine cortisol

Figure. Algorithm for management of adrenal incidentaloma

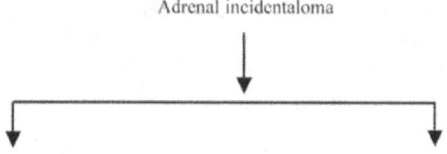

Adrenal incidentaloma

<4 cm with benign characteristics (homogeneous, regular borders, HU <10 on noncontrast CT scan)

≥4 cm on CT scan, indeterminate or malignant

Hormonally active (PAC/PRA; plasma-free metanephrines and normetanephrines; and overnight 1-mg dexamethasone suppression test)

Adrenalectomy after hormonal evaluation

Yes, adrenalectomy

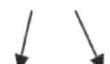

✱No, follow patient with repeat CT scan and biochemical evaluation

- **Follow-up**
    - Optimal follow up strategy is not clear
    - Can consider repeat in 6 months and then annual imaging for 4-5 years

OSTEOPOROSIS

- **Risk Factors**
    - Low BMI (<21)
    - Alcohol use (>3 drinks/d)
    - ↓Vitamin D or Ca
    - Smoking
    - Female
    - Parenteral history of hip fracture
    - ↑age (>65)
    - Chronic steroids
- **Screening**[168,169]
    - Women: ≥65 or >50 with ≤10 year risk of fracture of >9.3% based on FRAX tool
    - Men: >70 or at increased risk

Intervals of Screening	
15 years	For those with normal BMD (T-score ≥−1.0) or mild osteopenia (T-score <−1.0 and >−1.5)
5 years	For those with moderate osteopenia (T-score <−1.5 and >−2.0)
1 year	For those with advanced osteopenia (T-score <−2.0 and >−2.5)

- **Risk Factors**
  o Family history
  o Low body weight (<127#)
  o Systemic steroids, diuretics, SSRI, Depo-Provera
  o Low BMI
- **Imaging**
  o DEXA scan q5y (or q10y) of the lumbar hip and spine for screening
  o DEXA scan q1-2y if osteopenia/porosis
- **Labs**
  Current evidence is insufficient to support routine laboratory testing in patients with osteoporosis to identify possible secondary causes.
  o CBC
  o 25-OHD (goal >30 ng/mL) but conflicting data regarding utility of testing for this
  o TSH
  o PTH
  o CMP
    - Serum calcium
    - Serum creatinine
  o *Specialized labs*
    - Iron, ferritin (r/o hemochromatosis)
    - Testosterone (men; r/o hypogonadism)
    - SPEP/UPEP (r/o MM)
    - Urine free cortisol (r/o Cushing's)
    - Transglutaminase (r/o Celiac)

Diagnosis/Interpretation of DEXA Report	
Diagnosis	T-score
Normal	>−1.0
Osteopenia	−1.0 to −2.5
Osteoporosis	<−2.5 -or- osteopenia+fragility fracture
Severe osteoporosis	<−2.5 plus fragility fractures

- BMD gives your bone mineral density - the number of grams per centimeter of bone.
- Numbers of +1.0 or above are good.
- T score shows how your bone mineral density compares with women in their 30's, the peak bone density years.
- Calculated using the formula: (patient's BMD − young normal mean)/SD of young normal.
- Scores between -1 and -2.5 indicate Osteopenia (thin bones).
- Several large studies have shown an unacceptably high risk of fracture in postmenopausal women who have T-scores of −2.5 and below.
- Z score compares your bone mineral density with others of your own age.
- Are calculated similarly to the T-score, except the patient's BMD is compared with an age-matched (and race- and gender-matched) mean, and the result expressed as a SD score.
- In premenopausal women, a low Z-score (below −2.0) indicates that bone density is lower than expected and should trigger a search for an underlying cause.

- **Treatment**

The goal of treatment is to prevent disabling fractures.
- **Osteopenia**
  - **FRAX**
    - In patients not meeting diagnostic criteria for osteoporosis, use the http://www.shef.ac.uk/FRAX/tool.jsp to determine who would benefit still due to increased risk
    - FRAX was developed by the WHO to be applicable to both postmenopausal women and men aged 40 to 90 years.
    - It is validated to be used in **untreated** patients only and technically when BMD testing (DEXA) is unavailable.
    - NOF recommends **treating patients** with FRAX 10-year risk scores of ≥3% for hip fracture or >20% for major osteoporotic fracture, to reduce their fracture risk.
      - T-score of <-2.5 –or- osteopenia (-1 to -2.4) with **FRAX risk of at least 20% for major osteoporotic fracture of hip fracture of 3%**
- **Known Osteoporosis (T<-2.5)**
  - Offer pharmacologic treatment to women with <u>known</u> osteoporosis to reduce the risk for hip and vertebral fractures
    - Alendronate, risedronate, zoledronic acid, or denosumab may be used. See table for more information.
    - Combine with calcium/vitamin D supplementation
  - Avoid alcohol, tobacco, excessive caffeine
  - Weight-bearing Exercise
    - Jogging, walking, stair climbing can ↑ BMD by more than 5% from baseline
    - Duration has to be 30-60 min at least 3x/week
  - Medications
    - *ERT*
      - Not endorsed by ACP
      - When used, doses are as follows:
        - Conjugated estrogens in dosages of 0.625 and 1.25 mg per day
        - Transdermal estrogen (a weekly patch containing 0.05 mg) are equally effective in reducing bone loss in postmenopausal and oophorectomized women
    - *Calcium/Vitamin D Supplementation*
      - Combined calcium and vitamin D supplementation at prudent doses should be recommended in older institutionalized patients and community-dwelling older adults with inadequate dietary intake.
      - Elemental Ca (1g/d if <50; 1.2g/d >50) and Vitamin D (600IU if <70; 800-1000IU if >70)
        - Or have patient take one MVI (400U Vitamin D) with two tablets of calcium/vitamin D (600mg calcium and 200IU vitamin D)
        - Goal vitamin D (25-OHD) is ≥75 nmol/L
          - Repeat testing 3-4 months to ensure adequate level
    - *Bisphosphonates*
      - Indicated for women with osteoporosis, osteopenia (if FRAX major osteoporotic fracture probability is ≥20%, or if hip fracture probability is ≥3%), and low bone mass with fragility fracture.
      - Can be given after fragility fracture (4-6 weeks post fracture as long as patient can sit upright for >30 minutes)
      - Take 30 minutes prior to laying down/eating/taking other medications with plenty of water
      - Drug Holiday

- Therapy for known osteoporosis should last 5 years (if PO) or 3 years (if IV); **no need** to monitor BMD during this time. After this time period, re-evaluate fracture risk by repeating DEXA *(FLEX trial)*. See section below (Follow-up).
    - Mild risk of fracture: treat for 3–5 years, then stop. The 'drug holiday' can be continued until there is significant loss of BMD (i.e. more than the least significant change as determined by the testing center) or the patient has a fracture, whichever comes first.
    - Moderate risk of fracture: treat for 5–10 years, offer a 'drug holiday' of 3–5 years or until there is significant loss of BMD or the patient has a fracture, whichever comes first.
    - High risk of fracture (fractures, corticosteroid therapy, very low BMD): treat for 10 years, offer a 'drug holiday' of 1–2 years, until there is significant loss of BMD or the patient has a fracture, whichever comes first.
        a. A nonbisphosphonate treatment (e.g. raloxifene or teriparatide) may be offered during the 'holiday' from the bisphosphonate.
- In women aged ≥65 with osteopenia and at high fracture risk, treatment initiation is based on patient preference, fracture-risk profile, benefits, harms, and price of medications.

Pharmacologic Treatment of Osteoporosis

Medication	Dosing	Comment
Alendronic Acid *FIT*	10mg/d or 70mg/w (unless GFR<35) for 5 years (mild risk) or 6-10 years (high risk) 5mg/d for prevention purposes in patients only 7.5mg/d of prednisone for >3 months	Primary option for Osteoporosis
Risedronate *VERT-NA, VERT-MN*	35mg/w or 150mg/m	Alternative option if patient cannot tolerate Alendronic Acid
Ibandronate	PO 150mg/month or IV 3mg q3m	Once a month dosing or every 3 months
Zoledronic acid *HORIZON-PFT*	IV 5mg/year	Good for those who do not want to take PO medications
Denosumab *FREEDOM*	SQ 60mg q6m	Good to prevent vertebral and hip fx (unlike bisphosphonate and zoledronic acid); alternative to bisphosphonate in initial tx for high-risk post-menopause women Good for CKD stages 1-4 May cause hypocalcemia
Raloxifine	PO 60mg/d	SERM that acts similarly to ERT, lower breast cancer risk than ERT; It can be considered in the treatment and prevention of osteoporosis in postmenopausal women with high risk for invasive breast cancer. Due to the risk of DVT, PE, or stroke (especially in postmenopausal women at risk for coronary heart disease), it must be weighed against the benefits
Teriparatide *FPT*	SQ 20mcg/d for <2 years	Recombinant PTH; useful for those who suffer from fragility fractures despite tx

- **Follow-up**
  - At each yearly exam, determine...
    - **(1) Continuing bisphosphonate treatment**
      - Total of 3 years if low risk; *BMD<-2; no risk factors*
      - Total of 5 years if mild-moderate risk; *BMD≥-2-2.5 but stable, FHx of hip fx*
      - Up to 10 years if on PO tx; 6 years if IV) in patients at high risk; *see below*)
    - **(2) Starting drug holiday**[170]
      - May be done after 3-5 years of therapy
      - No clear data regarding this, based on *FLEX* and *HORIZON-PFT* trials
      - Goal is to maintain fracture risk at a low level while avoiding therapy as some data has suggested no benefit of bisphosphonate therapy >5 years and bisphosphonates themselves are associated with long-term safety risks.
      - Re-assess fracture risk (see next section for specific variables to monitor) after pre-defined ranges above in patients who:
        - Have had no hip, spine, or multiple or other osteoporotic fx
        - BMD in the osteopenia or normal range
        - Not at high fx risk (BMD≥-2.5; history of recent hip or spine fx, ongoing high-dose steroid tx
      - <u>Reasonable to stop therapy in patients at low-moderate risk for fracture who have been on therapy for 3-5 years and meet criteria above. Patients at high risk should continue therapy or change treatments and have re-assessment in another 2-3 years.</u>
    - **(3) Changing pharmacologic treatment**
      - If decrease in BMD≥4% in the spine or hip noted or new fracture occurs during holiday
      - Consider switching to Raloxifine
  - Monitoring Drug Holiday
    - Obtain DEXA (to calculate FRAX), vitamin D, and calcium levels
    - Ask about history of recent fractures
    - Ask about high dose steroid use
    - A treatment-induced BMD increase can only be detected in general after 2 years; goal is for stability or increase in T-score
      - Can ↓ to 1 year if patient on long-term steroids
      - Decline ≤3% is considered stable
    - Expressed as SDD, a BMD change should exceed 0.02 g/cm2 at the total hip (3.56%) and 0.04 g/cm2 at the spine (5.60%) before it can be considered a significant change.
  - Referral Criteria
    - If there is uncertainty regarding whether a patient will benefit from pharmacotherapy for fracture prevention
    - when to resume medication after a drug holiday
    - Which medication should be used after a drug holiday
    - In patients with intolerance to standard drug treatments or those in whom treatment failure is suspected.
    - Consultation with orthopedic or physical medicine and rehabilitation specialists is often required for management of patients presenting with an acute fracture.
- **Other Helpful Factors**
  - ↑Exercise
  - HRT not indicated unless patient has moderate to severe post-menopausal symptom

SEXUAL DYSFUNCTION

- **Types**[171,172]
  - Libido
  - Ejaculation
  - Erectile function - inability to achieve or maintain an erection of enough duration and firmness to complete satisfactory intercourse through vaginal penetration
  - Combination of the above
- **Symptoms**
  - Osteoporosis
  - Anemia
  - Muscle weakness
  - Depression
  - Sexual dysfunction
- **Features Consistent with Testosterone Deficiency**[173]
  - Incomplete sexual development
  - ↓libido and potency
  - ↓early-morning erection
  - Gynecomastia
  - ↓2/2 sexual characteristics (i.e. ↓shaving frequency)
  - Small testicles (normal adult: length of 4-7cm and volume 20-25cc)
  - Hot flashes (severe)
  - Low sperm count
  - Osteoporosis
- **Causes**
  - Psychologic – underlying depression, anxiety, fear of sexual failure (often sudden onset ED is a clue to this)
  - Primary Hypogonadism
    - Chronic steroid use or other known medication s/e
    - Mod-Sev COPD
    - T2DM
    - Infertility
    - HIV associated weight loss
    - ESRD
  - OSA
  - Hyperprolactinemia
  - Social – tobacco, EtOH
  - Systemic illness
  - Post-Surgical – colon, radiation therapy to prostate
  - Vascular – irradiation, peripheral vascular disease, T2DM, HTN
  - Neurologic – TBI, stroke, seizure d/o, demyelinating disease, T2DM c/b neuropathy, RLS
  - Hormonal - ↑prolactin or ↓testosterone; hypothyroidism, adrenal insufficiency, Cushing's
  - Medications (SSRI), antihistamines, decongestants, BB, spironolactone
- **History**
  - Loss of AM erections may be a sign of no REM sleep, not necessarily organic pathology
    - Presence of AM erections almost always points to psychologic causes
  - Longer duration of symptoms may mean that psychologic issues may cause persistence of symptoms even if pharmacologic therapy is initiated

ENDOCRINOLOGY

- **Physical Exam**
  - BP
  - Secondary Sexual Characteristics
    - Gynecomastia
  - Thyroid
  - Scrotal formation, size, consistency, nodules
  - DRE
- **Screening neurologic exam**
- **Labs**
  - Hormones: LH, FSH, SHBG, Prolactin
    - Testosterone → if low on 2 measurements then obtain LH/FSH to determine Primary or Secondary
      - [19–39 years] 264 to 916 ng/dL
      - [40-49 years] 208 to 902 ng/dL
      - [50-59 years] 192 to 902 ng/dL
      - [60-79 years] 190 to 902 ng/dL
      - [80-99 years] 119 to 902 ng/dL
  - CBC (HCT>52% is relative contraindication to testosterone replacement therapy)
  - CMP (evaluate kidney function)
  - TSH
  - Lipid Panel
  - Fasting Glucose
  - PSA (if likely to start testosterone therapy)
- **Diagnosis (hypogonadism specifically)**
  - AM testosterone low per reference lab standards (if no reference, then use 300)
    - Repeat testosterone to confirm
  - FSH/LH low: secondary hypogonadism (pituitary-hypothalamic)
    - Obtain PRL, MRI sella imaging
  - FSH/LH high: primary hypogonadism (testicular)
    - Obtain karyotype imaging to rule out Klinefelter's
- **Treatment**
  - CBT
  - If applicable, optimization of glucose and blood pressure
  - Tobacco cessation (see page 722)
  - Treatment of hyperlipidemia
  - ↓ EtOH
- **Testosterone Replacement Therapy**
  - Average age studied: 66
  - Outcomes of treatment:
    - *May improve:* sexual function
    - *No effect:* physical function, CVD, depression, energy, cognition.
    - *Evidence for long term benefits or harms are lacking*
  - Side Effects
    - General: hepatotoxicity, cardiotoxicity, polycythemia, ↑LDL, ↑BP, gynecomastia, testicular atrophy, acne, skin striations, depression, reduced fertility
    - Gel: skin irritation, transfer to partner
    - IM: deep tissue infection, mood fluctuations, ↑↑HCT
  - Contraindications to Therapy
    - Known history of Breast or Prostate Cancer
    - Prostate nodule palpated
    - PSA>4 ng/ml (or 3 if high risk such as AA)
    - Uncontrolled CHF

- HCT>50% or known polycythemia
- Severe OSA
- Threshold for Treatment
  The testosterone level to initiate treatment is unclear; most trials included patients with levels < 300.
  - US Endocrine Society: T (total) <300 ng/dL or T (free) lower limit of normal
  - Joint Societies: T (total) <230 ng/dL or T (free) <65 pg/mL
  - EAU: T (total) <230 ng/dL or T (free) <60 pg/mL
  - Italian Society of Endocrinology: T (total) <230 ng/dL
- Before initiating therapy, evaluate for OSA, BPH (do a DRE), prostate cancer (DRE), and PCV (obtain a CBC as above)
- Evaluate within **1 to 3 months** after starting therapy, then every **6-12 months** thereafter. Can increase interval after 12 months if stability noted.
  - Improvement should be seen in 3 months, if not, consider alternative diagnosis
- Testosterone Supplementation Options
  - *Management*
    Recommend testosterone therapy for symptomatic men with classical androgen deficiency syndromes aimed at inducing and maintaining secondary sex characteristics and at improving their sexual function, sense of wellbeing, and bone mineral density.

Management Options for Hypogonadism

Medication	Dosage	Advantages	Side Effects
IM (long acting)	Testosterone enanthate 50-100 mg qweek or 100-200mg q2weeks or 250mg q3w Testosterone cypionate 50-100mg qweek or 100-200mg q2w	Recommended as first line due to lower cost vs. transdermal. Corrects symptoms of androgen deficiency; relatively inexpensive if self-administered. flexibility of dosing	Requires IM injection, peaks and valleys without consistent levels. Avoid cypionate if soy allergy.
IM (extra-long acting)	Testosterone undecanoate 1000mg initially f/b 1000mg @ 6 weeks then 1000mg every 10-14 weeks	Less frequent dosing among IM preparations	Must monitor patients 30m after dosing; risk for anaphylaxis
1% Gel (i.e. Fortesta)	5-10g of gel applied to thighs daily	Corrects symptoms of androgen deficiency, provides flexibility of dosing, ease of application, good skin tolerability	Transfer to female partner, skin irritation
Patch	2-6mg/day (initial: 4mg) applied once a day at night to dry intact skin of back, abdomen or upper thigh	Easy to use; corrects symptoms of deficiency	May remain in the low-normal range; these men may need application of 2 patches daily; skin irritation at the application site occurs

					frequently in many patients. Cannot use same site for 7 days.
Oral		40-80mg; 2 to 3 times/day after meals		Oral	GI s/e; variable clinical and biochemical response

- o Imaging
  - DEXA scan qyear
- o Labs (Testosterone, HCT)
  - Re-evaluate 3-6 months after treatment initiation then annually with repeat testosterone levels, CBC (monitor HCT)
  - *Lab test timing based on formulation*
    - Oral: 3-5 hrs. after ingestion
    - Long-acting IM: midway between injections
    - Extra-long acting IM: before the next dose
    - Dermal: 3-12 hours after application
    - Gel: any time after at least 2 weeks of treatment
  - *Goal testosterone is in the mid-normal range of reference lab*
    - If HCT>54% then stop therapy until level <50%
    - Consider monitoring PSA yearly (>1.4 ng/mL in a year or increase in 0.4ng/dL after 6 months)
- o Weaning Off
  - *Medications*
    - Weaning testosterone is a lot like weaning glucocorticoids, there is no firm data to guide you.
    - Start by cutting the dose by 25% sequentially over a few weeks. E.g. Fortesta 4 pumps x 3 weeks, 3 pumps x 2 weeks, 2 pump x 3 weeks, 1 pump x 3 weeks.
      - The interval of how many weeks will depend on testicular mass and how long they have been on it
        - o If they have normal testis and have been on testosterone for under 6mo, they can wean sooner, e.g. 2 weeks.
        - o If longer or with atrophy then longer, in general it can take up 4-6months for the HPG axis to reset.
        - o If they are normal at any time after stopping testosterone, you are done.
    - Can consider co-administration of a SERM:
      - Clomiphene citrate 25mg/QOD x 10 weeks then decrease dose to 50% for total of 4 months
        - o This is off-label and documentation must note this!
  - *Labs*
    - After 4 weeks

DIABETES MELLITUS

- Diagnosis[174,175,176]

Glucose Testing and Interpretation			
	Normal	High Risk	Diabetes
Fasting	<100 mg/dL	100-125 mg/dL	≥126 mg/dL
Post-Prandial	<140 mg/dL	140-199 mg/dL	≥ 200 mg/dL
A1c	<5.5%	5-6-6.4%	≥ 6.5%

- Glucose Measurement[177]
    - *A1c*
        1. Ethnic and biological variation in values present
            - African Americans have falsely elevated levels (0.5% higher than actual glucose)
        2. Altered by changes in erythrocyte life span:
            - Falsely elevated (due to ↑erythrocyte life span): ↓Fe, ↓B12, ↑TRIG, uremia, chronic EtOH,
            - Falsely low (due to ↓erythrocyte life span): hemolysis, blood loss
    - *Fasting Plasma Glucose*
        1. Inexpensive
        2. Problem is it varies widely throughout the day and requires fasting of ≥8h
    - *Oral Glucose Tolerance Test*
        1. Considered the 'gold' standard but more cumbersome to obtain
        2. Sensitive indicator of the risk for developing diabetes
- Diagnosis typically requires symptoms and elevated glucose values
    - The diagnostic cutoff point for diabetes is a fasting plasma glucose level of **126** mg per deciliter (7.0 mmol per liter); the diagnosis requires confirmation by the same or the other test.
        1. Impaired fasting glucose (pre-diabetes) is 100-125 mg/dL; higher risk was considered to be A1c between **5.7-6.4%**
        2. Fasting value determined in the morning after absence of caloric intake at least 8 hours.
        3. Symptoms of DM (polyuria, polydipsia, unexplained weight loss with glucosuria and ketonuria) plus a random plasma glucose > 200 mg/dL or 2H post prandial 75g load of >200. (Whole blood values are lower by 10-15 mg/dL). Of note, symptoms are most commonly absent.
            - **A second test is always required if patients do not present with classic symptoms and >200mg on glucose level (i.e. fasting >126, A1c>6.5 require confirmatory test)**
- Additional Labs
    - Type 1 or 2: CMP, TSH, lipids, C-peptide can help differentiate between DM1 and DM2 (<5 microU/mL suggests type 1 whereas >1 ng/dL suggestive of Type 2)
    - Type 1: anti-insulin, glutamic acid decarboxylase antibodies (GAD) and anti-islet antibodies (ICA) within 6 months of diagnosis
        1. May suggest earlier need for insulin therapy if positive
    - DKA: ABG, urine ketones, beta-hydroxybutyrate, CMP for HCO3
    - Albuminuria: check spot prot/cr ratio; diagnosis can only be made with 2 of 3 checks elevated over a 3-6-month period
        1. 30-299 mg/g = microalbuminuria
        2. 300+ mg/g = macroalbuminuria
- Gestational
    - Overt: ≥ 126 mg/dL
    - Gestational: Fasting 92-125 mg/dL | 1-h post load ≥ 180 mg/dL | 2-h post load 153-199 mg/dL

- **Treatment**
  - Hypertension: debates, but ADA recommends a goal of <140/90
  - Prediabetes (FG 100-125; A1c 5.7-6.4%)
    - Primary goal is weight loss
    - No medications are FDA approved solely for pre-diabetes use; metformin and acarbose can ↓ risk of overt diabetes by up to 30%
    - Preventative metformin can be considered if patients are in this range and obese (BMI >35), <60 YO, or fail to respond to decrease their risk through lifestyle change (150 min activity/week and 5-7% weight loss)
  - Neuropathy
    - TCA
    - Duloxetine
    - Capsaicin cream
    - Gabapentin
  - Outpatient
    - Type 2
      - Lifestyle modification
      - A1c
        - <7.5%: Metformin 500-1000mg BID
        - 7.5-8.9%: dual therapy with metformin and SGLT-1/GLP-1 per table below
        - ≥ 9.0%: dual or triple therapy with metformin+GLP-1 or SGTL-2
          - Insulin should always be used for **symptomatic** hyperglycemia, A1C≥10, and/or BG ≥300 mg/dL.
      - Sulfonylureas
        - Not recommended unless patient preference (cost)
        - Glimepiride has longer half-life (once daily dosing) while Glyburide and Glipizide are BID dosing and thus have ↓ onset of hypoglycemia
        - See page 249 for oral medication options.
      - Insulin
        - See next section
        - Consider after 2 oral medications on board and A1c remaining above 8
    - Targets[178]
      - Reasonable glycemic targets would be:
        - A1C
          - <6.5% in healthy older adults with long life expectancy
          - <7.0% in patients with concomitant illness and at risk for hypoglycemia
        - Glucose Levels
          - Fasting: 80-130 mg/dL
          - 2 hour post prandial: <180 mg/dL
      - Nonpregnant adults
        - <7%
        - <6.5% if can be obtained safely without risk for hypoglycemia or significant comorbidities; see below for more information under *Preventive Medicine*)
        - Fasting/Pre-prandial 80-130 mg/dL
        - Post-prandial <180 mg/dL
    - **Monitoring**
      - Frequency of monitoring can be done with random glucose, post-prandial, and A1c (q3m)
        - PO medications: check once daily
        - Insulin: check TID

ENDOCRINOLOGY

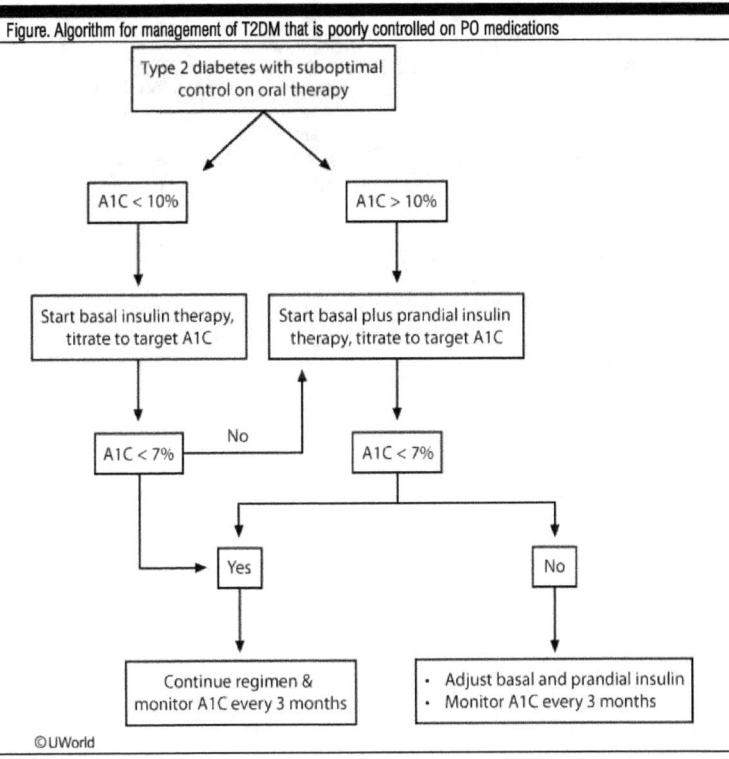

Figure. Algorithm for management of T2DM that is poorly controlled on PO medications

Oral Agents for Glycemic Patients (T2DM)			
Agent	Initial Dosing (mg)	Max Dosing	Usual Dosing
Biguanides			
Metformin	500 once or 850 daily with meal	2550mg	1500-2000 mg divided (BID)
Metformin ER	500-1000 mg daily with evening meal	2500mg	1500-2000 daily or divided
Sulfonylureas			
Glimepiride	1-2mg daily	8mg	4mg daily
Glipizide	IR: 2.5-5mg ER: 5mg	40mg ER: 20mg	10-20mg BID ER: 5-20mg daily or BID
Glyburide	2.5-5mg	20mg	5-20mg daily or BID
TZDs			
Pioglitazone	15-30mg	45mg	15-45mg
Rosiglitazone	4mg/d or BID	8mg/d	4-8mg/d or BID
Alpha-glucosidase inhibitor			
Acarbose	25mg w/food	300mg	50-100mg TID before meals
Miglitol	25mg w/food	300mg	25-100mg TID
Non-sulfonylurea insulin secretagogues			
Repaglinide	0.5mg w/meals	16mg	0.5-4 AC to QID
Nateglinide	60-120mg w/meals	360mg	60-120 AC
DPP 4 Inhibitors			
Sitagliptin	50-100mg daily	100mg	100mg daily
Saxagliptin	2.5-5mg daily	5mg	2.5-5mg daily

Linagliptin	5mg daily	5mg	5mg daily	
Alogliptin	25mg daily	25mg	25mg daily	
(SGLT2) Inhibitors				
Canagliflozin	100mg daily	300mg	100mg daily before first meal	
Dapagliflozin	5mg daily	10mg	5mg in AM	
Empagliflozin	10mg daily	25mg	10-25mg daily	
Combination formulations				
Glipizide/metformin (Metaglip)	2.5/250mg daily 2.5/500mg BID 2.5/500-5/500mg BID	10/2000 or 20/2000	Titrate to effective dose	
Glyburide/metformin (Glucovance)	1.25/250mg daily-BID 2.5/500mg BID 5/500mg BID	10/2000 20/2000	2.5/500 to 10/1000 daily-BID	

Injectable Agents for Glycemic Patients (T2DM)

Agent	Class	Onset of Action	Peak	Duration
Incretin Mimetic				
Exenatide (Byetta)	GLP-1	1 hr	2.1 hrs.	10 hrs.
Exenatide ER (Bydureon)	GLP-1	2 weeks	6-7 weeks	10 weeks
Liraglutide (Victoza)	GLP-1	<8 h	8-12 hrs.	24 hrs.
Dulaglutide (Trulicity)	GLP-1		24-72hrs	
Albluglitide (Tanzeum)	GLP-1		3-5 days	
Ultra-Rapid Acting Insulin				
Aspart (FIAsp)	N/A	2.5 min	1.5-2 hrs	5-7 hrs
Rapid Acting Insulin (give 15 minutes before or immediately after meals)				
Lispro (U100, U200)	N/A	15 min	0.5-2.5 hrs.	3-5 hrs.
Aspart (Novolog)	N/A	15 min	1-2hrs	3-5 hrs.
Glulisine (Apidra)	N/A	20 min	1-2 hrs.	5-6 hrs.
Short-Acting Insulin (give 30 minutes before meals)				
Regular (Humulin R)	N/A	30-60 min	2-3 hrs.	3-6 hrs.
Intermediate-Acting Insulin (within 30-60 min before a meal)				
NPH (Humulin N)	N/A	1-2 hrs	4-12 hrs	14-24 hrs
>70/30 Regular		30 min	1-2 hrs / 6-10 hrs	18-24 hrs
>70/30 Rapid acting		15-30 min	1-4 hrs	18-24 hrs
>70/25 Rapid acting		15-30 min	1-6.5 hrs	12-24 hrs
Detemir (Levemir)	N/A	3-4 hrs.	6-8 hrs.	6-23 hrs.
Long-Acting Insulin				
Glargine (Lantus)	N/A	2-4hrs	None	20-24 hrs.
Glargine (U300 Toujeo)	N/A	6 hrs	None	>30 hrs
Degludec (U100, U200; Tresiba)	N/A	1 hrs	9 hrs	>42 hrs
Concentrated, Intermediate Acting				
U500 Regular		30 min	1.5-3.5 hrs	Up to 24 hrs.

SGLT-2 vs GLP1*

Class	Fasting Glucose	Dyslipidemia	CV Effect Noted
SGLT-2	↓	↑ ↔	Started after 12 weeks on therapy
GLP-1	↔ ↓	↓	Started after 12 months

*both SGLT-2 inhibitors and GLP-1 agonists are recommended after metformin as second and third line medications for T2DM

Pharmacologic Options in the treatment of T2DM

Order of Initiation	Class / A1c↓	Dose	Pathophysiology	S/E	Points of Consideration
Non-insulin injectables					
- If after 3 months patient's glucose is not at goal with therapy started, add second/third agent/insulin. *- Consider dual-therapy if A1c ≥ 7.5% (understand a third agent is unlikely to help with A1c of 8 or more)* *- Consider injectable (insulin, GLP-1) if A1c > 9% and patient symptomatic* *- Initial therapy is always lifestyle modification with activity goal of 150 min/week and weight loss of 7% body fat*					
1	Biguanide 1% to 2%	**Metformin/Metformin ER** INITIAL: 500 to 850 mg in divided doses INITIAL ER: 500 mg every evening MAX INITIAL: 2,550 mg/day MAX ER: 2000mg/d	Inhibits hepatic glycogenolysis, gluconeogenesis and enhances insulin sensitivity in muscle and fat. Decreases the sugar that comes from the liver.	Nausea, diarrhea, abdominal pain. Lactic acidosis but GFR lower limits have been relaxed: must be at least 30 cc/min Add B12 if neuropathy develops If patient received IV contrast, restart after **48 hours**	• Promotes modest weight loss • Low risk of hypoglycemia • Newer data suggests it is okay to use even in the face of CHF, LF, CRF[179] • Do not start in patients with eGFR<45 but can be maintained if eGFR>30 • Do NOT stop use even if patient is now on insulin. It has been shown to decrease MACE, can lead to overall decrease in insulin requirements (6.6U/d) • Monitor B12 levels in patients with anemia or peripheral neuropathy

Pharmacologic Options in the treatment of T2DM

Order of Initiation	Class / A1c↓	Dose	Pathophysiology	S/E	Points of Consideration
2	**GLP-1 receptor agonist** 0.5-1%	**Liraglutide** *(Victoza)* INITIAL: 0.6 mg **SC** once daily x 1 week, then increase to 1.2 mg SC daily. MAX: 1.8 mg/day Aim for 3mg SQ/d for weight loss **Exenatide** *(Byetta)* INITIAL: 5 mcg SC BID within 60 min of a meal with 6h b/w meals. ↑ to max dose after 1 month. MAX: 10 mcg SC BID Exenatide extended-release *(Bydureon)* INITIAL: 2 mg SC once weekly MAX: 2 mg SC once weekly Albiglutide *(Tanzeum)* INITIAL: 30mg/week MAX: 50mg/week Dulaglutide *(Trulicity)* INITIAL: 0.75mg/week MAX: 1.5mg/week Lixisenatide INITIAL: 10 mcg SQ daily MAX: 20 mcg SQ daily	Stimulates GLP-1 receptors which increases production of insulin in response to high blood glucose levels, inhibits postprandial glucagon release, slows gastric emptying. (GLP-1 is an incretin hormone.)	Headache, **nausea**, diarrhea. May be associated with pancreatitis. May be associated with renal insufficiency.	• Transient n/v • **Continue in patients on insulin** • Once weekly doses take 5 half-lives to reach steady state: lower total insulin levels by 20-30% when starting • Causes weight loss • Injectable that sometimes is considered last line in combination **with insulin** especially if fasting levels are controlled by A1c remains high • **Contraindicated if severe kidney disease present (GFR<30) or FHx of medullary thyroid cancer** • Greater glucose reduction in daily preparations vs. weekly however those patients also had more s/e • Liraglutide had greater glucose reduction than exenatide • **Significantly lower risk of cardiovascular death, nonfatal MI, or nonfatal stroke than placebo in *LEADER* trial** • ↓BP, no hypoglycemia

Pharmacologic Options in the treatment of T2DM

Order of Initiation	Class /A1c↓	Dose	Pathophysiology	S/E	Points of Consideration
3	**SGLT2 inhibitor**[180] 0.7% to 1%	**Empagliflozin *(Jardiance)*** INITIAL: 10-25g/d MAX: Canagliflozin *(Invokana)* INITIAL: 100 mg PO once daily MAX: 300 mg/day Dapagliflozin *(Farxiga)* INITIAL: 5 mg PO once daily MAX: 10 mg/day	Sodium-glucose co-transporter 2 inhibitor reduces reabsorption of filtered glucose and lowers the renal threshold for glucose, resulting in increased urinary glucose excretion.	**Genital fungal infections** (male and female), urinary tract infection, increased urination, hypo-tension, ketoacidosis ↑risk for DKA when combined with insulin in T1DM patients Canagliflozin had ↑ risk for amputations	• Causes weight loss • ↓all-cause mortality and morbidity in HF patients (dapagliflozin) • **Good option to ↓ CVD in those with pre-existing dz,** • ↓ hospitalization in HF patients, and those with CKD (*EMPA-REG OUTCOME*) • **May delay onset of new HF in patients with DM (*DECLARE-TIMI 58 CV*)** • Causes slight reduction of BP. • Reduced incidence of ESRD in those with proteinuria (A:Cr >300 mg/g) and GFR ≥30 (*CREDENCE*) • Check BMP 1 week after starting therapy • May increase LDL • Stop 24 hours prior to surgery • Can cause positive urinary glucose test. • Can help decrease overall insulin required if concomitant insulin is used

Pharmacologic Options in the treatment of T2DM

Order of Initiation	Class / A1c↓	Dose	Pathophysiology	S/E	Points of Consideration
					o Reduce insulin level by 20-30% when starting
	DPP-4 0.5% to 1%	**Sitagliptin *(Januvia)*** INITIAL: 100 mg PO once daily Alogliptin *(Nesina)* INITIAL: 25 mg PO once daily Linagliptin *(Tradjenta)* INITIAL: 5 mg PO once daily *Saxagliptin (Onglyza)*: INITIAL: 2.5 mg/day MAX: 5 mg/day	Inhibits degradation of endogenous incretins which increases insulin secretion, decreases glucagon secretion (glucose-dependent).	May be associated with pancreatitis. Alogliptin and saxagliptin are associated with heart failure, but sitagliptin is likely not.	• Weight neutral. • Should not be used in patients with history of cardiac disease as it may increase risk of heart failure (alogliptin and saxagliptin only) • Contraindicated in **severe kidney disease (GFR<50)** but can reduce dose. • Low risk of hypoglycemia. • Dosage modification with renal impairment needed with sitagliptin, saxagliptin, and alogliptin. • Combination with metformin showed lower risk for all-cause death, MACE, stroke, and hypoglycemia[181]
	Meglitinide 0.7-1.1%	**Repaglinide *(Prandin)*** INITIAL: 0.5mg TID/meals or 1-2mg TID if already on hypoglycemic med MAX: 4mg TID/meals Nateglinide *(Starlix)* INITIAL: 120mg TID/meals but can start	Simulate insulin secretion	Avoid in patients with liver dysfunction	• Good option if patient is (1) intolerant to metformin +/- sulfonylurea and have CKD or (2) need add-on therapy to metformin • Rapid onset, short duration • ↑weight • Risk of hypoglycemia

Pharmacologic Options in the treatment of T2DM

Order of initiation	Class / A1c↓	Dose	Pathophysiology	S/E	Points of Consideration
		at 60mg if close to A1c goal MAX: 120mg TID/meals Exenatide INITIAL: IR-5mcg BID within 60 min of AM or PM meal; ↑ to 10mcg BID p̄ 1 month ER-2mg/week with or without foods			• Great for patients who have erratic eating schedules (you only take it with meals) or late postprandial hypoglycemia on sulfonylurea
4	Sulfonylurea 0.7-1.5%	Glimepiride *(Amaryl)* INITIAL: 1-2 mg/d USUAL: 4mg/d MAX: 8mg/d Glyburide *(DiaBeta)* INITIAL: 2.5-5mg/d USUAL: 5-20mg/d or BID MAX: 20mg/d Glipizide *(Glucotrol)* INITIAL: 2.5-5mg/d USUAL: 10-20mg/d MAX: 40mg/d	Stimulates the pancreas to put out more insulin over several hours.	Hypoglycemia ↑Weight	• Higher risk for hypoglycemia • Patients cannot skip meals • Avoid in patients with known sulfa allergies

Diabetes Medications Compared

	Metformin	GLP-1	SGLT-2	DPP-4	Metaglinide	Insulin	Sulfonylurea	TZD
Hypolycemia	↕	↕	↕	↕	Mild	Moderate/Severe	Moderate/Severe	↕
Weight Δ	↓	↓↓	↓↓	↕	↕	↑	↑	↑
Renal or GU dz	C/I if GFR<30	Exenatide C/I Liraglutide a benefit	Avoid if GFR<45 ↑genital mycotic infection Empaglifozin a benefit	Dose adjustment ↓albuminuria	Higher hypoglycemia	Higher hypoglycemia	More hypo risk	
GI Sx	↑↑	↑↑	↕	↕	↕	↕	↕	↕
Cardiac								
-CHF	Neutral	Liraglutide ↓MACE	Empaglifozin ↓CV mortality Canaglifozin ↓ MACE	↑hospitalization in CHF	↕	↑CHF risk	↑ASCVD	↓CVA
-ASCVD					↑ASCVD risk	↕		
Bone	↕	↕	↑ fx risk	↕	↕	↕	↕	Mod ↑fx
Ketoacidosis	↕	↕	DKA can occur in various stress settings	↕	↕	↕	↕	↕

liraglutide approved to prevent MACE
empaglifozin reduces CV mortality. Canaglifozin reduces MACE
more CHF exacerbations with alolgliptin and saxagliptin

Combination T2DM Medications

Name/Generic/A1c	Class	Dose	Pathophysiology	S/E	Points of Consideration
Combination Oral Medications					
Glucovance Glyburide+Metformin	Sulfonylurea +Biguanide	Initial: 5/500mg/BID	Stimulates pancreatic insulin secretion	Hypoglycemia ↑weight Nausea Abdominal pain Diarrhea	• Hypoglycemia • ↑Weight
Metaglip Glipizide+Metformin 0.7-1.3%		Initial: 20/2000mg/BID			
Actoplus Met Pioglitazone+Metformin 0.8-0.9%	Thiazolidine +Biguanide	Initial IR: 15/500mg BID 15/850mg daily ER: 15/1000mg daily 45/2000mg daily	Increases insulin sensitivity in muscle and fat	Edema ↑weight Nausea Abdominal pain Diarrhea CHF risk ↑ risk of bladder CA	• ↑weight • Edema • ↓ dosing if CHF
Janumet Sitagliptin+Metformin 0.5-0.7%	DPP-4 inhibitor +Biguanide	Already on Metformin: 100/(daily metformin) Not on Metformin: 100/1000mg daily	Increases insulin secretion in response to elevated blood glucose, decreases glucagon secretion, increases sense of fullness, and slows gastric emptying	Hives (if allergi) Nausea GI upset Diarrhea	• Risk of hives • Pancreatitis • Weight neutral • May ↑ risk for CHF • May ↑ joint pains

Combination T2DM Medications

Name/Generic/A1c	Class	Dose	Pathophysiology	S/E	Points of Consideration
Invokamet Canaglifozin+Metformin	SGLT-2 inhibitor +Biguanide	<u>Initial:</u> 100/1000mg daily (divide total BID if IR formulation) <u>Max:</u> 300/2000mg daily max	Blocks glucose reabsorption in the kidney, and increases urinary excretion of glucose	Nausea Abdominal pain UTI Yeast infections Dehydration	• Risk of UTIs higher • Dehydration risk • Empaglifozin use in patients with CVD for about three years may reduce CV disease
Glyxambi Empaglifozin+Linagliptin 0.4-0.7%		<u>Initial:</u> 10/5mg daily <u>Max:</u> 25/5mg daily			

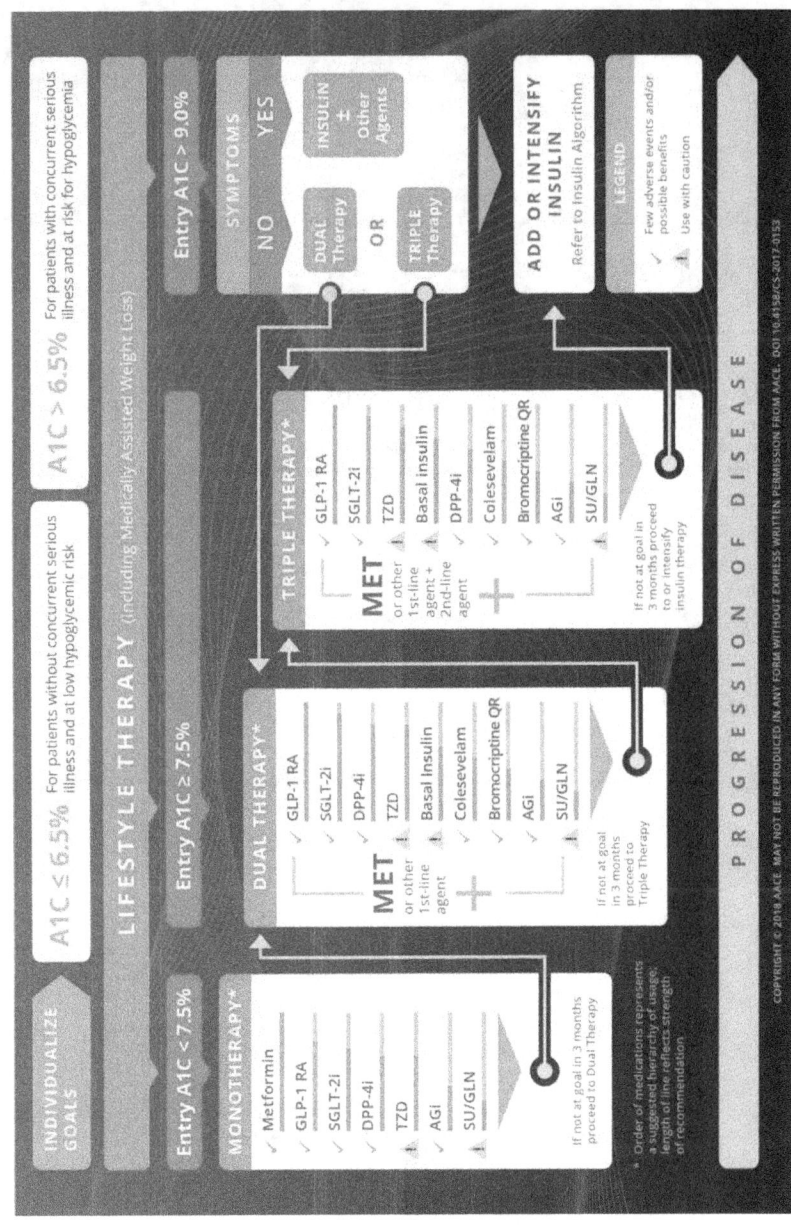

ENDOCRINOLOGY

Feeding Options

Feeding Method	Plan
PO/ Bolus Tube Feeds	Check BS AC and HS Basal: 50% of TDD during each feeding Premeal: 1/3 of ½ of TDD
Enteral/Continuous Tube	Check BS q4h Basal: 20% of TDD Premeal: 80% of TDD divided into 6 doses given equally q4h Hold if TF interrupted for >2 hours or if BS<100 mg/dL
Fasting/Clear Liquid/TPN	Check BS q4h Basal: 40-80% of TDD q4h Premeal: none

Ordering Outpatient Diabetes Supplies

Device	Purpose
Glucometer	Tests blood sugar level
Lancing Device	Device that pricks their finger to test blood sugar level
Lancets	Small needle that is loaded into the lancing device
Test strips	holds the blood and plugs into the glucometer to get a reading of the blood sugar
Insulin delivery mechanism	may be a preloaded pen or syringes Syringes -Volume (30, 50, 100cc) -Length: aim for 4mm (↑ length if burning reported)

- Inpatient
  - See feeding options above
  - **Target**:
    1. In critically ill patients - aiming for a target range of 140-180 mg/dL
    2. Non critically ill patients - goals of pre meal glucose < 140 mg/dL and random < 180 mg/dL
    3. Preoperative - ≤ 200 mg/dL
- **Gestational Diabetes**[182]
  - Preconception
    1. Women already on insulin should be treated with multiple daily doses of insulin or continuous SQ insulin infusion in preference to split-dose, premixed insulin therapy
    2. Women with diabetes successfully using the long-acting insulin analogs insulin detemir or insulin glargine preconceptionally may continue with this therapy before and then during pregnancy.
    3. Beginning 3 months before withdrawing contraceptive measures or otherwise trying to conceive, a woman with diabetes take a daily folic acid supplement to reduce the risk of neural tube defects
  - Treatment
    1. Target values as close to normal as possible
       - Pre-prandial Goal: ≤ 95 mg/dL
       - 1 h after meal: ≤ 140 mg/dL
       - 2 h after meal: ≤ 120 mg/dL

2. Initial treatment will always be dietary, however insulin (lispro, aspart as rapid acting along with long acting detemir or glargine) or glyburide are the only approved pharmacologic therapies in pregnancy (metformin can be added after first trimester)
- All women should track glucose via 1 or 2 hour post prandial, bedtime, and 3am levels

- **Treatment in Hospital**
  - Discharge Orders[190]
    - If newly diagnosed diabetic, needs glucometer, oral medications, and close follow-up
    - Consider the following regimen in newly diagnosed patients:
      - Begin low-dose metformin (500 mg) once or BID w/meals (breakfast and/or dinner)
      - After 5–7 days, if GI s/e have not occurred, ↑ dose to 850–1,000 mg before breakfast and dinner.
      - If gastrointestinal side effects appear as doses advance, decrease dose to the previous lower dose and try to advance at a later time.
      - The typical therapeutic dose is 850 mg twice daily. Higher doses, up to 2,550 mg daily, can be used but tend to be associated with more significant side effects and are not recommended as starting doses.

Microvascular vs Macrovascular Complications	
Microvascular	Macrovascular
Retinopathy	Atherosclerosis/CVD
Neuropathy	CVA
Nephropathy	HTN
ED	PVD
Autonomic dysfunction	Liver disease

- **Preventive Medicine**[183]
  - Microvascular Disease
    - The Diabetes Control and Complications Trial (DCCT), a prospective randomized controlled trial of intensive versus standard glycemic control in patients with relatively recently diagnosed type 1 diabetes, showed definitively that improved glycemic control is associated with significantly decreased rates of microvascular (retinopathy and diabetic kidney disease) and neuropathic complications.
      - Follow-up of the DCCT cohorts in the EDIC study demonstrated persistence of microvascular benefits in previously intensively treated subjects, even though their glycemic control approximated that of previous standard arm subjects during follow-up.
      - Achieving glycemic control of **A1C targets of <7%** has been shown to **reduce microvascular** complications of diabetes and, in patients with **type 1 diabetes**, mortality. If implemented soon after the diagnosis of diabetes, this target is associated with long-term reduction in macrovascular disease.
        - Retinopathy: annual exam (q2y if no evidence of retinopathy is found); associated with hyperglycemia and hypertension.
        - Nephropathy: Annual assessment of SCr, eGFR, and albumin/creatinine ratio. No benefit in T1DM with ACEi to prevent progression however clear prevention associated in T2DM. Progression linked to hyperglycemia and HTN.
          - UACR < 30 normal
          - UACR 30-299 is an early predictor for kidney complications; defined as microalbuinuria

ENDOCRINOLOGY

- UACR ≥ 300 mg/g are likely to develop ESRD; defined as macroalbuinuria/proteinuria
- Neuropathy: 5 years after diagnosis then annual assessment thereafter with 10g monofilament testing. Primarily associated with hyperglycemia. Symptoms mostly at night. Pain noted in the thighs with weakness may be sign of diabetic amyotrophy. Can manage with duloxetine or pregabalin.
  - Diabetic Autonomic Neuropathy – constipation, gastroparesis, diarrhea, anhidrosis, bladder dysfunction, ED, resting tachycardia, SCD.
- Hypertension: <130/80
  - PM administration of losartan (vs daytime) has found to be beneficial in preventing onset of new type 2 diabetes[184]
- Vaccinations
  - Hepatitis B vaccination if 19+ YO and no prior vaccination on record
  - Pneumococcal (13+23V) if >65
- Lipids: <100 if no ASCVD, if ASCVD also present then target <70
- Smoking cessation
- Labs: LFT, spot urine protein/creatinine, SCr, GFR
- Podiatry visits annually
- Nutrition consultation (target 7% loss in body fat)
  - Patients who are obese (BMI≥30) that had prediabetes (FS 100-125 mg/dL; A1c 5.7-6.4%) were found to have lower progression to overt diabetes if they took Liraglutide (Saxenda) at 3mg/d (SQ) for 160 weeks.[185]
  - Bariatric surgery for adults with BMI >35 kg/m and T2DM
  - FDA approved medications for weight loss: orlistat 60-120mg TID, Belviq 10mg BID

INSULIN MANAGEMENT

- **Considering Initiation (see chart on next page)**
- **Calculating dose to start**
  - Guidelines to starting insulin glargine (Lantus)
    - Multiple methods are utilized to convert to long-acting insulin after insulin requirements stabilize
    - Recommend giving 0.1-0.2 units/kg if A1c is <8% (0.2-0.3 U/kg if A1c >8%) with 50% of dose as Lantus and 50% as nutritional dose divided qAC. Then titrate dose as needed.
      - Starting points:
        - Basal: 10U
        - Adjustments:
          - Fixed dose: add 2U to TDD every 2-3 days
          - Adjustable regimen:
            - FBG >180: add 20% of TDD

Figure. Algorithm for initiation of insulin therapy

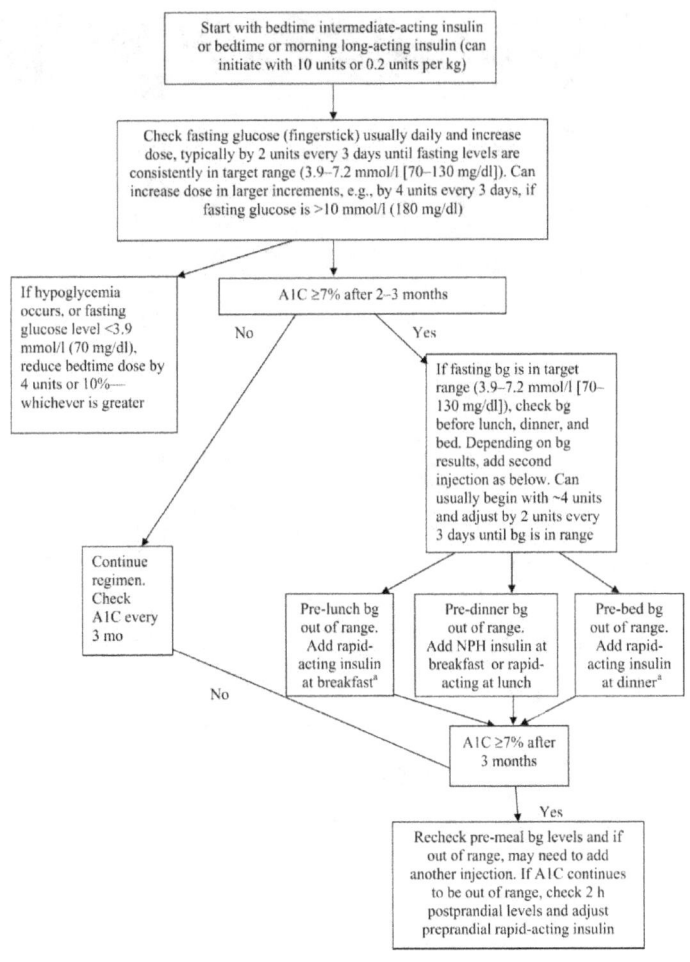

- FBG 140-180: add 10% of TDD
- FBG ≤139: add 1U to TDD
- Prandial: 4U/day
  o Typically, 50% of TDD divided into three meals
  o Adjustments:
    - Increase prandial dose by 10% or 1-2 units if 2h postprandial >140
    - Can add GLP-1 or SGLT-2 as well
- Goals: A1c<7% (<6.5% if very healthy)
  □ Fasting and Pre-prandial: 90-130 mg/dL
  □ Postprandial (2 hrs): <180 mg/dL
  □ Bedtime/overnight: 90-150 mg/dL

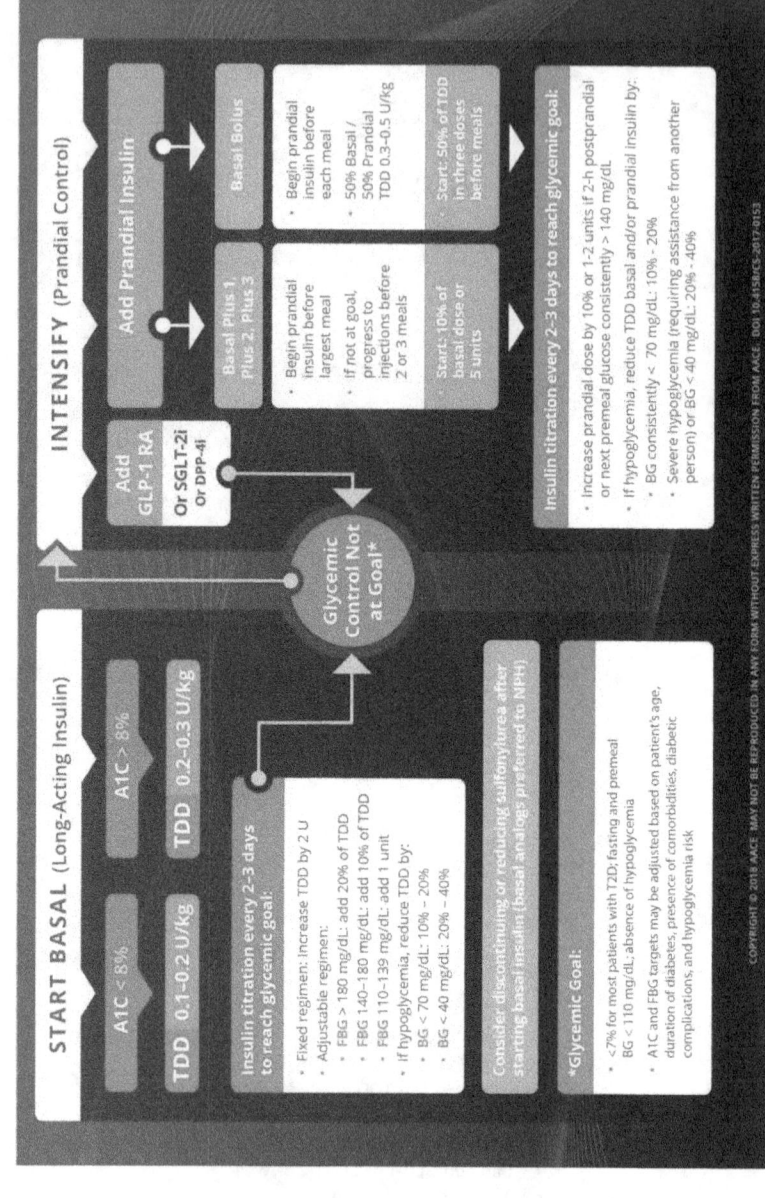

Managing Insulin in Diabetes

Unknown TDD	Known TDD	Known TDD (Premix)

1. Use medical history / body type to determine the TDD:
Malnourished/No h/o DM/Elderly/Frail
TDD = weight (kg) x (0.2 or 0.4)
Understand in insulin-naïve patients, you will likely have to work up to 0.6-0.7U/kg/d)
 	
Lean (BMI <25) T2DM, T1DM, 2/2 steroids
TDD = weight (kg) x 0.4
Overweight (BMI 25-30)
TDD = weight (kg) x 0.5
Obese (BMI>30), T2DM+steroids
TDD = weight (kg) x 0.6
 	
Renal impairment: Reduce total daily dose by 50% if creatinine clearance of <30ml/min
 	
2. Divide this # by 2 (or by 3 if you are doing pure short acting replacement before each meal)
   a. Half will be given as Lantus qhs and another half will be given pre-prandial as NovoLog
   b. Or consider 4U/d as a starting point
3. Now fine-tune your rapid acting
 	
MDI regimen (basal + rapid)
- Basal, long-acting insulin once or twice a day
	- TDD =
	   o Total # units for 24 hour period
	   -or-
	   o (Avg hourly insulin drip rate over 6 hrs) x 20 which comes out to be about 80% of the daily infusion dose
	
	Renal impairment: Reduce total daily dose by 50% if CrCl <30ml/min
	
	Analogue Insulin
	- Consider TDD of 10U as a starting point for basal insulin
	- Divide this # by 2 (or by 3 if you are doing pure short acting replacement before each meal)
	   o Half will be given as Lantus qhs and another half will be given pre-prandial as NovoLog (consider 4U/d as a starting point)
	   o Patients on TF should have this dose split into 4 and given as regular insulin q6h
	   o Add sliding scale on top of this to determine how much correction was needed
	- The following day, make changes as necessary to your regiment
	- Use the fasting AM glucose (0500-0700) to determine changes needed to **basal** insulin
	- Post meal insulin should then be used to adjust the **pre meal** insulin
	
	Split Mixed Human Insulin[186]
	- Using TDD above, divide by 3
		1. Add up all doses of premix given in 24 hours
		2. Give half as basal
		3. Divide pre meals by 1/3

- Prandial, short-acting insulin based on:
  - # of carbohydrate portions (e.g., 1:10, meaning 1 U of insulin for every 10 g of carbohydrate to be eaten)
  - Correctional short-acting mealtime insulin based on premeal blood glucose level (subtract target blood glucose level and divided by sensitivity factor)
  - Preset sliding scale utilized which you then add to prandial dosing the following day based on totals: If your patient required 15U total of SSI throughout the day then add this to your TDD and repeat step (2)
    - 2/3 given in AM before bfast (2/3 of NPH, 1/3 regular)
    - 1/3 given in PM before dinner (1/2 of NPH, 1/2 regular)

CSII regimin (insulin pump)
- May use regular insulin or rapid-acting insulin analogues
- Insulin is infused continuously at a preset rate, and bolus doses are given with meals as above.

ENDOCRINOLOGY

- **Options**

Insulin Adjuncts

Type	Onset	Peak	Duration	Timing of Dose	Dosing
Rapid Acting					
Lispro (*Humalog*)	5-15min	30-90min	3-5h	15 min before meal	U-100 Kwik pen
Aspart (*Novolog*)	15min	30-90min	4-6h	15 min before meal	PenFill U-100 FlexPen U-100 U-100 vial
Glulisine (*Apidra*)	30min	30-90min	5.3h	15 min before meal	SoloStar U-100 U-100 vial
Short to Intermediate Acting					
Regular 100u/mL (*Humulin R; Novolin R*)	30-60min	2-4h	6-12h	30-45min before meal	U-100 vial
Regular 500u/mL (*Novolin R or Humulin R*)	30-60min	2-4h	6-10h	30-45min before meal	U-500 vial Kwik pen U-500
Intermediate					
NPH (*Humulin or Novolin*)	1-2h	4-12h	10-24h	Twice a day	KwikPen U-100 U-100
Basal/Long					
Degludec (*Tresiba*) (U100/U200) (lower risk for hypoglycemia)	1h	No peak	42h	Once a day	Type 1: 0.2-0.4 U/kg Type 2: 10U SC/d U-100 Vial FlexTouch Pen
Glargine (*Lantus*)	1h	No peak	24 hours	Once a day	KwikPen U-100 SoloStar U-100
Glargine (*Toujeo*)	6h	No peak	24-36h	Once a day	SoloStar U-300 Max SoloStar
Detemir (*Levemir*)	2h	None	12-24 hours	Once or twice/day	

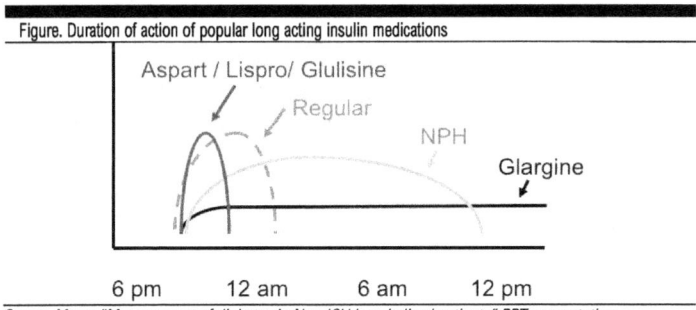

Figure. Duration of action of popular long acting insulin medications

Styner, Maya. "Management of diabetes in Non-ICU hospitalized patients" PPT presentation

- **Titration of Insulin**

ENDOCRINOLOGY

Insulin Titration

Fasting Glucose (mg/dL)	AACE/ACE	ADA
>180	↑20% TDD	Increase dose 10-15% or by 2-4U
140-180	↑10% of TDD	
110-139	↑1U	
<70	↓10-20%	Determine cause, if not clear, ↓ by 10-20% or
<40	↓20-40%	2-4U

- Insulin Sensitivity Ratio (ISF) estimates the point drop in mmol/L per unit of rapid- or short-acting insulin.

> 1700* / Total Daily Dose of Insulin = ISF →amount 1U of insulin will drop BS

- Now you know how much insulin to add to the pre meal insulin dose

or

- To use the insulin sensitivity factor, calculate the difference between the current blood sugar (glucose) and the desired blood sugar. Then divide the result by the sensitivity factor. The result is the amount of insulin that needs to be added or subtracted from the pre meal insulin dose.

> (CURRENT BG − IDEAL BG) = X
>
> X / ISF = INSULIN ADDED TO PREMEAL DOSE

- **Insulin Sliding Scale**
  - Check patients' blood glucose qAM and qHS if NPO
  - **Type 1**: type 1 patients require less insulin than type 2's. They need basal insulin (even when NPO) to prevent DKA and extra insulin with each meal. If patients are carbohydrate counting, allow patient to help determine meal insulin bolus. Sample type 1 pre-meal scale along with basal insulin (e.g. NPH 8 U SQ BID). Again, this scale is not intended for bedtime insulin coverage or patients that are not eating.
  - **Type 2**: for an average type 2 patient on orals meds as an outpatient consider the following sliding scale pre-meals (do not use these levels of insulin at bedtime) along with 5-10 units NPH qhs
- **Insulin Drip**
  - Indications
    - DKA
    - Hyperosmolar hyperglycemic state
    - Very poorly controlled diabetes despite Sub-Q insulin (BG >300-350 x 2 over 6-12 hr)
    - TPN
    - Type I DM who are NPO, periop, or in L & D
    - Post-MI with hyperglycemia

- ICU pt with hyperglycemia
- Suspect poor subQ absorption of insulin
o Transition
- When put back on Sub-Q insulin, give lispro 1-2 hr or long acting insulin 2-3 hr prior to stopping drip

DIABETIC KETOACIDOSIS (DKA)

Diagnosis of HHS and DKA

	Mild DKA	Mod. DKA	Severe DKA	HHS
Plasma Glucose	>250	>250	>250	>600
Venous or Arterial pH	7.25-7.30	7.00-<7.24	<7.00	>7.3
Serum Bicarb	15-18	10-15	<10	>18
Urine or Serum Ketones	+	+	+	Small
Effective Serum Osmolarity	Variable	Variable	Variable	>320
Anion gap	>10	>12	>12	Variable
Mental Status	Alert	Alert/Drowsy	Stupor/Coma	Stupor/Coma

- **Pearl**[187,188,190]
  o Mainstay of treatment is **insulin** rather than fluids (HHS)
- **Diagnosis**
  o Glucose > 250
  o pH < 7.30
  o low HCO3- (<18)
  o high anion gap (>12)
  o positive ketones
- **Useful calculations**
  o Anion gap = Na - (Cl + HCO3) –or– ALBUMIN x 3
  o Corrected Na = Na + [(glucose - 100)/100] x 1.6
  o Effective osmolality = {2 [Na + K]}/18 + glucose/2.8 + BUN
  o Evaluation for pure metabolic acidosis:
    - pCO2 = the last two numbers of pH
    - pCO2 = 1.5 [serum HCO3] + 8
- **Monitoring**
  o Daily ECG (↑K)
  o Vitals
  o Q1H glucose
  o Can follow anion gap to ensure resolution (do not follow ketones)
  o Q2-4H CMP alternating with glucose checks
- **Labs**
  o ICU panel q2h to monitor glucose, K, PO4, AG
    - Increase to Q4H when BS <200
  o FS q1hour
  o Serum and urine ketones one time
  o ABG x 1
  o Diet: NPO, but advance as tolerated

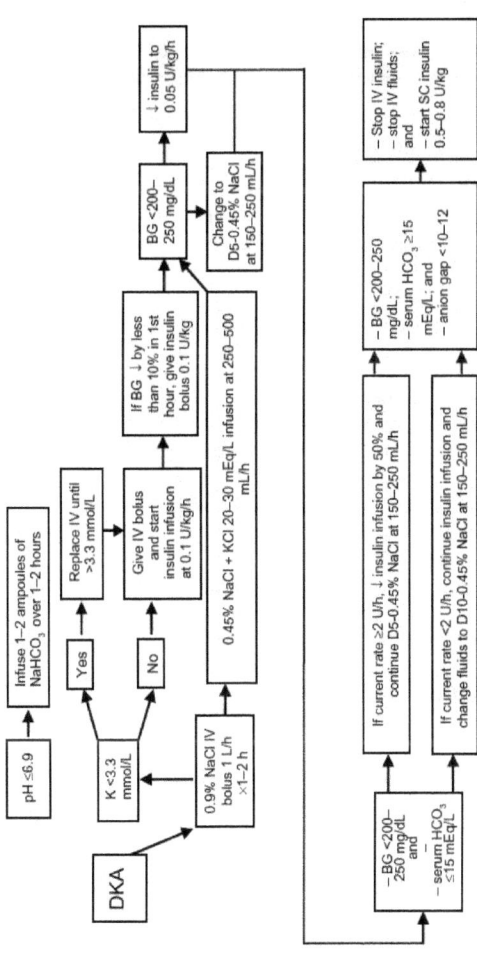

- **Treatment**
  - Fluids/Electrolytes
    - **Fluids**: assume about 10% dehydration (100 ml/kg) with deficit of 5-10L to be corrected over 36-48 hours
      - *If hypotensive* – 1L 0.9NS over 5-10 minutes (bolus) then 500 cc/hour (7.5 cc/kg/hr) for the next 2-4 hours →100-250 cc/hour
      - *If normotensive* – 1L 0.9NS over 60 minutes, then 500 cc/hour (7.5 cc/kg/hr) for the next 2-4 hours →100-250 cc/hour
      - Change to D5NS or D51/2NS when BG < 200 mg/dl
        - During therapy, hyperchloremic non-gap acidosis may develop as ketones cleared and bicarbonate deficit replaced with chloride ions from saline.

Hours	Volume
30min-1 hour	1L
2nd hour	1L
3rd hour	500cc-1L
4th hour	500cc-1L
5th hour	500cc-1L
Total 1-5hrs	3.5-5L
6-12th hours	200-500cc/hr

  - **Potassium** replacement: potassium will initially be falsely elevated due to acidosis and hypovolemia, but can drop quickly (deficit usually 200-1000 mEQ)
    - Wait until potassium is <5.3 mEq/L, then begin replacement aggressively:
      - Potassium < 3.3
        - Consider holding insulin drip until K at least 3.3
        - *Peripheral access:*
          - KCl 40mEq in 500mL over 4 hours
          - KPhos 30 mmol in 500 mL over 4 hours (consider if phos is <2.5)
        - *Central access:*
          - KCl 40mEq in 100mL over 1-4 hours (recommend 1-4 hour infusion)
          - KPhos 30 mmol in 250 mL over 1-4 hours
      - Potassium 3.3 – 4, add KCL 40 mEq / L to maintenance IVF
        - 0.45% NS 1L + potassium chloride 40mEq IV
        - 0.9% NS 1L + potassium chloride 40mEq IV
      - Potassium 4.1 – 5, add KCL 20 mEq / L to maintenance IVF
        - 0.45% NS 1L + potassium chloride 20mEq IV
        - 0.9% NS 1L + potassium chloride 20mEq IV
    - Max KCl administration rate: central line – 20 mEq/hour, peripheral line – 10 mEq/hour.
  - **Phosphate** replacement: generally, replacement not recommended despite anticipated fall during days 1 and 2.
    - may administer only if serum PO4 < 1.5 mg/dL
      - Use sodium phosphate (3 mmol PO4/cc; 4 mEq Na/cc)
      - Or K_2PO_4 at 0.5cc/hr
    - Give 0.3-0.6 mmol PO4/kg/day. Give phosphate ordered in millimole over 6 hours.
    - Do not use if patient has hypercalcemia or renal failure. Monitor Ca, PO4, and Na.
  - **Magnesium**: administer only if serum Mg < 1.8 mg/dL or if patient has tetany.
  - **Bicarbonate**: generally, replacement not recommended.

- For pH 6.9 - 7: Sodium Bicarbonate 50mEq IV in 0.45% NS 250mL IV over 1 hr
- For pH < 6.9: Sodium Bicarbonate 100mEq IV in 0.45% NS 500mL IV over 2 hr
- The non-gap acidosis that occurs in the recovery phase of DKA generally does not require management (2/2 to ↑Cl)

o **Insulin**
- Initialization ONLY if K > 3.3 mEq/L and 1L has already been given!
  - 0.1u/kg regular insulin, single bolus IV push *then*
  - 0.1 u/kg/hr regular insulin continuous IV drip (usually 5 – 7 u/hr)
- If glucose does not fall by 10% in the first hour, rebolus with insulin 0.14U/kg IV then continue previous infusion rate
- BS<=200 and tolerating PO intake, AG<12, HCO3>15
  - Switch to SQ insulin when BS reaches 200-250 and resolution of anion gap, patient tolerating PO inake, HCO3 >15, serum/urine ketones are low or absent
  - Either be sure acidosis has resolved on repeat ABG or check that there are no urine ketones.
  - Begin subcutaneous insulin appx 1-2 hrs before stopping IV insulin. There are no guidelines for this, here are some options[189]:

> Average insulin drip rate over previous 6 hours x 24 = TDD
>
> TDD x 60% = Basal insulin dose
>
> TDD x 10% = Preprandial dose
> Usually 0.5-1.3 u/kg/d divided 2/3 AM and 1/3PM with each dose divided 2/3 NPH and 1/3 R
>
> -or-
> Restart home dosage
> -or-
> Lantus (.1U/kg x ½)

- Keep IV insulin on board (1/2 normal rate or appx 0.02-0.05U/kg/hr) for 4 hours if you started Lantus, 2 hours if NPH
  - Start either prior dose of insulin or if starting on insulin then calculate long acting + short acting based on dose of 0.5-0.8 U/kg/d.
  - Add SSI for correction as needed
  - Fluids should be changed to D51/2NS from 0.9NS and maintain at 150-250 cc/hr
  - Maintain glucose at 150-200

Management of DKA

Glucose	Insulin Drip	IV Fluids	Potassium Repletion
To begin: - Fluids: Administer 0.9NS or 0.45NS at 500-1000cc/hr during the first 1-2 hrs depending on serum Na level - First give insulin bolus at 0.1 U/kg of regular insulin - Start IV insulin gtt at 0.1 U/kg/hr and check glucose levels q1-2h			
>500	Increase drip by 4 units/hr (or 25 %, which ever increase is less)	Na >135: 0.45NS Na <135: 0.9NS	K > 5: none K 4.1 - 5: add 20 mEq/L K 3.3 - 4: add 40 mEq/L K <3.3: use an IVPB
251-500	Do not adjust rate if blood glucose is decreasing by 50-75 mg/dL/hr If blood glucose is NOT decreasing by 50-75 mg/dL/hr, then increase the drip rate by 2 units/hr	Na >135: 0.45NS Na <135: 0.9NS	K > 5: none K 4.1 - 5: add 20 mEq/L K 3.3 - 4: add 40 mEq/L K <3.3: use an IVPB
151-250	When the plasma glucose reaches **200** mg/dl in DKA, decrease the insulin infusion rate to 0.05 - 0.1 unit/kg/h (or 3–6 units/h) to maintain serum glucose of 150-200 mg/dl	Change to Na >135: D5W-0.45NS Na<135: D5W-0.9 NS	K > 5: none K 4.1 - 5: add 20 mEq/L K 3.3 - 4: add 40 mEq/L K <3.3: use an IVPB
101-150	Decrease insulin drip by 50%	Na >135: D5-0.45NS Na<135: D5-0.9 NS	K > 5: none K 4.1 - 5: add 20 mEq/L K 3.3 - 4: add 40 mEq/L K <3.3: use an IVPB
71-100	Hold insulin drip for 1 hour	Na >135: D5-0.45NS Na<135: D5-0.9 NS	K > 5: none K 4.1 - 5: add 20 mEq/L K 3.3 - 4: add 40 mEq/L K <3.3: use an IVPB
<70	Hold insulin drip (if not already held). Give D50, 12.5 IV Recheck FS in 15 minutes	Change to D10W	K > 5: none K 4.1 - 5: add 20 mEq/L K 3.3 - 4: add 40 mEq/L K <3.3: use an IVPB

- **Resolution**
  - Glucose <200-250
  - Anion Gap <12
  - Serum Bicarb at least 19
  - Patient tolerating PO intake
  - Absent or low serum/urine ketones but not necessary as they can often be falsely elevated

Figure. Algorithm for management of adult patient with DKA

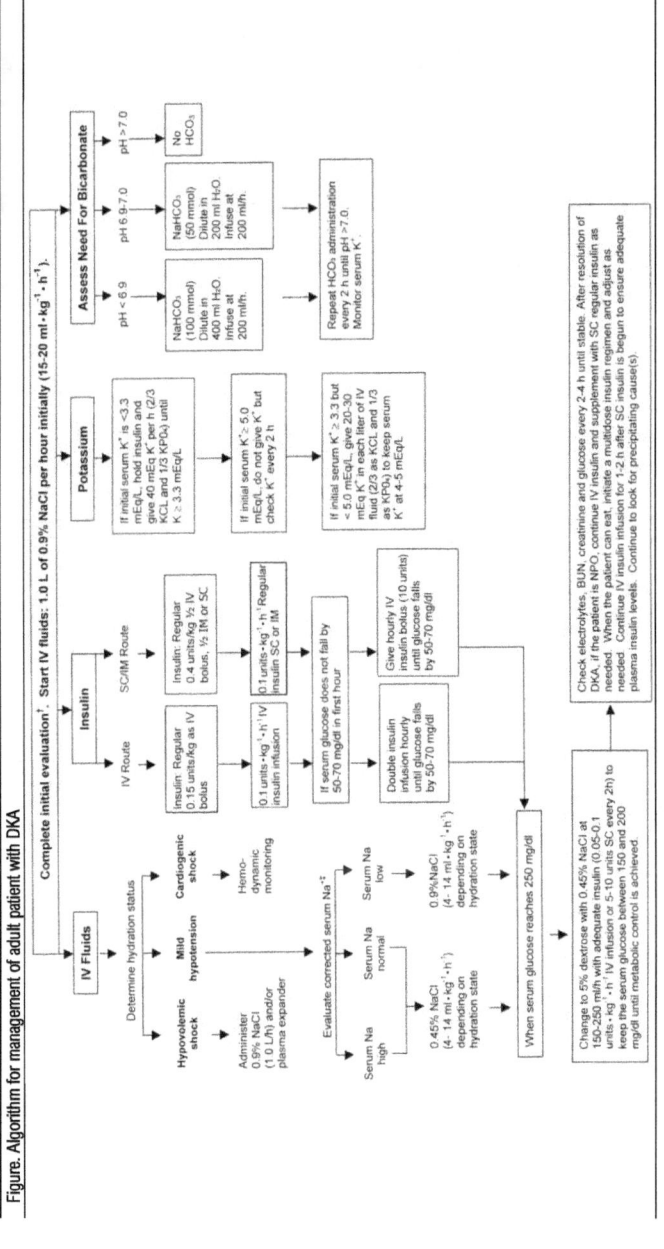

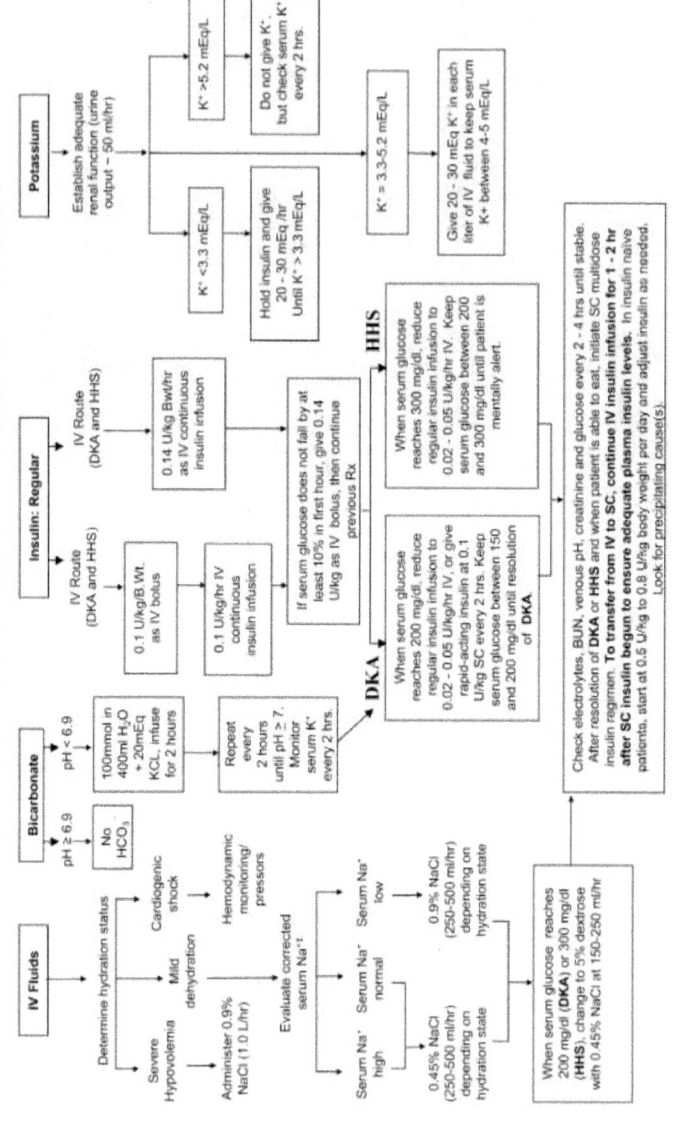

HYPEROSMOLAR NONKETOTIC COMA

- **Pearls**[190]
  - Mainstay of treatment is fluids rather than insulin (DKA); fluid deficit can be up to 10L
  - Often will have hyponatremia; need to correct for hyperglycemia!
- **Pathogenesis**: decreased insulin, increased stress hormones, usually precipitating event
- **Characteristics**: hyperglycemia, water deficit, hyperosmolarity, mental status changes
- **Diagnosis**: serum glucose > 600-800, Osm > 350, mental status changes, absent to low ketones, no acidosis
- **Symptoms**: polyuria, polydipsia, fatigue, weakness, lethargy, drowsiness, anorexia, mental status changes, seizures, aphasia, hemiplegia
- **Precipitants**: infection, CVA, pneumonia, MI, acute pancreatitis, drugs (phenytoin, diuretics, steroids, immunosuppressants)
- **Physical Exam**: orthostasis, tachycardia, tachypnea (shallow), fever, dry skin, myoclonus, hyperreflexia, positive Babinski sign, altered mental status/coma, sensory deficits, volume contraction, no Kussmaul breathing
- **Labs**: CBC, chemistry panel, glucose, serum/urine ketones, RUA, ABG, CXR, ECG, blood cultures
- **Treatment**:
  - <u>IV fluids</u>: start with rapid repletion NS 2-3 liters, replete 1/2 estimated deficit within 6 hours (usual total deficit is 8-10 L), then change to 0.45NS. Given the large amount of fluid administered, very careful monitoring of fluid status is imperative.
  - <u>Insulin</u>:
    - Initial loading dose of Regular Insulin 0.1U/kg (max 10U) f/b infusion at 0.1U/kg/hr
    - Titrate to decrease glucose 100 mg/dL/hour, use regimen described above for DKA
    - **Only give insulin after fluid deficit is starting to be replete** and potassium level normalized
      1. Low K can precipitate arrhythmias
      2. Often patient's glucose will normalize with fluids alone
  - Consider antibiotics if infection suspected

Figure. Algorithm for management of adult patients with HHS/HNK

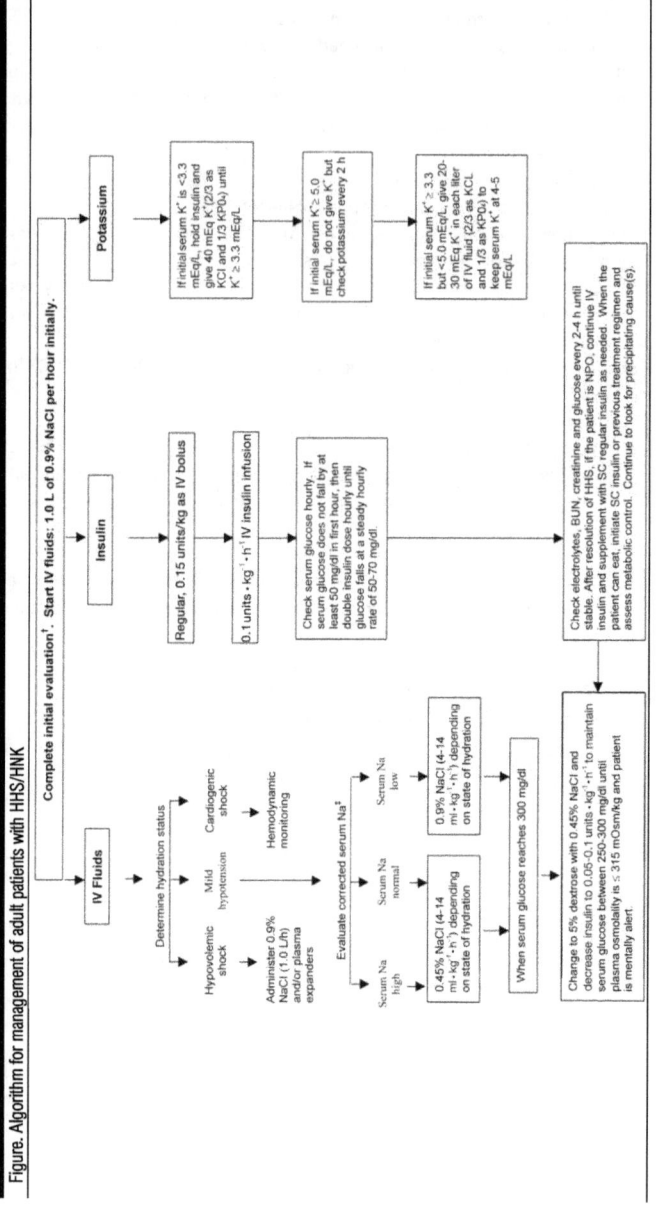

ENDOCRINOLOGY

HYPOGLYCEMIA

Hormone levels in Hypoglycemia

	C-Peptide	Proinsulin	Serum Insulin	Circul. PO Hypoglycemic Agent
Exogenous Insulin	↓	↓	↑	Negative
PO Hypoglycemic agents	↑	↑	↑	Present
Insulinoma	↑	↑	↑	Negative

Interpretation of Labs

Test	Normal	Insulinoma	Factitious (insulin injection)	Factitious (oral hypoglycemic)
Insulin	<3	Norm-High	Very High	Norm to High
C-peptide	<0.2	Norm-High	Low	Norm to High
Oral hypoglycemic screen	Negative	Negative	Negative	Positive
Proinsulin	<5	High	Low	High

- **Pearls**[190]
  - Sulfonylureas and meglitinide increase insulin secretion/activity and can cause hypoglycemia unlike metformin
    - ½ life often 14-16 hours
  - Consider naloxone and thiamine for patients with AMS and concern for need for intubation (see page 438 on *Unresponsive Patient*)
    - Injectable @ 800mcg >INH
- **Treatment**
  - Check BS q20m
- **Treatment**
  - If pt alert
    - Give 15-30g carbs via:
      - 8 oz juice/soda = 30 g carbs
      - ½ cup of juice
      - ½ cup of regular soft drink
      - 2 graham cracker squares = 10 g carbs
      - 3-4 glucose tablets
    - 15 g carbs will increase BG by 25-50 mg/dL
  - Non-alert pt
    - Give 25 g dextrose IV (1 amp D50) or 1 mg glucagon IM if no IV access and recheck BG after 5-10 min
    - If severe or recurrent hypoglycemia
      - Use D5 or D10 drip
      - When BG>90: Wait 1 hour, Recheck BG
      - If BG still >90: Restart infusion at 50% of most recent rate

HYPERTHYROIDISM

- **Etiology**[191]
  - Graves' disease (60-80%)
  - ABs: +TSI or TBII, anti-TPO, antithyroglobulin, ANA
  - Thyroiditis (either the thyrotoxic phase of subacute thyroiditis or painless)
  - Painful thyroid to palpation

ENDOCRINOLOGY

- o +TPO Ab
- o Toxic adenoma (single or multinodular)
- o Rx: amiodarone
- **History**
  - o Ask about h/o cancer, radiation exposure, pregnancy and family history of thyroid d/o.
- **Clinical Presentation**
  - o Restlessness, sweating, tremor, ↑HR, ↓weight, moist skin, diarrhea, ↑reflexes
  - o Consider storm in patients with delirium, ↑Temp, ↑HR, ↑BP with wide gap, GI sx
  - o Goiter
  - o Ophthalmopathy (seen in only 50%)
  - o Pretibial myxedema

Causes of Hyperthyroidism				
Disease	FT4	FT3	Uptake Scan (RAIU)	Others
Graves	↑	↑ (T3>T4)	Increased + homogenous	High TSI or thyrotropin receptor Ab
Silent Thyroiditis	↑	↑	Low uptake	Thyroid peroxidase Ab +
Painful subacute thyroiditis	↑	↑	Low uptake	Thyroid-related Ab usually negative
Exogenous Ingestion	↑	↑	Low uptake	Serum thyroglobulin very low or absent
Toxic multinodular goiter	↓/normal/↑	↑	Increased/patchy	Thyroid-related Ab usually -
Solitary nodule	↓/normal/↑	↑	Increased focal uptake, suppression within surrounding gland	Thyroid-related Ab usually -

- **Thyroid Storm**
  - Precipitants
    - o MI
    - o Infection
    - o Surgery
    - o DKA
  - Symptoms/Diagnosis
    - o Use SAALE point system
      - Storm likely with >45 points
      - Impending storm if point total 25-44
      - Unlikely storm if <25 points
  - Treatment
    - o *Medications*
      - Propranolol @ 240mg or higher (vs. atenolol due to ↑ reduction of T4→T3 conversion)
      - PTU>MMI (↑ reduction of T4→T3 conversion)
      - +/- steroids (suspected concomitant adrenal insufficiency)
      - +/- iodine (SSKI, Lugol) to inhibit further hormone release
      - Acetaminophen
    - o *Endocrinology consult*
- **Labs**

- o ↓TSH ↑FT4 and ↑FT3
    - Normal TSH often excludes hyperthyroidism
    - ↑ FT4 or FT3 confirms thyrotoxicosis. If FT4 elevated no need to check FT3, diagnosis is already confirmed.
    - if ↓ or normal FT4 and ↓ TSH, measure FT3; use T3 if FT3 assay not available
    - Normal FT4 and FT3 suggests subclinical hyperthyroidism, lab error, hypothalamic or pituitary disease, nonthyroidal illness, or medication effects.
- o ↑calcinuria
- o ↑Ca
- o Anemia
- o Consider measuring thyroid antibodies and serum thyroglobulin if the etiology is still unclear after a thyroid scan
- **Imaging**
    - o US
        - Useful in distinguishing cystic from solid nodules (benign vs. malignant)
        - If a solitary or dominant nodule, do FNA to r/o cancer
    - o Scintigraphy
    Scanning should not be performed in a woman who is pregnant (with the exception of a molar pregnancy) or breastfeeding. Perform scanning if patients do not have classic Graves (exophthalmos or symmetrically enlarged thyroid)
        - Iodine-123 (123 I) or technetium-99m (99m Tc) can be used for thyroid scanning.
        - Normally, the isotope distributes homogeneously throughout both lobes of the thyroid gland.
        - In patients with hyperthyroidism, the pattern of uptake (e.g., diffuse vs nodular) varies with the underlying disorder.
        1. Normal: 2-26% (@ 24 hours 8-25%)
        2. Increased (40-100%) and homogenous/diffuse: diffuse toxic goiter (Graves)
        3. Single/Multiple Foci of Increased Uptake: toxic thyroid adenoma or toxic multinodular goiter
        4. Decreased (<2%): thyrotoxic phase of subacute thyroiditis or a nonthyroidal source of thyroid hormone
        Less Common Forms
        5. Decreased (<25%): iodide-induced thyrotoxicosis, metastatic thyroid carcinoma or struma ovarii

ENDOCRINOLOGY

Medications for treatment of Hyperthyroidism

Drug	Dosing	Comment
Propylthiouracil	500–1000 mg load, then 250 mg every 4 hours	Blocks new hormone synthesis Blocks T4 → T3 conversion
Methimazole	60–80 mg/day	Blocks new hormone synthesis
Propranolol	60–80 mg every 4 hours	Consider invasive monitoring in congestive heart failure patients Blocks T4 → T3 conversion in high doses Alternate drug: esmolol infusion
Iodine (saturated solution of potassium iodide)	5 drops (0.25 mL or 250 mg) orally every 6 hours	Do not start until 1 hour after antithyroid drugs Blocks new hormone synthesis Blocks thyroid hormone release
Hydrocortisone	300 mg intravenous load, then 100 mg every 8 hours	May block T4 → T3 conversion Prophylaxis against relative adrenal insufficiency Alternative drug: dexamethasone

- **Treatment**
  - Pregnancy Specific Goals
  - Thyroid function testing q4w
    - Goals:
      - Maintain mild hyperthyroid state with TSH 0.1-0.3, FT4 just above trimester specific ranges, and TT3/TT4 1.5x nonpregnant range
  - Treatment includes symptom relief, antithyroid pharmacotherapy, radioactive iodine-131 (131I) therapy (the preferred treatment of hyperthyroidism among US thyroid specialists), or thyroidectomy.
  - Antithyroid medications are **not effective** in thyrotoxicosis in which scintigraphy shows **low uptake** of iodine-123 (123I), as in patients with subacute thyroiditis, because these cases result from release of **preformed** thyroid hormone.
  - Patients should be given written or documented verbal instruction to the effect that if they develop high fever (>100.5°F) or a severe sore throat, they should stop the medication and seek medical attention.
  - Many of the neurologic and cardiovascular symptoms are relieved with propranolol.
  - Anti-Thyroid Medications
    - Drug dose should be titrated every 4 weeks until thyroid functions normalize.
    - Best in patients with Graves' disease (or can use radioactive iodine)
    - Some patients with Graves' disease go into a remission after treatment for 12-18 months, and the drug can be discontinued.
      - 1/2 of the patients who go into remission experience a recurrence of hyperthyroidism within the following year.
      - Nodular forms of hyperthyroidism (i.e., toxic multinodular goiter and toxic adenoma) are permanent conditions and will not go into remission.
    - Methimazole
      - *Dosing*: 10-20mg PO once daily (in divided q8h dosing) or dose by symptoms severity:
        - mild, 15 mg/day
        - moderate, 30-40 mg/day
        - severe, 60 mg/day
      - *Pregnancy*: use lowest dose to keep free T4 at or slightly above ULN for nonpregnant women; assess monthly and adjust dose as required.

- □ *Duration* - taper or discontinue if TSH levels are normal after 12-18 months if for tx of Grave disease
- □ *S/E*: risk for agranulocytosis; check LFTs, WBC, TSH
- Propylthiouracil
  - □ *Dosing* – 50-150 mg PO TID; may ↑ to 400 mg/day for severe hyperthyroidism, very large goiters, or both.
  - □ *Duration*: as above
  - □ *Pregnancy*: used in thyrotoxicosis due to Graves' disease in the first trimester only (otherwise switch to MMU for 2nd and 3rd. Use lowest dose to keep mother's total thyroxine (T4) and triiodothyronine (T3) levels slightly above normal range for pregnancy, keep TSH suppressed.
  - □ *S/E*: risk for hepatocellular necrosis; best in pregnancy; check LFTs, WBC, and TSH

HYPOTHYROIDISM

- **Etiology**
  - o Hashimoto's, iodine deficiency, drugs (lithium, iodide, propylthiouracil, sulfonamides, amiodarone), infiltrative disease (*e.g.* sarcoid), genetic enzyme defects, after therapy for other thyroid disease, and secondary to hypopituitarism.
- **Classic Symptoms**: fatigue, sluggishness, hoarse voice, constipation, delayed distal tendon reflexes, and skin changes
- **Screening**
  Done with TSH only
  - o Women reaching age 50 YO
  - o Those at risk given hx of neck radiation, family history, hx of autoimmune disease, patients with goiter
  - o Use third generation TSH assays starting at 35 q5y or more frequent/early if high risk conditions such as pregnancy, female>60, T1DM, h/o neck radiation
- **Diagnosis**
  - o Screening: TSH, often elevated above 10, then get FT4 which should be low in hypothyroidism
    - If patient has elevated TSH (often <10) but normal FT4, this is termed **subclinical hypothyroidism** and data is mixed in whether to treat these patients. All pregnant patients with SCH should be treated
      1. If FT4 is normal can get anti-TPO antibody to determine risk of progressing to clinical hypothyroidism
    - Thyroglobulin AB (Tg Ab) is often also found in patients with Hashimoto's hypothyroidism (along with anti-TPO AB)
    - Other labs: ↑cholesterol, ↑AST/ALT
  - o Hospital - Should not be done due to high likelihood of SES (see next topic)
  - o Pregnant patients: FT4, Total T4, TSH (> 2.5 milliunits/L in the first trimester, > 3 milliunits/L in the second trimester, or > 3-3.5 milliunits/L in the third trimester)

ENDOCRINOLOGY

Thyroid Hormone Profiles

Hormone Profile	Associated Condition
↑TSH ↓T4	Hypothyroidism
↑TSH normal T4	Treated hypothyroidism or subclinical hypothyroidism
↑TSH ↑T4	TSH secreting tumor or thyroid hormone resistance
↑TSH ↑T4 and ↓T3	Slow conversion of T4→T3 or thyroid hormone AB artifact
↓TSH ↑T4/↑T3	Hyperthyroidism
↓TSH normal T4/T3	Subclinical hyperthyroidism
↑TSH ↓T4	Central hypothyroidism (r/o pituitary source)
↓TSH ↓T4 and ↓T3	Sick euthyroidism or pituitary disease

- **Types**
  - Primary – 95% of cases; ↑TSH ↓FT4
  - Secondary – due to insufficient stimulation of TSH (due to ↓TRH) caused by either pituitary or hypothalamic issue. Consider this diagnosis in patients with known mass lesion in the pituitary or multiple hormonal deficiencies are also present
- **Causes**
  - Hashimoto's
    - Most common cause in adequate iodine intake countries (whereas iodine deficiency is the most common cause in those countries where deficiency remains)
    - Form of autoimmune thyroid disease
    - +thyroid peroxidase ab
- **Treatment**
  - Levothyroxine: start *low* and go *slow* (↓ risk of AF or MI). Consider starting with 50mcg/d (1.5-1.7 mcg/kg of IBW which is about 100-125mcg/d in healthy adults or 1.0mcg/kg if elderly) taken ½ to 1 hour **before breakfast** with at least 3-4 hours between taking any other medications or 3 hours **after dinner**. Alternatively, patient can take the medication at nighttime as long as it is 3h after dinner. Patients with known cardiac disease should be started at lower dose of 12.5-25 mcg/d
    - **Always take on an empty stomach**
      1. Absorption affected by: coffee, soy, calcium, phosphate binders, raloxifene
    - Full replacement dose can be started initially (no titrating up required) in healthy and young patients (ATA does not define 'young')
      1. If elderly or h/o ischemic heart disease, start at ¼ - ½ the level and increase every 6 weeks
      2. Mild to moderate can often be treated with solely 50-75mcg
    - First labs obtained after starting therapy should be done after **at least** 2 months!
    - Goal TSH is 2-3 mIU/L → after reaching goal, check every 6 months then every 12 months
    - Often takes 4-6 weeks for TSH levels to reflect effects of therapy.
    - Sole treatment with L-T4 remains first line therapy as T4 is converted peripherally to T3 if sufficient T4 is given
    - Concurrent h. pylori, celiac disease, or gastritis may require higher doses
  - Myxedema coma: levothyroxine 5-8 mcg/kg IV load, then daily 50-100 mcg IV, consider adrenal insufficiency, treat underlying precipitant
  - **Hypertension** – classically patients will have ↑diastolic pressure and ↓pulse pressure.
  - Suggestion of whether the true ULN of TSH is inadequate, and patients should be treated to TSH of 1.0-1.5 mU/l
  - **Thyroidectomy**
    - Risks include voice loss or change in voice
    - TSH is the only pre-surgery lab value required
- **Monitoring**

- o TSH is best to use as a monitoring lab; T4 only checked if concerned of central hypothyroidism
    - Normal TSH considered 0.3-3.0 mIU/mL but up to 5.0 in older adults
- o If checking labs, make sure patient did not take their replacement therapy yet
- o Patients will often have ↑diuresis and weight loss with successful changes in therapy
- **Maintenance Changes**
    - o Most common reason for changes is **noncompliance**
    - o 12.5-25mcg changes at any time
    - o May take 6-8 weeks to note change.
        - Consider obtaining T3 and T4 to look for immediate changes while waiting for TSH to eventually respond
        - TSH can then be used once the T4 and T3 return to normal range
    - o Catch-up doses can be taken at the end of the week to maintain a weekly level
- **Adding T3 therapy (aka combination therapy)**
    - o Long held belief that those that have normal T4 levels should theoretically have normal T3 levels due to the physiologic conversion from T4→T3 to maintain homeostasis
    - o Animal models have shown those with primary hypothyroidism on L-T4 monotherapy is not sufficient to normalize systemic thyroid levels
    - o Debate ongoing between ATA and AACE due to s/e reported (↑ risk of AF, angina, MI)
    - o ATA previously advised against combination therapy, but more recently changed their stance to "insufficient evidence to support"
    - o Numerous studies have addressed potential benefits of combined therapy of triiodothyronine with LT4. Results of these studies have failed to support a potential benefit of combined therapy
    - o Suggestion of benefit was raised from question if LT4 alone is sufficient to treat hypothyroidism
    - o Presence of genetic polymorphism may suggest which patients on treatment may benefit from treatment with T3 as well.
        - Symptoms suggestive of the presence of this include patients with high free T4/free T3 ratio
        - Most physicians consider this route when patients on LT4 remain symptomatic
    - o Levothyroxine remains first-line therapy (effective in 80-90% of patients)

Figure. Evaluation of hypothyroidism

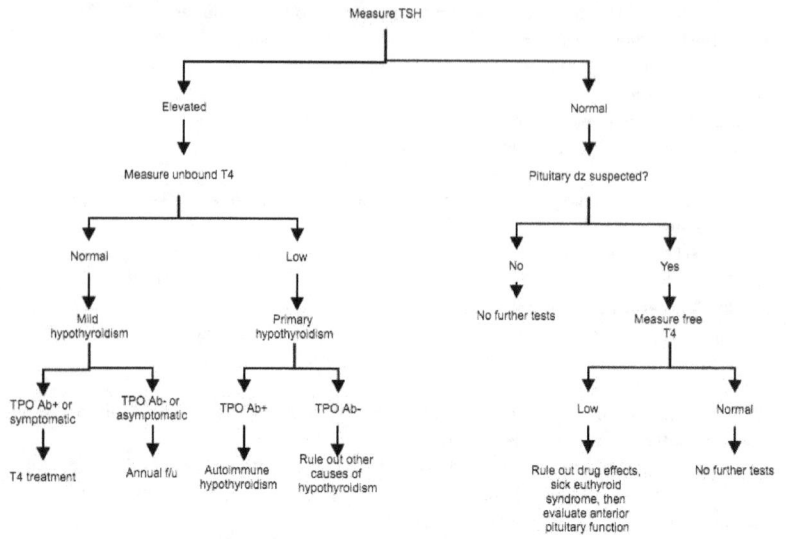

PITUITARY INCIDENTALOMA

- **Overview**[192]
  - Occur in up to 10% of patients undergoing MRI
  - All patients, no matter the size, should undergo clinical and laboratory workup for function
  - All patients with visual complaints (normally bitemporal hemianopsia) undergo formal visual field (VF) testing
- **Labs**
  - Hypersecretion:
    - Prolactin (PLCT)
    - GH/IGF-1
    - ACTH (if clinically indicated, routine measurement is not necessarily recommended)
  - Hyposecretion
    - Prolactin
    - TSH
    - Free T4
    - AM Cortisol
    - Testosterone
    - LH
    - FSH
    - IGF-1

Figure. Evaluation and treatment of pituitary incidentalomas

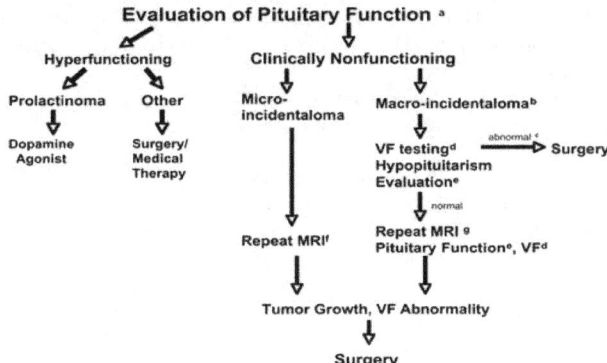

- **Management**
  - <10mm (*microadenoma*): if 2-4mm and no function (nml PLCT), then no further testing. If 5-9mm, then repeat MRI in 12 months (then 2 years if unchanged, then q3y, etc.)
  - >10mm (*macroadenoma*): check for pituitary hyper/hypo function with visual field testing. If positive, do surgery. If not positive, follow and do surgery if increasing in size over time and repeat imaging in 6 months (then 1 year if unchanged, then q2y, etc.)
  - Surgery
    - VF deficit
    - Compression on the optic nerve (or close to the chiasm if planning on pregnancy)
    - Unremitting headaches
    - Pituitary apoplexy
    - Hypersecreting adenomas
    - Clinically significant growth

STEROIDS

Steroid formulations				
Agent	Dose (mg)	Potency	Mineralcort. potency	Half life
Cortisone	25	0.8	0.8	8-12
Hydrocortisone	20	1	1	8-12
Prednisone	5	4	0.8	18-36
Prednisolone	5	4	0.8	18-36
Methylprednisolone	5	5	0.5	18-36
Dexamethasone	0.75	25	0	35-54

- **Emergency Steroids**
  - Immediate high-dose IV hydrocortisone 100 mg bolus followed by infusion of 100-200 mg over the next 24 hours or intermittent IV dosing at 100 mg q6-8 hours.
  - "Stress dose steroids" typically means at least 200-300 mg of hydrocortisone per day dosed as 100mg bolus followed by 50mg IV every 6 hours (or continuous infusion of 200mg/d). Decrease the dose the following day to 100mg over the entire day with complete tapering back to baseline dose in 3-4 days
- **Taper**[193]

- o Physiologic doses of steroids (Hydrocortisone 30 mg (20 mg qAM, 10 mg qPM) OR Cortisone 37.5 mg (25 mg qAM, 12.5 mg qPM) OR prednisone 7.5 mg (5 mg qAM, 2.5 mg qPM)) are around 5-10 mg/day thus any dose of this will not require a taper.[194]
- o When providing therapy of ≥20 mg for more than 20 days (20/20 rule) a taper is required to ↓ risk for withdrawal
- o If rx is <= 40, cut by half, if greater, then cut by 25%
- o All tapers are different, one example is as such:
  - First Method
    - □ Decrease dose by 10mg every other week until reaching 20 mg
    - □ Decrease dose by 5 mg every week until finished
  - Second Method
    - □ Rx for 40 mgs or above: a reduction of up to 10 mgs every few weeks is acceptable
    - □ Rx is between 20 and 40mgs: tapering of no more than 5 mgs every few weeks is standard
    - □ At 20 mgs, taper down in increments of 2.5 mgs every four weeks, and when the dosage gets down to 10 mgs per day, tapering in 1 to 2 mgs every four weeks is best.
  - Third Method
    - □ Decrease the dose the following day after surgery to 100mg over the entire day with complete tapering back to baseline dose in 3-4 days

THYROID NODULE

- **Differential Diagnosis**[195,196]
  - o Thyroid cancer (↑ risk if: family hx, excessive radiation exposure, sx such as hoarse voice, dysphagia)
  - o Benign adenoma
  - o Colloid cyst
  - o Metastasis

Types of Thyroid Nodules		
Adenomas	Carcinoma	Colloid Nodule
Macrofollicular adenoma (simple colloid)	Papillary (75%)	Dominant nodule in a multinodular goiter
Microfollicular adenoma (fetal)	Follicular (10%)	
Embryonal adenoma (trabecular)	Medullary (5-10%)	
Hurthle cell adenoma (oxyphilic, oncolytic)	Anaplastic (5%)	
	Other (i.e. Lymphoma 5%)	
Atypical adenoma	Cyst	Other
Adenoma with papillae	Simple cyst	Inflammatory thyroid disorders (i.e. subacute thyroiditis, chronic l lymphocytic thyroiditis, granulomatous dz)
Signet-ring adenoma	Cystic/solid tumors (i.e. hemorrhagic, necrotic)	
		Developmental abnormalities (i.e. dermoid, rare unilateral lobe agenesis)

- **Diagnosis/Evaluation**
  - o Obtain TSH
    - ↑TSH:
      - □ Likely cold nodule
      - □ Obtain US in all thyroid nodules

- Based on the ATA, obtain FNA if ≥1cm and at least one of the following suspicious signs:
  - **Nodule**: microcalcifications, hypoechogenicity, irregular margins, taller than wider
  - **LN**: microcalcifications, hyperechogenicity, peripheral vascularity, rounded shape, cystic aspect
- Or if solid isoechoic/hyperechoic ≥1 cm without the above findings or cystic and ≥2cm
  - Often requires 2-4 passes to have diagnostic significance in 80% cases
  - Calcitonin should only be sent for if patient has family hx of medullary thyroid cancer or MEN-2
  - If results confirm cancer, then proceed to RAIU to determine if nodule is functioning.
    - If functioning nodule (↑uptake, hot), can avoid surgery
    - If nonfunctioning nodule (↓uptake, cold) surgery is indicated
      - Monitor with f/u US if <1cm
    - Normal TSH:
      - Likely cold nodule
      - See above
    - ↓TSH:
      - Suggests hot nodule (toxic adenoma)
      - RAIU scan to confirm if hot
      - Hot? Treat with I131
      - Cold? Likely malignant, obtain FNA
- **Treatment**
  - Functioning nodule, ↑ Ca risk – hemithyroidectomy
  - Benign functioning nodule – radioiodine
  - Nonfunctioning nodules – ethanol injection if solid, therapeutic aspiration if cystic
  - Surgery – indications include features suggestive of cancer, symptoms 2/2 to nodules presence (hoarse voice, dysphagia); high risk of complications (such as hypoparathyroidism)
  - Levothyroxine – goal is to tx to obtain TSH of 0.3 to ↓ further growth however recent studies have shown better reduction if TSH is at 0.1 however ↑ adverse risks (atrial fibrillation, ↓bone density)
  - Radioiodine – tx of choice for functioning benign nodule; often implemented in cases of functioning nodule (↑uptake on RAIU), c/l in pregnant females, highest complication is hypothyroidism (test TSH yearly post operatively and continue to monitor for ↑ nodule size)
  - Ethanol injection – indicated in non-functioning nodules, cysts, benign functioning nodules by inducing coagulative necrosis and small-vessel thrombosis, higher efficacy with multiple treatments.

ENDOCRINOLOGY

Figure. Work up of a patient with a thyroid nodule

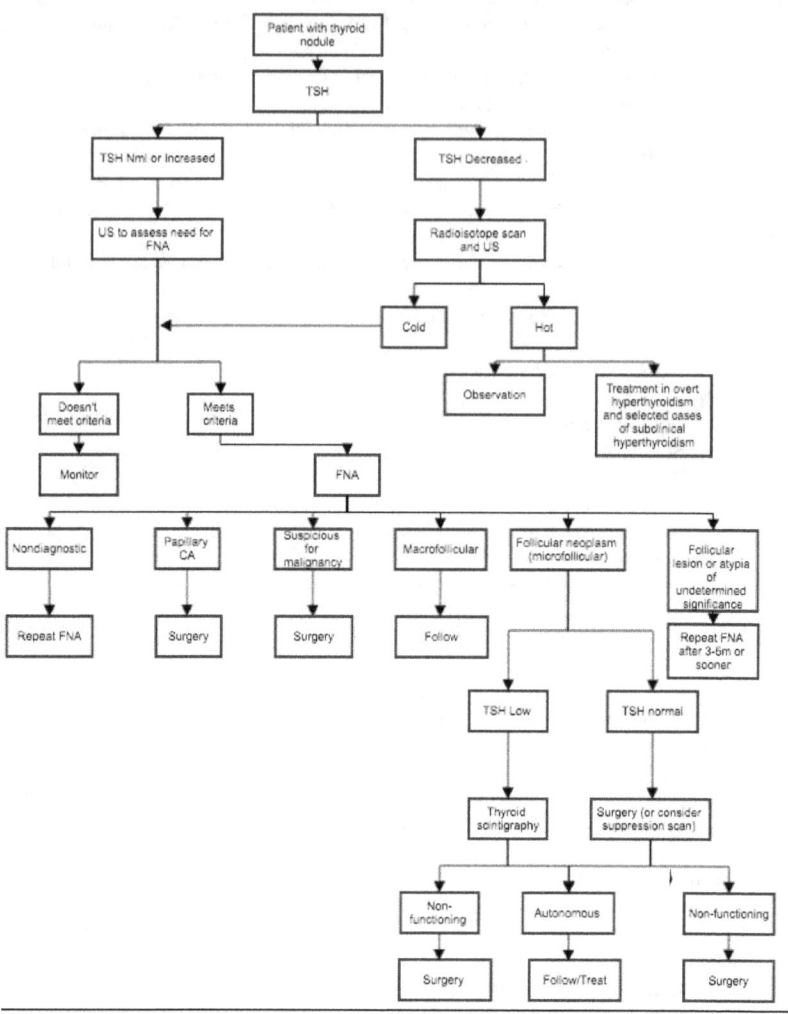

VITAMIN D DEFICIENCY

- **Who should be tested**
  - Evidence of severe deficiency:
    - Low 24-hour urine calcium excretion
    - ↑PTH
    - ↑ALKP
    - ↓Ca or PO4
    - Nontraumatic fractures
    - Osteopenia
- **Risk Factors**

- o Age>65
- o ↓ PO intake (malnutrition)
- o Low sun exposure
- o GI malabsorption (short bowel, celiac, pancreatitis, IBD, amyloidosis)
- o CKD
- **Symptoms**
  - o Bone discomfort/pain
  - o Generalized pain (may mimic fibromyalgia)
  - o Proximal muscle weakness
  - o Symmetric low back pain
  - o HA
  - o N/V
- **Other Labs**
  - o In severely low levels (<10), consider Ca, PO4, ALKP, PTH, BMP, transglutaminase
- **Diagnosis (Canadian Guidelines)**
  - o Deficiency: <10 ng/mL
  - o Insufficiency: 10-30 ng/mL
  - o Normal: >30 ng/mL
  - o Too High: >100 ng/mL
- **Testing/Normals**
  - o Total 25(OH)D is optimal
    - Goal 25-OHD: ≥30 ng/mL
- **Treatment**

  In patients that are nonobese and without malabsorption, for every 100 units of vitamin D3, serum 25(OH)D concentrations increase by approximately 0.7 -1.0 ng/mL (1.75 to 2.5 nmol/L).
  - o Commonly combined with 1000mg of Ca
    - If using oscal, comes with 25mcg of Vitamin D (1000IU) → raises serum levels by 6-10 ng/mL
    - Need 1200mg if age>71 or women 51-70 YO (d/t menopause)
  - o Dose needs to be increased by 2.5x if patient is obese or has malabsorption syndrome
  - o Contraindications: sarcoidosis, tuberculosis, metastatic bone disease, Williams syndrome
  - o Repletion:
    - *25(OH) <10 ng/mL*
      - Ergocalciferol (D3) 50,000IU (1250 mcg) PO once/week or 6000IU/d (150mcg/d) for 8w; after finishing you should start daily therapy with cholecalciferol 800-1000IU (max 2000IUj/d)
        - Recheck Vitamin D after 3 months
        - Maintenance: 800IU/d of VD3 thereafter
    - *25(OH) 10-20 ng/mL*
      - Ergocalciferol 800-1000IU (20-25mcg) daily; repeat lab after 3 mo
    - *25(OH) 20-30 ng/mL*
      - Ergocalciferol 600-800IU (10-15mcg) daily; repeat lab after 3 mo
    - *Malabsorption*
      - High doses of vitamin D of 10k-50k international units (250 to 1250 mcg) daily may be necessary.
  - o Long-term monitoring: if 25(OH)D levels remain low, consider UVB light therapy
    - Check 25-OHD levels only in patients with known osteoporosis, check 3-4 months after starting supplementation.
- **Prevention**
  - o Non-aged based: 1500-2000IU/d (37.5-50mcg/d)
  - o Low risk (<50 YO)

- 10-25mcg (400-1000IU) daily
- Moderate risk (>50 YO) or known osteoporosis
- 20-25mcg (800-1000IU) daily but up to 50mcg safe

Bibliography

[167] Zeiger et al. "American Association of Clinical Endocrinologists and American Association of Endocrine Surgeons Medical Guidelines for the Management of Adrenal Incidentalomas." Endocrine practice vol 15 (suppl 1) july/august 2009

[168] A. El Maghraoui and C. Roux. "DXA scanning in clinical practice" QJM (2008) 101(8): 605-617 first published online March 10, 2008 doi:10.1093/qjmed/hcn022

[169] South-Paul, Jeanette. "Osteoporosis: Part II. Nonpharmacologic and Pharmacologic Treatment." American Family Physician. March 15, 2001 / volume 63, number 6

[170] Lyles KW.Have we learned how to use bisphosphonates yet? J Am Geriatr Soc 2017 Sep; 65:1902. (http://dx.doi.org/10.1111/jgs.14948)

[171] AACE Male Sexual Dysfunction Task Force. AMERICAN ASSOCIATION OF CLINICAL ENDOCRINOLOGISTS MEDICAL GUIDELINES FOR CLINICAL PRACTICE FOR THE EVALUATION AND TREATMENT OF MALE SEXUAL DYSFUNCTION: A COUPLE'S PROBLEM–2003 UPDATE.

[172] Qaseem A, Horwitch CA, Vijan S, et al, for the Clinical Guidelines Committee of the American College of Physicians. Testosterone Treatment in Adult Men With Age-Related Low Testosterone: A Clinical Guideline From the American College of Physicians. Ann Intern Med. 2020; [Epub ahead of print 7 January 2020].

[173] Tsametis CP, Isidori AM. Testosterone Replacement Therapy: for whom, when and how?" Metabolism. 2018 Mar 9. pii: S0026-0495(18)30073-8.

[174] Schnipper JL. Chapter 149. Inpatient Management of Diabetes and Hyperglycemia. In: Lawry GV, Matloff J, Dressler DD, Brotman DJ, Ginsberg JS, eds. Principles and Practice of Hospital Medicine. New York: McGraw-Hill; 2012.

[175] AACE. "American Association of Clinical Endocrinologists' Comprehensive Diabetes Management Algorithm 2013." Endocr Pract. 2013;19:327-336.

[176] American Diabetes Association. Older adults. Sec. 10. In Standards of Medical Care in Diabetesd2016. Diabetes Care 2016;39(Suppl. 1):S81–S85.

[177] Sacks DB. Diabetes Care. 2011.

[178] Summary of revisions for the 2013 clinical practice recommendations. Diabetes Care. January 2013 vol. 36 no. Supplement 1 S3.

[179] Qaseem A, Barry MJ, Humphrey LL, Forciea MA; Clinical Guidelines Committee of the American College of Physicians. Oral Pharmacologic Treatment of Type 2 Diabetes Mellitus: A Clinical Practice Guideline Update From the American College of Physicians. Ann Intern Med. 2017 Jan 3.

[180] Ingham M, Lefebvre P, Pilon D, et al. Glycaemic control, weight loss, and use of other antihyperglycaemics in patients with type 2 diabetes initiated on canagliflozin or sitagliptin: a real-world analysis. Paper presented at: European Association for the Study of Diabetes (EASD) 53rd Annual Meeting 2017; September 11-15, 2017. Lisbon, Portugal. http://www.abstractsonline.com/pp8/-1/4294/presentation/5259. Accessed on September 18, 2017.

[181] Ou SM, Shih CJ, Chao PW, et al. Effects on clinical outcomes of adding dipeptidyl peptidase-4 inhibitors versus sulfonylureas to metformin therapy in patients with type 2 diabetes mellitus. Ann Inter Med. 2015;163:663-672. doi:10.7326/M15-0308.

[182] Ian Blumer, Eran Hadar, David R. Hadden, Lois Jovanovič, Jorge H. Mestman, M. Hassan Murad, Yariv Yogev; Diabetes and Pregnancy: An Endocrine Society Clinical Practice Guideline, The Journal of Clinical Endocrinology & Metabolism, Volume 98, Issue 11, 1 November 2013, Pages 4227–4249, https://doi.org/10.1210/jc.2013-2465

[183] Fowler, Michael. Clinical Diabetes. 2011.

[184] Hermida RC, Ayala DE, Mojón A, Fernández JR. Bedtime ingestion of hypertension medications reduces the risk of new-onset type 2 diabetes: a randomized controlled trial. Diabetologia. 2016 Feb;59(2):255-65. Erratum in: Diabetologia. 2016 Feb;59(2):395. PMID: 26399404.

[185] le Roux CW, Astrup A, Fujioka K, et al. 3 years of liraglutide versus placebo for type 2 diabetes risk reduction and weight management in individuals with prediabetes: A randomised, double-blind trial. Lancet. 2017;389:1399-1409. doi:10.1016/S0140-6736(17)30069-7.

[186] Shubrook, Jay. Doing the Math: Converting Analogue to Human Insulin. Medscape: Internal Medicine. June 12, 2019.

[187] USMLEWorld

[188] Kitabachi et al. "Hyperglycemic Crises in Adult Patients With Diabetes. DIABETES CARE, VOLUME 32, NUMBER 7, JULY 2009.

[189] Schmeltz, Lowell. "Management of Inpatient Hyperglycemia." Lab Med. 2011;42(7):427-434.

[190] McNaughton et al. "Diabetes in the Emergency Department: Acute Care of Diabetes Patients." Clinical Diabetes April 2011 vol. 29 no. 2 51-59

[191] Oxford Handbook of Clinical Medicine 10th edition and Pocket Medicine 6th Edition

[192] Freda et al. "Pituitary Incidentaloma: An Endocrine Society Clinical Practice Guideline." JCEM. July 02, 2013.

[193] Pazderska A, Pearce SH. Adrenal insufficiency - recognition and management. Clin Med (Lond). 2017;17:258-262

[194] http://www.mayoclinic.com/health/prednisone-withdrawal/AN01624

[195] Welker, Mary Jo. "Thyroid Nodules" AAFP Practical Therapeutics. FEBRUARY 1, 2003 / VOLUME 67, NUMBER 3

[196] Hegedus, Laszlo. "The Thyroid Nodule." NEJM 2004; 351:1764-71

GERIATRICS

Dementia 292
Mild Cognitive Impairment 301
End of Life Management 301

DEMENTIA

- **Defined** - decline in 2 or more cognitive capacities that causes impairment in function but not alertness or attention.
  - Consider in patients with memory difficulty that interferes with **independence**, daily function, unexplained functional decline, deterioration in hygiene, poor adherence to medical therapy, new-onset psychiatric symptoms, and new or repeated hospitalizations.
- **Overview**[197]
  - Aging — most significant r/f for Alzheimer disease and dementia in general
  - Pure Lewy body dementia or vascular dementia more common in younger patients
- **Most Common Types**
  AD, FTLD, LBD, VD, TBI, SUD, HIV, prion, PD, HD
  - Alzheimer's (AD)
    - *Diagnosis*: symptoms that...
      - Interfere with the ability to function at work or in usual activities
      - Represent a decline from previous levels of function
      - Are not due to delirium or a major psychiatric disorder
      - Are diagnosed through history, clinical examination, and a standardized instrument
      - Involve ≥2 cognitive domains
    - *Presentation*: short-term memory loss most common presenting symptom; immediate memory also affected; subtle language variants (e.g., logopenic [difficulty repeating or retrieving word]) and visual variants (e.g., inability to find objects in visual field) also seen; other symptoms — executive dysfunction; apathy; reactive irritability; most patients with dementia have **delusions** and **disorientation** late in disease. Poor performance on animal fluency suggests medial temporal or temporal lobe disorder.
    - *Notes*
      - Earliest presenting symptoms may be paranoid delusions or depression
      - Neurologic signs, such as falls, tremor, weakness, or reflex abnormalities, are not typical early in the disease and suggest alternative diagnosis.
  - Frontotemporal lobe (FTLD)
    - *Presentation*: executive dysfunction and behavioral changes; minimal memory loss; apathy and poor insight; cortical dysfunction, particularly involving language; behavioral disturbances; behavioral and aphasic are the main variants
  - Lewy Body (LBD)
    - *Presentation:* psychosis early in disease suggests LBD. Difficulty with executive functioning and visuospatial skills (i.e. clock drawing) more than issues with memory loss (more problems with processing speed). Will perform well on delayed recall. poor performance on animal fluency suggests medial temporal or temporal lobe disorder (e.g., AD), Poor performance on letter fluency more suggestive LBD. Insight often intact, so depression common; early visual hallucinations strongly correlated with LB pathology.
    - *Notes*
      - Accounts for up to 20% of dementia cases
      - Look for mild parkinsonism
      - Unexplained falls, hallucinations, delusions
  - Prion - sporadic — rapidly progressive; can occur in different sites in brain, so presentation variable; often presents with psychiatric disturbances and painful dysesthesias.

- Vascular (VD) – stepwise worsening of memory; often in combination with vascular disease; may co-occur with AD, LBD, and other disorders
- Parkinson's Disease Dementia (PD)
  - *Presentation:* Difficulty with executive functioning and visuospatial skills (i.e. clock drawing). Will perform well on delayed recall. poor performance on animal fluency suggests medial temporal or temporal lobe disorder (eg, AD), Poor performance on letter fluency more suggestive of PD.

- **Step by Step Approach**
  1) Pre-diagnostic Testing (look for risk factors, medical history of comorbid cardiovascular disease, prior labs such as CBC, glucose, thyroid, B12, RPR, LFTs, UA)
  2) Assess their performance (see screening below)
  3) Asses their daily functioning (determine the level of independence, and degree of disability with ADLs)
  4) Assess behavioral symptoms (NPI-Q, look for drug toxicity, psychiatric diagnoses that may be contributing)
  5) Identify caregiver needs
- **Protective from Dementia (*FINGER*)**
  - Nutrition
  - Exercise
  - Cognitive Training
  - Social Activity
- **Risk Factors for AD**
  - Female>male
  - Prior head trauma
  - Family history of AD
  - Obesity
  - HTN
  - DM
  - ↑Age
  - Smoking
- **History**
  - Warning signs associated with AD
    - Memory loss
    - Difficulty performing familiar tasks
    - Problems with language
    - Disorientation to time and place
    - Poor or ↓ judgement
    - Problems with abstract thought
    - Misplacing things
    - Changes in mood/behavior
    - Changes in personality
    - Loss of initiative
- **Screening**[198,199]
  - ACE v2
  - MMSE
  - Mini-Cog
  - SLUMS
  - MoCA

Memory screening and assessment tools

Tool	Key Features	Time	Cut off Score	Sensitivity/Specificity
MMSE	Costly Quick and easy Can be used to track progression of decline Insufficient evaluation of short term memory (STM)	5-10 minutes	23-24 / 30	79/95
Mini-Cog	Very short (only 3 items) Similar sens/spec to MMSE Poor evaluation of non-AD dementias	3 minutes	Probably normal/ possibly impaired	76/89
MoCA	Best to screen for MCI d/t high sensitivity. (look for delayed recall) Free Not good at detecting moderate/severe dementia More evaluation of executive function and STM Look at pattern rather than score	10 minutes	≤25	100/87

- **Diagnostic Testing**
  o Labs
    - Most will be WNL
    - *Initial Labs:* CBC, CMP, TSH, B12
    - *Consider*
      - HIV
      - RPR
      - ESR
      - Heavy metal screen
      - Thiamine level
      - UA (r/o infxn)
      - Paraneoplastic panel
      - Vitamin-D (unclear association b/w ↓ levels and ↑ risk for PD)
    - Presenilin-1 and amyloid precursor protein testing in patients with young-onset dementia and strong family history.
    - If dementia strongly suspected, biomarkers may be obtained to strengthen diagnosis of AD (through examination of cerebrospinal fluid [CSF] for β-amyloid [Aβ] and phospho-tau [P-tau], or amyloid imaging)

CSF evaluation/interpretation

	Aβ-amyloid	phospho-tau [P-tau]
Alzheimer's	↓↓ (<400 pg/mL)	↑↑ (≥60 pg/mL)
Lewy-Body	↓↓	↔
Parkinson's Disease	↓↓	↔
Fronto-Temporal	↔	↔
Creutzfeldt-Jakob	↔	-- (Tau levels ↑↑)

  o Imaging
    - CXR: r/o mass/tumor

- MRI better for identifying vascular disease
    - FTD: often shows more atrophy than expected; look for asymmetry
    - LBD: mild atrophy
    - Prion: cortical ribboning
    - VD: hyperintensities in >25% of white matter; multiple large-vessel infarcts; ≥2 basal ganglia and white matter lacunas
- Amyloid imaging – may ↑ diagnostic accuracy (more important for early-onset dementia)
- FDG-PET:
    - AD: parietal and posterior cingulate hypometabolism
    - FTD: frontal hypometabolism and relatively preserved parietal or posterior cingulate metabolism
    - LBD: hypometabolism in occipital region; scan not highly sensitive.
- o Consults
    - Neuropsych testing helpful in early cases or those that are atypical presentations.
- **Dementia with Behavioral Disorders**
    - o >95% of patients with dementia will experience behavioral disturbances over a 5 year span
    - o Evaluation
        - H&P
        - Screening tool: NPI-Q (can be used at baseline and after treatment to determine if rx is effective)
        - Consider MRI
            - Evaluate for cerebral atrophy, hippocampus involvement
        - Labs to r/o reversible cause
            - B12, folate, CBC, CMP, LFT
            - Optional: syphilis (RPR), HIV, Paraneoplastic ab (r/o autoimmune encephalitis), CSF proteins (tau, P-tau, 14-3-3) to r/o CJD
    - o Treatment[200]
        - Pharmacotherapy: see table on page 299
        - Psychosis
            - Changes in:
                - Mood: seen early, presents with depression, anxiety, mania, apathy
                - Thinking/Perception: seen early and late, presents with SI, delusions, suspiciousness, hallucinations
                - Activity: seen early and late, presents with agitation, verbal and physical attacks, aggression, disordered eating, altered sleep, inappropriate behaviors.
                - In general, look for: jealousy, paranoid delusions, auditory hallucinations, sreaming, agitation
            - Treatment
                - Nonpharmacologic: distract, leave room, light therapy, music/pet therapy, acupuncture, hand massage, CBT
                - Pharmacologic: no clear standard of care; consider starting when sx are severe, dangerous, or cause significant distress to patient
                - Nonemergency antipsychotic medication should only be used in treatment of agitation/psychosis when symptoms are severe, dangerous, and/or cause significant distress to the patient.[201]
                    - Use of any antipsychotics is off-label in the US (black box for increased risk of death compared to placebo; high risk for EPS); in Europe only risperidone is licensed for ≤6 weeks
                    - Always obtain an EKG to evaluate QTc

- Stop if no response noted within 4 weeks; taper off after 4 months of effective tx as they have been shown to worsen cognitive decline (*CATIE-AD)*.
  - Concluded that **olanzapine and risperidone** show equal and best effects with minimal side effects (↑ risk of stroke, gait abnormalities) in comparison to quetiapine and placebo
  - Can consider using Aripiprazole as well[202]
- Treatment Options:
  - Quietiapine (studied at 50mg/d; typically start at 12.5mg)
  - Olanzapine 5-10mg (5.5mg studied)
  - Risperidone 1mg (however better to start low at 0.25mg daily; studied @ 1mg)
  - Aripiprazole 2.5-10mg/d
  - Citalopram 10mg/d increased over 3 weeks to 30mg/d (nml max 20mg)
  - Parkinsons Disease Psychosis → Nuplazid
  - Pseudobulbar Affect → Neudexta
- *Monitoring Treatment*[203]
  - Baseline measurements:
    - Persona/Family history
    - Weight
    - Waist circumference
    - BP
    - Fasting glucose
    - Fasting lipids
  - Every 4-8 weeks: check weight
  - Every 12 weeks: Check weight, BP, glucose, lipids
  - Every Quarter: Check weight
  - Once a year: check personal history, wasit circumference, BP, glucose
- Agitation
  - APA recommends that in patients with dementia with agitation or psychosis, if there is no clinically significant response after a **4-week trial** of an adequate dose of an antipsychotic drug, the medication should be tapered and withdrawn.
  - In patients with dementia who show adequate response of behavioral/ psychological symptoms to treatment with an antipsychotic drug, an attempt to taper and withdraw the drug should be made **within 4 months of initiation**, unless the patient experienced a recurrence of symptoms with prior attempts at tapering of antipsychotic medication.
  - Options:
    - Citalopram 10mg/d→30mg/d over 3 weeks
    - Trazodone (limited data, beware sedation, falls)
    - Quietiapine 25mg qHS titrated to maximum 150mg BID (morning, evening)
    - Prazosin 1mg daily → increase to 1mg BID (max dose 9mg/d)
- Depression
  - Seen in up to 30% of patients with AD; often begins before the diagnosis of AD
  - Citalopram was the only antidepressant that showed benefit @ 10mg/d
  - Other options include Remeron (15mg/22.5mg/30mg)
- **Rapid Onset Dementia**
  - Defined – no specific timeline noted in literature, however considered decline in 1 or more cognitive domains in less than 1 or 2 years however, most occur over weeks to months when they are seen in the medical setting.[204]
  - Differential

- *CJD* (look for concomitant myoclonus, sleep difficulties, and psychiatric presentation, MRI of the brain will often show a pattern of increased intensity in the DWI of the basal ganglia and cortex)
- *HIV encephalopathy*
- *Lyme disease*
- *Neoplasm*
- *Frontotemporal dementia*
- *Dementia with Lewy bodies*
- *Progressive supranuclear palsy*
- *Vascular dementia*
- *Neurosyphilis*
  - Diagnostics
    - Imaging
      - Brain MRI (T1, T2, DWI, FLAIR, with and without contrast)
      - CXR
      - Others to consider: CT head, CT C/A/P, MRA/V, Mammogram, FDG-PET CT, TTE, testicular/pelvic US
    - CSF with
      - 14-3-3 (CJD)
      - Tau (CJD)
      - West Nile Virus
      - Cell count and differential
      - Culture
      - Glucose
      - Protein
      - IgG index
      - Oligoclonal bands (MS)
      - VDRL
      - Neuron specific enolase
      - Cryptococcal antigen
      - <u>Others to consider</u>: Whipple PCR, metagenomic deep sequencing, phosphorylated tau, B2-microglobulin and EBV PCR, amyloid-beta-42
    - EEG
      - Periodic sharp wave complexes seen with CJD
    - Labs
      - HIV
      - CBC with differential
      - LFTs
      - RPR
      - Rheumatologic screen (ESR, C-RP, ANA)
      - TSH
      - VB12
      - Appropriate medication levels (i.e. digoxin, phenytoin, lithium)
      - BMP/CMP
      - UA with culture
      - Urine toxicology
      - Heavy metal screen (urine)
      - Cultures: urine, blood, viral PCR, cytology

      Additional Labs to Consider
      - SPEP/UPEP
      - Blood smear
      - INR/PT/PTT

- Homocysteine
- Lyme AB
- Cortisol
- Antithyroglobulin, Anti-TPO
- ANCA, anti-ds-DNA, anti-Smith, SCL-70, SSA/SSB, RF, C3, C4, CH50

Figure. Suggested work up for rapidly progressive dementia

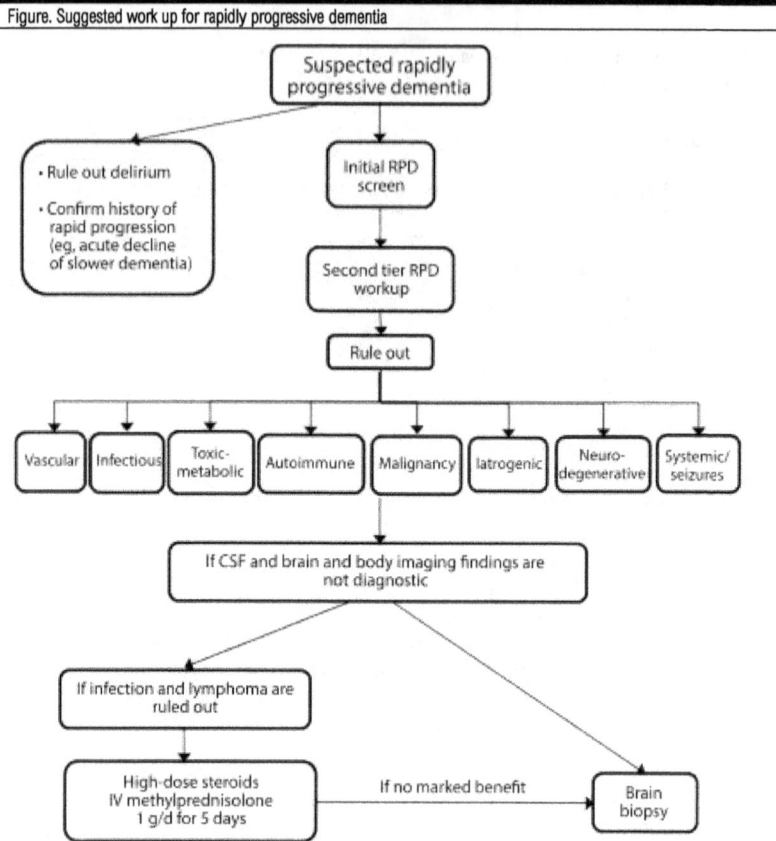

Treatment Options in Dementia

Class	Dosing	S/E	Be Aware...	Indications
Cholinesterase inhibitors (ACHEI)				
Donepezil (Aricept)	Initially, 5 mg q.d.; after 1 month→increase to target dose of 10 mg qd	Nausea Vomiting Diarrhea Anorexia Bradycardia	Substrate of CYPs 2D6, 3A4	Class 1A indication; no meaningful difference between drugs within this class; efficacious in mild/mod/severe AD. Duration may be from 4-7 years per studies.	Combination of NMDA antagonist and cholinesterase inhibitors has been shown to decrease rates of institutionalization
Rivastigmine (Exelon)	*Take during breakfast* Start at 5 mg/d. Increase by 5 mg/d every week until target of 10 mg twice daily	Fatigue Vivid dreams **Insomnia**		
NMDA receptor antagonist				
Memantine (Namenda, Namenda XR)	Immediate-release: Initially, 5 mg q.d. May increase to 10 mg bid. Extended-release: Initially, 7 mg q.d. May increase to target dose of 28 mg qd	Headache, dizziness, drowsiness, constipation	Caution with severe hepatic disease. Decrease dose with CrCl<30	Small benefit in **moderate-severe AD**; no benefit in mild AD or vascular dementia
Atypical antipsychotics[205]				
Olanzapine (Zyprexa, Zyprexa Zydis)	Initially, 2.5 mg qHS Maximum dose 10 mg qHS	Hyperprolactinemia Causes weight gain Sedation Orthostatic Hypo. EPS	Caution with CKD. Substrate of CYPs 1A2, 2D6	
Quetiapine (Seroquel)	Initially, 12.5 mg qHS. Effective/max dose 200 mg qHS	Hypothyroidism, hepatotoxicity Maybe less EPS Sedation, Ortho Hypo.	Caution with CKD. Periodic eye exams. Substrate of CYP3A4	First line
Risperidone (Risperdal)	Initially, 0.25-0.5 mg qHS but most effective @ 1-2 mg qHS	Hyperprolactinemia Less weight gain Osteoporosis	Decrease dose with CKD. Substrate of CYP2D6	

Drug	Dose	Side effects	Comments
Aripiprazole (Abilify)	Initially, 2mg/d but increase to max 10-15mg/d	Orthostatic Hypo Mild somnolence Minimal weight change Less QT effects	Insufficient literature to support use in elderly
Ziprasidone (Geodon)	Initially, 10mg/d IM Max: 20mg/d		Insufficient literature to support use in elderly
Other			
Haloperidol (Haldol)	0.25-5 mg total daily dose, dosed q.d.-bid	Drowsiness, dizziness, other CNS side effects, orthostatic ↓BP, QT prolongation and TdP, anticholinergic effects, hematologic toxicity, hyperprolactinemia, skin hyperpigmentation, photosensitivity, ocular toxicity, EPS, NMS, TD	Increased mortality in elderly patients with dementia related psychosis. Avoid abrupt withdrawal, extreme temperature, severe hepatic disease. Caution with pregnancy, seizure disorder, cardiac disease, pulmonary disease. Metabolized by CYPs 2D6 and 3A4
Agents for sleep disturbances			
Trazodone	Initially, 25 mg qHS. Maximum dose 100 mg qHS	↓BP, anxiety, blurred vision, priapism	Decrease dose w/elderly, hepatic disease, potent CYP3A4 inhibitors. Caution with cardiac disease, CKD
Zolpidem (Ambien)	Initially, 5 mg qHS. Maximum dose 10 mg qHS	CNS side effects, anterograde amnesia, sleep-related behaviors (e.g. sleep-talking and sleep-walking	Decrease dose by 1/2 with: hepatic disease, elderly. Caution with depression, respiratory disorders, history of substance abuse, CYP3A4 inhibitors or inducers. Avoid abrupt withdrawal after >2 weeks use	Second-line

GERIATRICS

MILD COGNITIVE IMPAIRMENT

- **Overview**[206]
  - For patients for whom the patient or a close contact voices concern about memory or impaired cognition, clinicians should assess for MCI and not assume the concerns are related to normal aging
  - For patients for whom screening or assessing for MCI is appropriate, clinicians should use validated assessment tools to assess for cognitive impairment. For patients who test positive for MCI, clinicians should perform a more formal clinical assessment for diagnosis of MCI
  - For patients with MCI, clinicians should assess for the presence of functional impairment related to cognition before giving a diagnosis of dementia
  - For patients diagnosed with MCI, clinicians should perform serial assessments over time to monitor for changes in cognitive status

Cognitive Impairments	
Normal Aging	• Slight decrease in ability to process new information • Normal functioning of ADLs
MCI	• Mild decline in ≥1 cognitive domain(s) • Normal functioning in ADLs
Dementia	• Significant decline in ≥1 cognitive domain(s) • Irreversible global cognitive impairment • Marked functional impairment • Chronic and progressive, months→years • To r/o Alzheimer's, consider CSF testing for Aβ42 peptide (will be ↓) and ↑ tau protein and p-tau levels.

- **Reversible Causes**
  - Sleep deprivation
  - Depression
  - General medical conditions
  - Medication side effects
- **Treatment Options**
  - <u>Pharmacologic</u> – no promising medications have been shown to be effective in decreasing progression to AD
  - <u>Non-Pharmacologic</u> – treatment with exercise training for 6 months is likely to improve cognitive measures

END OF LIFE MANAGEMENT

- **Palliative Care**[207]
  - Focuses on providing relief from the symptoms and stress of serious illness
  - Does not seek to make a diagnosis
  - Goal is to improve quality of life for both the patient and family
- **Key Symptoms of Management**
  - Nausea
    - Non-specific: Haldol 1mg PO or 0.5mg SQ/IV q6-8h
    - Others: prochlorperazine, Zofran, scopolamine, meclizine

GERIATRICS

- o Delirium
    - Haldol 1-2mg PO or 1mg SQ/IV q2h prn until settled then q6-h (consider ↓ dose by 50% in elderly)
    - Second generations: risperidone, quetiapine (use in patients with PD), olanzapine (causes sedation), aripiprazole
    - Lorazepam
- o Airway secretions
    - Scopolamine
    - Glycopyrrolate 0.2mg SQ q4-6h / 0.2-0.4mg PO q8h / TD q72h with 1.5mg patch
- o Fatigue anorexia
- o Anxiety/Depression
    - Anxiety
        - Lorazepam 1mg PO/SQ/IV q6h prn
        - Midazolam
- o Pain
    - Morphine 10mg/5ml, 5mg po Q2H prn dyspnea.
    - Morphine 20mg/ml, 5mg SL Q2H prn dyspnea.
    - Morphine 2mg IV Q2H prn dyspnea
- **Advanced Care Planning**
    - o Encourage patients to appoint a health care proxy or surrogate decision maker
    - o Patients who discuss EOL concerns with a physician earlier are more likely to take a comfort-focused approach to care at the EOL

Bibliography

[197] "Mini-mental state." a practical method for grading the cognitive state of patients for the clinician. Journal of Psychiatric Research, 12(3): 189-198, 1975.

[198] Sink et al. Pharmacological Treatment of Neuropsychiatric Symptoms of Dementia: A Review of the Evidence. JAMA, February 2, 2005—Vol 293, No. 5 (Reprinted)

[199] Kao, Amy. Fast Five Quiz: Test Your Knowledge on Key Aspects of Alzheimer Disease - Medscape - Sep 14, 2017.

[200] ACP Smart Medicine. "Dementia."

[201] APA 2016: The American Psychiatric Association Practice Guideline on the Use of Antipsychotics to Treat Agitation or Psychosis in Patients with Dementia

[202] Maglione et al M, Ruelaz Maher A, Hu J, et al. Review No. 43.

[203] ADA, APA, AACE, NAASO Diabetes Care 2004; 27:596-601

[204] Geschwind, Michael D. "Rapidly Progressive Dementia." Continuum 2016; 22(2): 510-537.

[205] Subramoniam et al. World J Psychiatry. 2014 Dec 22.

[206] Ronald C. Petersen, Oscar Lopez, Melissa J. Armstrong, Thomas S.D.Getchius, Mary Ganguli, David Gloss, Gary S. Gronseth, DanielMarson, Tamara Pringsheim, Gregory S. Day, Mark Sager, JamesStevens, Alexander Rae-Grant. "Practice guideline update summary: Mild cognitive impairment." Neurology Jan 2018, 90 (3) 126-135; DOI: 10.1212/WNL.0000000000004826

[207] Buss, Mary K. Mayo Clinic Proceedings. 92(2). 280-286.

HEMATOLOGY/ONCOLOGY

Section Editor: Bhavani Suryadevara, MD

The CBC	304
Anemia	305
Breast Cancer Screening	313
Blood Transfusion	314
Screening for Bleeding Disorders	324
Disseminated Intravascular Coagulation	326
Elevated INR	327
Hemolytic Anemia	328
Heparin-Induced Thrombocytopenia	328
Neutropenia	331
Neutropenic Fever	332
Supportive Care of Cancer Patients	339
Venous Thromboembolism	340

THE CBC

Background

Pluripotent stem cells form two distinct linages in the bone marrow to produce myeloid and lymphoid progenitors. Myeloid progenitors differentiate further into the granulocytes and monocytes. When the monocytes enter the tissues, they enlarge, develop large numbers of lysosomes and are then called macrophages. Myeloid progenitors also give rise to erythrocytes and megakaryocytes. Megakaryocytes in the bone marrow produce platelets.

Lab Analysis[208,209]

Element	Description	Differential
Left shift/Bands	A presence of **immature** cells with one or two nuclear lobes is called a "shift to the left" as the more lobes that are present, the older the cell is. "**Bands**" are the immature forms of PMNs (more mature are designated as "segs" and thus have more lobes). A left shift is present in the CBC when > **10–12% bands are seen (nml is 2-4%)**	Infection toxemia hemorrhage myeloproliferative
Reticulocyte Count	Indicator of erythropoietic activity. Reticulocytes are juvenile RBCs. The presence of these cells is suggested by basophilia of the RBC cytoplasm on Wright stain (polychromasia). Basophils are commonly seen with CML, s/p splenectomy, PC.	High levels may indicate a bleed (>2%), low levels suggest chronic disease, bone marrow suppression, or marrow failure (<2%).
Leukocytes	One of the body's chief defenses against infection that become active in sites of infection or inflammation by crossing the wall of venules and migrating into the tissues. Two major types: granulocytes and agranulocytes. About 70% of circulating leukocytes are mature neutrophils which are the first leukocytes to arrive at sites of infection. **Be aware of blasts**	Increased Smoking, Infection, inflammation (RA, allergies) leukemia, severe stress (physical and emotional), postoperative state (physiologic stress), severe tissue damage (e.g., burns), steroids. Decreased BM failure, 2/2 cytotoxic medication, VB12 or folate deficiency, r/o autoimmune disorder
Eosinophils	Eosinophils make up only about 4% of leukocytes and function in killing parasitic worms, and release chemokines and cytokines with allergies. Counts greater than 1500 warrant heme/onc consult.	Increased Allergies, parasites, skin dz, cancer, asthma. Decreased Steroids, ACTH
Basophils	Make up only 1% at most of leukocytes. Granules contain histamine and have surface receptors for IgE. With rapid degranulation → vasodilation occurs → anaphylaxis → sudden ↓ in BP	Increased Allergies, myeloproliferative neoplasm
Monocytes	↑ #'s occurs in the early phase of inflammation following tissue injury. Chronic inflammation can lead to excessive tissue damage.	Increased Inflammation, infection, in older patients think CMML Decreased Immunosuppression, BM failure, chemotherapy
Lymphocytes	White blood cells which include B-cells and T-cells; counts above 5000 warrants heme/onc consult. More likely to be benign in children than adults.	Increased Viral processes, lymphoproliferative disorder (lymphoma), leukemia, parasites, syphilis, autoimmune

HEMATOLOGY / ONCOLOGY

Neutrophils	Most abundant type of WBC that respond quickly to an infection (see Left Shift above), especially bacterial.	Decreased Immunosuppression, HIV, BM failure, chemotherapy Increased Infection, intense exercise, leukemia, stress, steroids Decreased (Leukopenia) Causes are either congenital or acquired: -Congenital: ethnic, benign familial, cyclic, constitutional -Acquired: infxn (post-infxn, sepsis), drug induced (agranulocytosis, mild PMNia), AI (primary, secondary, Felty's), malignancy (leukemias, MDS, myelopathies), dietary deficiencies (B12, folate)

RBC Morphology Differentials

Appearance	Differential
Basophilic Stippling	Lead or heavy-metal poisoning, thalassemia, severe anemia
Spherocytes	Hereditary spherocytosis, immune hemolysis, severe burns, ABO transfusion reaction
Target Cells	Thalassemia, hemoglobinopathies, liver disease, any hypochromic anemia, aftermath of splenectomy
Nucleated RBCs	Severe bone marrow stress (e.g., hemorrhage, hemolysis, hypoxia), marrow replacement by tumor, extramedullary hematopoiesis
Schistocytes	DIC, microangiopathic anemia, severe burns, drug effect (i.e. tacrolimus)
Polychromasia	Bluish red cell on routine Wright stain suggests reticulocytes
Helmet Cells	Microangiopathic hemolysis (TTP, HUS, HELLP syndrome), hemolytic transfusion reaction, transplant rejection
Howell–Jolly Bodies:	Asplenia
Acanthocytes	Severe liver dz; ↑ levels of bile, fatty acids, or toxins
Heinz Bodies	Drug-induced hemolysis

- **Basics behind analysis of the CBC**
  - Absolute counts are more important than percentages
  - Use flow-cytometry if suspected LAD of uncertain etiology and patients with an absolute lymphocyte count > 5000
  - Three things that matter when concerned about infection: total WBC, neutrophil count, and bands

ANEMIA

Anemia lab analysis[210211]

Category	Disease	CBC	Smear Clues	Other
Microcytic (MCV<80)	Iron Deficiency Anemia	↓Ferritin ↑TIBC ↓Iron Sat ↓Iron	Anisocytosis Poikilocytosis Elliptocytosis	↑Transferrin ↓MCV ↓MCHC ↓Reticulocytes ↓ferritin

HEMATOLOGY/ONCOLOGY

Microcytic (MCV <80)	ACD	↑Ferritin ↓TIBC ↓Iron Sat ↓Iron	Polychromasia Target Cells Basophilic stippling	↑ESR/CRP ↔MCHC ↔ RDW ↑ferritin ↑hepcidin
	Thalassemia *(Mentzer index (MCV/RBC) < 13*	↑Ferritin ↓TIBC ↓MCHC ↑Iron Sat ↑Iron ↓↓MCV	Target cells Polychromasia	↑↔RDW ↑↔ RBC ↑reticulocyte
	Lead poisoning	↓MCHC	Basophilic stippling	Elevated blood lead Peripheral neuropathy
Normocytic (MCV 80-100)	Hemolysis	Hemoglobinuria	Polychromasia Spherocytes Schistocytes Bite Cells	↔ ↑ RDW ↑reticulocyte count ↑indirect bilirubin ↑LDH Splenomegaly
	ACD	↓TIBC ↓iron	Unremarkable	↔RDW ↑ferritin ↓reticulocyte
Macrocytic (MCV>100)	Drug-induced	Marked or mild macrocytosis	Oval macrocytes	↑RDW
	MDS or BM disorder	N/A	Dimorphic RBC Oval macrocytes	↑RDW ↓Reticulocyte
	Liver Disease / EtOH	N/A	Round macrocytes Target Cells	↑RDW ↓PLT
	Hypothyroidism	N/A	Round macrocytes	↔RDW ↓PLT
	VB12 Deficiency	N/A	Hypersegmented	↓PLT ↓PMN ↑MMA ↑LDH
	Folate deficiency	N/A	Hypersegmented	↓PLT ↓PMN ↑Homocysteine ↑LDH

**↓↔Iron, ↓↔ferritin, and ↓TIBC suggestive of ACD with concurrent IDA

- **Defined** – pathologic state which occurs as a result from an insufficient number of RBCs to deliver oxygen to organs and tissues. Can result from blood loss, underproduction of RBCs, destruction of RBCs, or a combination of these factors.
- **History**
    - Bleeding episodes (esp. with surgery, brushing teeth)
    - Systemic illness
    - Medications
    - Exposures
    - EtOH
    - Family history of bleeding
- **Approach**
    - First step is to obtain MCV and characterize as microcytic, normocytic, or macrocytic
        - If microcytic → check ferritin, if low then IDA. If normal, and chronic, then likely thalassemia and get hemoglobin electrophoresis. If acquired/new, then consider ACD.
        - If normocytic →
            - Check reticulocyte count
                - <2% (Hypoproliferative)
                    - Leukemias

- o Aplastic anemia
- o BM syndromes
- o PRBC aplasia
- >2% (Hyperproliferative)
  - o Hemolysis w/u via haptoglobin, LDH, indirect bili, smear with (spherocytosis, schistocytes), and retic count. No e/o hemolysis suggests ACD or primary bone d/o such as MDS.
  - o Hemorrhage
  - If macrocytic → r/o drug causes, r/o b12 and folate then consider liver dz, EtOH, thyroid, bone marrow d/o. MDS can occur with MCV<110 but more common if greater than 110.
- **General Labs**[212,213]
  - o MCV, MCHC, RDW
  - o Reticulocyte count
  - o Smear
  - o Iron panel, B12, Folate, TSH
  - o LDH, Haptoglobin, Reticulocyte count, Differential with observation for schistocytes
  - o Soluble transferrin receptor index
- **Decreased Production**
  - o Low MCV (<80fL) /Microcytic
    - Iron Deficiency Anemia
      - o ↓ferritin
      - o ↑TIBC
      - o ↓Fe
      - o ↓Iron Saturation
      - o ↑RDW (newer RBCs are smaller therefore there is a larger spread of cell widths present)
      - o ↑soluble transferrin receptor index (falsely elevated however in hemolysis and recent blood loss)
      - o Reactive thrombocytosis
      - o Treatment: every other day of PO iron
        - 10cc of iron elixir (ferrous sulfate) mixed in one-fifth of a glass of orange juice and taken 30 minutes prior to breakfast. This will provide 88mg of elemental iron
        - Ferrous sulfate 325mg contains 65mg of elemental iron per tablet
    - Thalassemia
      - o Normal iron studies
      - o Basophilic stippling
      - o ↑reticulocyte count
      - o Abnormal hemoglobin electrophoresis
      - o Mentzer index
        - MCV/RBC >13 = IDA
        - MCV/RBC <13 = Thalassemia
    - Anemia of Chronic Inflammation/Anemia of Kidney Disease
      - o *Pathophysiology*: IL-6 leads to ↑hepcidin production and ↓iron absorption from the enterocyte. IL-6 also blunts erythropoietin response to anemia which leads to a blunted reticulocyte count (in relation to the degree of anemia)
      - o *Smear*: typically shows a normocytic normochromic anemia with eventual microcytosis over time, echinocytes (burr cells) with concurrent uremia
      - o Labs:
        - ↓Fe
        - ↓TIBC

- ↑ferritin
- Fe/TIBC > 18%
- Sideroblastic Anemia (uncommon)
    - ↑Fe
    - ↔ TIBC
    - ↑Ferritin
    - Basophilic stippling
    - Ringed sideroblasts on BM Bx
- Normal MCV (80-100fL) / Normocytic
    - Anemia of Chronic Disease, Anemia of Kidney Disease
    RA, COPD, ESRD, Connective tissue diseases, Sideroblastic anemia, PRBC aplasia
        - ↑ferritin
        - ↓TIBC
        - ↓Fe
        - ↓iron saturation
- High MCV (>100 fL) / Macrocytic
    - Causes
        - *Megaloblasts on smear:*
            - Due to large immature RBCs (megaloblasts) and hypersegmented PMN
            - B12 deficiency (pernicious anemia from autoimmune gastritis and ↓IF, **malabsorption** 2/2 IBD, bacterial overgrowth, gastric bypass, vegan diet), drug induced, ↓bioavailability (age related gastric achlorhydria, PPI)
                - ↓B12 leads to ↓wt, glossitis, "Lemon yellow" skin, jaundice appearance. When severe, may be associated with dorsal column neurologic sx (loss of viratory sense, loss of proprioception, spastic ataxia)
                - Labs
                    - ↓B12: ↑methylmalonic acid, ↑homocysteine level
            - Folate deficiency (malnutrition, EtOH, impaired absorption), rapid turnover state (pregnancy, hemolysis, desquamating skin disorders), drugs (methotrexate, phenytoin, triamterene), small bowel disorder (celiac, IBD, amyloidosis)
                - Labs
                    - ↓folate: nml methylmalonic acid, ↑homocysteine level
        - *No megaloblasts on smear:*
            - EtOH elevation, thyroid disease (may cause falsely low ferritin in hypothyroidism), bone marrow disease (MDS), liver disease, congenital bone marrow failure syndromes
        - Medications (OCP, purine analogs, methotrexate, TMP-SMX, anti-convulsants)
- **Increased Destruction**
    - ↑reticulocyte count (>2%)
    - Obtain haptoglobin, LDH, reticulocyte count, TBILI, peripheral smear
    - Reticulocyte count
        - "Poor man's bone marrow aspirate"
        - Measures RBC production
        - >2%: acute blood loss, hemorrhage, acute hemolytic anemia (hereditary such as G6PD, SSA, thalassemia, hereditary spherocytosis, PNH vs acquired such as MAHA, prosthesis, malaria, hypersplenism, Wilson's)
        - <2%: aplastic anemia, BM infiltration, sepsis (BM failure), disordered RBC maturation (↑B12/folate/iron)

HEMATOLOGY/ONCOLOGY

Differential based on reticulocyte count			
Low reticulocyte	RDW		Conditions
	↓	↔	Iron deficiency, Thalassemia, ACD, Sideroblastic
MCV	↔	↔	Acute bleed, hemolysis, ACD, liver dz, sideroblastic, ↓thyroid, MDS, aplastic
	↑	↔	B12 deficiency, folate deficiency, drug cause, liver dz, ↓thyroid, MDS
High reticulocyte	RDW		Conditions
	↑	>2%	AIHA, MAHA, PNH, sickle cell, spur cell, G6PD
LDH/BILI	↔	>2%	Subacute bleed, splenic sequestration, liver sequestration

- **Treatment**[214]
  Indications for treatment include symptomatic anemia (weakness, HA, ↓exercise tolerance), pica, and RLS
  - B12 deficiency:
    - PO: 1000-2000mcg daily for chronic supplementation
    - SC/IM: 1000mcg/d for 5 days then 1000mcg weekly for 5 weeks then 1000mcg monthly
    - Supplementing folate may improve anemia but not neurologic sx
  - Folate deficiency
    - PO: 1mg daily
    - SC/IM: 1mg daily
  - Anemia of Kidney Disease
    - In CKD patients (not ESRD), KDIGO recommends HGB≥11 g/dL therefore patients with a level between 9-10 should have an ESA started (stop if HGB approaches 11.5) often with concurrent iron supplementation (325mg TID)
      - ESA: 300U/kg/d SC for 10 days before surgery and 4 days after surgery
      - See also page 545
    - Anemia with ESRD associated with ↑mortality.
      - IV Fe supplementation: HGB<10g/dL + %SAT≤30 and ferritin≤500ng/mL or HGB>10 with %SAT≤20 and ferritin≤200
        - Start ESA if HGB<10 despite loading dose of IV Fe
      - ESA only if HGB<10 and %SAT>30
  - IDA
    - Iron supplementation to target saturation of 20-50% and ferritin of 200-500 ng/dL taken every other day rather than daily.
    - Dosing to replenish stores is dependent on severity of deficiency, age, etc.
      - In general, rule of thumb is to replace 1000mg of elemental iron for parental formulations
      - A 50-kg woman whose hemoglobin is 9 g/dL (75% of normal assuming 12 g/dL is normal) has an iron deficit of 0.25 × 27 mL/kg × 50 kg = 337.5 mL of red blood cells (or 337.5 mg of iron).
        - 0.25 is calculated by subtracting the % normal (75% from 100% to find deficit)
        - 27 cc/kg calculated as this the appx RBC volume in women (men is 30 cc/kg)
        - The parenteral iron dose is the iron deficit plus (usually) 1 extra gram to replenish iron stores and anticipate further iron loses, so in this case 1.4 g
      - Another, simpler, formula is

        Total dose of iron(mg) = Whole blood hemoglobin deficit (g/dL) × body weight (lbs.)
        i.e. Total dose to correct = weight × (16 − HGB level)
        To replete stores, add 1g for men and 600mg for women to the above result

    - If treating for CHF, may not respond well to PO formulation

- *PO administration* start Ferrous Sulfate 325mg TID (but given every other day - for example MWF) **not** with food unless the patient has GI s/e in which case can take with food.
  - Taken with vitamin C (orange juice; 200mg) can improve absorption.
  - Don't take iron pills concurrently with H2 or PPI.
  - Typical dose daily is 100mg-200mg of elemental iron.
- *IV administration* is often done in patients who cannot tolerate PO s/e, want quicker repletion (1-2 doses), or have on going blood loss. Watch PO4 levels, iron isomaltoside associated with less hypophosphatemia than ferric carboxymaltose.[215]

Oral Iron Replacement Preparations			
Name	% Elemental iron	Dose	Elemental Iron (mg/dose)
Ferrous sulfate	20	**325mg TID**	65
Ferrous gluconate	12	300mg TID	36
Ferrous fumarate	33	100mg TID	33
Iron polysaccharide complex	46	150mg BID	150
Carbonyl iron	100	50mg BID-TID	50

HEMATOLOGY/ONCOLOGY

IV Iron Replacement Preparations

Name	Indication	Cumulative Dosing
Iron sucrose (Venofer) 20 mg/mL elemental iron	IDA in non-dialysis dependent CKD patients	Goal is a total of 5 doses over 14 days. CKD (non-dialysis): 200 mg (10cc) IV over 2-5 min daily for 5 days total over a 14 day period Dialysis: 300mg IV over 1.5h x2 separated by 14 days f/b single infusion of 400mg over 2.5h 14 days later
Ferric carboxymaltose (Injectafer) 50mg/mL elemental iron	IDA where PO administration has failed (cannot tolerate or did not respond) **and patients with non-dialysis dependent CKD**	<50kg: 15mg/kg IV x 2 (separated by 7 days) ≥50kg: 750mg IV over 7.5min and repeat after 7 days for 2 total doses
Iron dextran/LMW ID (INFeD) 50 mg/mL elemental iron	IDA where PO administration has failed	Dose should be calculated using formula above 100mg IV over 2 min x 10 dialysis sessions (or replete based on deficit calculated above) Always give 0.5mL IV over 30s prior to the first dose as a test dose while observing the patient. If no reaction, give the rest of the dose over 1 total hour
Ferric gluconate (Ferrlecit) 1cc = 12.5mg elemental iron	IDA	125mg IV q1w for 8 weeks (max dose total is 1g)
Ferumoxytol (Feraheme) 30mg/mL elemental iron	IDA	510 mg over 15 min; given as 2 doses 3-8 d apart Observe patient for at least 30 min after administration. Serious hypersensitivity reactions have been observed with rapid IV injection (<1 min).
Sodium ferric gluconate complex in sucrose (Ferrlecit)	IDA in adult hemodialysis (except peritoneal)	1 amp (5cc) per 2.5g of bicarbonate concentrate for preparation of hemodialysate

Consider pre-treatment in patients with h/o asthma, multiple drug allergies, inflammatory arthritis. Options include 125mg methylprednisolone given IV prior to infusion, and possible short course of prednisone for 4 days after if they have arthritis. **Avoid antihistamines in treatment. Consider treating concomitantly with **Vitamin C supplementation**

Figure. Anemia workout flow chart

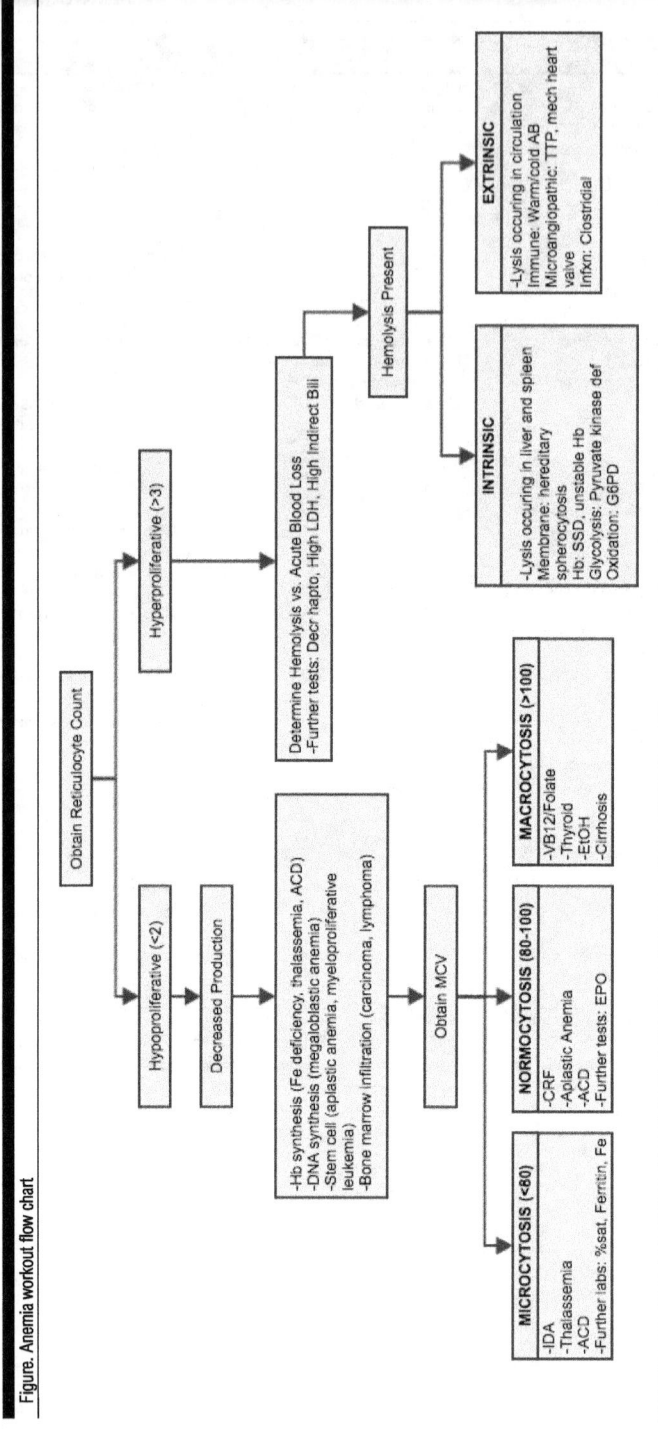

BREAST CANCER SCREENING

Screening with magnetic resonance imaging may be considered in high-risk women, but its impact on breast cancer mortality is uncertain. [216]

Screening Guidelines (Average Risk)	
Age	Recommendations
25-40	• For women with an estimated lifetime breast cancer risk of more than 20 percent • Have a BRCA mutation -or- • Age that is five to 10 years younger than the earliest age that breast cancer was diagnosed in the family
40-49	The risks and benefits of screening should be discussed, and the decision to perform screening should take into consideration the individual patient risk, values, and comfort level of the patient and physician. • The ACS recommends annual screening starting at 45 until 55 then every 2 years thereafter • USPSTF recommends every 2-year from 40-49. • ACOG recommends annually starting at 40 with concurrent clinical breast exam • ACR recommends yearly mammograms
50-74	There is general agreement that screening should be offered at least biennially to women of this age group however ACR and ACOG recommend yearly from 50-54 (with addition of CBE by ACOG)
>75	Information is lacking about the effectiveness of screening (USPSTF, AAFP) but can continue screening if woman is in good health and life span > 10 years (ACS) and stop if life expectance is <5-7 years (ACR)

- **Women with Dense Breasts**
  - Unclear benefit of breast US, MRI, digital breast tomosynthesis but can consider addition of US to mammography (ACR)

**High risk family history includes
(1) Two first degree relatives with breast cancer, including 1 relative before age 50
(2) Three or more 1st or 2nd degree relatives with breast cancer
(3) 1st or 2nd degree relative with breast & ovarian cancer
(4) 1st degree relative with bilateral breast cancer
(5) Breast cancer in male relative

- **Women at higher risk**
  - Start screening at age 40
  - Start with yearly mammogram, per ACR, can add MRI
  - Per ACOG, if BRCA positive, do twice/yearly CBE and annual self breast exams
  - If chest irradiation history between 10-30 years of age, then do annual mammogram with annual MRI starting 8 years after treatment except if 25 or younger

- **Medications for Primary Prevention**
  - Treatments may increase risk of hot flashes
  - Tamoxifen - for pre- or postmenopausal women. Benefit may last up to 8 years after completing therapy. Start at 20mg/d
  - Raloxifene - only for postmenopausal women, especially those with osteoporosis as it lowers risk of vertebral fx. Start at 60mg/d

HEMATOLOGY/ONCOLOGY

- o Anastrazole – only for postmenopausal women without osteoporosis as it can lower bone density. May increase stroke risk. Start at 1mg/d.

BLOOD TRANSFUSION

PRBCs - 4cc/kg will increase Hb 1gm/dl
Platelets – 1U (6-pack) will increase count by 30,000; 10-60min after transfusion
Fresh Frozen Plasma - 10 ml/kg round up/down to closest unit
Cryoprecipitate - 1 bag / every 5-10kg (Source of fibrinogen and factor VIII)

- Logistics[217,218,219,220]
    - o Blood Bank phone: _____ - _____.
    - o Informed consent must be obtained once during each hospital stay using forms present in patient's chart
    - o Blood must be infused within 4hrs. It can be split into smaller aliquots.
    - o A unit of blood that has been issued and allowed to warm to 10 C but not used cannot be reissued.
    - o Blood must not be stored in un'monitored refrigerators
    - o Standard blood filters have a pore size of 170 microns.
    - o Proper patient identification is essential, mislabeled specimens will not be accepted

Transfusion Guidelines

Component	Threshold/Goal	Indication	Guideline
HGB	Liberal: >10 g/dL Restrictive: >7 g/dL	Hospitalized and Critically Ill, But Hemodynamically Stable **without history of** Coronary Artery Disease	AABB 2016, NICE 2014, BCSH 2012, TRICC, FOCUS
	<10 g/dL	↑ESBL	AABB 2016
	> 8 g/dL	Cardiac or Orthopedic Surgery Patients or <u>Any</u> <u>Patient with Preexisting</u> <u>Cardiovascular Disease</u>	AABB 2016
	> 8 g/dL	Patients with Acute Coronary Syndrome	BCSH 2012 NICE 2014 TRICC FOCUS
	Early resuscitation: >9 g/dL	Critically Ill Patients with Sepsis	BCSH 2012
	Late resuscitation: >7-9 g/dL		
	> 10 g/dL	Symptomatic anemia	AABB 2016
PLT	>20k	CVC placement	AABB 2015
	>50k	Lumbar puncture	
	>50k	Major non-neuraxial surgery Neuraxial surgery	AABB 2015
	>80k		
	Insufficient evidence	ICH	AABB 2015
	>100k	Active bleeding	

HEMATOLOGY/ONCOLOGY

>5k	ITP
>20k	DIC, hepatic + renal failure, splenomegaly

Basic Understanding of Transfusion Thresholds:
- Hgb<10: transfuse only if either symptomatic, or large ESBL prior to surgery
- Hgb<8: transfuse only if orthopedic or cardiac surgery, or if patient has history of CAD
- Hgb<7: all others

- **Components**
  - Whole blood: 40% hematocrit; used primarily in hemorrhagic shock.
  - RBC Transfusion
    - *Indications*:
      1. Active bleeding and one of the following:
      2. Blood loss > 500cc or 15% of blood volume (70 cc/kg body weight)
      3. SBP < 100 mmHg or 20% fall in SBP
      4. Pulse > 100 bpm
      5. General anesthesia and Hgb < 9 g/dl
      6. Chronic, symptomatic anemia (generally Hgb < 9g/dl)
      7. Chronic transfusions to suppress endogenous Hgb in selected patients with sickle cell disease

      8. Hgb < 8 g/dl in patients with known coronary artery disease, unstable angina, or acute MI
         - the myocardium is more sensitive to anemia d/t ↑ oxygen requirements
      9. Hgb < 8 g/dl – undergoing orthopedic surgery, cardiac surgery, and those with pre-existing cardiovascular disease
      10. Hgb < 7: in hospitalized patients without cardiovascular disease who are hemodynamically stable

    - *Dose effect*: 1 unit PRBC (volume = 225-350 cc) should raise Hgb by about 1 g/dl
    - *Complications*
      1. Hypocalcemia is most commonly seen in patients with renal or hepatic impairment
      2. This is due to their inability to metabolize citrate which is included in the transfusion; the citrate is normally metabolized to lactate
      3. The continued presence of citrate binds to calcium causing ↓Ca, however regular calcium testing will be normal, must check **iCa**
      4. Prophylactic administration of 10cc of 10% calcium gluconate recommended

Indications for Specialized Transfusions[221]	
Irradiated	Indicated for patients at risk for transfusion associated graft vs host disease (TA-GVHD) (rare but fatality rate >90%)
	Fetal and neonatal receipitents of intrauterine transfusion
	Bone marrow transplant recipient
	Acquired or congenital cellular immunodeficiency
	Hodgkin's Disease
	Treatment with purine analogue and purine antagonist drugs (bendamustine, alemtuzumab, antithymocyte globulin, fludarabine, cladribine)
	Blood components donated by 1st or 2nd degree relative
	Hematologic malignancies (acute leukemias)

HEMATOLOGY/ONCOLOGY

Leukoreduced	NHL, HL Patients on immunosuppressive medications (**except** HIV, aplastic anemia) *Indicated to decrease frequency of recurrent febrile NH transfusion reactions and HLA alloimmunization* Chronically transfused patients CMV seronegative at-risk patients (i.e. AIDS, transplant) Acute and chronic leukemia Solid tumor malignancy potentially treated with HRC Thalassemia Potential transplant candidates Previous febrile nonhemolytic transfusion reaction
Washed *(shelf life: 24h)*	*Indicated to remove unwanted plasma when it contains constituents that predispose patients to transfusion reactions* IgA deficiency Complement-dependent autoimmune hemolytic anemia Continued allergic reactions (i.e. hives) with RBC transfusion despite antihistamines At risk for hyperkalemia (↑K)
Volume reduced *(shelf life: 24h)*	*Removes excess plasma thereby reducing unwated plasma proteins, including antibodies; more commonly in pediatric and in-utero transfusions* Thalassemia major SSD CHF Infants with impaired cardiac function

Klein et al.[222]

- o Platelets
    - One unit of apheresis platelets will increase platelet count 30,000/mm^3; usual dose is 1 unit of platelets per 10 kg body weight; single-donor platelets obtained by apheresis are equivalent to 6 platelet concentrate; platelets are stored at room temp; ABO compatibility is not mandatory.
    - A normal platelet count is 150,00-440,000/mm^3.
        1. Thrombocytopenia is defined as <150,000/mm^3.
    - Intraoperative bleeding increases with counts of 40,000-70,000/mm^3, and spontaneous bleeding can occur at counts <20,000/mm^3.
        1. During surgery platelet transfusions are probably not required unless count is less than 50,000/mm^3.
    - *Indications for transfusion*
        1. Platelet count < 5-10K in ITP, significant purpura, life threatening bleeding
        2. Platelet count < 10K in J patients, or patients not predisposed to spontaneous bleeding
            - No change in bleeding events in RCT when compared to < 20K as transfusion threshold
        3. Platelet count < 20K and a clinical factor that would be associated with risk of spontaneous bleeding
            - Temperature > 38.5°C
            - Infection
            - Concomitant coagulopathy
            - Disseminated intravascular coagulopathy (DIC)
            - Hepatic or renal failure
            - Marked splenomegaly
        4. Platelet count < 50K and invasive procedure (LP, indwelling lines, liver or transbronchial biopsy, epidural puncture), surgery, or post-op bleeding
        5. Platelet count < 100K with active bleeding
    - *Premedication*: Tylenol 650 mg p.o. × 1, Benadryl 25-50 mg p.o. OR IV × 1

- Post Transfusion
    1. 10-60 minutes after transfusion, recheck platelet level
        - Adequate response → recheck 24 hours later, if count lowers back to original then consider in the differential: sepsis, DIC, medications (vancomycin, heparin, amphotericin)
        - Inadequate response → consider alloimmunization due to presence of antibodies on transfused platelets (HLA-1). Screen patient (HLA) and transfuse HLA-matched platelets
- Fresh frozen plasma (FFP): 250 cc/bag; **contains all coagulation factors** except platelets; 10-15 mL/kg will increase plasma coagulation factors to 30% of normal; fibrinogen levels increase by 1 mg per mL of plasma transfused; acute reversal of warfarin requires 5-8 mL/kg of FFP. ABO compatibility is mandatory.
    - *Indications*
        1. Active bleeding or risk of bleeding if PT and/or PTT> 1.5-1.8x normal.
        2. Patient with massive bleeding at high risk for clotting factor deficiency while coags pending.
        3. May help in 2/3 of cirrhotics (worsens coagulation in 1/3)
        4. Common causes of factor deficiency: liver disease, vitamin K deficiency, DIC, hemorrhage, TTP (MAHA+↓PLT; treatment with plasma exchange)
        5. Reversal of warfarin therapy
            - Minimal evidence that FFP can correct mildly elevated INR (< 1.8).
        6. Management of patients with rare specific plasma protein deficiencies such as C1 inhibitor when recombinant products are unavailable
        7. Management of patients with selected coag factor deficiencies, congenital or acquired for which no specific coag concentrations are available
    - *Initial Dosage*
        1. 10cc/Kg (round up to nearest 200cc) = #units FFP / 200 cc/unit FFP
            - One unit of FFP contains:
                o 200-250 cc volume (if apheresis, then 400-600 cc)
                o 400 mg fibrinogen
                o 200 units of other factors (factors V, VII, XI, ATIII, Protein C, Protein S)
    - *Common Parameters*

Recommended Coagulation Parameters for Common Procedures		
	Platelet Count*	INR
Lumbar Puncture	≥50,000	≤1.5
Paracentesis	≥30,000	≤2.0
Thoracentesis	≥50,000	≤1.5
Transbronchial Lung Bx	≥50,000	≤1.5
Subclav/IJ Line	≥30,000	≤1.5
Renal Bx	≥50,000	≤1.5
Liver Bx	≥50,000	≤1.5

- Cryoprecipitate: 10-20 mL/bag; contains 100 units factor VIII-C, 100 units factor vWF, 60 units factor XIII, and 250 mg fibrinogen.
    - *Indications*
        1. hypofibrinogenemia, von Willebrand disease, hemophilia A and preparation of fibrin glue; ABO compatibility not mandatory.
        2. Fibrinogen < 100 mg/dl (as in DIC)
        3. Preparation of topical fibrin glue for surgical hemostasis

4. Concentrated factor VIII and von Willebrand factor are preferred treatments of Hemophilia A and von Willebrand's disease since cryoprecipitate not virus inactivated, thus carrying a higher risk for virus transmission.
5. May be considered for control of uremic bleeding after other modalities have failed

- Albumin: 5% and 25% (heat treated at 60 degrees C for 10 hrs.)
- 4-Factor Prothrombin Complex Concentrates (50U/kg)[223]: (contains factors 2, 7, 9, 10) for patients who have life-threatening hemorrhage and are within 3–5 half-lives of the last dose of factor Xa inhibitor in intracranial hemorrhage with INR $\geq$ 1.4 then repeat testing of INR 15-60 m after PCC administration and serially q6-8h for the next 24-48h. Any further corrections required if INR remains >1.4 done with FFP

Blood products

Component/Product	Composition	Volume (ml)	Indications	Expected Change	Formula for transfusion volume
Whole Blood	RBCs (HCT 40%), plasma; WBCs; platelets	500	Increase both red cell mass and plasma volume (WBCs and Platelets not functional); plasma deficient in labile clotting Factors V and VIII	1 unit will ↑ HGB 1gm/dl or HCT 3%	
Red Blood Cells (PRBC)	RBCs (HCT 75%); reduced plasma; WBCs; platelets	250-350	Increase red cell mass in symptomatic anemia (WBCs and platelets not functional)	1 unit will ↑ HGB 1gm/dl or HCT 3%	Packed cells (mls) = wt (kg) x Hb rise required(g/L) x 0.4
PRBC, Adenine-Saline Added	RBCs (HCT 55-65%); reduced plasma; WBCs; platelets; 100ml of additive solution	330	Increase red cell mass in symptomatic anemia (WBCs and platelets not functional)	1 unit will ↑HBG 1gm/dl or HCT 3%	
PRBC, Leukocytes Reduced (prepared by filtration)	>85% original vol. of PRBCs; <5 x 10^6 WBC; few platelets; minimal plasma	225	Increase red cell mass; <5 x 10^6 WBCs to decrease the likelihood of febrile reactions, immunization to leukocytes (HLA antigens) or CMV transmission	1 unit will increase hgb 1gm/dl or Hct 3%	

Blood products

Component/Product	Composition	Volume (ml)	Indications	Expected Change	Formula for transfusion volume
PRBC, Washed	RBCs (HCT 75%); <5 x 10^8 WBC; no plasma	180	Increase red cell mass; reduce the risk of allergic reactions to plasma proteins	1 unit will ↑ HGB .8gm/dl or HCT 2.5%	
PRBC, Frozen & PRBC Deglycerolized	RBCs (HCT 75%); <5 x 10^8 WBC; no plasma, no platelets	180	Increase red cell mass; minimize febrile or allergic transfusion reactions; used for prolonged RBC storage	1 unit will increase HGB 1gm/dl or Hct 3%	
Platelets	Platelets (>5.5 x 10^{10}/unit); RBC; WBC, plasma	50	Bleeding due to thrombocytopenia or thrombocytopathy	6-pack will increase PLT by 30,000	(5 - 10 ml/kg will raise platelet count by 50 - 100x 109 /L)
Platelets, Apheresis	Platelets (>3 x 10^{11}/unit). RBC; WBC; plasma	300	Bleeding due to thrombocytopenia or thrombocytopathy; sometimes HLA matched	1 unit will increase platelet count by 30,000-60,000	

Blood products

Component/Product	Composition	Volume (ml)	Indications	Expected Change	Formula for transfusion volume
Platelets, Leukocyte Reduced	Platelets (>3 x 10^{11}/unit). <5 x 10^6 WBC per final dose of pooled Platelets	300	Bleeding due to thrombocytopenia or thrombocytopathy; <5 x 10^6 WBCs to decrease the likelihood of febrile reactions, immunization to leukocytes (HLA antigens) or CMV transmission (see below) In CMV seronegative recipients who are at risk for severe CMV infections such as: pregnant women and their fetus, low birth weight infants, hematopoietic progenitor cell transplant recipients, severely immunocompromised receipients, and HIV infected patients.	1 unit will increase platelet count by 30,000-60,000	
Fresh Frozen Plasma (FFP)	Plasma; all coagulation factors; complement; no platelets	200-250	Treatment of bleeding due to deficiency in coagulation factors	10-20ml/kg (4-6 units in adults) will increase coagulation factors by 20%	
Cryoprecipitate	Fibrinogen; Factors VIII and XIII; von Willebrand factor	20-50	Deficiency of fibrinogen and/or Factor VIII; Second choice in treatment of Hemophilia A and von Willebrand's disease	1 unit will increase fibrinogen by 5mg/dl	

2. **Orders:**
   o Type, cross match and transfuse __ units with H&H 1 hour after 2nd and 4th units.
     - Do H&H 1 hour after every 2 units of blood given
     - Cross match
       1. Use when transfusion is expected
       2. ABO-Rh, screen, and crossmatch; 99.95% compatible.
       3. Crossmatching confirms ABO-Rh typing, detects antibodies to the other blood group systems, and detects antibodies in low titers.
     - Screen
       1. Use when transfusion is a possibility
          - Blood is set aside for that pt and is returned to bank if not used; best one to order, unless you know pt will use the blood
       2. Hematocrit is determined, if normal, the blood is typed, screened for antibodies, and tested for hepatitis B, hepatitis C, syphilis, HIV-1, HIV-2, and human T-cell lymphotropic viruses I and II. ALT is also measured as a surrogate marker of nonspecific liver infection.
   o Lasix 20 mg IV daily or 20 mg PO prior to each unit of packed RBCs (if concern for hypervolemia)
   o Benadryl 50 mg IV daily-for itch
   o Tylenol 650 mg PO Q 6 hours prn fever greater than 100.4

Figure. Transfusion reactions

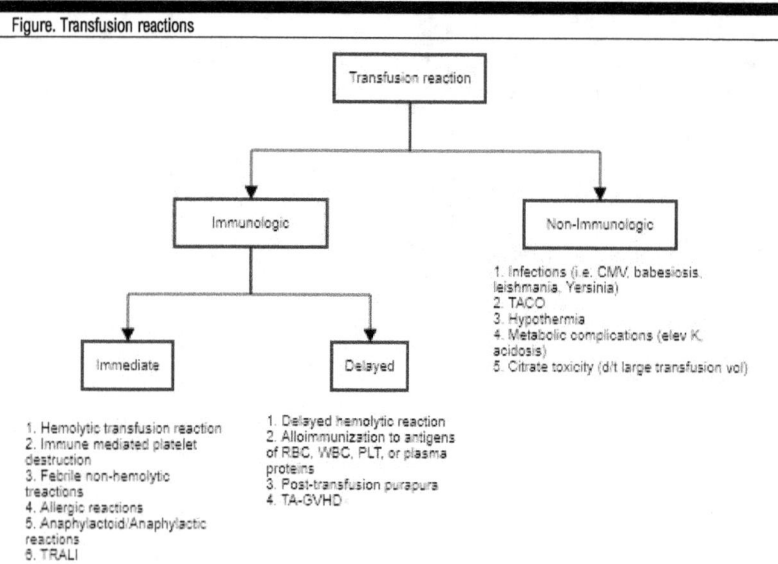

3. **Reactions**
   o **Hemolytic reactions**
     - Acute hemolytic reactions
       1. Occurs when ABO-incompatible blood is transfused resulting in acute intravascular hemolysis; severity of a reaction often depends on how much incompatible blood has been given.
       2. Symptoms include fever, chills, chest pain, anxiety, back pain, dyspnea; in anesthetized patients, the reaction is manifested by rise in temperature, unexplained tachycardia, ↓BP, hemoglobinuria, and diffuse oozing from surgical

site. Free hemoglobin in the plasma or urine is presumptive evidence of a hemolytic reaction. Abnormal bleeding or shock also can be seen.
3. Risk of fatal hemolytic transfusion reaction: 1:600,000 units.
4. Labs: hemoglobinemia, hemoglobinuria, ↑serum unconjugated bilirubin, DAT positive
5. Treatment
    - Stop transfusion and notify blood bank immediately
        o May require post reaction blood sample, preferably drawn from a site other than transfusion access site
    - Vigorous hydration with **NS**
- Delayed hemolytic reactions
    1. Occurs because of incompatibility of minor antigens (e.g., Kidd, Kelly, Duffy, etc.) are characterized by extravascular hemolysis.
    2. The hemolytic reaction is typically delayed 2-21 days after transfusion, and symptoms are generally mild, consisting of malaise, jaundice, and fever. Treatment is supportive.
o **Non-hemolytic reactions**
- Febrile reactions
    1. Most common non-hemolytic reaction (0.51.0% of RBC transfusions and up to 30% of platelet transfusions); due to recipient antibodies against donor antigens present on leukocytes and platelets; treatment includes stopping or slowing infusion and antipyretics.
- Urticarial reactions
    1. Characterized by erythema, hives, and itching without fever.
    2. Occur in 1% of transfusions and are thought to be due to sensitization of the patient to transfused plasma proteins.
    3. Treated with antihistaminic drugs (cetirizine 10mg, fexofenadine 180mg, loratadine 10mg all taken up to QID)
- Anaphylactic reactions
    1. Anaphylactic reactions are rare; about 1:500,000.
    2. Patients with IgA deficiency may be at increased risk of the presence of anti-IgA antibodies that react with transfused IgA.
    3. Cause: recipient antibodies react with donor plasma forming immune complexes which activate complement. Reported in patients with congenital IgA deficiency and high titers of anti-IgA IgG.
    4. Signs: sudden onset flushing, and hypertension followed by ↓BP, edema, respiratory distress, shock.
    5. Workup: none (no evidence of RBC incompatibility)
    6. **Treatment**
        - *See page 461*
    7. Prevention: patients with history of anaphylaxis to blood should receive components depleted of plasma (saline washed RBCs).
- Transfusion related acute lung injury (TRALI)
    1. Due to transfusion of antileukocytic or anti-HLA antibodies that interact with and cause the patient's white cells to aggregate in the pulmonary circulation.
    2. Risk is 1:6000.
    3. Leading cause of transfusion related mortality.
    4. Defined clinically and radiologically as acute lung injury (b/l infiltrates) within 6 hours of transfusion leading to hypoxemia without hypervolemia
    5. Exam: dyspnea, hypoxia, fever, chills, ↓BP with CXR showing b/l pulm infiltrates.

6. Treatment is supportive, mimicking the treatment of ARDS.
- Transfusion Associated Circulatory Overload (TACO)
  1. 1-8% of transfusion recipients
  2. Risk factors: bimodal (young and elderly), h/o cardiac disease, kidney disease, h/o reception of multiple transfusions d/t chronic severe anemia (i.e. myelodysplastic patients), rapid administration rate.
  3. Defined as respiratory distress within 6 hours with known positive fluid balance, ↑BNP, ↑CVP, CXR with pulmonary edema.
  4. Treatment: stop transfusion, diuresis, supportive care.
  5. When restarting transfusion, keep rate at 1 mL/kg/hr.
- Graft-vs-host disease
  1. Most commonly seen in immunocompromised patients.
  2. Cellular blood products contain lymphocytes capable of mounting an immune response against the compromised host.
- Posttransfusion purpura
  1. Sudden development of self-limited thrombocytopenia (7-10 days after transfusion)
  2. Due to the development of platelet alloantibodies; the platelet count typically drops precipitously 1 week after transfusion.
  3. Rare syndrome, r/o more common causes of purapura
  4. Treat with high dose IVIG
- Immune suppression
  1. Transfusion of leukocyte-containing blood products appears to be immunosuppressive (can improve allograft survival following renal transplants).
  2. Blood transfusions may increase the incidence of serious infections following surgery or trauma.
  3. Blood transfusions may worsen tumor recurrence and mortality rate following resections of many cancer.

SCREENING FOR BLEEDING DISORDERS

- **Overview of hemostasis**
  - Platelets normally circulate in inactivated state, when they do become activated (disruption in vascular endothelium (d/t release of VWF, etc.) or due to molecules (TxA2, ADP) released by other activated platelets) they gain ability to adhere to one another
  - This allows for the facilitation of platelet and college adhesion to allow for formation of occlusive plug
  - Second set of reactions activate the coagulation cascade leading to thrombin formation
  - This allows for stabilization of the thrombus
  - Thrombin then converts fibrinogen → fibrin monomers

Expected Lab Changes with Specific Bleeding Disorders			
	Mechanism Tested	Normal	Where Abnormal
PT	Extrinsic and common pathways (Factors VII, X, V, II)	<12 sec	Defect in vitamin K-dependent factors, liver diseases, DIC, oral anticoagulants
aPTT	Intrinsic and common pathways (Factors XII, XI, IX, VIII, X, V, II)	25-40 sec	Hemophilia, von Willebrand's disease, heparin therapy, DIC, deficient XII, XI, IX circulating anticoagulant

HEMATOLOGY/ONCOLOGY

Thrombin time	Fibrinogen-fibrin conversion	10-15 sec	Third-stage anticoagulant, fibrin split products, DIC, severe hypofibrinogenemia
Bleeding time	Primary hemostasis platelet function	3-7 min	Platelet dysfunction, von Willebrand's disease, thrombocytopenia
INR	Derived from dividing the PT of patient by control	<1.1	Warfarin, liver disease

Corresponding factor deficiencies and assay results	
Assay Result	Suspected Deficiencies
↑aPTT; normal PT	VIII, IX, XI, XII, VWD (if severe and Factor VIII is very low), heparin exposure
↑PT; normal aPTT	VII deficiency, DIC, Vitamin K deficiency, liver disease, warfarn
↑PT and ↑aPTT	II, V, X, fibrinogen, heparin overdose, DIC, Vitamin K deficiency, severe liver disease, warfarin toxicity

- **Hemophilias (A, B)**
  - Genetics
    - Deficiency of factor VIII and IX respectively
    - X linked, primarily found in males
    - Female offsprings of men with hemophilia are obligate carriers
    - Severity - mild, moderate, or severe according to circulating factor levels
  - Clinical presentation – spontaneous hemarthrosis or bleeding into deep muscles or excessive or delayed bleeding after trauma; recurrent hemarthrosis
  - Labs: ↑aPTT (corrects in mixing study), nml PT and CBC
    - Assay of individual factor VII and IX to confirm dx
    - VWF must be measured in Hemophilia A to r/o type 3 VWD
  - Treatment: manage bleeding (give factor concentrates), desmopressin for mild hemophilia A which stimulates release of preformed factor VIII from endothelial cells, aminocaproic acid + TXA act as antifibrolytic agents in those with uncontrolled bleeding from dental procedures.
- **VWD**
  - Most common hereditary bleeding disorder; deficiency/ineffective VWF
    - Type 1: partial def of VWF, most common; sx when VWF levels < 30%
    - Type 2: Qualitative defect in VWF (subtypes A, B, M, N)
    - Type 3: rare, complete def. of VWF
  - Labs
    - aPTT ↑ or nml
    - Prolonged PFA-100 clot-time
  - Diagnosis: confirmed by ↓VWF ristoceitin cofactor assay
  - Management
    - Type 1: desmopressin IV prior to surgery or intranasally PRN in outpatient setting
    - Type 2B: should not receive depressin because it inducese platelet aggresgation leading to secondary thrombocytopenia, use VWF
    - Type 3: desmopressin ineffective, use VWF
    - Can use antifibrinolytic therapy after surgery or with menorrhagia to prevent against delayed bleeding
- **Thrombophilia Work-Up**
  - Activated protein C resistance
  - Factor V Leiden
  - Prothrombin gene mutation
  - Antiphospholipid antibodies[224]
  - Patients will have prolonged aPTT, ↓PLT
  - Beta-2 glycoprotein I antibody, IgA

HEMATOLOGY/ONCOLOGY

- Cardiolipin antibody, IgA
- DRVVT
- Prothrombin Ab
- Lupus inhibitor
- Antithrombin deficiency
- Protein C deficiency
- Protein S deficiency

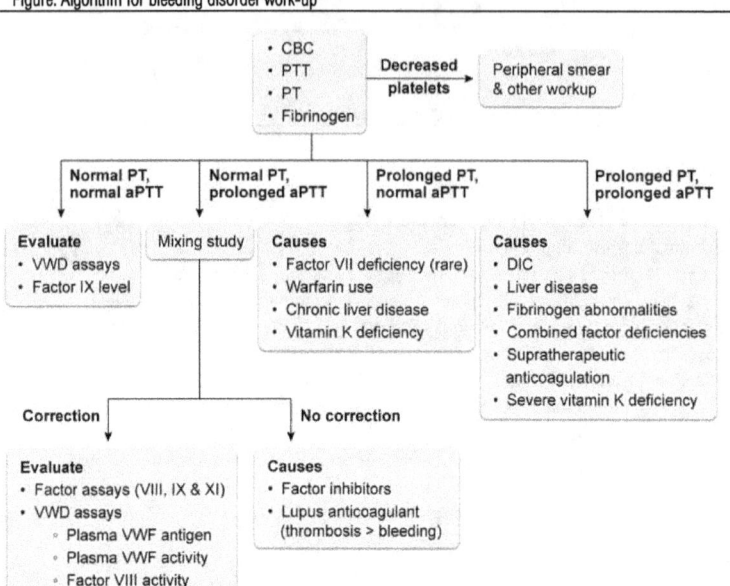

Figure. Algorithm for bleeding disorder work-up

DISSEMINATED INTRAVASCULAR COAGULATION

- **Overview**[225,226]
    - Characterized by the consumption of plasma coagulation factors and platelets after exposure to antigen (i.e. infection) due to the over-formation of fibrin with secondary fibrinolysis leading to prethrombotic state and increased bleeding due to consumption of platelets
    - ↑PT, ↑Thrombin Time (TT), and ↑PTT
    - Thrombotic events due to deposition of thrombin in microvasculature
    - Often seen in patients with malignancy, infection (esp. GN) and post-surgical
    - Most often affects the liver, kidney (ATN), brain, heart (endocarditis)
- **Diagnosis**
    - Exam
        - Hemorrhage at multiple sites to include mucosal surfaces
        - Petechiae, ecchymosis

HEMATOLOGY/ONCOLOGY

Labs in DIC

Test	Abnormality	Causes Other Than DIC Contributing to Test Result
Platelet count	Decreased	Sepsis, impaired production, major blood loss, hypersplenism
Prothrombin time	Prolonged	Vitamin K deficiency, liver failure, major blood loss
aPTT	Prolonged	Liver failure, heparin treatment, major blood loss
Fibrin degradation products	Elevated	Surgery, trauma, infection, hematoma
Fibrin	Elevated	
D-dimer	Elevated	
Factor VIII	Low	Can help distinguish superimposed DIC in patients with underlying liver failure

- Labs
  - PT, PTT, TT
  - CBC (↓platelets due to thrombin generation)
  - Fibrinogen level (↓due to fibrinolysis; what actually deposits in microvasculature)
  - Blood smear (schistocytes due to trauma experienced by presence of fibrin strands)
  - Fibrinogen degradation products (↑Fibrin D-Dimer assay due to circulating plasmin that degrades fibrin)
  - D-dimer (increased; due to ↑FDP)
- Imaging
  - Consider LE duplex US (to r/o DVT)
- **Treatment**
  - Cryoprecipitate (replaces fibrinogen if <50) → goal ↑100 mg/dl
  or
  - FFP (replaces coagulation proteins/factors, most notably 5 and 8) → may not be necessary with normal liver function
  - Platelets (1-2U per 10kg per day)
  - IV Heparin @ 5000U bolus then 500/h (due to risk of thrombotic events) for first 24 hrs, ↑ to 10U after 24hrs if no improvement in fibrinogen and FDP levels **not supported by experimental data**

ELEVATED INR

Bleeding Patient[227,228]

	Action	Comment
Any INR	1. Hold warfarin 2. Vitamin K 5-10mg IV 3. Give Factor-4 prothrombin complex concentrate (PCC) 25-50 u/kg 4. Repeat INR in 30min	FFP can be substituted for PCC at 15cc/kg Factor VIIa or 4f-PCC can be considered in urgent situation
INR <4.5	1. Lower Warfarin dose or omit dose 2. Monitor more frequently 3. Resume at lower dose when INR therapeutic	
INR 4.5 - 10	1. Hold 1-2 doses of warfarin 2. Monitor INR frequently 3. Vitamin K not recommended	
INR >10	1. Hold warfarin 2. Give vitamin K 2.5-5mg PO 3. Monitor INR frequently	Vitamin K not routinely recommended if no evidence of bleeding Vitamin K can be used if urgent surgery needed

HEMOLYTIC ANEMIA

- **Defined** – premature destruction of RBCs due to the development of autoantibodies or secondary to medications, cancer, or a hereditary condition.
- **Types**
  - Intravascular: ↑↑LDH, ↓↓haptoglobin
  - Extravascular: splenomegaly
- **Symptoms**
  - Fatigue, jaundice, mild splenomegaly
- **Conditions**
  - G6PD, SSA, HS, PNH, AIHA (warm with IgG vs cold with IgM), MAHA
- **Risk Factors** – autoimmune disorder, prosthetic heart valve, PNH, recent Abx exposure (think PCN, ceph) or NSAIDs
- **Labs**
  - Bilirubin (↑indirect)
  - Coombs (DAT) → differentiates autoimmune from drug-induced
    - drug induced (consider ABx; -DAT, ↑LDH)
    - autoimmune (+DAT, spherocytes)
  - Smear (spherocytes; schistocytes)
  - CBC (↓HGB, MCHC)
  - ↑LDH
  - Urinalysis (hemoglobinuria→ no RBCs, +blood)
  - ↓Haptoglobin
  - Reticulocyte count (↑ in HA; >2%)
  - Others to Consider
    - LFTs
    - SCr
    - Flow cytometry (CD55, CD59)
    - ANA
- **Treatment**
  - Coombs Positive (+DAT) → suggestive of autoimmune hemolytic anemia (AIHA)
    - Corticosteroids
    - Consider plasmapheresis +/- splenectomy (give rituximab prior to splenectomy)
  - Coombs Negative (-DAT) → suggestive of drug induced cause
    - Stop offending agent
    - Start steroids
  - Steroids +/- discontinuation of drug if DAT-

HEPARIN-INDUCED THROMBOCYTOPENIA

- **Defined**
  - HIT is as an antibody-mediated activation of platelets with heparin exposure that results in thrombocytopenia, and in some cases, venous or arterial thrombosis.
  - HIT causes thrombosis by activating platelets to release pro-thrombotic substances via a complex (combining) of heparin, platelet factor 4 (PF4), and antibody (usually IgG) leading to thrombin generation.
- **Statistics**
  - Seen in approximately 8% of patients placed on anticoagulation with up to 5% developing thrombotic events
  - UFH associated with 10x higher risk than LMWH
  - Higher incidents in major post-surgical and orthopedic patients (knee replacement)

- **Defined**
    - Type 1 – 10%; benign; no ↑ risk of thrombosis; unknown pathophysiology; mild transient thrombocytopenia (>100k) seen early in administration and recovers quickly after stopping heparin
    - Type 2 – immune mediated with ↑ **risk of thrombosis**; occurs 5-15 days after heparin exposure or within 24 hours of re-exposure; typically see fall in PLT of 50k-70k.
- **Pathophysiology**
    - Immune response (type 2) associated with an antigen in the form of the heparin/PF4 complex (PF4 is a molecule found on platelets). When platelets get activated, PF4 gets released and binds to the platelets and heparin then binds to the PF4 (opposite charges, attract).
    - This complex then causes the formation of an IgG AB against the heparin-PF4-plt complex by binding to another region on the platelet. When the AB binds to this Fc region, it causes more activation of platelets and aggregation which ultimately bind to a tissue surface which activates the coagulation system leading to thrombosis
    - Can cause false positives as it is also seen in patients simply exposed to heparin without clinical symptoms
    - False positives are highest in first 85 days (length of duration for PF4 antibodies to leave circulation)
- **DDx**
    - Decreased production: liver disease (decreased thrombopoietin), bone marrow hypoplasia (from meds, toxins, infections, pregnancy), ineffective erythropoiesis (megaloblastic anemia, MDS), and bone marrow infiltration (cancer, infection, myelofibrosis)
    - Increased destruction: hypersplenism, ITP, the thrombotic microangiopathies (TMAs), and HIT
- **Clinical**
    - Exposure to heparin or LMWH leads to low platelet count (<150,000) or a decrease of 50% or more from baseline with thrombosis resulting in up to 50% of patients
        - Platelets rarely drop <10,000 or cause bleeding
    - Onset is often 5-10 days from initiation of medication (no hx of exposure) or within **hours** if they have been exposed in the past (due to presence of the circulating PF4-heparin ABs
    - 4T Score

    The 4T score includes the degree of thrombocytopenia, the timing of platelet decrease, the presence of thrombosis, and considering the likelihood of other etiologies of thrombocytopenia. A low score effectively excludes HIT.

The 4T's of HIT

	2 points	1 point	0 point
Thrombocytopenia	PLT count fall >50% and PLT nadir >20k	PLT count fall 30-50% or PLT nadir 100-19k	PLT count fall <30% or PLT nadir <10,000
Timing of PLT count fall	Clear onset between days 5-10 or PLT fall < 1 day (prior heparin exposure within 30 days)	Consistent with days 5-10 fall, but not clear (i.e. missing PLT counts); onset after day 10, or fall <1 day (prior heparin exposure 30-100 days ago)	PLT count fall <4 days without recent exposure
Thrombosis or other sequelae	New thrombosis (confirmed); skin necrosis, acute systemic reaction post IV UFH bolus	Progressive or recurrent thrombosis; non-necrotizing (erythematous) skin lesions; suspected thrombosis	None
Other causes for thrombocytopenia	None apparent	Possible	Definite
Score	0-3 No further w/u; HIT effectively excluded	4-5 Check anti-PF4	6-8 ELISA If OD>2.0 then check SRA and if positive→tx; if SRA neg then not HIT

- **How to objectively diagnosis**
  - The resulting clinical probability scores were divided into high (6–8 points), intermediate (4–5 points), and low (<3 points) groups.
    - Low suspicion – no testing
    - Intermediate – check anti-PF4
    - High/Intermediate suspicion – check ELISA
- **Laboratory confirmation**[14]
  - CBC
  - SRA – more specific; preferred; detects C-Serotonin release from activated platelets: Sn up to 100%, Sp up to 100%. If positive, treat, if negative, HIT has been excluded.
  - PF4 – more sensitive; detects circulating IgG, IgA, and IgM antibodies: Sn 97%, Sp 86%
    - High titer of ≥1.5 confirms diagnosis
  - Heparin-induced platelet aggregation
- **Treatment**
  - <u>Adequate alternatives:</u>
    - Two classes to choose from: direct-thrombin inhibitors or heparinoids. These should be initiated when you **suspect** HIT and then send for above labs to confirm.
      1. DTI: argatroban, or bivalirudin good options for quick on/off
         - Argatroban – significant ↓ risk of death, amputation, and thrombosis.
         - Bivalirudin – patient's s/p PCA at high risk of HIT
      2. DOAC (recommend rivaroxaban): slow on/off preferred
      3. Argatroban: dosed 2 mcg/kg/min to an aPTT goal of 1.5-3x/baseline (reduce dose to 0.5 mcg/kg/m if hepatic dysfunction)
      4. Once you have confirmed the diagnosis (labs have returned), you can switch to a vitamin K antagonist (warfarin) or alternate anticoagulant for 3 months (only after PLT>150k)
    - Duration of therapy

1. No hx of thrombosis – until platelet counts recover to stable level or baseline with switch to warfarin for additional 4-6 weeks
2. Hx of thrombosis – allow platelet counts to recover to 150,000 then transition with bridging to warfarin (5 day bridge) and keep until INR is therapeutic for 48 hours then stop after 3 months
    - Not adequate alternatives:
        - Warfarin monotherapy d/t s/e such as venous gangrene and skin necrosis
        - ASA
        - IVC filter
        - LMWH – AB often cross-react
    - Patients often recover in 4-14 days after discontinuation of heparin

NEUTROPENIA

- **Definition**: absolute neutrophil cell count (ANC) < 1500 cells/mm^3 and graded as:
    - Mild – 1000-1500 cells/mm^3
    - Moderate – 500-1000 cells/mm^3
    - Severe – <500 cells/mm^3 (very high risk for serious infections)

> ANC = WBC Count × (total % of PMN)
> ANC = WBC Count × (% segmented PMN + % bands/100)
>
> **automated analyzers do not distinguish bands from segmented neutrophils, the percent neutrophils calculated by automated analyzers includes both stages

- **Types**
    - Bone Marrow
        - *Benign ethnic neutropenia*- congenital neutropenia seen in blacks, Asians and those of Mediterranean descent (ANC as low as 1200). These patients have good neutrophil reserve and are not prone to infections.
        - *Cyclic neutropenia*- rare, congenital condition leading to reduction in PMN counts every 21 days. PMN counts can get low enough that patients develop recurrent infections every 21 days.
    - Non-Bone Marrow
        - *Aplastic anemia*
        - *Drugs* (chemotherapeutic agents, NSAIDs, phenytoin, carbamezapine, propylthiouracil, psochotropics, TMP-SMX)
        - *Hypersplenism*
        - *Auto-immune* (SLE, Felty Syndrome, HIV)
        - *Infections* (viral, bacterial -- gram positive and gram negative, fungi – *Candida and Aspergillus*, ricketsial)
- **Complications**
    - Risk of serious infection ↑ dramatically when ANC falls below 1000.
- **Management**: when ANC reaches 500 or less, or in patients with impending neutropenia (i.e. patients receiving conditioning chemotherapy with ANC 1000 or less and dropping), institute:
    - Myeloid growth factors (i.e. filgastrim, sargramostim) – facilitate PMN recovery; can use single dose or chronically (daily or QOD) in patients with cyclic or congenital neutropenias.
        - Prophylactic use may decrease risk of febrile neutropenias

- o Neutropenic precautions (hand washing for all contact with patient; masks, gowns or gloves are not necessary unless the health care worker in contact with the patient is ill, i.e. has a cold or URI)
- o Neutropenic diet (low bacterial, i.e. no fresh fruits or vegetables)
- o Gut sterilizers (pre-printed antibiotic form)
  - Norfloxacin 400 mg p.o. BID
  - Clotrimazole troche 10 mg to dissolve in mouth 4x daily OR nystatin swish and swallow 5 cc 5x daily
  - Nystatin powder to apply to axilla and groin TID
  - Nystatin tablets 1 million units p.o. 4x daily
- o Patients at high risk for febrile neutropenia (*see next page;* AML/MDS, hematopoietic stem cell recipients) should be considered for antibiotic and antifungal prophylaxis with fluoroquinolone and oral triazole in conjunction with ID consultation.

NEUTROPENIC FEVER

- **Pearls**
  - o Start broad spectrum Abx at the first sign of fever in a neutropenic patient (within hour of documented fever)
  - o Normal gut and mucosal flora may shift from predominantly gram positive to gram negative in sick patients
- **Definition**[229,230,231]
  - o ANC <=500/mm^3 or an ANC expected to ↓<500 in next 48 hours
    - Remember there are grades with mild defined as <1500
  - o 100.4F temp (38.3C) x 2 hours –or– any recorded temp of 101F
  - o If caused by chemotherapy regimen, consider nadir of ANC to likely occur 12-14 days from day one of therapy
- **Etiology**
  - o The majority of documented infections are due to bacterial pathogens derived from the patient's own normal bacterial microflora that colonize the mucosal surfaces of the gastrointestinal tract, the upper and lower respiratory tract, the genitourinary tract, and skin.
  - o Damage to these surfaces due to cytotoxic therapy or invasive procedures permits colonizing microorganisms to gain access to deeper tissues.
  - o Cytotoxic therapy–induced damage to the patient's cellular defenses allows rapid, unimpeded microbial proliferation
- **Pathogens**
  - o GN (E. coli, Pseudomonas, Klebsiella, Enterobacter) and GPC (S. aureus)
  - o Viruses (HSV, CMV, VZV, EBV, HHV-6)
    - Respiratory (influenza, RSV, coronavirus, rhinovirus)
  - o Fungi (candida, aspergillus, mucor, trichosporon, fusarium)

HEMATOLOGY/ONCOLOGY

Multinational Association for Supportive Care in Cancer Score (MASCC)	
Characteristic	Points
Burden of febrile neutropenia symptoms	
No or mild symptoms	5
Moderate symptoms	3
Severe or morbid symptoms	0
No ↓BP (SBP<90)	5
No COPD	4
Solid or hematologic cancer with no previous fungal infection	4
No dehydration necessitating parenteral fluids	3
Outpatient status on onset of fever	3
Age<60	2

- **Outpatient vs. Inpatient Management**
  MASCC or CISNE can be used.
  - MASCC[232]
    - MASCC score < 21 or significant comorbidities with ANC<500 = hospitalization
      1. High Risk Features:
         - Age > 70 years
         - Mucositis greater than grade 2
         - Poor performance status (ECOG)
         - Initial ANC < 0.1×10^9 cells/L
         - Patients with active comorbidities, such as congestive cardiac failure or renal insufficiency
         - Patients with sepsis or septic shock syndrome
         - Documented infection with a defined clinical focus, such as pneumonia (*e.g.*, community-acquired pneumonia), cellulitis, or intra-abdominal sepsis syndrome
    - MASCC score ≥ 21 or no comorbidities with ↑ANC = outpatient treatment → oral fluoroquinolone + amoxicillin
      1. If patient re-fevers or continues to fever on tx in 48 hours, should return for hospitalization
  - CISNE[233]- more specific than MASCC
    - Use in adult outpatients with solid tumor, T≥100.4F x 1h, ANC≤500 or 1000 and expectation to be decreasing to 500).
    - Not applicable if patient has acute organ failure (AKI, CHF, arrythmia, delirium, acute abdomen, ARF defined as SaO2<90%), severe infection, SBP<90, septic shock
    - Scores
      - 0 points – low risk, consider discharge with PO Abx. 1.1% chance of complications
      - 1-2 points – intermediate risk, clinical judgement for admission. 6.2% chance of complications
      - ≥3 points – high risk; admit for further investigation, obtain BCx. 36% chance of complications.
- **Workup**
  - Labs
    - CBC
    - HFP
    - Cultures (bacterial, fungal, urine, sputum with viral culture) and from any indwelling lines or 2 separate venipuncture sites
    - If Pneumonia:
      - S.pneumo

- Legionella
- RSV
- Influenza
- Viral Culture
- UA with culture
- Lactate (r/o sepsis)
- Diarrhea
- Stool culture
- Enterovirus RNA
- Fecal leukocytes
- CMV (if s/p transplant)
- C.diff (w/ diarrhea)
  - Imaging/Procedures
    - CXR
    - LP if AMS
    - CT of the liver/spleen indicated in patients with persistent or recurrent fever at the time of recovery from neutropenia to r/o hepatosplenic candidiasis
- **CLABSI**
  - S. aureus and Pseudomonas
  - Require 14d treatment
    - 4-6-week treatment if complicated by deep tissue infection, endocarditis, thrombosis, or bacteremia x 72 hrs. **after** catheter removal
  - Remove catheter
    - Other indications to remove catheter include sepsis without resolution of fever for 72 hours, endocarditis, septic thrombosis.
    - Can remain if documented source is **coagulase negative staph**
- **Prophylaxis**
  - Leukemia
    - ABx: Moxifloxacin 400mg PO daily + Amoxicillin 500mg PO TID (start on day 5)
    - Antifungal: Voriconazole or Posaconazole susp 200mg PO TID or 300mg PO daily
    - Antiviral: Valacyclovir 500mg PO BID or Acyclovir 800m PO BID
  - Lymphoma
    - ABx: Moxifloxacin 400mg PO daily
    - Antifungal: Fluconazole 200mg PO daily
    - Antiviral: Valacyclovir 500mg PO BID or Acyclovir 800m PO BID

Figure. Fever with neutropenia work-up

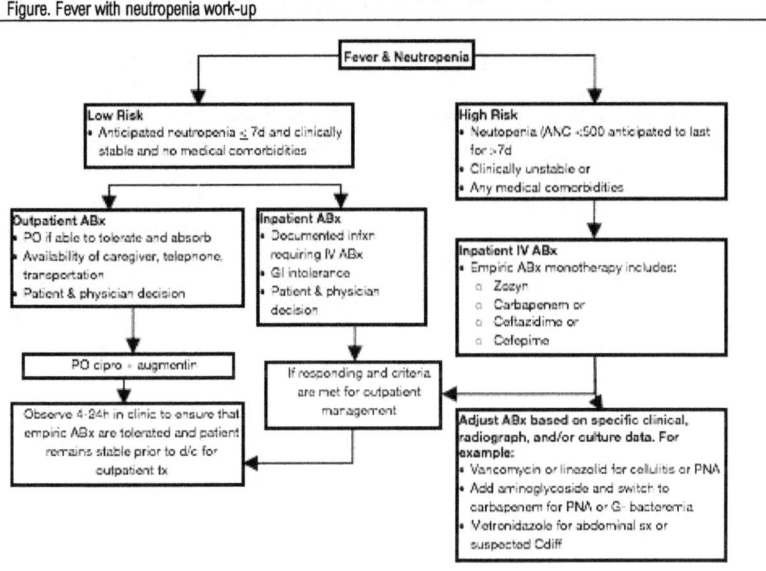

- **Treatment**
  - <u>GSF</u> – not typically used in treatment unless patient has either persistent fever despite abx treatment or severe neutropenia (ANC<100) which is expected to last > 7 days
  - <u>Antibiotics</u>
    - *Administration* - Antibiotics given through a triple lumen should be rotated to give Abx through different lumen each day.
    - *Treatment Options*
      - See table on next page
      - Add empiric antifungal therapy if neutropenic patient remains febrile after 4-7d of broad-spectrum ABx
    - *Monitoring Response*
      - Re-evaluate at 72h and at 5 days for:
        - Fever
        - Clinical deterioration
        - New microbiologic finding from cultures
        - Clinical progression
        - Medication intolerance
      - Persistent fever/neutropenia (4-7d after initiating treatment)
        - Continue empiric ABx and add anti-fungal therapy
    - *Duration of Treatment*
      1. Should be continued until the patient has been afebrile for 4 to 5 days, on the basis of clinical trial definitions of treatment response
         - MASCC → low risk and no documented source → minimum of 7 days duration of therapy
         - MASCC → high risk (↓PMN for >7d prior to fever) and no documented source or invasive candidiasis cx → minimum of 10 days duration of therapy
      2. Controversy however as some say ABx can be withdrawn with the resolution of fever + neutropenia (or ↑ to more than 0.5×10^9 cells/L which is typically after 72h. (*ANTIBIOSTOP*)

3. Transition to PO ABx if patient clinically stable

Neutropenic Fever Treatment

Antibiotic regimen

Monotherapy

Cefepime or Ceftazidime 2 gm IV q8hrs
Meropenem 1-2g IV q8h or Imipenem 500 mg IV q6hrs

Or if allergic to PCN:

Zosyn 4.5g IV q6-8h

**Vancomycin not typically used unless suspected CLABSI, SSTI, PNA, known MRSA colonization, or hemodynamically unstable

PLUS

Any of the following depending on the situation

G+, Catheter related infection, SSTI	Vancomycin, linezolid
Pneumonia:	Fluoroquinolones, Vancomycin
VRE	Linezolid, daptomycin
G-	Carbapenem (or switch to ESBL if G- cultured while on broad spec)
ESBL (E. coli, K.pneumonia)	Carbapenem, meropenam-varborbactam, ceftazidime-avibactam
Severe sepsis	Vancomycin
Hemodynamic Instability	Vancomycin
Necrotizing gingivitis	Add clindamycin or metronidazole to empiric therapy
Vesicular/ulcerative lesions	Add HSV coverage with Valacyclovir
Sinus tenderness/nasal ulcers	Suspect fungal infection with *Aspergillus* or *Mucor*
Acute abdominal pain	Suspect typhlitis and add anti-anaerobic coverage (or meropenam)
Focal resp lesion with neutropenia	*Aspergillus* and perform bronch+bx or tx with voriconazole

Antifungal Treatment

Consider addition of antifungal agent if > 4-7 days of fever on antibacterial agents (50% patients will have resolution of febrile neutropenia s/p initiation of antifungals) and expected neutropenia > 7 days

Any of the following:

Micafungin 100 mg IV q24h if sinus or head CT **not** suggestive of fungal infection
Voriconazole 6 mg/kg q12h for 2 doses, then 4 mg/kg q12h **if** chest CT suggestive of fungal infection

Other Options:

Caspofungin 70 mg IV for 1 dose, then 50 mg IV q24h Anidulafungin 200 mg IV for 1 dose, then 100 mg IV q24h
Amphotericin B liposomal complex 3 mg/kg q24h
Posaconazole 20 mg PO q6h for 7d, then 400 mg PO q12h
Itraconazole 200 mg IV q12h for 2d, then 200 mg IV or PO q24h for 7d, then 400 mg PO q24h thereafter
Vancomycin + Meropenem 1 g IV q8h + Amikacin

Complicated case or antibiotic resistance present
(clinically unstable and/or persistent fevers despite appropriate ABx and anti-fungal coverage)

Step Down Therapy for discharge
Ciprofloxacin 750mg PO BID + Augmentin 875mg PO BID
-or-
Moxifloxacin 400mg PO daily

HEMATOLOGY/ONCOLOGY

SUPPORTIVE CARE OF CANCER PATIENTS

Section Editor: Ashley Allemon, DO

Treatment Options

Condition	Treatment Options	Be Aware/Other

Oral Care and Mucositis [234,235]	**Preventitive**
	• Routine oral care
	• Remove dentures and clean with soft toothbrush head and rinse mouth with salt/baking soda (1/2 tsp salt and 1 tasp baking soda in 1 qt water) solution every 4 hours, rinse oral cavity - cryotherapy
	• Swish ice chips orally for about 30 minutes
	• If received FU-containing chemotherapies
	  o Palifermin IV 60 mc/kg/day for 3 days before and 3 days after starting chemotherapy in preparation for HSCT
	  o Peridex 15 cc PO swish and spit QAC and QHS
	
	Treatment
	• Routine oral care
	• Remove dentures and clean with soft toothbrush head and rinse mouth with salt/baking soda (1/2 tsp salt and 1 tasp baking soda in 1 qt water) solution every 4 hours
	• "MMX" Susp, 10 cc PO swish and spit/swallow QAC, QHS, prn (Mylanta/Maalox, Mycelex, Xylocaine)
	• Viscous Lidocaine 2%, 10 cc PO swish and spit/swallow QAC, QHS, prn
	• Hurricane Spray to mouth/throat QAC, QHS, prn
	• Topical Cocaine 2-4% swish or swab Q4hr prn
	• Carafate Susp/tab 1 gm swish and swallow/PO QAC, QHS
		Neutropenic mouth care, antibacterial and antifungal activity
		Consider IV Narcotics for pain control

Nausea and Vomiting	Compazine 10 mg IV/PO Q6 hr prn (ATC if needed)
	Haloperidol 1 mg PO or 0.5 mg subq/IV q6-8h prn
	  • if > 65 yo, 0.5 mg PO or 0.25 mg subq/IV q8h prn
	  • lower and less frequent dosing than with delirium
	  • no more than 6 mg PO or 3 mg subq/IV in 24 hours
	
	Droperidol 0.625-1.25 mg IV Q4hr prn2
	Reglan 10 mg IV/PO QAC, QHS, or Q6hr prn (ATC if needed)
	Phenergan 25 mg IVPB Q6 hr prn
	Ativan 0.5-2 mg IV/PO/SL Q4hr prn
	Decadron 4-8 mg IV/PO Q12-24hr prn
	Marinol 2.5-5 mg PO Q4hr prn
	Zofran 4 mg IV or 8 mg PO Q4hr prn (ATC if needed)
		Beware of EPS with dopaminergic antagonists
		
		Consider anti-emetics ATC to prevent sxs.

Diarrhea	Imodium 2 mg PO after each loose stool, max 8 tabs per day (16 mg) Lomotil 2.5 mg PO after each loose stool, max 8 tabs per day (20mg) Tincture of Opium 0.5-1 cc PO Q4hr prn Metamucil 5 cc PO TID Questran 4 gm PO TID Lactinex 1 tab/packet PO TID Octreotide 100-500 mcg Sub-Q Q8hr	Anti-motility agents Probiotic Antisecretory
Constipation	**Softner** Colace 100mg BID **Osmotic Agent** Polyethylene Glycol 17g daily-BID Glycerin supp PR daily prn Magnesium Citrate 150-300 cc PO daily prn	Onset 24-72 hours Onset 1-2 hrs Onset 30-60 minutes

	Sorbitol 30 cc PO daily prn, Lactulose 30 cc PO daily prn	Onset 24-48 hrs
	Stimulant Laxative	
	Senokot 2 tabs PO daily prn (up to 4 tabs BID), Cascara 5-10 cc PO QHS prn	Onset 6-10 hrs
	Dulcolax 10 mg PO/PR daily prn	Onset 30-60 minutes
	Cascara 300mg once a day (no longer than 6 days)	
	Bulk Forming Laxative	
	Psyllium 3.4g up to TID	Onset 12-72 hrs
	Metamucil 5-10 cc PO daily prn	Onset 12-24 hrs
	Lubricant Laxative	
	MOM 30 cc PO Q6hr prn	Onset 3-6 hrs
	Mineral Oil 30 cc PO prn	Onset 6-8 hrs

VENOUS THROMBOEMBOLISM

- **Defined** – VTE is a spectrum involving either the thrombosis of the deep veins (DVT) and/or pulmonary veins (PE). [236]
- **DVT Location**
  - Distal lower extremity DVT – calf or peroneal veins
  - Proximal lower extremity DVT – popliteal, femoral and iliac veins **more dangerous
  - Upper extremity DVT – axillary and subclavian veins
- **PE Types**[237,238]
  - <u>Low-Risk</u> – no hemodynamic instability, no changes on ECG/CT/TTE
    - *Subsegmental PE*: poor data to recommend for or against treatment
  - <u>Submassive/Intermediate-Risk</u> – no hemodynamic instability but TTE/CT/ECG evidence of RV strain or dysfunction or TROP leak indicative of myocardial necrosis
    - TTE – look for RV dilatation, strain
    - CT – same as above
    - ECG – T wave inversions, ST depressions
  - <u>Massive/High-Risk</u>– ↓BP (SBP<90 x 15min) +/- bradycardia
- **Strong Risk Factors**
  - Current infection
  - Age >50
  - Cancer (kidney, pancreas, lung, colon)
  - History of VTE
  - Hospitalization for HF or AF in past 3 months
  - MI in last 3 months
  - Spinal cord injury
  - Immobility
  - Trauma/Surgery
    - Fracture of lower limb
    - Hip/knee replacement
  - Pregnancy (equal risk through all 3 trimesters)
- **Differential**
  - Muscle strain, lymphangitis, venous insufficiency, cellulitis
- **Physical examination**
  - DVT
    - Palpable cord, calf/thigh pain, unilateral edema
    - Pain at the iliac vein (May Thurner Syndrome)
    - Look for calf circumference difference or absence of calf swelling **only 2 factors shown to help r/o **
    - In pregnant patients, m/c to have L>R VTE
  - PE
    - Tachycardia

HEMATOLOGY / ONCOLOGY

- SOB
- DOE
- Sharp chest pain
- **Scoring Systems** – used to determine what labs/imaging should be performed
  - rGeneva *(see table below)*
  - PERC rule for Pulmonary Embolism (rules out PE if **no** criteria are present)
  - Wells Criteria
  - Simplified Pulmonary Embolism Severity Index (sPESI)
    - 0 points: 30 day mortality risk 1%
    - ≥1 point: 30 day mortality risk 10.9%

PE Scoring/Risk	
Revised Geneva (simplified version)	
Age>65 (+1)	
Surgery or lower limb fx in last month (+1)	
Unilateral lower limb pain (+1)	Low Risk: 0-1
Tachycardia (75-94 is +1; >95 is +2)	Moderate Risk: 2-4 → consider d-dimer
Hemoptysis (+1)	High Risk: ≥5 → consider CT or US
Previous history of DVT or PE (+1)	
Active cancer (+2)	
Pain on limb palpation (+1)	

PE likely if score ≥3

- **Disposition (Inpatient vs. Outpatient)**

HESTIA criteria
If at least one of the questions is answered with "yes," then the patient should be admitted to hospital.
Hemodynamic instability?
Thrombolytic or embolectomy therapy needed?
Active bleeding or at high risk for bleeding?
Oxygen needed for _24 hours to keep O2 saturation _90%?
PE developed while on anticoagulant therapy?
Intravenous pain medication needed for _24 hours?
Medical or social reason for admission?
Renal impairment (creatinine clearance _30 mL/min)?
Severe liver impairment?
Pregnancy?
H/o HIT?

- **Risk Stratification/Mortality**
  - High Risk: hemodynamic instability (SBP<90 or vasopressors required to achive SBP≥90 with end organ dysfunction such as AMS, cold U/LE, oliguria/anuria, ↑lactate) with RV dysfunction, +TROP → ICU for fibrinolysis/TPA, NE, ECMO
  - Intermediate to High Risk: no hemodynamic instability but **+TROP**, +RV dysfunction, sPESI ≥1 or HESTIA ≥1 → consider reperfusion therapy, consider ICU
  - Intermediate to Low Risk: no hemodynamic instability, **-TROP**, - RV dysfunction, sPESI ≥1 or HESTIA ≥1→ hospitalize
  - Low Risk: no hemodynamic instability or RV dysfunction, -TROP, low PESI and HESTIA→ early discharge if close f/u and social support, otherwise hospitalize
- **Labs**
  - CBC, coagulation panel, UA, ICU panel
    - ↑SCr and ↓GFR related to 30 day all-cause mortality
    - ↓Na associated with increased in-hospital mortality
  - D-dimer
    - Should be age adjusted: (age x 10 mcg/L) as cut-off for those >50 YO

- Low/medium/high probability from Well's score will determine if d-dimer required (*YEARS*)
- Troponin (c/w RV strain, worse prognosis in acute phase of PE
- BNP (can help evaluate severity of RV dysfunction; adverse outcome in levels ≥600)
- Lactate (levels ≥2 associated with severe PE)
- Screening for hypercoagulable state:
  Only should be done in patients with intermediate risk for progression d/t transient risk factors such as small travel, OCP, minor surgery, pregnancy. Should not be done on first episode, unprovoked VTE. (SOME trial)
  - Coagulation panel
  - Protein C and S activity, free protein S
  - Activated protein C → if abnormal then Factor V Leiden gene mutation
  - Prothrombin mutation
  - Antiphospholipid AB (APLAS) with cardiolipin AB (IgG, IgM), DRVVT (lupus anticoagulant), and B2-glycoprotein
    □ Presents as a prothrombotic disorder with either (1) vascular thrombosis or (2) pregnancy complications. Bleeding is uncommon and if present, is usually secondary to significant thrombocytopenia, dysfunctional platelets, hypoprothrombinemia, or an underlying disease. Often see ↑PLT and ↑APTT levels.
    □ If only one test is positive, repeat in 12 weeks and if it remains positive then diagnosis is confirmed.
  - Antithrombin activity (AT3)
  - Prothrombin gene mutation
    □ *Done mostly in those with no risk factors, family history, recurrent disease*
  - +/- SS trait
  - Homocysteine level
- **Imaging**
  - Duplex/compression US → if Wells Score is **high** and US negative, repeat in 7 days d/t chance of false negative
  - 2016 meta-analysis of prospective clinical trials that evaluated use of the Wells rule and D-dimer level to predict PE found that a more appropriate D-dimer threshold should be age adjusted.
    - For patients older than 50 years, the D-dimer threshold is (age × 0.01 μg/mL).
  - Venography only used if noninvasive testing unavailable
  - Pregnancy: duplex US, V/Q scan, or pulmonary angiogram
- **Treatment**
  - **Suspected PE with hemodynamic instability**
    - Bedside TTE → if RV dysfunction → CTPA
    - IV anticoagulation with UFH for high-risk PE
  - **Suspected PE without hemodynamic instability**
    - Start anticoagulation

- Oxygen: Supplemental oxygen should be administered if hypoxemia exists. Severe hypoxemia or respiratory failure should prompt consideration of intubation and mechanical ventilation
- Fluids: Intravenous fluid administration is first-line therapy if normal/low CVP. It may improve hemodynamic performance, as illustrated by a series of 13 patients with acute PE and a cardiac index <2.5 L/min/m^2. May over-distend RV, beware.
  - NS or LR ≤500cc over 15-30min
  - There are no randomized trials that definitively determine the optimal vasopressor for patients with shock due to acute PE
    □ Norepinephrine 0.2-1.0mcg/kg/min

- ▫ Dobutamine 2-20mcg/kg/min
- Vasopressors
  - NE 0.2-1.0 mcg/kg/m (↑RV inotropy and SBP)
  - Dobutamine 2-20 mcg/kg/m (↑RV inotropy, ↓filling pressure), avoid using without another vasopressor on board (aggravates arterial hypotension)
- Thrombolytic therapy/Fibrinolysis
  - Generally considered for patients with **massive PE**. PEITHO trial showed no mortality benefit in submassive PE patients.
  - Absolute contraindications:
    - ▫ H/O hemorrhagic CVA or cryptogenic stroke
    - ▫ Ischemic CVA in last 6 months
    - ▫ CNS neoplasm
    - ▫ Major trauma or surgery or head injury in last 3 wks
    - ▫ Bleeding diathesis
    - ▫ Acting Bleeding
  - Relative contraindications: TIA in last 6 months, on PO anticoagulation, current pregnancy or first post-partum week, non-compressible puncture sites, traumatic resuscitation, refractory hypertension (SBP >180), advanced liver disease, infective endocarditis, active peptic ulcer
  - Pharmacologic Options
    - ▫ rtPA 100mg over 2h (extreme situations, consider 0.6 mg/kg over 15m for max dose of 50mg; this is not officially approved)
    - ▫ Streptokinase 250kIU as loading dose over 30m f/b 100k IU/h over 12-24h
    - ▫ Urokinase 4400 IU/kg as loading dose over 10 min f/b 4400 IU/kg/h over 12-24h
- Embolectomy – **massive PE and thrombolytic therapy is contraindicated or** remain unstable after initiation of fibrinolysis
- Filter – patients with contraindications to anticoagulation or active bleeding or PE in setting of anticoagulation or patients who will likely die if they have another PE
  - After placement, if anticoagulation contraindication resolves, patients should be initiated on therapy
  - Most will get retrievable
  - Permanent are for those with long-term anticoagulation contraindications
- Anticoagulation - does not dissolve existing clots directly but limit further thrombus formation and allow fibrinolysis to naturally occur
  - **Isolated subsegmental PE** – no treatment if no concurrent DVT, no underlying malignancy, and no risk factors. *(VTE Guidelines Chest 2016)*
  - **Aspirin** - In patients with unprovoked VTE or PE, start ASA for further prevention after anticoagulation therapy has finished (*INSPIRE, ASPIRE*)
  - **IVC Filter** - indicated if you cannot anti-coagulate patient due to bleeding complications/risk
  - **OCP**: avoid injectable contraceptives. Should aim for progestin-releasing IUD
  - **Pregnancy**: LMWH (preferred) for 3-6m prior to delivery (may consider up to time of delivery and 6w post-partum)
    - ▫ Dosing based on early pregnancy body weight
    - ▫ D/c heparin at least 24-36h prior to delivery
    - ▫ D/c heparin 6h prior to epidural
    - ▫ Resume heparin 12h after delivery then switch to warfarin for 6w
  - **NOACs/Parental Therapy**
    In general, parenteral therapy with a transition to warfarin or DOAC is done unless choosing specific DOACs which do not require initial parental tx.
    - Parenteral options: UFH, LMWH, Fondaparinux
      1) Parenteral f/b Warfarin:

HEMATOLOGY/ONCOLOGY

- UFH – not favored in treatment except for high risk PE; used if GFR<30cc/min; BMI>40. Dosing as follows:
  - 80U/kg bolus f/b gtt @ 18U/kg/h target APTT 60-80s
- LMWH/Fondaparinux f/b Warfarin for 5 days (until INR ≥2.5 for at least 24 hours) for low or intermediate risk PE
  - Warfarin dosing
    a. <50kg: 5mg daily
    b. 50-100kg: 7.5mg daily
    c. >100kg: 10mg daily

2) Parenteral f/b DOAC:
- DOAC – non inferior to above regimen; see table below.
  - Non-Cancer Patients – see table below
  - Cancer Patients
    - 6 months duration; DVT and PE. Avoid in patients with PLT<50k[239]
      - Rivaroxaban 15mg PO BID x21d then 20mg/d (*SELECT-D*)
        **recommended per NCCN guidelines
      - Edoxaban 60/30mg PO daily after LMWH for ≥ 5 days (*Hokusai-VTE*)
        Appropriate alternative to rivaroxaban per ESC guidelines
      - Apixaban 10/5mg PO BID (*AMPLIFY, CARAVAGGIO, ADAM VTE*)
      - Dabigatran (*RE-COVER*)
    - If PLT<50k then consider LMWH/UFH (and consider platelet transfusion if high risk of VTE progression)
    - Avoid in patients of extreme weight
    - LMWH still recommended over NOAC in patients with GI malignancy d/t bleeding risk in NOACs
    - If recurrent VTE on LMWH, increase dose by 20-25%

Pharmacologic Anticoagulation Options in Non-Malignancy		
Medication	Dosage	Misc. Information/Good for...
LMWH	SQ 1mg/kg BID or 1.5mg/kg/d	Cancer; Co-existing liver disease; Pregnancy or risk thereof
UFH	80U/kg bolus then 18U/kg/hr ▫ Alternative dosing is 8k-10k SQ q8h or 15k-20k q12h	Adjust dosing for an APTT of 1.5-2.5x control
Apixaban (*AMPLIFY-EXT*) (*APLIFY*)	10mg BID x7d then... -5mg BID or -2.5mg BID if SCr >1.5 or age>80 or weight <60kg ≥6 Months of Therapy (no cancer): 2.5mg BID	Preferred DOAC Half-life 12h Less dyspepsia or GIB risk; Want to avoid any parental therapy initially; Efficacy in patients with PE was similar to that in the patients with DVT; Has been shown to be effective for the prevention of recurrent venous thromboembolism in patient's s/p 6 to 12 months of therapy
Rivaroxaban (*EINSTEIN DVT*) (*EINSTEIN EXT*)	15mg BID x3w then 20mg/d ≥6 Months of Therapy (no cancer):	Half-life 5-9h Want to avoid any parental therapy initially, Once daily therapy requested

VKA/Warfarin	10mg/d Start 5mg/d for 2 days and adjust to INR 2-3 x 48h	Preferred in patients with +thrombophilia w/u Start on same day as UFH gtt; Less dyspepsia or GIB risk; Once daily therapy requested; poor compliance expected; known severe renal disease (GFR<30)
Dabigatran *(REMEDY, RESONATE, RE-COVER)*	150mg BID	Requires initial parenteral therapy x5-10d unless transitioning from UFH gtt, warfarin (INR should be <2), or LMWH (within 2 hrs. of next dose)
Edoxaban *(Hokusai-VTE)*	60mg daily after 5 days of parenteral tx (30mg if < 60kg in weight; assuming normal SCr)	Requires initial parenteral therapy x5d

Use of NOACs in patients with VTE	
Patients to consider and discuss NOACs	Patients not to use NOACs
• NOACs are good choices in many patients with acute VTE or on long-term warfarin for VTE; the main reason to use a NOAC is one of patient convenience, not of efficacy or safety • In patients on long-term warfarin, NOACs are particularly attractive in those with (a) fluctuating/unstable INRs, or (b) a high "warfarin hate factor"	• Patients with renal impairment when GFR is 30 mL/min. • Patients at high risk for bleeding because there is no antidote or known reversal strategy for the NOACs • Patients with cancer because LMWH is the treatment of choice in these patients; however, if the patient cannot afford LMWH, then either warfarin or a NOAC are appropriate considerations • Significantly obese patients, such as those with a body mass index 40 kg/m2 or a body weight 140 kg because only a limited number of such patients were studied in the phase 3 clinical trials • Underweight patients, such as those with a body weight of 50 kg or body mass index of 20 kg/m2 • Patients on interfering drugs • Patients with moderate to severe liver disease • Sick inpatients because they may need procedural interventions (central venous lines, etc) • Patients with high copays for NOACs for whom the existing financial drug support mechanisms do not apply

- **Duration**
    - The risk of VTE recurrence is **greatest in the first 6 months after** the event and remains elevated indefinitely compared with the general population.
        - Patients should remain on anticoagulation for at minimum 6 months, can consider stopping after 6 months if no active malignancy noted *(ASCO)*
    - Risk for recurrence classified as high, intermediate, low based on risk factors present at time of index event (see table below)

Risk factors for recurrence based on initial cause of VTE		
Risk	% Risk of PE in a year	Examples
Low (major transient or reversible RF)	<3%	• Surgery with general anesthesia longer than 30 min • Hospital bed (only up to bathroom) for ≥3 days • Trauma c/b fx

Intermediate (transient or reversible RF; non-malignant RF)	3-8%		• Minor surgery lasting <30m • Hospital admission for <3 days • Estrogen therapy • Pregnancy • In bed (but not hospital) for ≥3 days due to illness • Leg injury w/o fx but c/b reduced mobility • Long flight • IBD or active AI dz
High	>8%		• Active cancer • 1+ episodes of VTE that were not a/w major RF • APAs

- ▫ Those with first PE/VTE secondary to a major transient/reversible risk factor, can d/c anticoagulation after 3 months
- ▫ Consider anticoagulation >3 months in those with:
  - First episode of PE and no identifiable risk factor
  - First episode of PE associated with a persistent risk factor other than antiphospholipid antibody syndrome
  - **If treating with NOAC for >6mo reduce dose according to table above**
- Lifetime recurrence rates for DVT ranges from 21% to 30%, depending on the population.
- D-Dimer
  - ▫ The d-dimer test has been used to stratify risk of recurrent VTE.
  - ▫ The d-dimer value is checked **one month after anticoagulation ends**, with an increased level indicating increased risk.
  - ▫ Consider serial D-dimer's in patients experiencing first unprovoked episode q2m starting 1 month after duration of anticoagulation therapy to determine risk of recurrence (PROLONG trial)
    - <500 ng/mL associated with 3.5% yearly risk of recurrence
    - >500 ng/mL associated with 8.9% risk in each of the first 2 years
- Unprovoked (idiopathic) VTE – at least 3 months; if no bleeding issues and tolerated well then consider extended therapy duration (6 months). Extended duration of DOAC therapy has been found to be superior to simply using ASA. The study specifically utilized higher dose Rivaroxaban 20mg (*Weitz et al. NEJM 2017 Mar 18*). Men have higher risk than women (1.75 fold) and a positive d-dimer doubles the risk of another event. If extended duration therapy is initiated, it should be re-assessed at least annually to decide if it remains required.
  - ▫ In females, risk stratification with HERDOO2 score can be done to help stop anticoagulation
- Antiphospholipid ABS → extended duration / possibly lifelong with VKA with increasing INR ranges depending on if clots continue to occur on tx.
- Cancer – LMWH for 3-6 months if GI malignancy, otherwise consider NOAC; consider extended treatment until cancer treated
- Proximal DVT – 3 months (but if no risk factors, asymptomatic may consider serial US w/o tx)
- Distal (below the knee) DVT – compression stockings

Situation	Management Recommendation
Unprovoked DVT (no cancer)	DOAC (dabigatran, rivaroxaban, etc.) over VKA for at least 3 months. Extended duration of therapy should be considered based on patient risk factors (low (0.8% risk of major bleed)/moderate (1.6% annual risk)/high

	(>6.5% annual risk) with re-evaluation of extended therapy done at least annually.
Provoked DVT d/t cancer	LMWH for duration of cancer therapy
Unprovoked UE DVT	Investigate for thoracic outlet syndrome

- **DVT Prophylaxis**
  Based on *Padua score (medical)* or *Caprini score (if non-ortho surgical patient)*
  o Leg pumps (PCDs) while in bed
  o Elastic compression stockings
  o Lovenox 40 mg SQ daily (unless GFR<30; then use Heparin 5000U SQ TID)
    - Post-operative:
      ▫ *Low Risk (outpatient surg, neurosurgery)*
        - PCD
        - Early ambulation
        - UFH until discharge
      ▫ *High Risk (Hx malignancy, ortho surg, hx VTE)*
        - LMWH x 5 weeks
          o Use 30 mg if renal impairment
          o Don't give if bleeding, thrombocytopenic or going to surgery
        - If Creatinine Clearance 30, use Heparin 5000 units SC Q 8 hours (7500 units SC Q 8 hours if obese)
    - *Orthopedic Surgery (REMODEL, RENOVATE, REMOBILIZE, RECORD2, EPCAT II)*
      ▫ *Knee Arthroplasty (TKA)*
        - Medications: apixaban 2.5mg BID, dabigatran 150mg or 220mg daily, rivaroxaban 10mg PO daily
        - Duration: 10-14 days but ACCP advises extending to 35 days
        - Rivaroxaban may have better outcomes but comes with higher bleeding risk
        - EPCAT II showed similar rates when using rivaroxaban for 5 days then completing 10-14 day course (TKA with ASA than using rivaroxaban for entire 14 days
      ▫ *Hip Arthroplasty (THA)* – as above, however if following EPCAT II may affect duration of anticoagulation (30 days)
        - Medications: apixaban 2.5mg BID, dabigatran 150mg or 220mg daily, rivaroxaban 10mg PO daily
        - Duration: 30-35 days
        - If using rivaroxaban, can consider starting with rivaroxaban for 5 days then finishing total 30-35 day course with ASA
      ▫ *Hip Fracture* – DOACs not approved
- **Recurrent VTE on Anticoagulation Therapy**
  o If patient is on warfarin (assuming therapeutic INR) → switch to treatment-dose LMWH
  o If patient is on LMWH → ↑ dose by 20-25%
  o If anticoagulation intensity cannot be safely ↑ due to bleeding risk → insert IVC

Primary VTE Prophylaxis in Orthopedic Patients[290]

Surgery	Treatment	Duration	Society Recommendation
Total Hip / Total Knee	LMWH (12h post-surgery)	10-14 days and up to 35 days	ACCP
	UFH		
	VKA		
	Fonadparinux 2.5mg/d		
	Apixaban 2.5mg/BID†		
	Dabigatran 150-220mg/d*		
	Rivaroxiban 10mg/d		
	ASA 75-100mg/d		
THR	LMWH -or- Fondaparinux 2.5mg/d	10 days then ASA for total of 28 days (1 month)	NICE
	Rivaroxiban 10mg/d	14 days	
	Apixaban 2.5mg/BID	35 days	
	Dabigatran 150-220mg/d*	14 days	
Hip Fracture	DOACs not approved		
	Lovenox	10-14 days and up to 35 days (28 days for SIGN except with warfarin)	ACCP, NICE, SIGN
	UFH		ACCP, SIGN
	Warfarin		ACCP
TKR	ASA 75-100mg Δ	14 days	NICE
	Rivaroxaban 10mg/d	>14 days	
	Apixaban 2.5mg/BID	12 days	
	Dabigatran 150-220mg/d*	12 days	

** start with ½ dose of dabigatran as first dose after surgery, then continue at dosing above
† Apixaban not recommended for hip fracture
Δ ASA not recommended by SIGN

HEMATOLOGY/ONCOLOGY

Figure. Anticoagulation recommendations based on probability of PE

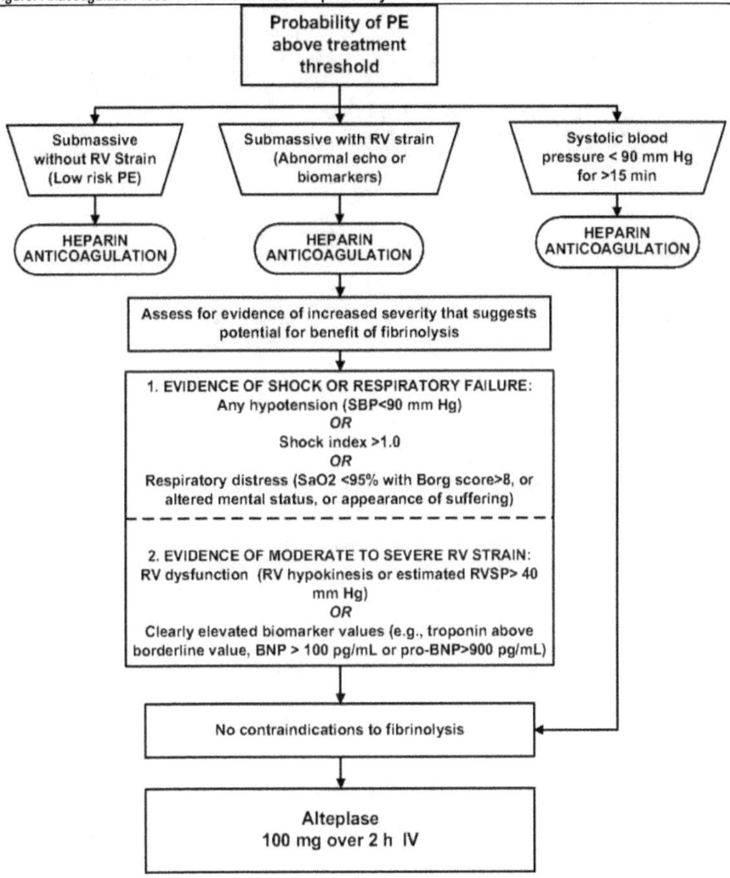

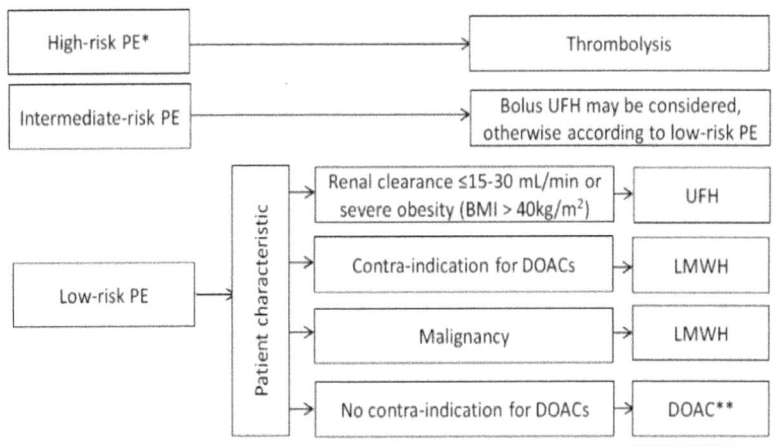

Bibliography

[208] Chapter 5. Laboratory Diagnosis: Clinical Hematology. In: Gomella LG, Haist SA. eds. *Clinician's Pocket Reference: The Scut Monkey*, 11e New York, NY: McGraw-Hill; 2007. http://accessmedicine.mhmedical.com/content.aspx?bookid=365&sectionid=43074914. Accessed November 10, 2018.

[209] Blood. In: Mescher AL. eds. Junqueira's Basic Histology: Text and Atlas.

[210] Ganz, Tomas. Anemia of Inflammation. N Engl J Med 2019;381:1148-57.

[211] Tefferi et al. Mayo Clin Proc (2005).

[212] Fischer, Conrad. "USMLE:Master the Boards Step 3." Kaplan Medical.

[213] Wan et al. "83-Year-Old Man With Chest Pain, Exertional Dyspnea, and Anemia." Mayo Clinic Proceedings Residents Clinic. November 2013;88(11):e129-e133

[214] Clinical Resource, Comparison of Oral Iron Supplements. Pharmacist's Letter/Prescriber's Letter. March 2017.

[215] Wolf et al. JAMA. 2020.

[216] Tirona, Maria Taria. Breast Cancer Screening Update. *Am Fam Physician*. 2013;87(4):274-278

[217] Ezekial, Mark. "Current Clinical Strategies: Handbook of Anesthesia" 2007-2008

[218] Carson JL, Reynolds RC. In search of the transfusion threshold. Hematology. 2005;10(Suppl 1):86-88.

[219] Carson JL, Duff A, Poses RM, et al. Effect of anemia and cardiovascular disease on surgical mortality and morbidity. Lancet. 1996;348(9034):1055-1060.

[220] Herbert. et al. "A Multicenter, Randomized, Controlled Clinical Trial of Transfusion Requirements In Critical Care." NEJM. 11FEB1999. 340(6).

[221] Federici et al. "Transfusion issues in cancer patients." Thrombosis Research. 2012. S60-5.

[222] Klein et al. "Red blood cell transfusion in clinical practice." The Lancet. Vol 370 (4AUG2007)

[223] Frontera et al. "Guideline for Reversal of Antithrombotics in Intracranial Hemorrhage." Neurocrit Care (2016) 24:6–46.

[224] Sangle et al. "Antiphospholipid Antibody Syndrome." Archives of Pathology and Laboratory Medicine. 135 (9/2011)

[225] Larson RA, Hall MJ. Chapter 71. Acute Leukemia. In: Hall JB, Schmidt GA, Wood LD, eds. Principles of Critical Care. 3rd ed. New York: McGraw-Hill; 2005.

[226] Habermann, Thomas M. Mayo Clinic Internal Medicine Concise Textbook. Edition 1. 2008

[227] PL Detail-Document, How to Manage High INRs in Warfarin Patients. Pharmacist's Letter/Prescriber's Letter. May 2012.

[228] Holbrook A, Schulman S, Witt DM, et al. Evidence-Based Management of Anticoagulant Therapy. Chest 2012. February 1, 2012;141(2 suppl):e152S-e84S.

[229] Freifeld et al. "Clinical Practice Guideline for the Use of Antimicrobial Agents in Neutropenic Patients with Cancer: 2010 Update by the Infectious Diseases Society of America"CID. 2011:52

[230] Bergstrom C, Nagalla S, Gupta A. Management of Patients With Febrile NeutropeniaA Teachable Moment. JAMA Intern Med. Published online February 12, 2018. doi:10.1001/jamainternmed.2017.8386

[231] Pizzo, Philip. "Management of Patients With Fever and Neutropenia Through the Arc of Time." Ann Intern Med. doi:10.7326/M18-3192.

[232] Mohindra et al. Am J Emerg Med. 2019.

[233] Carmona-Bayonas et al. Br J Cancer. 2011.

[234] Cedars-Sinai Medical Center Intern Survival Guide

[235] Oral Health in Cancer Therapy: A Guide for Health Care Professionals. 3rd Edition.

[236] Konstantinides et al. Eur Respir J. 2019.

[237] Jaff et al. Management of Massive and Submassive Pulmonary Embolism, Iliofemoral DVT, and Chronic Thromboembolic Pulmonary Hypertension. Circulation. 2011: 123; 1788-1830

[238] Jeikai Liang et al. "A 51-year-old woman with dyspnea" CCJM. August 2013: 80(8)

[239]

[240] Flevas et al. EFORT Open Rev. 2018

OPTHALMOLOGY

Eye Pain 352
Conjunctivitis 353
Corneal Abrasion 357

EYE PAIN

- **History**[241]
    - Ask about vision loss or vision changes → immediate referral (for other referral indications, see next page)
    - Photophobia or Foreign body sensation → likely corneal process, abrasion, retained foreign body
    - Ask about contact lens use → r/o bacterial and acanthamoeba keratitis
    - HA → r/o AACG, scleritis, cluster HA (usually unilateral), migraines
    - Stabbing pain → scleritis, uveitis, optic neuritis
    - ↓ vision → optic neuritis, scleritis, keratitis, uveitis, AACG, cellulitis
- **Exam**
    - Functional assessment
        - Vision check with Snellen chart @ 20'
        - Visual Fields - confrontation testing with wiggle test from boundary of visual field
        - Extraocular movements – have pt. keep head stationary and follow fingers
    - Structures
        - Look for eyelid swelling, erythema, lesions, ptosis, rashes, vesicles
    - Differentials
        - Conjunctival injection → conjunctivitis, uveitis, scleritis, keratitis, corneal abrasion
        - Eyelid swelling → hordeolum, orbital cellulitis, pre-septal cellulitis
        - Pain w/ extraocular mvmt → optic neuritis, cellulitis, scleritis, AACG
        - +Fluorescein stain → corneal abrasion (linear pattern), keratitis (dendritic pattern), superficial keratitis (punctate pattern)
- **Imaging**
    - MRI with gad in patients with suspected optic neuritis
    - CT orbits if suspecting orbital cellulitis
- **Management**
    - See red flags in next section for indications for urgent referral
    - Corneal abrasion treated with topical NSAID drops, with topical fluoroquinolone (FLQ) or aminoglycoside (AMG) drops in patients who were using contact lenses. See section dedicated to corneal abrasions below.
    - Viral and Bacterial conjunctivitis – see *Conjunctivitis* section below
    - Scleritis – NSAIDs
    - Bacterial keratitis – broad spectrum ABx if not wearing contact lenses, if using, then topical FLQ or AMG
    - Dry eye syndrome – artificial tears QID but refer if persistent
    - Orbital cellulitis – optho referral, inpatient admission, IV Vanco + (ceftriaxone, cefotaxime, Augmentin, or Zosyn)

OPTHALMOLOGY

Figure. Work up for the diagnosis of eye pain

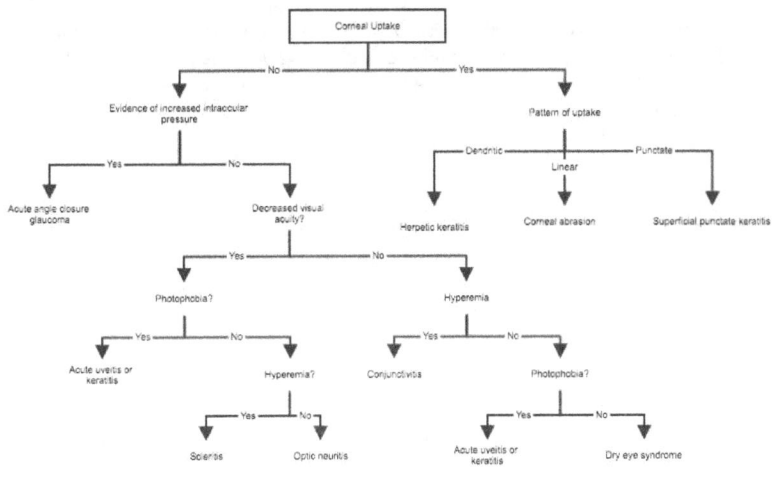

CONJUNCTIVITIS

- **General**[242]
    o The conjunctiva is a thin semitransparent membrane that covers the sclera.
    o Conjunctivitis is an inflammation of the conjunctival tissue due to infection or other irritants.
    o The three most common causes of conjunctivitis are:
        - viral (m/c due to adenovirus)
        - allergic
        - bacterial
- **Historical Features**
    o Patients with viral conjunctivitis present with foreign body sensation, red eyes, itching, light sensitivity, burning, and watery discharge.
        - Usually have a recent history of an upper respiratory tract infection or recent contact with a sick individual.
        - Visual acuity is usually at or near their baseline vision.
        - The conjunctiva is injected (red) and can also be edematous.
    o Patients with bacterial conjunctivitis present with all the above symptoms, **but with mucopurulent discharge and mattering of the eyelids upon waking**.
    o Red Flag Symptoms
        - Visual acuity change (usually one-line change)
        - Copious/muco purulent discharge
        - Photophobia
        - Foreign body sensation
        - Corneal opacity
        - Fixed pupil
        - Trouble keeping eye open
        - Severe HA w/ nausea
        - Pain

353

OPTHALMOLOGY

- Constant blurred vision
- **Management**
  - Viral – conservative tx
  - Bacterial – Moxifloxacin, Erythromycin or TMP+polymyxin; alternative is quinolone; azithromycin 1% applied every 2 hours for the first 1-2 days then decrease to QID for the next 5-7 days. If ABx hard to come by, consider povidone-iodine solution 1.25% ophthalmic solution.
  - Allergic – usually lasts <24 hours; can try Olopatadine if recurrent or prolonged course

Diagnosis / Differential of Conjunctivitis

	Viral	Bacterial	Allergic
Percentage	9-80%	18-57%	90%
Involvement	Unilateral, may progress to bilateral	Unilateral, may progress to bilateral	Bilateral
Stuck shut in morning?	Yes	Yes	Yes
Discharge	Watery; scant; serous	Purulent, green, white, or yellow; thick	Watery; scant
Discharge re-appears after wiping **can help distinguish bacterial from viral**	No	Yes	No
Other	Burning, sandy, gritty sensation, viral prodromal symptoms	Unremitting ocular discharge	Itching
Conjunctiva	Diffuse appearance	Diffuse	Diffuse
Causes	Adenovirus Herpes simplex Herpes zoster Enterovirus	S. aureus H. influenzae S. pneumoniae	Pollens
Treatment	• May take up to 3 weeks • Cold compress • Artificial tears QID • Antihistamines • Good hand hygiene	• Tobramycin ointment: 3 x/d for 1 wk • Ciprofloxacin ointment: 3 x/d for 1 wk Solution: 1-2 drops 4 x/d for 1 wk • Azithromycin: 2 x/d for 2 d; then 1 drop daily for 5 d • Trimethoprim/polymyxin B: 1 or 2 drops 4 x/d for 1 wk	• Azelastine 0.05%: 1 drop 2 ×/d A52 • Cromolyn sodium 4%: 1-2 drops every 4-6 h A52 • Ketorolac: 1 drop 4 x/d B53,54

- *Herpes Zoster*
  Oral famciclovir 500mg TID x7d or valacyclovir 1g TID x7d
- *Herpes Simplex*
  Topical acyclovir: 1 drop 9 x/d
- Gentamicin Ointment: 4 x/d for 1 wk Solution: 1-2 drops 4 x/d for 1 wk
- *2/2 Neisseria Gonorrhea*
  Ceftriaxone 1g IM
  Lavage of eye
  Azithromycin 250mg PO
- Naphazoline/pheniramine: 1-2 drops up to 4 x/d
- Olopatadine 0.1%: 1 drop 2 x/d

CORNEAL ABRASION

- **General**[243]
  - 3rd leading cause of red-eye behind conjunctivitis and subconjunctival hemorrhage
- **Differential Diagnosis**
  - Acute angle closure glaucoma
  - Conjunctivitis
  - Corneal Ulcer
  - Hyphema (blood in anterior chamber)
  - Dry Eye Syndrome
  - Infective Keratitis (HSV, fungal, bacterial)
  - Uveitis
- **Evaluation**
  - Look for evidence of penetrating trauma, infection, and significant vision loss,
    - Penetrating trauma should be suspected in any patient with extruded ocular contents, or who has a pupil that is dilated, nonreactive, or irregular.
  - In corneal abrasion, the pupil is typically round, and central, and conjunctival injection may be present.
  - The anterior chamber should be inspected for blood (hyphema) or pus (hypopyon).
  - After inspection, visual acuity should be documented.
    - Vision loss of more than 20/40 requires referral.
  - Extraocular movements should be tested and documented
  - Confirm presence of red reflex
- **Urgent Ophthalmology Referral Indications**
  - Penetrating Trauma
  - Corneal opacity
  - Foreign bodies
  - ↓vision >1-2 lines on Snellen
  - Worsening symptoms
- **Management**
  - Topical ABx usually prescribed to prevent superinfection.
  - Topical ABx are used for corneal abrasions caused by contact lens use, foreign bodies, or a history of trauma as there is a higher risk of secondary bacterial keratitis in these cases.
  - Consider providing sunglasses for protection
  - For uncomplicated abrasions, options include erythromycin 0.5% ophthalmic ointment, polymyxin B/trimethoprim (Polytrim) ophthalmic solution, and sulfacetamide 10% ophthalmic ointment or solution
  - Topical antibiotics are generally dosed **four times a day** and **continued until the patient is asymptomatic for 24 hours**.
  - Ointments provide better lubrication than solutions

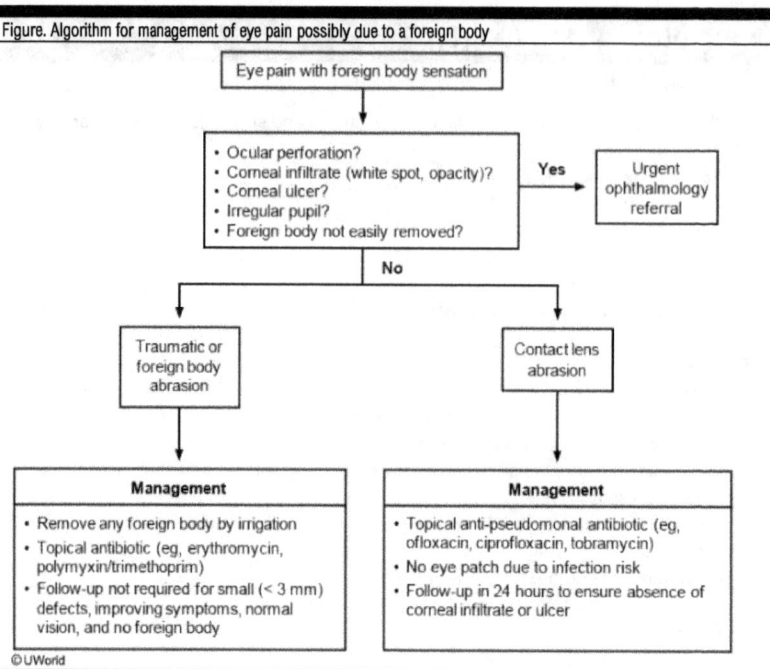

Figure. Algorithm for management of eye pain possibly due to a foreign body

Pharmacologic treatments for corneal abrasions	
Medication	Dosage
Antibiotics	
Erythromycin 0.5% ointment	0.5-inch ribbon, four times per day for three to five days
Polymyxin B/trimethoprim (Polytrim) solution	1 drop, four times per day for three to five days
Anti-Pseudomonal	
Ciprofloxacin 0.3% (Ciloxan) ointment	0.5-inch ribbon, four times per day for three to five days
Ofloxacin 0.3% (Ocuflox) solution	1 to 2 drops, four times per day for three to five days
NSAIDs	
Diclofenac 0.1% (Voltaren)	1 drop, four times per day for two to three days
Corneal Ulcer	
Ciprofloxacin/Ofloxacin	1 drop every 5 minutes for 3 doses; 1 drop every 15 minutes for 6 hours, then 1 drop every 30 minutes
Scopolamine 0.25% (pain)	1 drop BID
Foreign Body	
Proparacaine 0.5%	1 drop for anesthesia for better evaluation and removal

Bibliography

[241] Pflipsen et al. Am Fam Physician. 2016 Jun 15.
[242] Azari et al. "Conjunctivitis A Systematic Review of Diagnosis and Treatment." JAMA. 2013;310(16):1721-1729.
[243] Special Operations Forces Medical Handbook. 1 June 2001.

RADIOLOGY

CXR 360
Abdominal Film 366
Echocardiography 367

RADIOLOGY

CXR

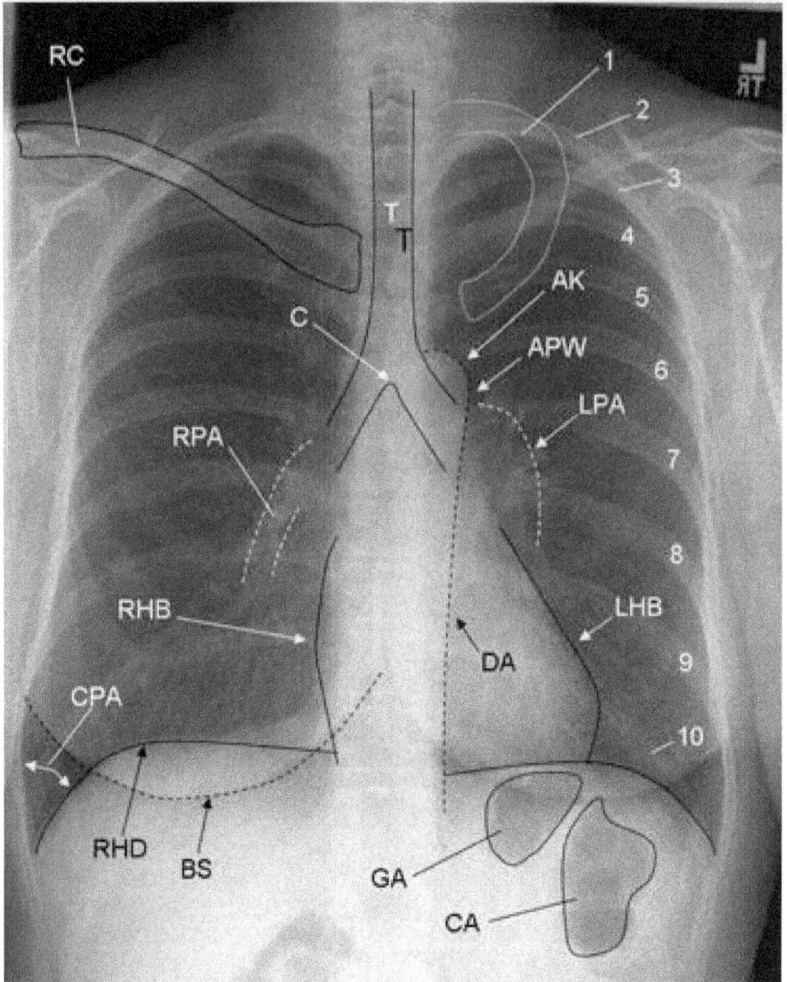

1 = first rib; 2–10 = posterior aspect of ribs 2–10; AK = aortic knob; APW = aortopulmonary window; BS = breast shadow (labeled only on right); C = carina; CA = colonic air; CPA = costophrenic angle; DA = descending aorta; GA = gastric air; LHB = left heart border (*Note:* Most of the left heart border represents the left ventricle; the superior aspect of the left heart border represents the left atrial appendage.); LPA = left pulmonary artery; RC = right clavicle (left clavicle not labeled); RHB = right heart border (*Note:* The right heart border represents the right atrium.); RHD = right hemidiaphragm (left hemidiaphragm not labeled); RPA = right pulmonary artery; T = tracheal air column.

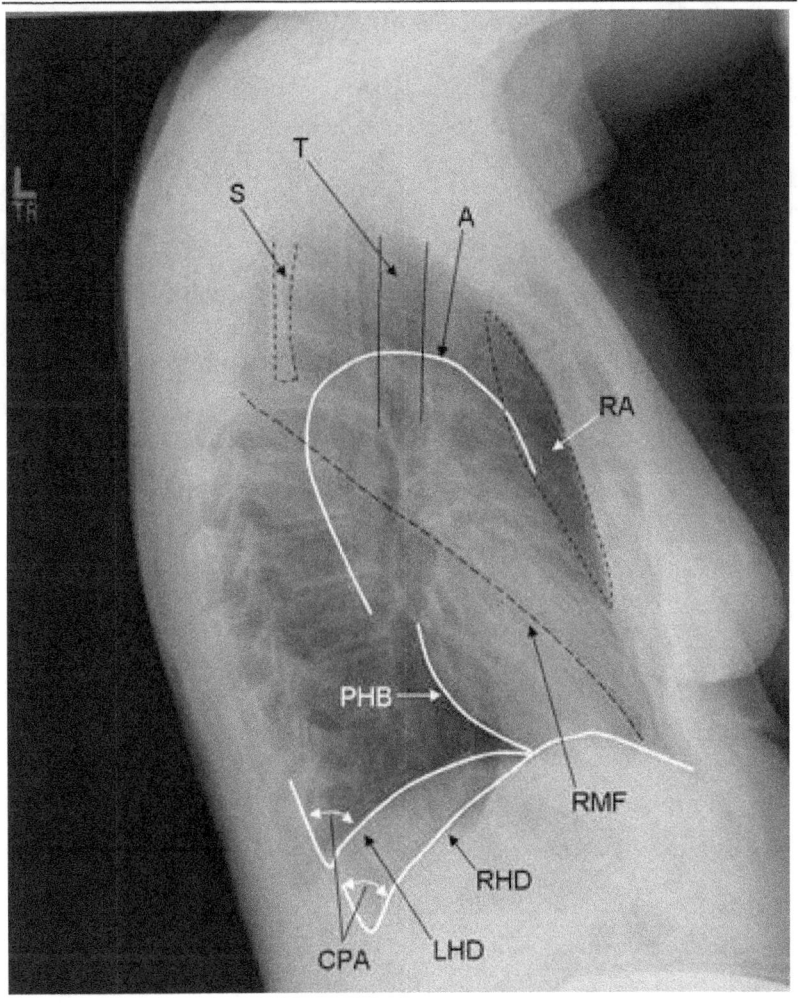

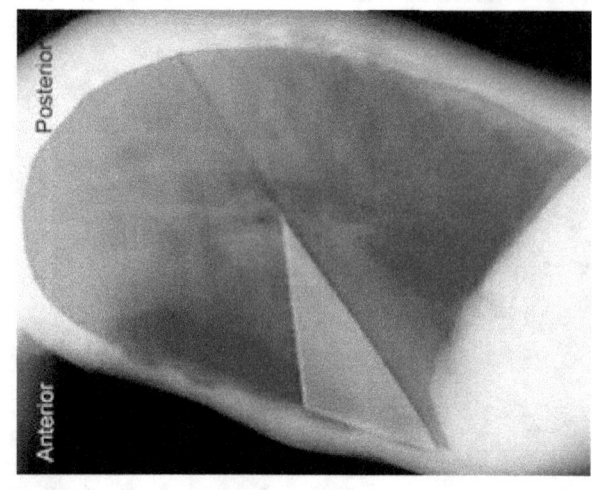

Left Upper Lobe
Major Fissure
Left Lower Lobe

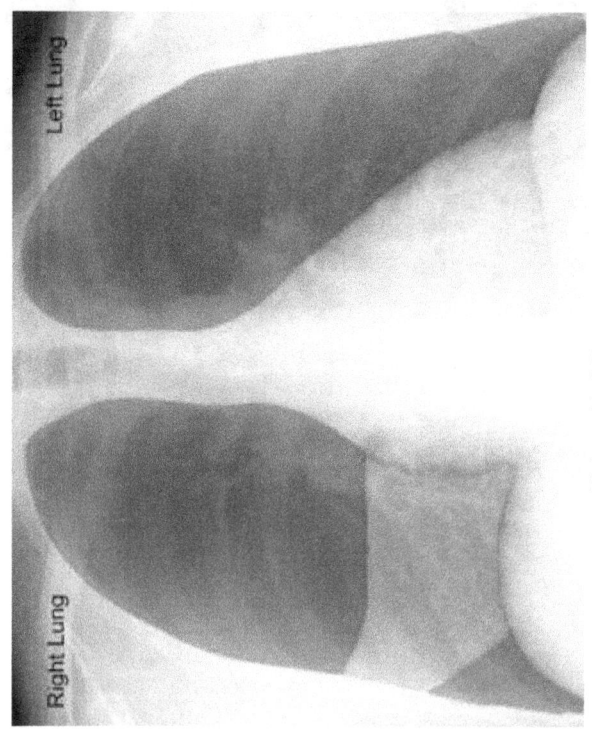

Right and Left Upper Lobes
Right Middle Lobe
Right and Left Lower Lobes

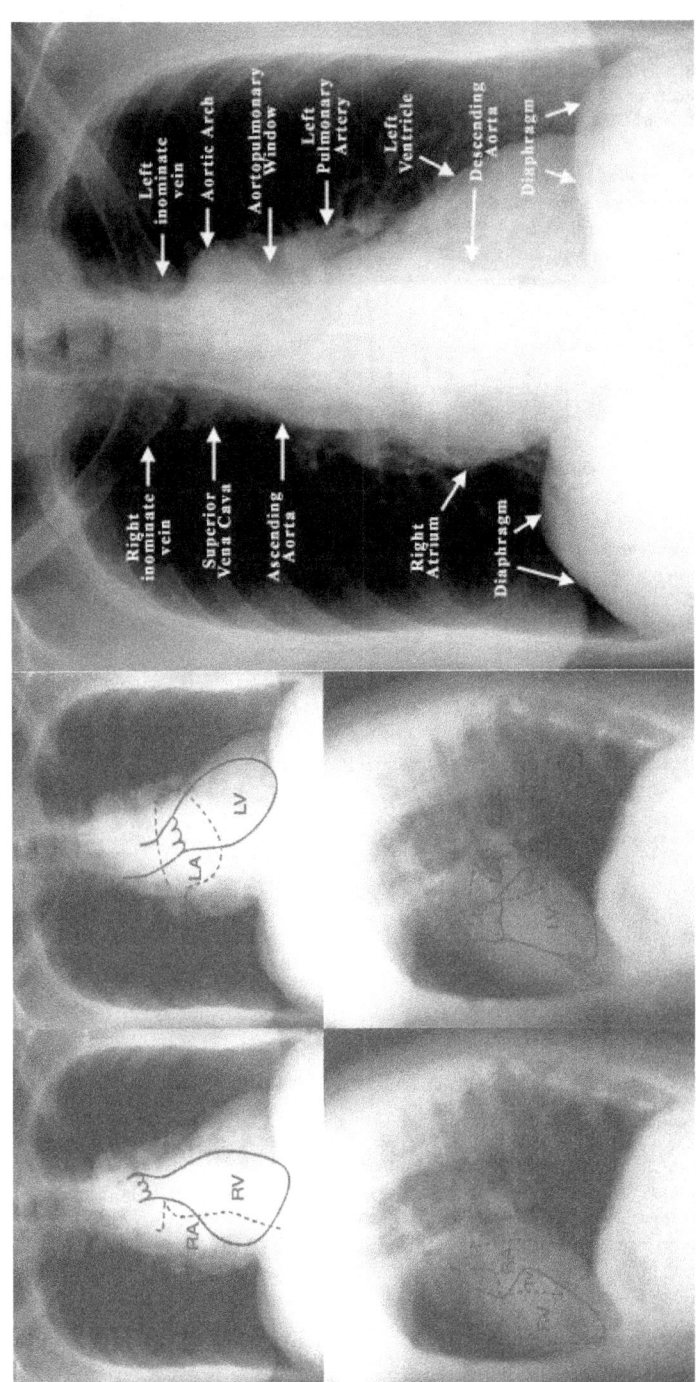

- **How to Read**[244]
  - Determine the Adequacy of the Film
    - Inspiration: Diaphragm below ribs 8–10 posteriorly and 5–6 anteriorly
    - Rotation: Clavicles are equidistant from the spinous processes
    - Penetration: Disc spaces are seen but bony details of spine cannot be seen
  - PA Film
    - Remember, the film is on the patient's chest and the x-rays are passing from back (posterior) to front (anterior).
    - *Soft Tissues*: Check for symmetry, swelling, loss of tissue planes, and subcutaneous air.
    - *Skeletal Structures*: Examine the clavicles, scapulas, vertebrae, sternum, and ribs. Look for symmetry. In a good x-ray, the clavicles are symmetrical. Check for osteolytic or osteoblastic lesions, fractures, or arthritic changes. Look for rib-notching.
    - *Diaphragm*: Sides should be equal and slightly rounded, although the left may be slightly lower. Costophrenic angles should be clear and sharp. Blunting suggests scarring or fluid. It takes about 100–200 mL of pleural fluid to cause blunting. Check below the diaphragm for the gas pattern and free air. A unilateral high diaphragm suggests paralysis (either from nerve damage, trauma, or an abscess), eventration or loss of lung volume on that side because of atelectasis or pneumothorax.
    - *Mediastinum and Heart*: The aortic knob should be visible and distinct. Widening of the mediastinum is seen with traumatic disruption of the thoracic aorta. In children, do not mistake the normally prominent thymus for widening. Mediastinal masses can be associated with Hodgkin's disease and other lymphomas. The trachea should be in a straight line with a sharp carina. Tracheal deviation suggests a mass (tumor), goiter, unilateral loss of lung volume (collapse), or tension pneumothorax. The heart should be less than one-half the width of the chest wall on a PA film. If greater than one-half, think of CHF or pericardial fluid.
      - **Differential Diagnosis of Mediastinal Mass**[245]
        - Anterior
          1. Thymoma
          2. Teratoma
          3. Terrible Lymphoma
          4. Thyroid mass
          5. Tumor
        - Middle
          1. Bronchogenic cyst or tumor
          2. Lymphoma
        - Posterior
          1. Aneurysm
          2. Esophageal diverticula, tumor
          3. Neurogenic tumor
    - *Hilum*: The left hilum should be up to 2–3 cm higher than the right. Vessels are seen here. Look for any masses, nodes, or calcifications.
    - *Lung Fields*: Note the presence of any shadows from CVP lines, NG tubes, pulmonary artery catheters, etc. The fields should be clear with normal lung markings all the way to the periphery.
      - The vessels should taper to become almost invisible at the periphery.
      - Vessels in the lower lung should be larger than those in the upper lung. A reversal of this difference (called cephalization) suggests pulmonary venous hypertension and heart failure.

- **Kerley's B lines**, small linear densities found usually at the lateral base of the lung, are associated with CHF. Check the margins carefully; look for pleural thickening, masses, or pneumothorax.
- If the lungs appear hyperlucent with a relatively small heart and flattening of the diaphragms, COPD is likely.
- Thin *plate-like* linear densities are associated with atelectasis. To locate a lesion, do not forget to check a lateral film and remember the "silhouette sign." Obliteration of all or part of a heart border means the lesion is anterior in the chest and lies in the right middle lobe, lingula, or anterior segment of the upper lobe. A radiopacity that overlaps the heart but does not obliterate the heart border is posterior and lies in the lower lobes.
- Examine carefully for the following:
  - Coin lesions: Causes are granulomas (50% which are usually calcified), (histoplasmosis 25%, TB 20%, coccidioidomycosis 20%, varies with locale); primary carcinoma (25%), hamartoma (<10%), and metastatic disease (<5%).
  - Cavitary lesions: Causes are abscess, cancer, TB, coccidioidomycosis, Wegener's granulomatosis.
  - Infiltrates: Two major types
    1. *Interstitial pattern.* "Reticular." Causes are granulomatous infections, miliary TB, coccidioidomycosis, pneumoconiosis, sarcoidosis, CHF. "Honeycombing" represents end-stage fibrosis caused by sarcoid, RA, and pneumoconiosis.
    2. *Alveolar pattern.* Diffuse, quick progression and regression. Can see either "butterfly" pattern or air bronchograms. Causes are PE, pneumonia, hemorrhage or PE associated with CHF.
- **Regions That Commonly Hide Pathology**
  - Apical
  - Paratracheal
  - Perihilar
  - CPA
  - Retrocardiac
- *Lines/Devices –*
  - ETT - If the patient is intubated, check the position of the endotracheal tube (ETT; should be a minimum of 2 cm above the carina with 3 to 5 cm being ideal). Good rule of thumb is it should be near the medial ends of the clavicles.
  - Central venous catheters - should follow expected venous courses and should generally terminate in the superior vena cava (SVC), near the level of the **carina** (cavo-atrial junction) along the right aspect of the mediastinum. The end of the catheter should travel along the long axis of the superior vena cava (vertically).
  - Nasogastric (NG) and enteric feeding tubes may be partially visualized. Ensure they do not coil in the esophagus or extend outward into the lung due to endobronchial placement.
  - Chest tubes –
    - More common in the ICU environment
    - Should lie between the visceral and parietal pleura with its position on the CXR determining its intent: anterosuperior for drainage of PTX while posteroinferior for pleural effusions.

- Verify function by ensuring all fenestrations in the tube are within the thoracic cavity. The last side-hole in a thoracostomy tube is indicated by a gap in the radiopaque line. If this interruption in the radiopaque line is not within the thoracic cavity or there is evidence of subcutaneous air, then the tube may not have been completely inserted.
    - Pacemakers –
        - *Single chamber* – look for the electrode tip in the right atrial (RA) appendage (if it is atrial paced) or the right ventricular (RV) apex (for ventricular paced).
        - *Dual chamber* – the electrode tips will be both in the RA and RV
        - *Biventricular* – electrode tips will be in the RA, RV, and coronary sinus (to stimulate the LV)
        - *ICD* – electrode tips in the apex of the RV

ABDOMINAL FILM

- **How to Read**[246]
    - Bones – start with the spine, then ribs then finish with the pelvis and upper femurs. Common pathology includes arthritis, fx, and osteolytic/osteoblastic lesions.
    - Lines/Tubes – NG/OG and other enteric tubes. These should terminate in the LUQ with appearance of the proximal port past the GE junction. Enteric tubes should farther, moving past the GE junction into the right abdomen then **crossing midline** to the left to terminate in the jejunum.
    - Soft Tissue – look for masses (fibroids in the uterus), calcifications (GB, pancreas, phleboliths), and free air under the diaphragm.
    - GI Structures
        - *Gastric bubble* (larger size may be suggestive of an obstruction)
        - *Bowel gas pattern* – common to see a small amount of air in the colon but is commonly absent in the SI. Large fecal burden in the colon may be seen in the elderly. If the colon is obstructed, it may distend. If there is loss of the haustral markings (do not completely cross the lumen), this is concerning (r/o toxic megacolon).
            - >6cm in colon is pathologic
            - >3cm in small intestine is pathologic
        - *Air fluid levels* - nonspecific

ECHOCARDIOGRAPHY

General[247248]

- Planes
  - 3 standard planes of cut: axial (transverse), sagittal (longitudinal), and coronal (frontal).
  - For most non-cardiac POCUS imaging, you will point the probe marker toward the patient's head for sagittal and coronal planes of cut, and toward the patient's right for the axial plane of cut.
  - Remember to remain aware of your probe marker's location to ensure orientation in each plane.

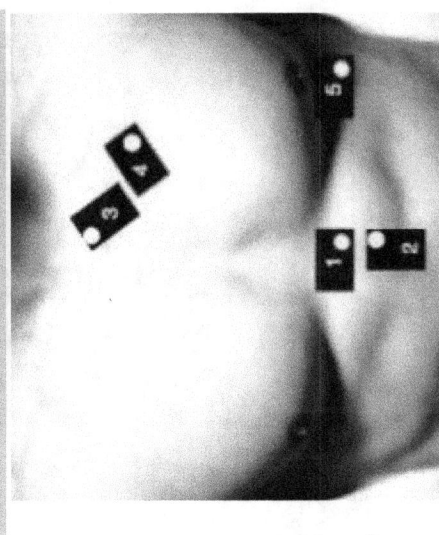

- Views (#'s correspond to image on right showing placement)
  1. Subcostal long axis (SLAX) - marker pointing to patients left
  2. Subcostal inferior vena cava (SIVC) - marker pointing down
  3. Parasternal long axis (PLAX) - marker pointing to right shoulder
  4. Parasternal short axis (PSAX) - marker pointing to left shoulder
  5. Apical 4 chamber (A4CH) - marker pointing directly to left
- Wall Motion - normal, hyperkinetic, akinetic, dyskinetic (bulges outward during systole), hypokinetic
- Volume Status - can be determined with SIVC view; look for IVC collapse of >50% during respiratory cycle. Can also use any chamber view and look for ventricular walls coming together suggestive of an EF>70%
- Hypertrophy - post wall thickness can be observed best on PLAX view and diagnosed with it exceeds 10mm

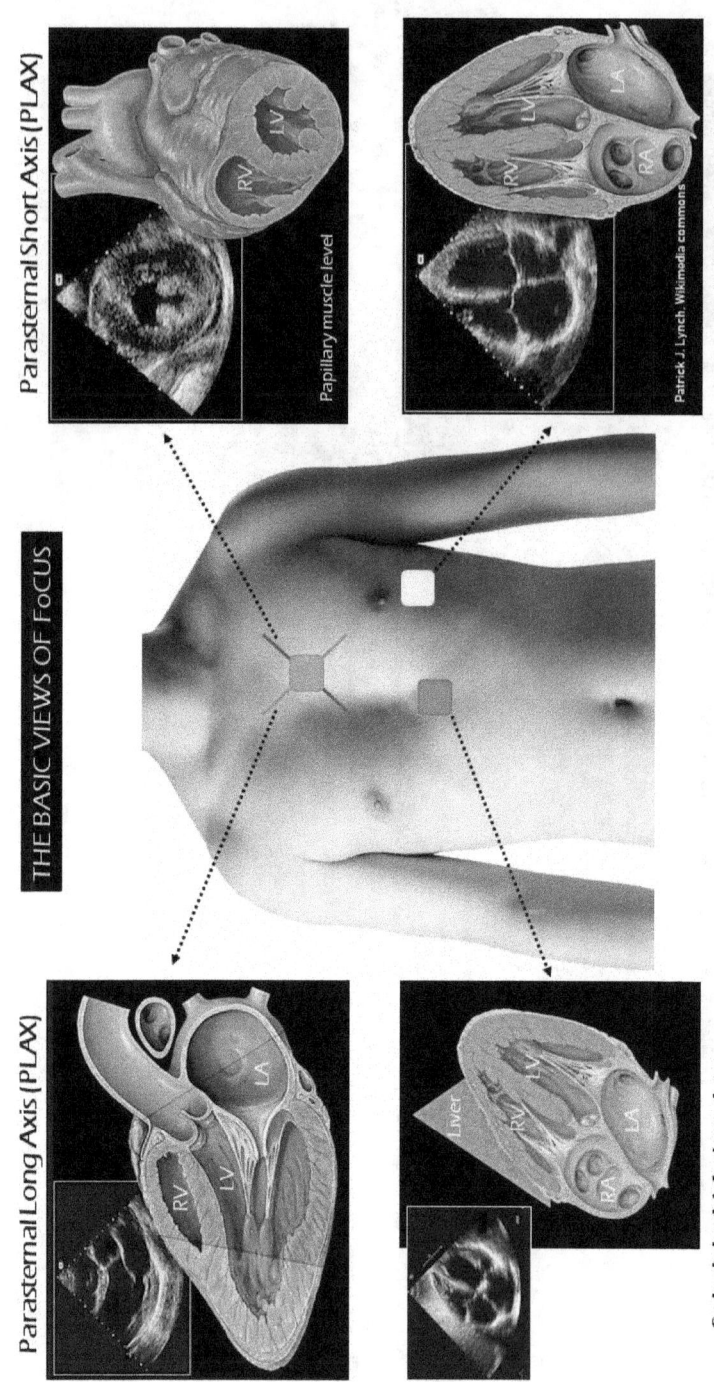

Parasternal Long Axis (PLAX)

- <u>Views</u>: aorta, left ventricle with function, chamber enlargement, left atrium, aortic valve, mitral valve, and pericardium
- <u>Patient position</u>: left lateral or decubitus
- <u>Transducer placement</u>: Direct the probe marker toward the patient's right shoulder, and place the probe in the 4th intercostal space, parasternally. In obese patients, you may need to use the 3rd ICS, and for COPD patients, try the 5th ICS.

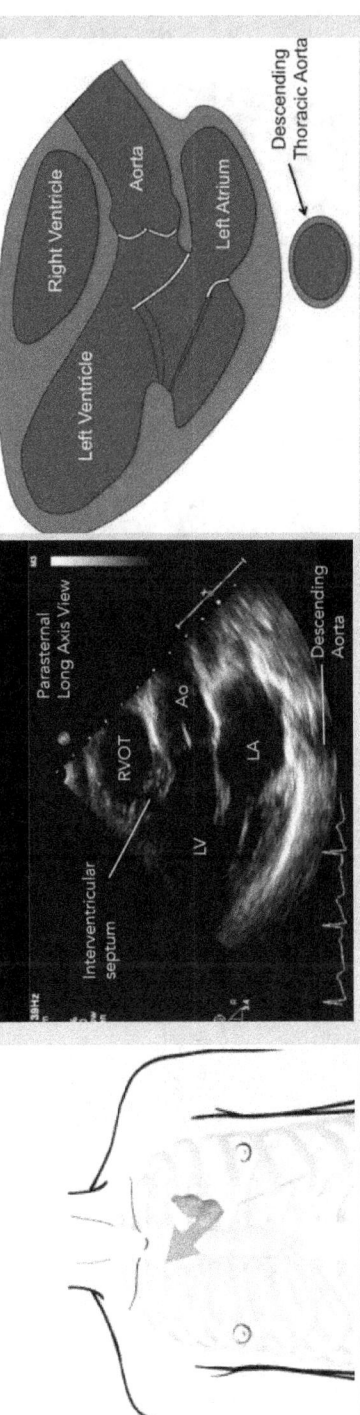

Parasternal Short Axis (PSAX)

- <u>Views</u>: shows cross sections of LV walls at level of AV, MV, and mid ventricle
- <u>Transducer placement</u>: Probe location same as PLAX, but rotated 90 degrees to the left shoulder

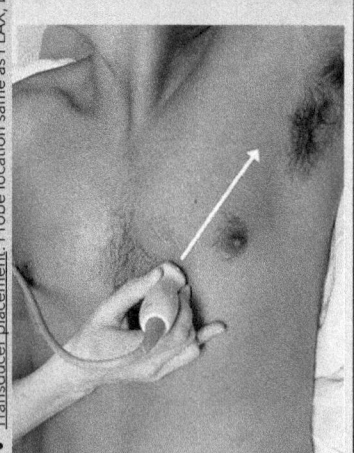
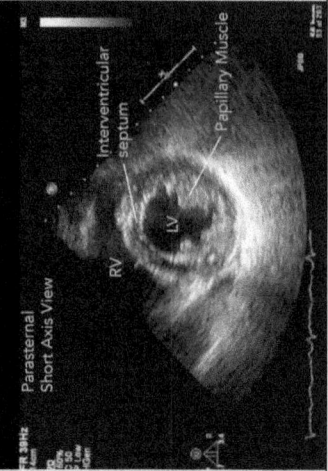
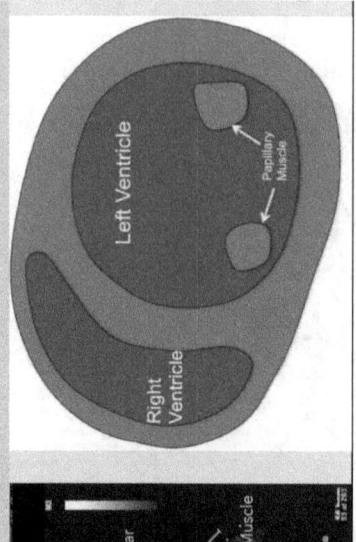

Subxiphoid/Subcostal 4-chamber

- <u>Views</u>: best all-around imaging view for identifying pericardial effusion and overall wall motion. Often bowel gas may obstruct your view, attempt to slide probe more towards the patient's right side, directed at their left shoulder to use the liver as a better acoustic window
- <u>Transducer placement</u>: ace the transducer under the xiphoid, slightly to the right of the sternum. The transducer marker should be to the patients left in the 3:00 position; the imaging plane should be directed upwards and to the left shoulder in slightly clockwise rotation. Ask the patient to inhale while you advance the transducer towards the heart. Inspiration fills the lungs and displaces the diaphragm and the liver caudally. This allows the heart to move closer to the transducer.

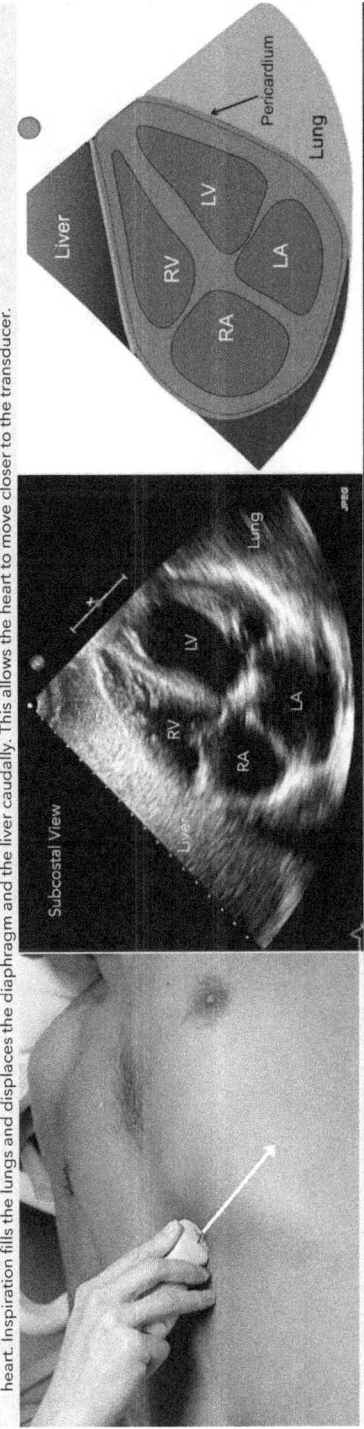
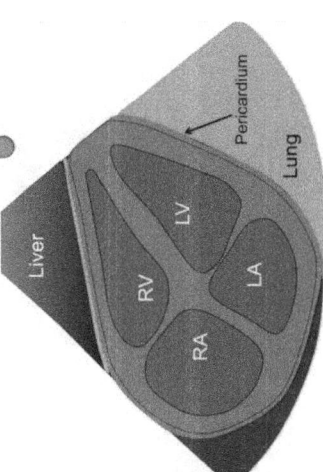

Apical (4 Chamber)

- <u>Views</u>: aorta, left ventricle with function, left atrium, aortic valve, mitral valve, and pericardium
- <u>Patient Position</u>: left lateral decubitus position or supine
- <u>Transducer placement</u>: Indicator toward left axilla. Slide from PSAX toward the point of maximum impulse (PMI) until septum is vertical, then fan until all anatomy is visible.

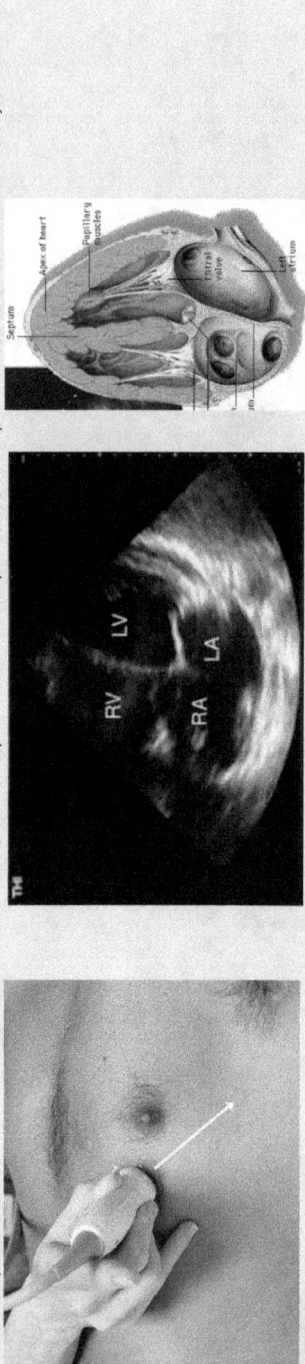

Subcostal Inferior Vena Cava

- <u>Views</u>: IVC, liver, RA, diaphragm. In this view, you can see the IVC draining into the RIGHT atrium. You can glean some information about volume status and right-sided pressures by viewing the IVC in this position.
- <u>Patient Position</u>: supine
- <u>Transducer placement</u>: The easiest way to obtain the subcostal view of the inferior vena cava is to start with a subcostal four-chamber view. Make sure the right atrium is in the center of the image. Then rotate the transducer counterclockwise and direct it to the patient's head. The subcostal view shows the vena cava inferior in a "long axis". The axis of the transducer is parallel to the cranio-caudal axis of the body.

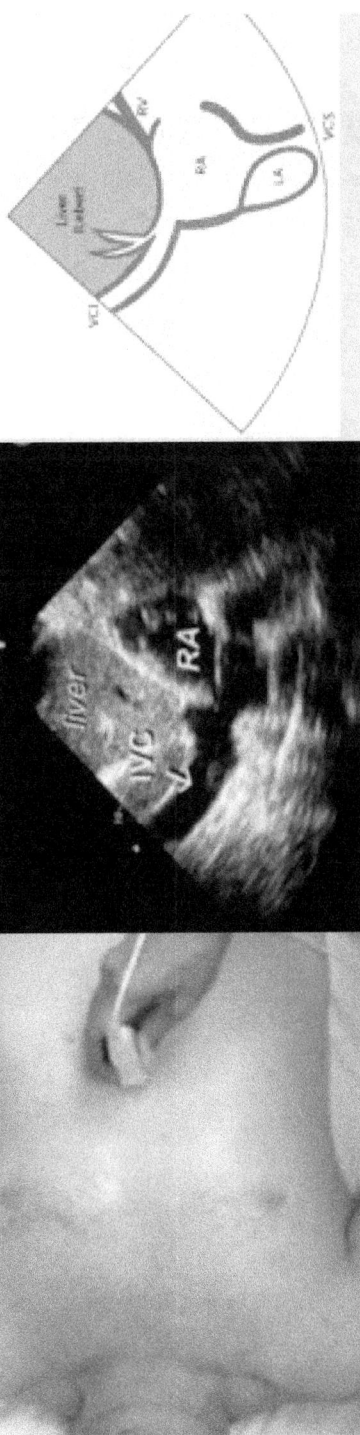

Bibliography

[244] Editorial Board. In: Gomella LG, Haist SA. eds. *Clinician's Pocket Reference: The Scut Monkey, 11e* New York, NY: McGraw-Hill; 2007.

[245] Quizlet Oncology Flashcards <http://quizlet.com/37408090/oncology-flash-cards/>

[246] De Fer et al. "Washington Manual Internship Survival Guide, The." 2013:4.

[247] Moore CL. Chapter 6. Echocardiography. In: Carmody KA, Moore CL, Feller-Kopman D. eds. *Handbook of Critical Care and Emergency Ultrasound* New York, NY: McGraw-Hill; 2011

[248] Cardiac Ultrasound. In: Baston CM, Moore C, Krebs EA, Dean AJ, Panebianco N. eds. Pocket Guide to POCUS: Point-of-Care Tips for Point-of-Care Ultrasound New York, NY: McGraw-Hill.

MUSCULOSKELETAL

Back Examination 376
Knee Examination 378
Knee Effusion 386
Leg/Ankle/Foot Pain Differential 388
Shoulder Examination 391

MUSCULOSKELETAL

BACK EXAMINATION

- **Duration**[249]
    - Acute (6-12 weeks) vs. Chronic (>12 weeks)
- **Types**
    - Nonspecific
    - With radiculopathy
    - 2/2 cause
- **Differential**
    - MSK
        - Herniation (Leg pain>back pain; anterior radiation is likely L1-3, past knee is L4-S1 → positive straight leg raise)
        - Strain (worse with movement, better with rest)
        - Spondylolisthesis (leg pain>back pain but better with flexion of spine, if better with extension consider spondylolysis)
    - Infection
    - Malignancy
    - Fracture
    - Osteoporosis
    - Inflammatory

Etiology of back pain based on exam findings		
Condition	History	Exam
Axial Pain		
SI Joint	Gluteal Pain Off-midline pain below L5 Worse with rising from seated position	Compression - Compression of the iliac crest in the lateral position Distraction - Downward pressure on the anterior superior iliac crest FABER - Flexion abduction external rotation of the thigh and hip Gaenslen - Hyperextension of the leg on the affected side Thigh trust - Adduction of the flexed hip on the affected side Fortin finger - Pain localized 1 fingerbreadth of the posterior iliac crest Gillet - Flexion of the leg toward the chest while standing
Facet Joint	Age>65 Pain worse with standing (load) Pain improves with sitting Paraspinal distribution	
Intervertebral Disk	Age<45 Worse with sitting Midline pain	
Spinal Stenosis	Age>65 Neurogenic claudication Improved with flexion Pain in buttocks/legs	+Romberg Wide-based gait No pain with spinal flexion Thigh pain with >30sec of back extension
Muscle/Ligament	Delayed onset Decreased mobility	Spasms palpable
Radicular Pain		

MUSCULOSKELETAL

Herniated Disk	Known traumatic event Onset 1-2 days after event Sharp/Burning sensation with clear dermatome Improved with sit/laying	Straight leg raising - Patient supine and hip flexed with knee extended Cross straight leg raising - Pain with passive extension of the contralateral Muscle weakness - During ankle dorsiflexion or extension of the great toe Impaired reflexes - Achilles tendon (S1 radiculopathy) Forward flexion - Pain with bending forward in the standing position

- **Examination**
  - Sciatica symptoms
    - Yes
      - Urinary retention, saddle anesthesia, motor weakness, b/l neuro findings
        - Yes → MRI
        - No → ↓activity, NSAIDS, f/u as outpatient
    - No
      - Red Flag Symptoms
        - Age>50
        - Hx of cancer
        - Wt loss
        - Pain >1 month
        - Pain @ HS
        - Not responsive to initial therapy
        - Neurological symptoms
        - Hx of IVDA
        - Recent UTI
      - Yes → Back XR + ESR and if abnormal then MRI
      - No → ↓ activity, NSAIDS, routine f/u and if not improved then do XR with ESR
- **Neurologic Exam**

Disk Herniation						
Nerve Root	Motor deficiency	Sensory deficiency	Reflex	Central	Paracententral	Lateral
L1	None	Inguinal	Cremasteric			
L2	Hip flexion Hip adduction	Proximal anterior/medial thigh	Cremastic			
L3	Hip flexion	Anterior/medial thigh	Patella	Above L2-L3	L2-L3	L3-L4
L4	Knee extension	Anterior leg/medial foot	Patella	Above L3-L4	L3-L4	L4-L5
L5	Dorsiflexion\great toe	Lateral leg/dorsal foot	Medial hamstring	Above L4-L5	L4-L5	L5-S1
S1	Plantar flexion	Posterior leg/lateral foot	Achilles tendon	Above L5-S1	L5-S1	

- **Treatment**
  - Non-Pharmacologic
    - Exercise
    - Pilates
    - Yoga

MUSCULOSKELETAL

- Heat therapy in conjunction with education or NSAIDs is more effective than education or NSAIDs alone at 14 days.
- PT: McKenzie method and spine stabilization
- TENS has not been shown in evidenced based literature to be effective for chronic LBP.
  - Pharmacologic
    - Nonsteroidal anti-inflammatory drugs, acetaminophen, and muscle relaxants are effective treatments for nonspecific acute low back pain.
      - Add the muscle relaxer or opiate for short term based on severity of pain
        - Moderate-quality evidence shows that non-benzodiazepine muscle relaxants (e.g. cyclobenzaprine [Flexeril], tizanidine [Zanaflex], metaxalone [Skelaxin]) are beneficial in the treatment of acute low back pain.
          - Skelaxin is non-sedating, 800mg TID
        - There is moderate-quality evidence that muscle relaxants combined with NSAIDs may have additive benefit for reducing pain.[250]
        - Most pain reduction from these medications occurs in the first 7 to 14 days, but the benefit may continue for up to four weeks.
      - Change NSAID type if repeat visits

KNEE EXAMINATION

- **History**[251]
  - Location
    - Anterior
    - Medial
    - Lateral
    - Posterior
  - Characterization of pain
    - Dull
    - Sharp
    - Achy
  - Mechanism of injury
    - Onset
    - Rapid
    - Insidious
  - Associated sounds heard during injury (i.e. popping associated with ligamentous injury)
  - Swelling immediately after injury
  - Recent infections
- **Historical Data**
  - Injury → suspect ligamentous or meniscal tear
  - Popping sensation → consider ACL tear
  - Swelling → within hours with ACL tear but if it occurs overnight then consider meniscal
  - Locking → meniscal tear
  - Buckling → quad weakness, trapped meniscus, ligamentous instability, patellar dislocation
  - Pain with climbing/descending stairs → PFPS
  - Squatting ↑ pain → meniscus tear
  - Jumping pain → patellar tendonitis
- **PMHx**
  - Gout (monosodium urate)

- o Pseudogout (calcium pyrophosphate)
- o Surgeries
- o RA
- o DJD
- **Differential**
  - o By Anatomy
    - Patellar Tendon
      - □ *Cause:* Commonly injured when patient has foot firmly planted in ground and flexes quadriceps
      - □ *Symptoms:* swelling and tenderness in the anterior portion of the knee; cannot bear weight
      - □ *Examination:* Unable to actively extend knee (d/t quadriceps requirement)
      - □ *Treatment:* orthopedic referral due to risk of quadriceps atrophy with ↓ROM of knee
    - Pes Anserine Bursitis[252]
      - □ *Risk:* m/c in long distance runners, DM
      - □ *Anatomy:* At point where sartorius, gracilis, and semitendinosus tendons meet
      - □ *Cause:* trauma
      - □ *Diagnosis: Purely clinical with on imaging required*
        - Pain at medial joint line anterior aspect, approximately 5cm distal to the medial joint line
        - Pain when going up stairs or downstairs
        - Sensitivity to palpation
        - Sometimes local swelling
      - □ *Treatment:* rest, cryotherapy, NSAIDS
    - ACL
      - □ *Cause:* direct trauma to anterior portion of knee
      - □ *Symptoms:* popping sensation, inability to ambulate directly after, ↑pain and laxity upon performance of the anterior drawer test or Lachman maneuver
      - □ *Examination:* Anterior drawer test with ≥1cm laxity in comparison to other knee
    - PCL
      - □ *Cause:* posterior directed force on flexed knee (dashboard being struck; hyperextension)
      - □ *Symptoms:* not associated with much pain or effect on ROM
      - □ *Examination:* posterior drawer test is positive
    - MCL/LCL
      - □ *Cause:* dramatic varus or valgus stress; uncommon
      - □ *Symptoms:* local tenderness
      - □ *Examination:* local tenderness over joint lines, abnormal valgus and varus stress testing
    - Meniscus
      - □ *Cause:* sudden twisting movement of knee when knee is firmly planted in ground
      - □ *Symptoms:* locking sensation to knee
      - □ *Examination:* McMurray's test (place one hand over the anterior aspect of the knee, with fingers and thumb on the medial and lateral joint lines. Grasp the patient's heel with the other hand and externally rotate the tibia, using the first hand to apply valgus force at the knee during passive flexion and extension. The maneuver is repeated when applying internal rotation and varus stress to test the lateral meniscus) shows popping sensation with audible click/pop during extension
      - □ *Treatment:* Active rehabilitation is as effective as arthroscopy for improving pain and function in patients with nontraumatic medial meniscal tears and is as

good as meniscectomy for improving physical function in patients with meniscal tears and osteoarthritis
- Prepatellar Bursitis
  - Inflammation of the bursa sac d/t direct pressure to the patella
  - Trauma directly to knee or a fall or continuous kneeling
- Patellofemoral Syndrome
  - M/c in W>M age <45
  - Sx: worsened with climbing stairs, extended sitting
  - DDx: patellofemoral compression test (medial and lateral pressure onto the patella with knee in extension → pain)
- Osteoarthritis[253]
  - *Treatment*
    - PT and exercise are the foundation of therapy
    - If locking or catching sensation → likely meniscal tear requiring ortho referral
    - If BMI> 25 then lose weight through monitored exercise program
    - Otherwise, treat with Tylenol (1300mg TID) +/- NSAIDs with addition of Tramadol/Injections/Brace if ineffective. If continued pain, can consider opiates or ortho referral.
  - By Mechanism Of Injury
    - Varus stress → LCL damage
    - Valgus stress → MCL damage
    - Deceleration with twisting/pivoting motion → ACL
    - Twisting while pivoting on knee → Meniscal tear
- **Exam**
  - Duck walk – to perform successfully, must have intact ligament system, no meniscal damage, no OA
  - Standing – look for resting deformities
- **Imaging (to r/o fracture)**
  Ottawa Knee Rules
  1) Age>55
  2) Tenderness @ head of fibula
  3) Isolated patellar tenderness
  4) Cannot flex > 90 degrees
  5) Cannot bear weight and/or complete 4 steps
  if suspect osteoarthritis then obtain weight bearing films

Figure. Superficial landmarks on knee examination

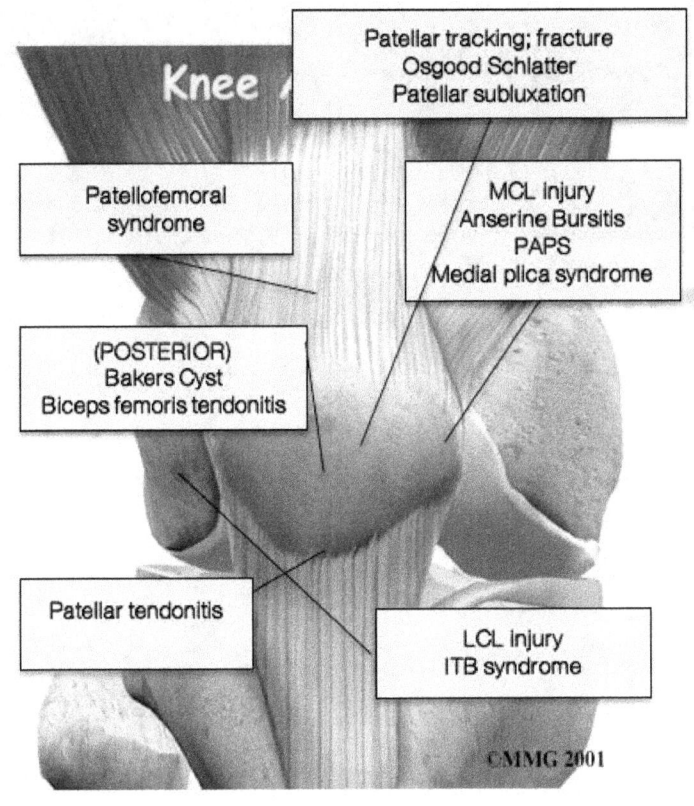

Evaluation of knee pain based on location of pain

Location	Pathology	Mechanism	Symptoms	Evaluation	Treatment
Joint Lines	Meniscal Tear	Sudden twisting or pivoting	"Locking" Slow onset effusion or recurrent Pain with squatting	• Tenderness of the joint line • McMurray's test (place one hand over the anterior aspect of the knee, with fingers and thumb on the medial and lateral joint lines. Grasp the patient's heel with the other hand and externally rotate the tibia, using the first hand to apply valgus force at the knee during passive flexion and extension. The maneuver is repeated when applying internal rotation and varus stress to test the lateral meniscus) shows popping sensation with audible click/pop during extension	• RICE • PT to strengthen the muscular support of the knee • Consider evaluation by Orthopedic Surgery (↑ likelihood in severe twisting injuries, concurrent ACL tear, knee locking, pain w/ McMurray, no improvement with 3-6 weeks of PT)
N/A	Ligament Tear	PAL: dashboard; hyperextension LAL: medial force MAL: lateral force AAL: twisting while planted foot; quick start and stop; hyperextension	"Popping" "Giving way" Immediate swelling <2hrs Cannot walk immed. after	ACL ▫ Anterior drawer test with ≥1cm laxity in comparison to other knee ▫ Lachman's test - The test is performed with the patient in a supine position and the injured knee flexed to 30 degrees. The physician stabilizes the distal femur with one hand, grasps the proximal tibia in the other hand, and then attempts to sublux the tibia anteriorly • PCL ▫ Posterior drawer test is positive • MCL/LCL ▫ Local tenderness over joint lines, abnormal valgus and varus stress testing	• RICE • PT • Surgical evaluation

Evaluation of knee pain based on location of pain

Location	Pathology	Mechanism	Symptoms	Evaluation	Treatment
Anterior	Patellofemoral (PFPS)	Overuse Training Errors Recent alteration in training program History of knee trauma or surgery	Pain with walking up and down stairs Squatting Kneeling "Giving way" Gradual onset anterior knee pain Theatre sign (prolonged knee flexion) Pain under/behind or around patella	Positive Patellar Grind Test - Accomplished by pressing the patella away from the femoral condyles while asking the patient to contrast the quadriceps muscles. A positive test is represented by sudden patellar pain and relaxation of the muscle. The opposite test involves lifting the patella away from the knee joint while passively bending and straightening the knee. If this relieves pain, the patellofemoral joint is likely the source. Other Tests – Pain with squatting, patellar tilt pain Patients often have more pain with rest and complain of giving-way sensation	Often caused by weak quadriceps, hip strengthening, hip flexors, and IT band 3x/week for 8 weeks PT, bracing (limited evidence to support the use of the lateral patellar buttress brace), patellar taping, normal gait biomechanics
Anterior Superior	Patellar Tendonitis (Jumper's Knee)	Jumping Uphill running Squatting Stand from sitting	Anterior knee pain that is tender on exam	Focal pain to the inferior pole of the patella and proximal tendon. Pain with single-leg decline squat is characteristic.	Rest NSAIDs NO STEROIDS! Surgery if not improved after 3 months
Medial	Medial Plica Syndrome	Genetic Overuse	Anterior knee pain Snapping sensation as the plica moves over the femoral condyle	Palpable band parallel to the medial border of the patella	MRI for diagnosis PT

Evaluation of knee pain based on location of pain

Location	Pathology	Mechanism	Symptoms	Evaluation	Treatment
	Pes Anserine Bursitis	Tendinous insertion of the Sartorius, Gracilis, and Semitendinosus get inflamed	Pain on medial knee Increased pain w/ flexion and extension	Tenderness to medial aspect of knee posterior and distal to the joint line No effusion Reproduced pain with valgus move	- Rest - Consider steroid injection
Lateral	IT Band Syndrome	Distance runners Analysts	Pain reproduced after reaching certain mileage	Noble compression test - The examiner applies pressure along the palpable iliotibial band approximately 2 cm proximal to the lateral femoral epicondyle while passively flexing the knee from 0 to 60 degrees. A positive result is pain at 30 degrees of flexion. Noble test - With the patient in a supine position, the physician places a thumb over the lateral femoral epicondyle as the patient repeatedly flexes and extends the knee. Pain symptoms are usually most prominent with the knee at 30 degrees of flexion.	Rest Decrease distance Changing shoes Stretching+NSAID combo Steroid injections
	Popliteus Tendinitis	Excessive use of quadriceps	Posterior lateral aspect of the knee Downhill running	Webb test - internally rotate the leg in the supine patient, the knee is flexed at 90 degrees, with the patient then forcing external rotation while the examiner provides resistance. A positive test produces pain with the maneuver.	Test NSAIDs

Knee Tests

Anterior Drawer	McMurray

Posterior Drawer	

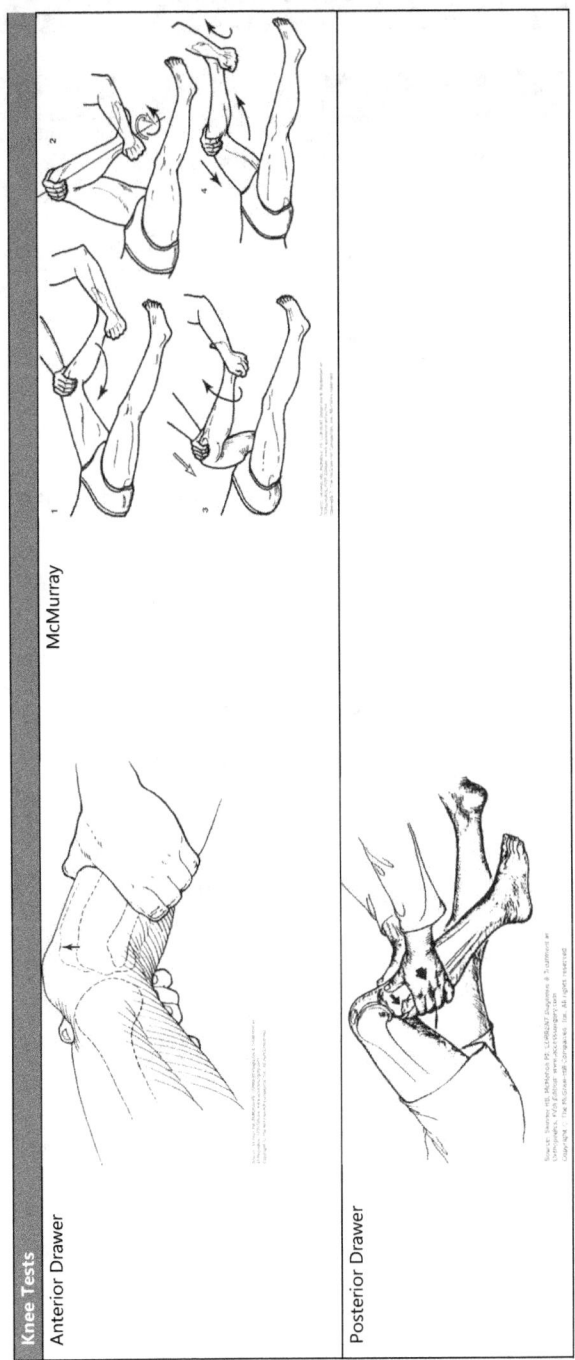

KNEE EFFUSION

Etiologies[254,255]

Hemorrhagic	Inflammatory	Infectious	Non-Inflammatory
Traumatic (ligament injury, meniscal injury, articular injury)	RA	Gonorrhea (younger patients)	OA
	Gout	Lyme	Cancer
Anticoagulants	Septic arthritis	TB	
Hemophilia	Reactive arthritis		

- **History and Physical**
  - Recent trauma → fracture (look for ecchymosis, deformity, acute swelling)
  - Knee 'gives way', unstable, or pivot movement → AAL tear (positive drawer sign, acute swelling <4 hrs. after incident)
  - Cannot squat, clicking/locking → Meniscal tear (joint line tenderness, +Apley's, +McMurray, acute swelling <4 hrs. after incident)
  - Repetitive causational movement → overuse syndrome
  - Recent sex, no trauma, fevers, chills→ Infectious (look for erythema, swelling, +joint aspiration)
  - History of prosthetic joint carries unique criteria for infection
    - C-RP>1, ESR>30, fluid WBC >3000, alpha-defensin >1
  - Night pain, fevers, weight loss → tumor (+imaging, joint aspiration)
- **Imaging**
  - Most common: AP, lateral, axial patellar. Get lateral @ 15-30 degrees flexion if effusion suspected
  - MRI not necessary to diagnose AAL/PAL tear, simple AP enough with PE
  - Ottawa Rules
    1) Inability to bear weight after incident or in ER (no more than 4 steps)
    2) Age 55+
    3) Isolated tenderness to the patella or head of fibula
    4) Cannot flex more than 90 degrees

Joint Fluid Analysis

Findings	Normal	Noninflammatory	Inflammatory	Septic	Hemorrhagic
Color	Clear	Yellow	Yellow to green	Yellow	Red
Clarity	Transparent	Transparent	Opaque	Opaque	Bloody
Viscosity	High	High	Low	Variable	Variable
WBC per mm^3	< 200	200 to 2,000	2,000 to 50,000	50,000 to 200,000 (>3k if prosthetic joint)	200-2500
PMNs	< 25%	< 25%	> 50%	> 75%	50-75%
Mucin clot	Good	Good	Good to poor	Poor	Unk
Protein g/dL	N/A	1-3	3-5	3-5	4-6
Glucose mg/dL	N/A	=blood	<blood	<<blood	=blood

Figure. Evaluation of the swollen knee

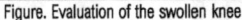

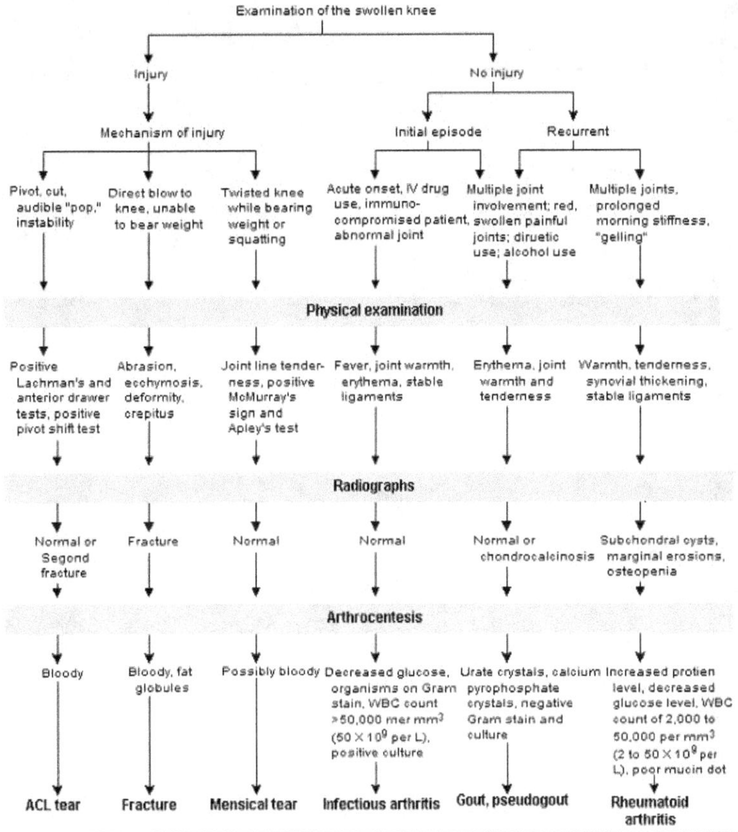

LEG/ANKLE/FOOT PAIN DIFFERENTIAL

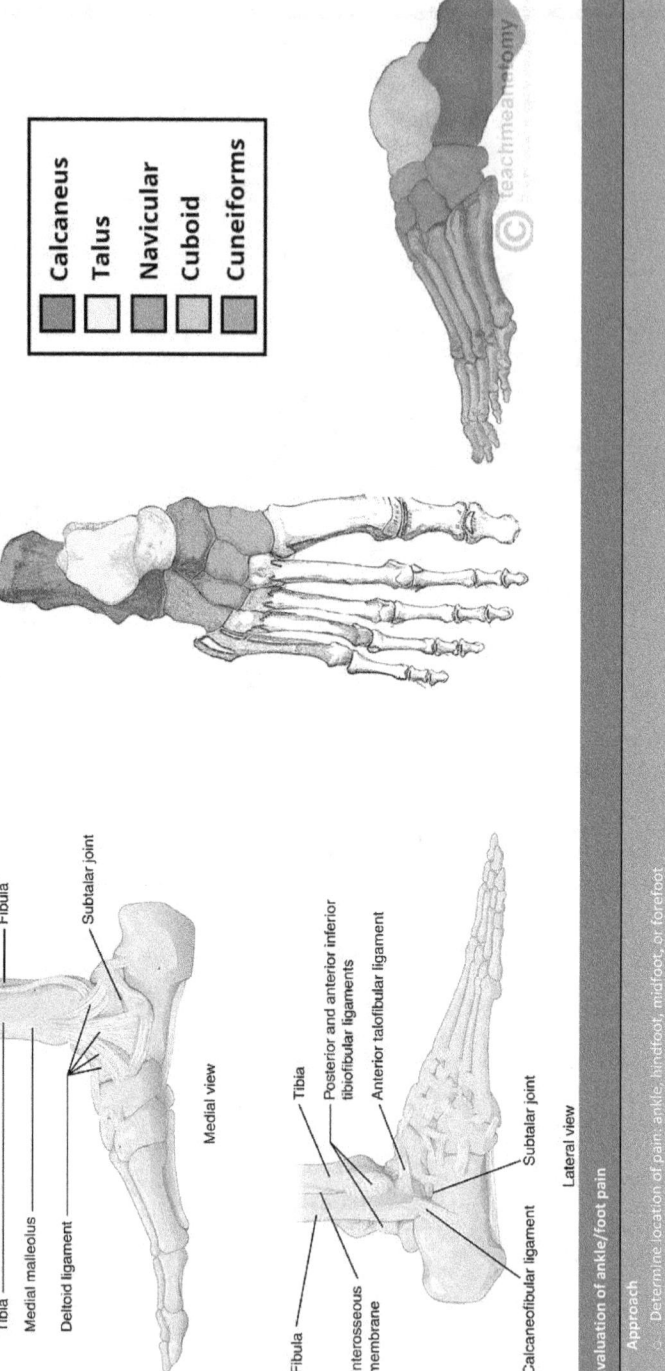

Evaluation of ankle/foot pain

- **Approach**
  - Determine location of pain: ankle, hindfoot, midfoot, or forefoot

- Ankle pain: red flags include deformity, neurovascular compromise, and concurrent nonankle injuries (distraction). Lateral pain: think peroneal tendinopathy (pain w/ eversion), ATFL, posterior tibial tendon dysfunction (pain w/ inversion). Imaging based on Ottawa ankle rules. Grading of sprain determined by following tests: anterior drawer, talar tilt, and syndesmosis evaluation.
- Heel pain: ddx includes Achilles tendonitis (pain w/ single calf raise; pain @ insertion site), heel bursitis, Achilles rupture (popping sensation → painful ambulation; immediate surgical referral required), calcaneal stress fx, Haglund's deformity (look for bump/prominence @ insertion of Achilles), plantar fasciitis (pain w/ 1st step in morning, +windlass test), tarsal tunnel syndrome
- Midfoot pain: ddx includes metatarsal stress fx (look for pain @ 5th metatarsal especially), navicular stress fx (!risk w/ jumping, sprinting, changing direction; pain @ "N" spot), Lisfranc (fleck sign on XR, surgery req'd)
- Forefoot pain: ball of foot pain; ddx includes Morton's neuroma, capsulitis, bursitis, Freiburg's disease, bunion

Location	Pathology	Mechanism	Symptoms	Evaluation	Treatment
Ankle	Achilles Tendinopathy	Overuse	Posterior heel pain	Pain/swelling/tenderness at 2-6cm above insertion into the calcaneus	Eccentric heel-lowering exercises performed with toes on a step so that the heel can be lowered below the toes
					Shock wave therapy has limited evidence of benefit, with improvement in patients with insertional tendinopathy but not for those with the more common midportion tendinopathy.
					Injections and surgical techniques have insufficient evidence of benefit.16,41
Foot	Plantar Fasciopathy (Plantar Fasciitis)		Pain typically located at the medial calcaneal tubercle and is worse with early morning ambulation,	Tenderness over the medial calcaneal tubercle that extends along the plantar fascia, often with crepitus, thickness, or swelling	Passive stretching of the plantar fascia (e.g., pulling back toes with a hand or towel and active strength training (e.g., heel raises) are recommended.
				Plantar fascia thickness of more than 4 mm on ultrasonography or plain radiography can support the diagnosis	

Leg Pain Differential

Location	Pathology	Mechanism	Symptoms	Evaluation	Treatment
Tibia	Medial Tibial Stress Syndrome (Shin Splints)	Overuse	Presents with pain over the middle or distal one-third of the posteromedial tibial border	and improves with activity. The Windlass test, in which the toes are passively extended, can elicit pain by stretching the fascia	A meta-analysis showed that foot orthoses with arch support led to improvement in pain and function after 11 weeks. Local steroid injections reduce pain at one month but not afterward.
Tibia	Tibial Stress Fracture	Rapid increases in activity	Present with pain and tenderness on palpation, most commonly in the middle to distal 1/3 of the anterior tibia	The most sensitive physical examination finding is tenderness to palpation over the posteromedial tibial border. XR is useful if a tibial stress fracture is suspected. MRI is more sensitive and specific than bone scans for dx. Patients with significant pain or difficulty walking should undergo MRI.	Treatment is conservative. Relative rest and calf stretching are recommended because evidence links tightness in the soleus and posterior tibialis to medial tibial stress syndrome. Temporary (6 to 8 weeks) vacation from running, with continued weight bearing unless walking is painful. Return to activity should be slow and dependent on pain levels. Surgery may be considered for failure of union.

SHOULDER EXAMINATION

- **History**[256,257]
  - Scapular winging, trauma, recent viral illness → Serratus anterior or trapezius dysfunction
  - Seizure and inability to passively or actively rotate affected arm externally → Posterior shoulder dislocation
  - Supraspinatus/infraspinatus wasting → Rotator cuff tear; suprascapular nerve entrapment
  - Pain radiating below elbow; decreased cervical range of motion → Cervical disc disease
  - Shoulder pain in throwing athletes; anterior glenohumeral joint pain and impingement → Glenohumeral joint instability
  - Duration (acute<6 weeks; subacute 6-12 weeks; chronic >3 months)
  - Pain or "clunking" sound with overhead motion → Labral disorder
  - Nighttime shoulder pain → tear
- **Examination**

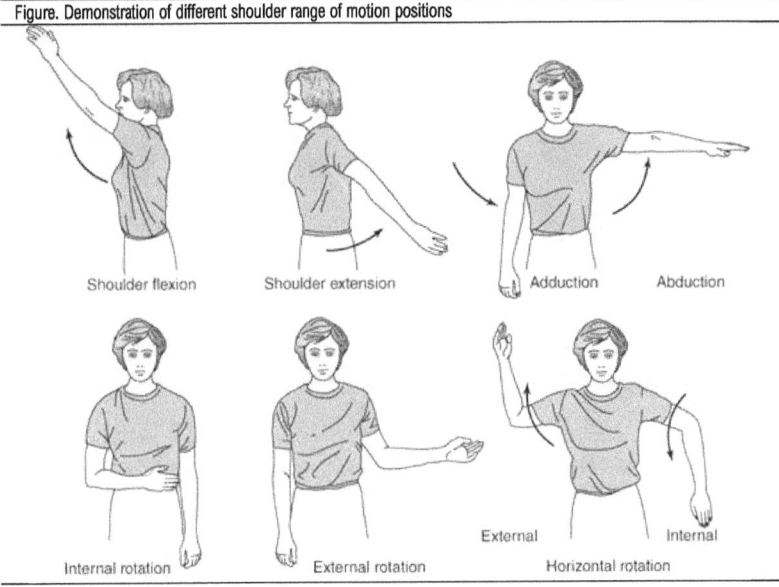

Figure. Demonstration of different shoulder range of motion positions

MUSCULOSKELETAL

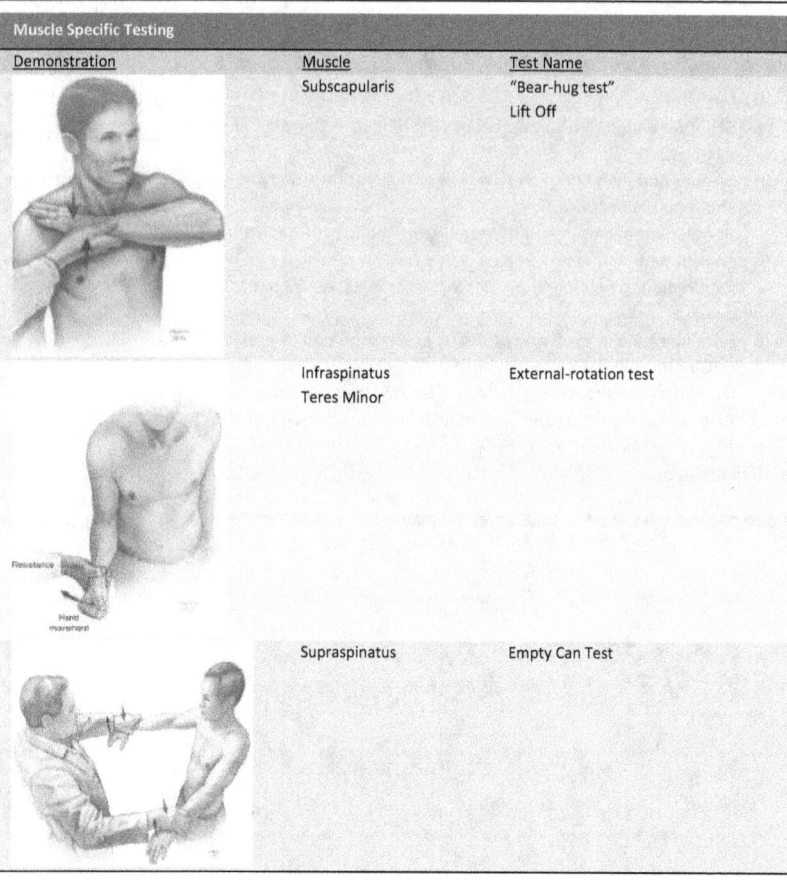

Muscle Specific Testing		
Demonstration	Muscle	Test Name
	Subscapularis	"Bear-hug test" Lift Off
	Infraspinatus Teres Minor	External-rotation test
	Supraspinatus	Empty Can Test

- **Common Diagnoses**
  - Impingement
  Lateral pain, subacute, worse with movement overhead. Neer and Hawkins are best.
    - *Subacromial Bursitis* - Pain occurs during arm elevation **beyond 90°** (impingement position) and is frequently referred down the upper arm (deltoid region) to the mid-humerus.
    - *Supraspinatus/rotator cuff tendonitis* - Pain occurs especially during active or resisted **abduction** and frequently radiates down the upper arm (deltoid region) to the mid-humerus.
  - Biceps tendonitis - Pain during forward flexion and forearm supination is usually felt anteriorly in the region of the bicipital groove.
  - Rotator Cuff Tear – sudden onset, drop arm positive, pain at night, weakness
  - Adhesive Capsulitis / Frozen Shoulder – distant injury with minimal ROM, inability to reach over head
  - GH arthritis
  - AC joint arthritis

- **Diagnosis (see next page)**

Imaging modalities for shoulder pain		
Imaging modality	Advantages	Disadvantages
MRI	95% sensitivity and specificity in detecting complete rotator cuff tears, cuff degeneration, chronic tendonitis and partial cuff tears No ionizing radiation	Often identifies an apparent "abnormality" in an asymptomatic patient
Arthrography	Good at identifying complete rotator cuff tear or adhesive capsulitis (frozen shoulder)	Invasive Relatively poor at diagnosing a partial rotator cuff tear
Ultrasonography	Accurately diagnoses complete rotator cuff tears	Less useful in identifying partial cuff tears Operator-dependent interpretation
MRI arthrography	Reliably identifies full-thickness rotator cuff tears and labral tears	Invasive
CT scanning	May be useful in diagnosis of subtle dislocation	Ionizing radiation

- **Treatment**
  - Impingement/RCD – ice/heat, analgesics, HEP, if no improvement after 3 months then referral to orthopedics
  - Tear – consider surgical referral

Systematic evaluation of the shoulder

Order	Test	Description
1	Appearance	Symmetry, bulk, deformities, atrophy above or below the scapular spine. Atrophy in the space below the scapular spine suggests RCD or injury to the suprascapular nerve.
2	Palpation	Sternoclavicular joint, clavicle, acromioclavicular joint, lateral acromion, biceps tendon in the groove between the greater and lesser tubercle of the humerus. Remember: some patients can be tender at many points, but you are trying to recreate the pain that they have been experiencing at home. The anterior joint line can be palpated.

3	ROM	ROM testing identifies limitations in ROM and localizes pain. Start with these basic ROM tests with the patient standing. Test active ROM first and add passive ROM if the patient has pain or limited motion. All maneuvers start from the anatomic position with arms at the side and palms facing forward.
		• Flexion – 160-180 degrees
		• Extension – 40-60 degrees
		• Abduction – raise arm from side to overhead; normal is 180 degrees.
		   - 0-90 is determined by supraspinatus and deltoid.
		   - After 90 degrees, trapezius and serratus anterior
		   - **Painful arc** is 60-120 and is indicative of subacromial impingement
		   - 120-180 is due to AC joint pathology
		• Adduction – 45 degrees
		• External Rotation – hold arms in front of body with elbow bent 90 degrees and palms facing in moving away from center. Normal is 55-80 degrees. Pain here localizes to teres minor and infraspinatus.
		• Internal Rotation – hold arms in front of body with elbow bent 90 degrees and palms facing in and move towards center. Normal ROM is 45 degrees. Pain here localizes to the subscapularis.

| 4 | Impingement/RCD | 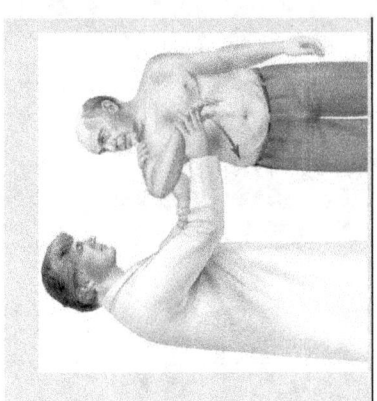 • Hawkins-Kennedy - Patient holds arm at 90 flexion with elbow at 90 flexion. Place downward pressure on the forearm and passively internally rotate the arm.

Positive test: Tear
Muscle: supraspinatus/teres minor/infraspinatus
Movement – internal rotation |

- **Neer's** - The patient internally rotates their hand (thumb toward the ground). Place your hand on the back of the patient's shoulder to stabilize the scapula. Forward flex the patient's straight arm by grasping just below the elbow and lifting.

  Muscle: No specific group
  Movement: Flexion
  Positive test: Impingement subacromial structures to humeral head

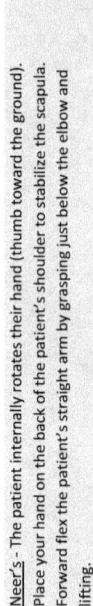

- **Empty Can** - Patient starts with a straight arm at 90 abduction. The arm is then brought forward 30 toward center on the horizontal plane and the thumb rotated toward the floor. Apply gentle pressure downward above the elbow while patient attempts to resist this pressure. Pain suggests impingement of the **supraspinatus**. Weakness suggests a partial- or full-thickness tear.

  Muscle: Supraspinatus
  Movement: adduction
  Positive test: Tear

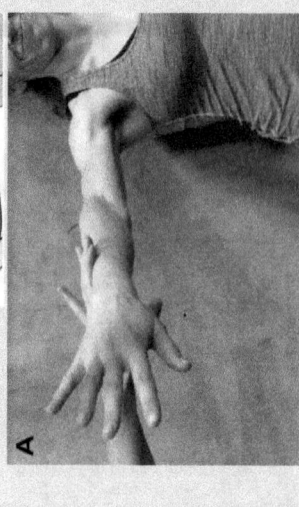

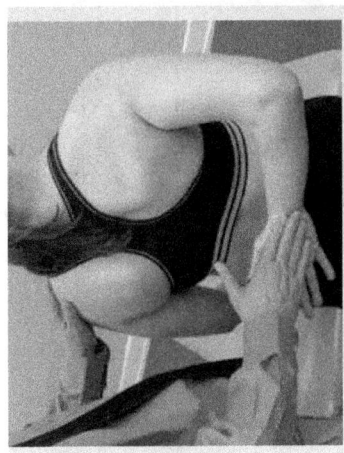 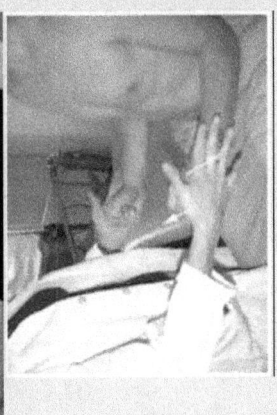

- **Lift Off** - Patient internally rotates shoulder. Place the back of their hand against the small of the back. Internal rotation against resistance. Examiner resists patient's attempt to force their hand away from their back. Weakness suggests a subscapularis muscle tear or impingement

  Muscle: Subscapularis
  Movement: Internal rotation
  Positive test: Impingement

- **External Push Off** - Placing the patient's arm at the side in neutral rotation and with the elbow flexed. Support the elbow and instruct the patient to maintain this position while you apply moderate to firm pressure at the distal forearm, attempting to internally rotate the arm.

  Positive test: Impingement
  Muscle: Infraspinatus + Teres minor

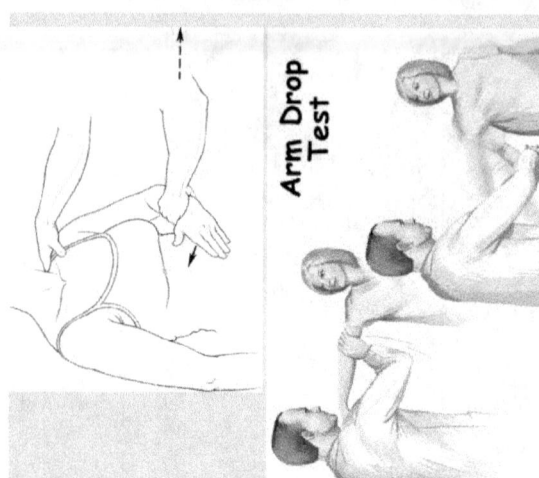

- <u>Belly Press</u> - A positive "belly-press" test is the inability to hold the elbow in front of the trunk while pressing down with the hand on the belly. A positive belly press test indicates subscapularis tendon insufficiency.

  Muscle: Subscapularis
  Movement: Internal rotation
  Positive test: Impingement

- <u>Drop Arm</u> - Passively abduct shoulder to 160 degrees. Once at the position, the patient will now attempt to slowly bring arm back to their side by adducting. If the arm suddenly drops, or gives way with a tap, consider rotator cuff tear

  Positive test: Tear

5	Other tests if not suspecting impingement or RCD	*Concern for biceps pathology* • <u>Speed's</u> - Forward flex arm to 50 degrees. Keep palm up. Elbow should be slightly flexed at 15 degrees. Provide resistance against patient trying to keep shoulder up (examiner pushes down). Pain suggestive of biceps tendonitis • <u>Yergason's</u> - The patient flexes their elbow to 90. Provide resistance to supination. A positive test is pain in area of bicipital groove.

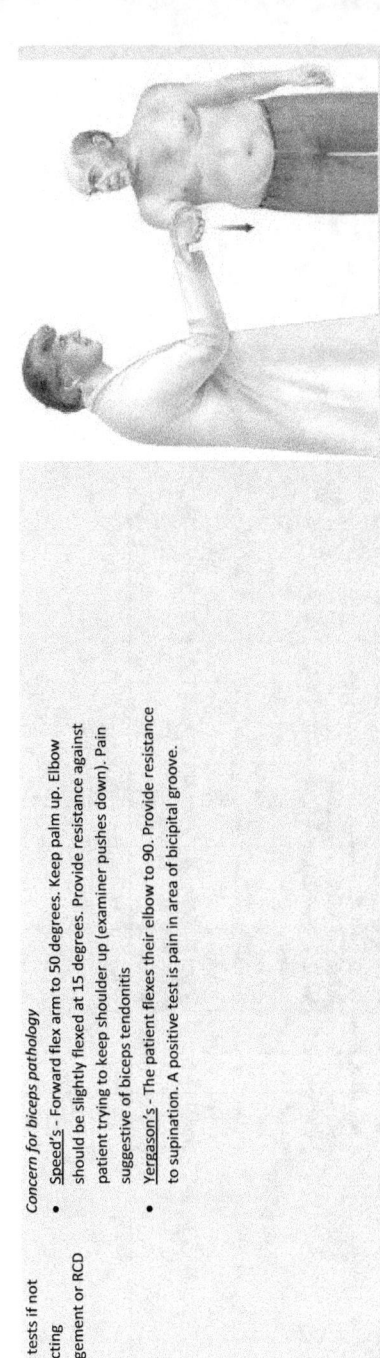

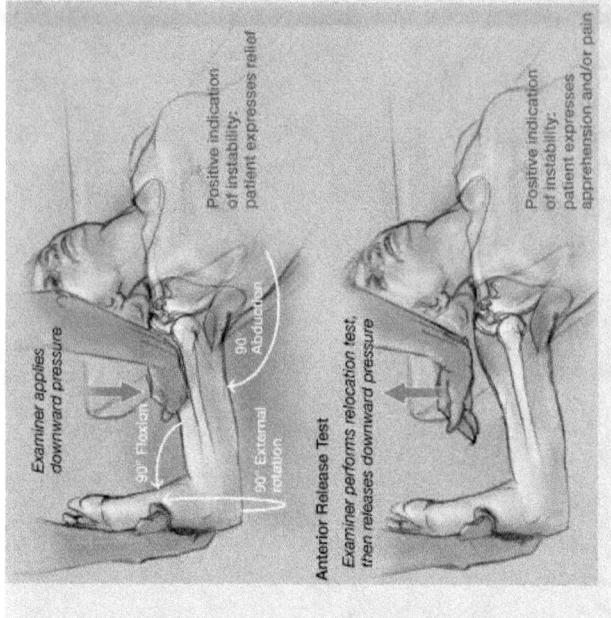

*Concern for **labral** tear (lateral or anterior shoulder pain)*

- O'Brien - Performed to rule out labral cartilage tears that often occur following a shoulder subluxation or dislocation. The test involves flexing the patient's arm to 90 degrees, fully internally rotating the arm so the thumb is facing down (palm down) and adducting the arm to 10 degrees. Once positioned properly, the clinician applies downward force and asks the patient to resist. The test is then repeated in the same position except that the patient has his arm fully supinated (palm up). A positive O'Brien test for labral tear is pain deep in the shoulder with palm down more than the palm up.

  The O'Brien test can also be used to identify AC joint pathology. The patient would typically complain equally of pain directly over the AC joint with the palm down or up.

  o Speed's - examiner places the patient's arm in shoulder flexion, external rotation, full elbow extension, and forearm supination; manual resistance is then applied by the examiner in a downward direction. The test is considered to be positive if pain in the bicipital tendon or bicipital groove is reproduced.

  o Crank - This test is usually performed with the patient in sitting but can also be performed with the patient in supine or standing. The examiner flexes the patients elbow to 90 degrees and elevates the patient's arm to approximately 160 degrees in the scapular plane. In this position, the examiner applies a gentle compressive force on the glenohumeral joint along the axis of the humerus while simultaneously moving the humerus into internal and external rotation

Bibliography

[249] Hooten et al. "Evaluation and Treatment of Low Back Pain: A Clinically Focused Review for Primary Care Specialists." Mayo Clin Proc. 2015;90(12):1699-1718.
[250] Van Tulder MW, Touray T, Furlan AD, Solway S, Bouter LM. Muscle relaxants for non-specific low back pain. *Cochrane Database Syst Rev.* 2003;(2):CD004252.
[251] Schraeder et al. Clinical Evaluation of the Knee. N Engl J Med 2010;363(4):e5.
[252] Helfenstein et al. "Anserine syndrome" Bras J Rheumatology. 2010; 50(3). 313-27
[253] Jones et al. "Nonsurgical Management of Knee Pain in Adults." Am Fam Physician. 2015 Nov 15;92(10):875-883.
[254] McGahan JP, Shoji H. Knee effusions. J Fam Practice 1977;4:141-4
[255] Johnson MW. Acute knee effusions: a systematic approach to diagnosis. Am Fam Physician. 2000 Apr 15;61(8):2391-400.
[256] Woodward TW, Best TM. The painful shoulder: part I. Clinical evaluation. Am Fam Physician. 2000 May 15;61(10):3079-88.
[257] Greenberg, Deborah. "Evaluation and Treatment of Shoulder Pain." Med Clin N Am 98 (2014) 487–504.

NEUROLOGY

Neurological Exam	404
Syncope	407
Altered Mental Status	411
Concussion	413
Headaches	417
Migraine Headaches	421
Parkinson's Disease	427
Sensory/Motor Deficits	429
Seizure	430
Unresponsive Patient	438
Stroke	439
Transient Ischemic Attack	454
Vertigo	456

NEUROLOGY

Figure. Anterior dermatomes

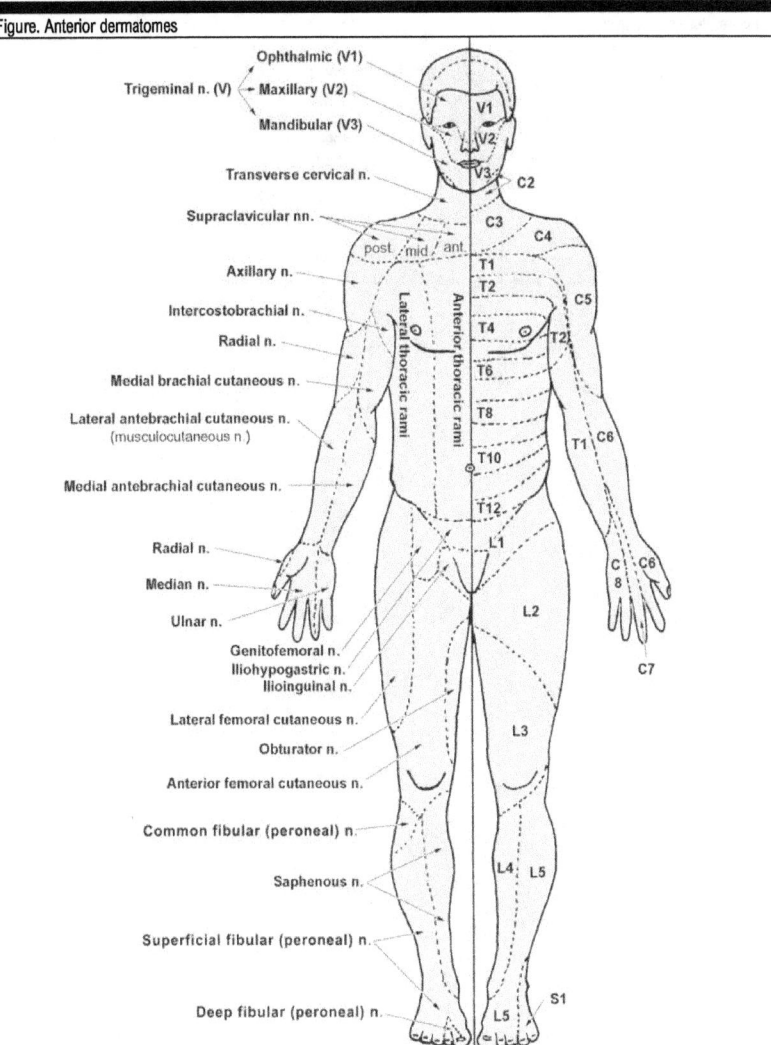

Figure. Posterior dermatomes

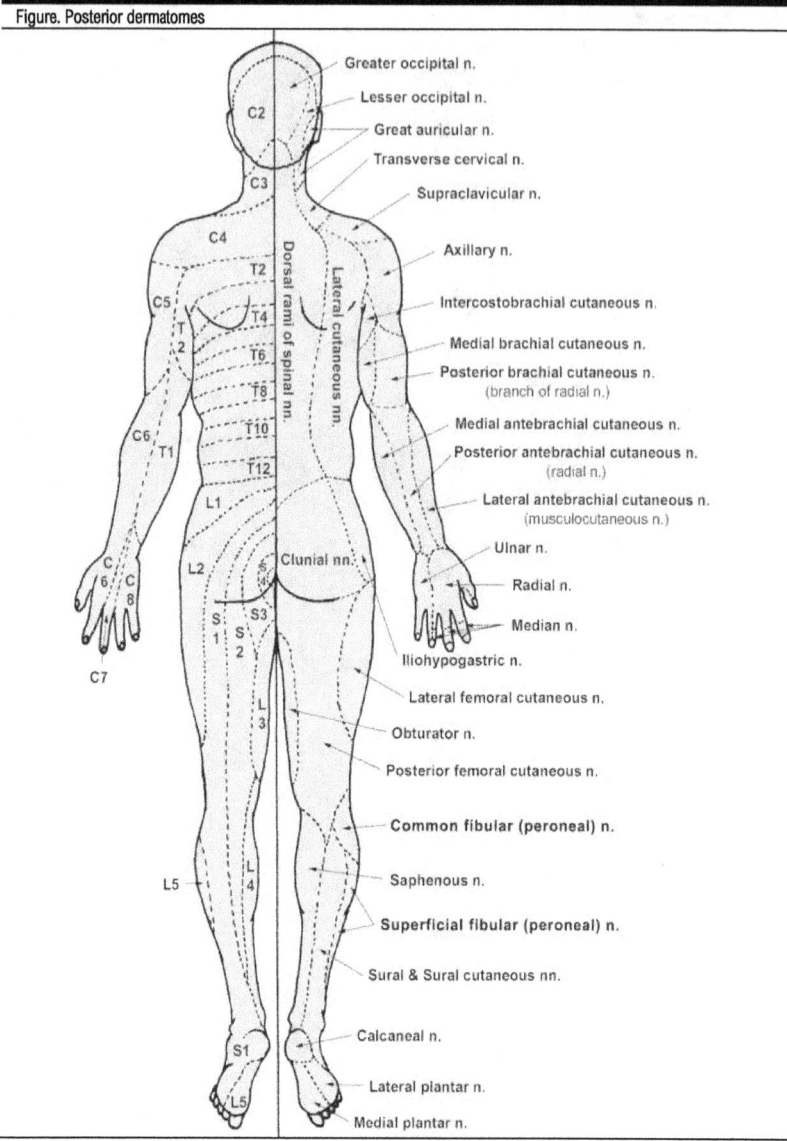

NEUROLOGICAL EXAM

- <u>General Appearance</u>: LOC, hygiene, posture, motor activity
  - Chorea – sudden movements
  - Dystonia – sudden tonic contractions (tongue, neck, mouth)
  - Akathisia – writhing, repetitive movements
  - Tremor – intention vs. resting

- o LOC/Mental Status: Alertness, interaction, responsiveness to command, orientation. Consider noting a Glasgow Coma Scale score in comatose patients and Mini-Mental State Examination score (MMSE) or Montreal Cognitive Assessment (MoCA) in patients with cognitive problems. AA&Ox3, appropriately interactive, normal affect
- Attention: WORLD backwards, MOY backwards, digit span 4 forwards, 3 back
- Speech: fluent w/o paraphasic error, repetition, naming, reading, writing intact
- Calculations: 9 quarters = $2.25
- Praxis: Able to mimic brushing teeth and blowing out match with either hand.
- Cranial Nerves
  - o CN I – *olfactory*, sense of smell (can use alcohol swab), test each nare separately
  - o CN II – *optic*, visual acuity, confrontation

    Confrontation Testing
    1. Tested by facing the patient one foot away, at eye level. Select one eye to cover and cover it with the same side hand.
    2. As the instructor, now you cover the ipsilateral eye (should be opposite of patient) with your hand
    3. While the patient looks you in the eyes, outstretch your opposite arm (to the side of the eye being covered) and extend your arm and first 2 fingers out to the side as far as possible. Wiggle your fingers moving them closer towards the both of you.
    4. The patient should be instructed to tell you when the fingers enter from out of sight, into their peripheral vision, the patient. The patient should say "now" at the same time you see your own fingers.
    5. Repeat this a total of eight times per eye, once for every 45 degrees out of the 360 degrees of peripheral vision.
    6. Repeat the same maneuver with the other eye.
  - o CN III – *oculomotor*, "PERRLA" via light source (check for sluggish pupils, accommodation), optic discs sharp
  - o CN IV, VI – *trochlear, abducens;* have patient watch penlight without moving head; check for nystagmus, palsies, ptosis. "EOMI"
  - o CN V – *trigeminal;* sensation to b/l face (3 areas tested), masseters strong symmetrically. Often do not test corneal reflex.
  - o CN VII – *facial;* "face symmetric without weakness" by asking patient to raise their eyebrows, smile, puff out cheeks. Look for ptosis, loss of normal facial creases. Have the patient close their eyes and try and open them (against resistance)
  - o CN VIII – *vestibulocochlear;* "hearing grossly intact" assess by snapping your fingers on either side of the head. Can also perform Weber-Rinne testing.
  - o CN IX, X – *glossopharyngeal, vagus;* "voice normal, palate elevates symmetrically, gag intact"; have patient swallow and ask if they have any difficulty doing so. Have them say "AH" and note for equal rise of the uvula (should not be deviated to one side).
  - o CN XI – *accessory;* "SCM/trapezii 5/5"; have the patient shrug their shoulders against resistance as well as side bend their head against your resistance.
  - o CN XII – *hypoglossal;* "tongue protrudes midline, no atrophy or fasciculation"; have patient stick their tongue out and move it to both sides.
- Motor: assess bulk and tone, look for tremors, rigidity or bradykinesia. Evaluate for pronator drift which may be a sign of UMN disease.

  Pronator Drift
  1. Patient is asked to hold his or her arms outstretched with palms facing upward.
  2. The eyes are closed in order to accentuate the response, because without vision, the patient must rely on proprioception alone to maintain the position of the arms.

3. In the presence of an upper motor neuron lesion, the supinator muscles in the upper limb are weaker than the pronator muscles causing the palm to turn toward the floor.
- Cerebellar/Coordination
  - Rapid alternating (hands)
  - Point-to-point (FNF, HTS, TTF) movements
  - Scanning speech ("The British Constitution")
  - Heel-to-shin
  - Nystagmus
  - Rebound test (have patient flex an arm and pull the arm away from the patient, who should be resisting, then let go. With an intact cerebellum, the patient should be able to prevent their arm from suddenly hitting themselves, if it is affected, when you let go, they may hit themselves)
  - Hypotonia (after checking patellar reflex, an abnormal reaction would be for the leg to continue swinging multiple times after the impact)
  - Gait: wide based (abnormal) and falling to one side (abnormal, towards side of cerebellar infarction)
- Language: receptive and expressive language intact
- Visuospatial: normal clock-drawing
- Proprioception: Romberg (assessment of pts with disequilibrium or ataxia from sensory and motor disorders)
- Motor strength:
  - *Testing*
    - 5/5: movement against gravity with full resistance
    - 4/5: movement against gravity with some resistance
    - 3/5: movement against gravity only
    - 2/5: movement against gravity eliminated
    - 1/5: visible/palpable muscle contraction but no movement
    - 0/5: no muscle contraction
  - *Upper extremity*
    - Shoulder abduction (c5 – deltoid/supraspinatus)
    - Shoulder adduction
    - Elbow flexion (c5/c6 -biceps brachii – musculocutaneous nerve)
    - Elbow extension (c7 -triceps -radial nerve)
    - Wrist flexion (c7 – fcr/fcu – median/ulnar)
    - Wrist extension (c6 – ecr/ecu – radial nerve)
    - Finger adduction (t1-interossei-ulnar)
    - Thumb radial abduction (c7 – apl – radial nerve)
    - Thumb opposition (c8/t1 -opponens pollicis – median nerve)
    - Rapid hand exam
      - Median nerve = "a-ok" sign, try and pull fingers apart
      - Ulnar nerve = "fingers spread apart, try and squish together
      - Radial nerve = make a fist, push down on hand while they resist and pull upward. Alternative is have them make a stopping motion with hand (look for wrist drop).
  - *Lower extremity*
    - Hip flexion (l1/l2 – iliopsoas muscle)
    - Hip extension (l5/s1 – gluteus maximus muscle)
    - Knee flexion (l5/s1 -hamstrings -sciatica nerve)
    - Knee extension (l3/l4 -quadriceps femoris muscle -femoral nerve)
    - Ankle dorsiflexion (l4/l5 -tibialis anterior muscle -deep peroneal nerve)
    - Ankle plantarflexion (s1 – gastrocnemius muscle -tibial nerve)
    - Ankle eversion (l5/s1 -peroneus longus/brevis – superficial peroneal nerve)

- Ankle inversion (I4/I5 -tibialis posterior muscle – tibial nerve)
- Extensor hallucis longus (I4/I5 – ehl/edls – deep peroneal nerve)
- Flexor hallucis longus (s1 – fhl, fdls – tibial nerve)
- Reflexes:
  - *Anatomy*
    - Triceps (C7, radial)
    - Biceps (C5, musculocutaneous)
    - Brachioradialis (C6, radial)
    - Patellar (L4, femoral)
    - Achilles (S1, tibial)
    - Babinski (downward, no fanned toes)
  - *Testing*
    - +4/4: hyperactive with clonus (UMN)
    - +3/4: hyperactive
    - +2/4: normal
    - +1/4: hypoactive
    - +0/4: no reflex (LMN)
- Sensory:
  - Lateral spinothalamic – pinprick, temperature nl
  - Dorsal columns – proprioception nl
  - Cortical – graphesthesia nl, proprioception nl
  - Hand – test for median, ulnar, and radial nerves

SYNCOPE

- **Definition**[258,259]
  - Transient global cerebral hypoperfusion characterized by rapid onset, short duration, and spontaneous complete recover
  - *Presyncope* refers to the symptoms (nausea, LH, sweating, weakness, visual changes) that occur before syncope without actual LOC
- **Diagnosis** (requires all three)
  1) Transient loss of consciousness must be established
  2) Recovery must be complete and spontaneous
  3) Head trauma and epilepsy must be ruled out
- **Admission**
  - Admit:
    - HPI: chest pain
    - PMH: CAD, CHF, ventricular arrhythmia
    - PE: CHF, valvular disease, focal neurologic deficit or disorder
    - ECG: ischemia, arrhythmia, bundle branch block, prolonged QT
  - Strongly consider admission:
    - HPI: age > 70, exertional syncope, frequent syncope, cardiac disease suspected
    - PE: tachycardia, moderate to severe orthostasis, injury
- **Major Causes/Classification**[260]
  - Neurocardiogenic/Reflex
    - *Vasovagal* – noxious stimuli, fear, stress, heat, emotional distress
    - *Carotid Sinus Hypersensitivity* – head rotation, shaving, tight collar
    - *Situational* - cough, micturition, defecation, deglutition, post exercise
  - Orthostatic ↓BP
    - Medications (vasodilators, anti-depressants)
    - Hemorrhage, diarrhea, vomiting

- Autonomic failure 2/2 nervous system dysfunction - POTS, postural orthostatic ↓BP, MSA, MS. Secondary failure from DM, amyloidosis, etc.
  - Cardiac
    - Bradycardia (sinus node dysfunction, AV conduction disease)
    - Tachycardia (SVT, VT)
    - Structural (AS, ACS, HCM, tamponade, PE, dissection)
- **Evaluation**
  - HPI
    - Prodromal symptoms
    - Vasovagal syncope - typically preceded by warmth, diaphoresis, nausea, abdominal pain, lightheadedness, and/or ringing in ears
      - Symptoms are usually consistent from episode to episode for each patient
    - Cardiac syncope - may present with dyspnea, chest pain, pressure or tightness, or palpitations
      - Sudden-onset palpitations immediately followed by syncope favor a cardiac cause
      - Can also occur without any warning signs, especially in elderly people
    - Postdromal symptoms - in vasovagal syncope, symptoms such as fatigue and nausea can persist up to several hours
    - In cardiac syncope, postrecovery period is not usually marked by lingering malaise
  - Relevant PMHx
    - Previous cardiac disease (e.g., valvular dz, arrhythmia, cardiomyopathy) → cardiac syncope
    - H/o Parkinson disease or Addison disease → orthostatic hypotension triggering syncope, autonomic instability/neuropathy
    - T2DM → may indicate orthostatic hypotension due to autonomic neuropathy
  - Exam: Supine and standing BP, BP (look for unexplained ↓SBP below 90 mmHg), GIB on rectal exam, HR<40 bpm, new SEM
    - Orthostatics: abnormal ↓ in SBP by ≥20mmHg or DBP ≥10mmHg or overall ↓ in SBP to <90mmHg
    - Consider tilt table testing if orthostatic ↓BP suspected
  - Diagnostics: ECG, TTE if previous known heart disease present or concern for structural heart disease
    - *ECG findings*: look for bifasicular block, complete heart block or second degree type 2 block, ↑QRS duration, inappropriate sinus bradycardia (or slow AFib), ↑ST segment, LVH, Type 1 Brugada, SVT or NSVT, dysfunction in implanted pacemaker, QTc>460ms
    - *Carotid sinus massage*: ventricular pause >3s or a ↓ in SBP of >50mmHg concerning for carotid hypersensitivity (often seen with tight collars, shaving, rotating head history leading to syncope)
  - Labs: CBC, TROP, d-dimer, ABG, B-HCG
- **Initial Assessment**
  - ECG - rule out arrhythmias such as Brugada, VT, AF
  - Postural BPs
  - Optional
    - TTE
    - CT (if head trauma)

Figure. Differential diagnosis to consider for transient loss of consciousness

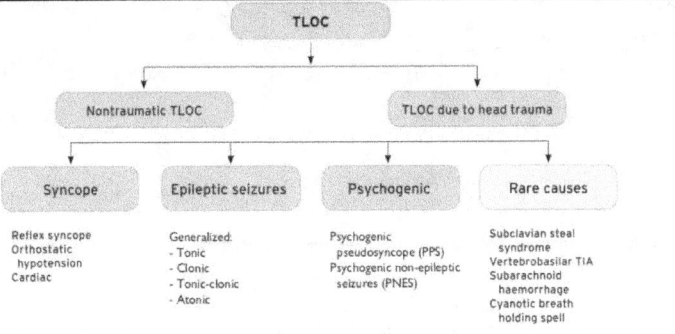

- **Mimics of syncope**
    - Metabolic: hypoxia, hypoglycemia, hyperventilation
    - Subclavian Steal
    - Intoxication
    - Epilepsy
    - Carotid TIA

NEUROLOGY

Causes of syncope	
Reflex	
Vasovagal	Emotional distress
Situational	Cough, sneeze
	GI stimulated (swallow, defecation)
	Micturition
	Post-exercise
	Post-prandial
Atypical	
Orthostatic Hypotension (Consider tilt table testing)	
Primary Autonomic Failure	MSA, Parkinson's disease, Lewy Body Dementia
Secondary Autonomic Failure	DM, amyloidosis, uremia, spinal cord injuries
Drug-induced	EtOH, vasodilators, diuretics, anti-depressants
↓Volume	Hemorrhage, diarrhea, vomiting
Postprandial Hypotension	Defined as drop in SBP by 20 or more points within 2 hours of eating; important to ask patient when the events occur (around mealtime); symptoms include dizziness, near syncope, syncope, weakness, angina. Mechanism is not fully understood. Patients at higher risk include those on BP medications, diuretics, low salt diet. Treatment includes avoiding sitting for long periods after eating, liberal salt intake if possible, with adequate fluids, avoid EtOH.
Cardiac	

Arrythmia	• Bradyarrhythmia
	   o Sinus node dysfunction
	   o AV conduction disease / Heart block
	• Tachyarrhythmia
	   o Supraventricular arrhythmia
	   o Ventricular arrhythmia (MOST important one to exclude risk of sudden cardiac death in patients with history of cardiac disease)
	• Other
	   o QT prolongation
	   o Brugada

Structural	Valvular disease (aortic stenosis, mitral stenosis, pulmonary stenosis), global ischemia, aortic dissection, obstructive cardiomyopathy, left atrial myxoma, prosthetic valve dysfunction, pulmonary embolus, pulmonary hypertension (careful cardiac auscultation and obtain ECHO)

- **Management**
  - Answer the following questions to determine management:
    - Is there a serious underlying cause that can be identified? Often r/o with above diagnostics and history/exam
    - What is the risk of a serious outcome?

High and Low risk symptoms in evaluation of syncope
High-risk (should be admitted)
Major
• New onset chest pain, SOB, DOE, abdominal pain, or HA
• Syncope during exercise or when supine
• Sudden onset palpitations leading to syncope
Minor (only considered high risk if below findings found with structural heart disease or ECG findings)
• No prodromal symptoms or short (<10 seconds) prodrome
• Family history of SCD at young age
• Syncope while sitting
Low-risk (typically can be sent home)
• Typical reflex syncope suspected based on hx (LH, warmth, sweating, n/v)
• Unpleasant sound, smell, pain leading to syncope
• Syncope after prolonged standing or in crowded place
• Syncope after meal

- Syncope after cough, defecation or micturition
- Syncope after rotating head or shaving
    - Should the patient be admitted to hospital?
        - *High risk* → admit and monitor for at least 24 hours in the hospital
        - *Mix of High and Low Risk* → admit and monitor for at least 24 hours in the hospital
        - *Low Risk* → can be d/c home
- **Treatment**
    - Reflex
        - lifestyle education
        - ↑fluids (2L/d)
        - ↑salt intake (2-4g/d)
        - ↓BP medications
        - pharmacologic meds
            - fludrocortisone 0.1-0.2mg/d
            - midodrine 5-10mg/TID can be helpful in vasovagal syncope (*STAND*)
        - pacemaker (if asystole was noted)
    - HOCM/ARVD/BBB/↑QTc/Sinus Node Disease → refer to Cardiology. Consider Holter or prolonged ECG if necessary. ICD may be required if cause was 2/2 structural heart dz
    - Seizure → refer to Neurology

ALTERED MENTAL STATUS

- **Defined** - refers to diffuse disturbance in cerebral function with change in behavior; AMS must be distinguished from somnolence, depression, organic disorder, psychosis, drug intoxication, established cognitive impairment, and history of traumatic brain injury
- **General**
    - Stabilize first, then diagnose
    - If received over the phone:
        - Obtain Vitals
        - Is the patient diabetic?
        - Order: accu-check, O2 sat, new set of vitals, ECG
- **Differential**

Causes of AMS
Structural
Traumatic contusions
Diffuse axonal injury
ICH
CVA
Tumors
Hydrocephalus
Anoxic brain injury
Metabolic
Electrolyte abnormalities (low Na, high Na, high ca)
ARF (often leads to electrolyte abnormalities)
Hyper or hypo-osmolarity
Acid-base disorders
Hypercapnia
Hypoxia
Hypo or hyperglycemia
Dialysis disequilibrium syndrome
Acute or chronic liver failure (hepatic encephalitis; obtain NH3, paracentesis)
Thyroid
Pituitary failure

NEUROLOGY

Nutrition
Thiamine deficiency (think alcoholics with Wernicke's)
Toxic
EtOH w/d or intoxication (check B12, thiamine often low)
illicit drugs (cocaine, opioids, PCP, amphetamines, sedatives)
Lithium
SS
Benzodiazepines
Infectious
Systemic infection
Sepsis
CNS infection (meningitis, encephalitis)
Others
Seizure
Autoimmune encephalitis
SLE
Paraneoplastic neurology syndromes
Sensory deprivation
Sleep disturbance
Hemorrhage
Delirium (hypoactive vs. hyperactive)

- **Exam**
    - Vitals
        - Hypertension: PRES, hypertensive encephalopathy
        - Temp
            - Hypothermia: sepsis, hypothyroidism, EtOH intoxication, sedation, adrenal crisis, sepsis
            - Hyperthermia: infection, thyroid storm, adrenal crises, ICH, tumor
    - Neurological exam *(see page 404)*
    - Skin – jaundice (liver failure), needle tracks (IVDA), sweating (hypoglycemia, thyroid)
- **Diagnostics**
    - Imaging
        - CT head
        - ECG
        - CXR
        - Consider LP if fever/meningeal/immunosuppressed
        - EEG
    - Labs
        - Bedside glucose measurement (give 1 amp D50 if suspected hypoglycemia)
        - TSH
        - CBC → look for anemia, new or ↑WBC
        - CHEM7 → electrolyte abnormalities, uremia
        - LFTs → look for acute liver failure
        - TSH
        - Cultures: BCx, UCx
        - ABG → hypo or hypercapnic resp failure
        - UDS
        - NH3 → encephalopathy however understand NH3 is not req'd for diagnosis
- **Diagnosis** - refers to change in baseline level of arousal or thought content; content refers to cortical functions of orientation, perception, executive function, and behavior; arousal means wakeful state
- **Treatment**
    - Protect airway prn (supplemental o2 +/- OPA)
    - If suspected alcoholic, give thiamine 100mg IV
    - Give 1 amp D50 if suspected hypoglycemia **after** giving thiamine

- o Narcan 0.4-2mg IV or IM if suspect narcotic overdose (if patient does not respond to initial dose, consider fentanyl as source which may require multiple doses)
- o Oxygen

CONCUSSION

- **Defined**: no standard universal definition of concussion or mTBI, diagnosis is based primarily on characteristics of immediate sequelae after the event.
  - o Generic definition is a condition in which there is a traumatically induced alteration in mental status, **with or without** an associated loss of consciousness (LOC).
  - o No single test score can be the basis of a concussion diagnosis.
  - o Each successive concussion results in additive damage to the cerebrum
- **Epidemiology**[261,262,263,264]
  - o Highest risk sports include hockey, rugby, football, and soccer
  - o Military highest risks with blast injuries
  - o 10% of patients do not lose consciousness
- **Symptoms**
  - o Exercise intolerance
  - o Headache
  - o Increased emotions
  - o Nausea
  - o Tinnitus
  - o Irritability
  - o Drowsiness
  - o Poor balance
  - o Slowed verbal output
  - o Noise/Light sensitivity
  - o Difficulty remembering
  - o Sleep disturbances
  - o Difficulty concentrating
- **Signs**
  - o LOC
  - o Altered heart rate (HR) and BP response to submaximal exercise
  - o Post traumatic amnesia
  - o Eye movement abnormalities
  - o Seizure
  - o If symptoms are worsening over time, alternative explanations for the patient's symptoms should be considered.
- **Examination**
  - o Vitals
    - Autonomic dysregulation - abnormal blood pressure (BP) control, temperature regulation, and disruption of endocrine, analgesic, and circadian functions may occur after head injury.
    - Orthostatic Hypotension – 20mmHg or greater reduction in SBP or 10mmHg drop in DBP with or without symptoms after standing
      - □ Obtaining: lay down for 2 minutes, obtain VS, then stand, wait for 1 minute, and re-do VS. Wait 2 minutes, and obtain a second set of VS
      - □ Lack of HR change is more concerning for underlying neurologic injury, whereas a change is c/w likely concurrent hypovolemia
      - □ In POTS there will be tachycardia without a change in BP
      - □ Seated position is not recommended to do
  - o Mental Status Exam
    - SCAT, SAC
    - Orientation
    - Immediate and delayed recall
    - Concentration, mood, affect, insight, judgement
  - o Neurologic Exam
    - CN 2-12 with CN 2, 3, and 7 being most often injured

- DTRs
- MSK Exam
  - Head and neck, ROM, TTP
  - Neck isometrics
  - Cervical proprioception with ROM
  - Jaw
  - Thoracic Spine
  - Spurling Test
- Balance
  - Static and/or dynamic balance assessment
  - In athletes, have them keep their eyes closed and do tandem gait with feet-together
- Vestibulo-occular
  - Screening ocular examination
  - Pupillary reactivity
  - Visual acuity
  - Nystagmus (vertical may lead to difficulty with jumping; horizontal may lead to difficulty tolerating car rides due to motion sickness)
  - Convergence (difficulty with near vision work)
  - Saccades
  - Smooth pursuits (difficulty may mean patient has issues reading or using electronic devices)

- **Diagnosis** - clinical diagnosis when more severe conditions (i.e. ICH) have been ruled out. Based solely on subjective symptoms. The GFAP blood test may be utilized in specific scenarios to assist in diagnosis.
- **Grading / Assessing**
  - Colorado Sports Concussion Grading Scale
    - Grade I: confusion without amnesia, no LOC
    - Grade II: confusion with amnesia, no LOC
    - Grade III: LOC
  - American Academy of Neurology Concussion Grading Scale
    - Grade I: transient confusion, no LOC, sx <15m
    - Grade II: transient confusion, no LOC, sx >15m
    - Grade III: LOC of any duration
  - Cantu Sports Concussion Grading Scale
    - Grade I: amnesia, no LOC, <30m
    - Grade II: amnesia lasting 30m-24h, LOC of <5m,
    - Grade III: LOC of >5m, amnesia lasting >24h
- **Diagnostic Testing**
  - Labs: The Banyan Brain Trauma Indicator measures the serum proteins UCH-L1 and GFAP within 12 hours of head injury. Levels of these proteins can help indicate whether a patient has a low probability of intracranial lesions and thus can eliminate the need for unnecessary CT imaging. Test results can take 3 to 4 hours.
  - The purpose of neuroimaging is to assess for other etiologies or injuries, such as hemorrhage or contusion that may cause similar symptoms but require different management.
  - Guidelines
    - *Canadian CT Head Rule* – CT imaging is required in the following situations:
      - The patient fails to reach a Glasgow Coma Scale score of 15—on a scale of 3 (worst) to 15 (best)—within 2 hours
      - There is a suspected open skull fracture
      - There is any sign of basal skull fracture
      - The patient has 2 or more episodes of vomiting
      - The patient is 65 or older

- The patient has retrograde amnesia (i.e., cannot remember events that occurred before the injury) for 30 minutes or more
- The mechanism of injury was dangerous (e.g., a pedestrian was struck by a motor vehicle, or the patient fell from > 3 feet or > 5 stairs).
- *The New Orleans Criteria* - CT imaging is required in the following situations:
  - Severe headache
  - Vomiting
  - Age over 60
  - Drug or alcohol intoxication
  - Deficit in short-term memory
  - Physical evidence of trauma above the clavicles
  - Seizure.
- Post-TBI dysfunction
  - LH
  - FSH
  - Testosterone (men), estradiol (women)
  - IGF
  - Free thyroxine, TSH
  - 0800 cortisol
- **Quick Assessments for Cognitive Dysfunction**
  - SCAT 5 – 10 minutes; for those ≥13 yo
  - MoCA – 10 minutes; for those ≥18 yo
  - ImPACT – 25 minutes; for those 12-59 yo
  - King-Devick – test for saccades, rapid number naming, takes 2 minutes
  - BESS – assesses postural stability, takes 10 minutes
  - SOT – postural control assessment; takes 15 minutes
- **Treatments**
  - Data suggests that most adults will recover in 2-4 weeks, if patients have symptoms that persist beyond **2 weeks** it may be indicative of a more severe injury.
  - Rest (physical and cognitive)
    - Initial therapy involves several days of cognitive and physical rest, followed by a gradual return to physical and cognitive activities.
      - The optimal period of rest suggested by recent studies is 3 to 5 days after injury, followed by a gradual resumption of both physical and cognitive activities as tolerated, remaining below the level at which symptoms are exacerbated.
  - Post-Traumatic Headache
    - Most common type is migraine, followed by tension
      - *PRN:* Analgesics (NSAIDs) are often used initially by patients to treat posttraumatic headache.
      - *Prophylactic:*
        - In adults, nortriptyline 20 mg or gabapentin 300 mg at night as an initial prophylactic headache medication, increasing as tolerated or until pain is controlled, though there are no high-quality data to guide this decision.
        - The ideal prophylactic medication depends on headache type, patient tolerance, comorbidities, allergies, and medication sensitivities. Gabapentin, amitriptyline, and nortriptyline can produce sedation, which can help those suffering from sleep disturbance.
  - Dizziness
    - Patients should be encouraged to begin movement—gradually and safely—to help the vestibular system accommodate, which it will do with gradual stimulation. It usually resolves spontaneously.

- Referral for a comprehensive balance assessment or to vestibular therapy should be considered if there is no recovery from dizziness **4 to 6 weeks after the concussion**.
  - Sleep Disturbances
    - Sleep hygiene education – minimize screen time, keep consistent sleep schedule, avoid naps, minimize use of nicotine, caffeine, and alcohol
    - Consider use of **melatonin** which can help in patients with TBI
    - Use of medications above for HA may also cause sedation s/e which can help with sleep
    - Order of treatment: sleep hygiene → melatonin → amitriptyline / nortriptyline → trazodone
  - Mental Fogginess
    - Amantadine may be helpful in recovery phase
    - Consider neuropsych consult for MoCA (≥18yo; takes 10 minutes), ImPACT (12yo-59yo; takes 25 minutes) to assess for cognitive dysfunction
  - Anxiety/Depression
    - Consider referral to BH
    - SSRI, SNRI and TCAs may improve depression after concussion

Return to Play Guidelines in Athletes with Concussion

Grade	Guideline
Grade I (confusion)	
First concussion	Remove from play; observe every 5 minutes for 20 minutes with neurologic examination; return to play if no signs or symptoms
Second concussion	Remove for 2 weeks consider CT
Third concussion	Remove for rest of season, obtain CT
Grade II (confusion + amnesia)	
First concussion	Remove from play for 1 week
Second concussion	Remove for 1 month, obtain CT
Third concussion	Remove for entire season, obtain CT, consider limiting any other contact sports
Grade III (confusion, amnesia, LOC)	
First concussion	Remove from play for 2 weeks if loss of consciousness <1 minute, otherwise 1 month; transport to hospital; CT scan; rule out any additional cervical spine injury
Second concussion	Remove from play from season, follow above guidelines; consider any further contact sport contraindicated

- **Returning to Activity** – physiologic recovery is delayed behind symptomatic recovery, thus, if patients are feeling better, their body may not be completely healed. This is the basis behind "return to play" protocols. Each stage lasts 24h, If symptoms begin to occur during this protocol, patients should be advised go back to the previous stage and attempt to advance again when asymptomatic for 24 hours

Return to Play Protocol

Stage	Aim	Activity	Goal
1	Symptom free activity	ADLs	Return to work/school as tolerated
2	Light aerobic exercise	Stationary bike/walking	↑HR
3	Sport-specific activities	Running, swimming, etc.	Incorporate movement
4	Noncontact practice	Resistance training; sports simulation without head injury potential	Exercise with coordination and thinking
5	Full contact practice	Simulation of sports activities, normal training	Build confidence, allow for assessment by athletic staff

| 6 | Return to sport | Game play | Unrestricted |

All Adults
- After the rest period, patients may gradually resume cognitive and physical activities while avoiding those that result in severe symptom exacerbation.
  - Recommended modifications include reduced workload, shortened workdays, and frequent breaks to allow provocable symptoms to improve and cognitive stamina to recover.
  - For those whose symptoms persist **beyond 1 month**, there is evidence that noncontact aerobic activity is helpful in promoting recovery.
- Light physical activity (typically walking or stationary bicycling), followed by more vigorous aerobic activity, followed by some resistance activities.
- Mild aerobic exercise (to below the threshold of symptoms) may speed recovery from refractive post-concussion syndrome, even in those who did not exercise before the injury.

Athletes
- Once aerobic reconditioning produces no symptoms, then noncontact, sport-specific activities are begun, followed by contact activities.
- Have patients return to the clinic once they are symptom-free for repeat evaluation before clearing them for high-risk activities (e.g., skiing, bicycling) or contact sports (e.g., basketball, soccer, football, ice hockey).

- **Referring Out**
  - Approximately 10% of athletes have persistent signs and symptoms of concussion beyond 2 weeks. If concussion is not sport-related, most patients recover completely within the first 3 months, but up to 33% may have symptoms beyond that.
  - Consults
    - Vestibular rehabilitation – sx of BPPV, cervicogenic dizziness
    - Visual rehabilitation – convergence insufficiency, light sensitivity
    - Cognitive rehabilitation – inattention, memory impairment, decreased reaction
  - If their recovery is prolonged (i.e., longer than 6 weeks), they likely need to be referred to a concussion specialist.
  - High risk for persistent symptoms:
    - High-force mechanism of injury
    - History of multiple concussions
    - Underlying neurologic condition
      - Intractable pain and emotional lability after initial injury

HEADACHES

- **Diagnosis**[265,266]
  - ≥4 Hours
    - *Migraine* – two of four pain features (unilateral, pulsatile, moderate-severe intensity, associated with routine activity) AND at least one of the following (nausea, photophobia/phonophobia). Often occur 1-5x/month lasting 4-72 hours at a time. F>M with + family history
    - *Hemicrania continua*
    - *Tension* – typically new onset HA in older pt
  - <4 Hours
    - *Cluster* – most often in males; 15min-3 hrs. duration, associated with rhinorrhea, tearing, often occurs multiple times throughout the day, periorbital.
    - *Paroxysmal hemicrania*

- Hypnic HA
- Primary cough HA
- Primary exercise HA
- **Types**
  - Primary
    - Tension
    - Migraine w/ or w/o aura
    - Cluster
    - Pseudotumor cerebrae
    - Trigeminal autonomic cephalgia
  - Secondary
    - Temporal arteritis / GCA – systemic sx, scalp tenderness, jaw claudication
    - Mass lesion – subacute onset of neuro sx, papilledema
    - ICH (SAH/SDH) – thunderclap, focal neuro sx, ↓LOC, concurrent anticoagulation
    - CVA - look for focal neuro sx, suspect posterior circulation involvement
    - Vascular malformation
    - Cardiac cephalgia – HA precipitated by exertion
    - Acute glaucoma – HA noted in dimly lit conditions
    - Cervicogenic HA – HA associated with neck movement
    - Post traumatic
    - OSA – AM headache, h/o OSA
- **Red Flags**[267]
  - First HA in patients >50 (or 40 if c/f SAH)
  - Witnessed LOC
  - Limited flexion of neck
  - Sudden onset with maximum intensity reached within 5 minutes
  - Pain worse with Valsalva type maneuvers (i.e. cough)
  - Recent head injury in the last 3 months
  - Associated with fever
  - PMHx of HIV or immunosuppression
  - Focal neurologic signs
  - Pain associated with local tenderness, e.g., region of temporal artery
  - Vomiting that precedes headache
  - Associated conjunctivitis
  - Papilledema
  - Positional in nature
  - Worsened with Valsalva
- **Diagnostics**
  - CT head (non-contrast; perform within 6 hours of symptoms c/f SAH)
  - Consider CTA of the head if LP cannot be performed if concerned for SAH
  - When to image:
    - For thunderclap headache, CT imaging of the head without contrast appropriate
    - For new headache with optic disc edema, MRI of the brain with or without contrast or CT head without contrast are appropriate
    - New or progressive headache with "red flags" (e.g., subacute head trauma, exertional headache, neurologic deficit, cancer, immunocompromise, pregnancy, age ≥50) warrants plain CT head or MRI brain with or without contrast.
    - New primary headache of suspected trigeminal autonomic origin (e.g., cluster headache) should be investigated with MRI brain with contrast.
    - For chronic headache with new features or progression, MRI brain with or without contrast is appropriate
- **Treatment**

- GCA – prednisone 1mg/kg (up to 60mg) and ASA 81mg; labs include ESR, CRP, CBC, temporal artery biopsy within 7 days of steroid initiation
- Cluster – 100% O2 at 6-12L/min using nonrebreather for 15min; can also give SQ sumatriptan or zolmitriptan nasal spray; prophylactic tx with verapamil/lithium/topiramate for prevention

Headache Types and Characteristics

Symptom	Migraine	Tension-type headache	Paroxysmal hemicranias	Hemicrania continua	Trigeminal neuralgia	SUNCT/SUNA	Cluster headache	Medication-overuse headache
Aura	Yes	No	No	No	No	No	No	No
Headache duration	4-72 hrs.	30m-7d	2-30min	Continuous	1-120 sec	1-600 sec	15-180m	Some or all of the day
Frequency	Episodic, variable	1-15 days per month, variable	>5 daily for more than ½ time	Continuous	Variable freq	>1 daily for more than ½ time	1 on alternate days to 8 per day, often for 7 days to 1 year when episodic	Daily >15d/month, for more than 3 months
Laterality	Unilateral	Bilateral	Unilateral	Unilateral	Unilateral	Unilateral; V1/V2>V3	Unilateral	Unilateral/Bilateral
Character of pain	Pulsating	Pressing/tightening (non-throbbing)	Variable	Variable	Neuralgiform	Neuralgiform	Knife-like, severe, excruciating	Pressing/tightening/pulsating
Severity of pain	Moderate/severe	Mild/moderate	Very severe	Mod-very severe	Very severe	Very severe	Severe/Very severe	Mild/moderate/Severe
Aggravated by movement	Yes	No	N/A	N/A	N/A	N/A	No	No
Eased by movement	No	No	N/A	+/-	N/A	N/A	Yes; restless	No
Nausea +/- movement	Yes	No	N/A	+/-	N/A	N/A	No	No
Photophobia/phonophobia	Yes	No	N/A	+/-	N/A	N/A	No	No
Red/watery eye	No	No	No	No	No	No	Yes	No
Autonomic sx	+/-	-	+++	+++	Sparse	+++	+++	-
Watery or blocked nose	No	No	+++	+++	-	-	Yes	No
Indomethacin response	+/-	+/-	+++	+++	-	-	-	-

- **Generic Treatment Options**
  - Tylenol 650 mg PO Q 4-6 hour prn HA
    - 15 mg/kg Q 6 hours
  - Naprosyn 500 mg PO bid prn HA
  - Diclofenac
  - Fioricet 2 tabs q4h **avoid in pts with hx of addiction
- **Headache Cocktail (EM)**
  - Combination of:
    - Toradol 30mg IV or 60mg IM
    - Benadryl (optional but encouraged)
    - Reglan 10mg IVP
    vs
    Prochlorperazine 10mg IVP
    - IV NS (1L)
    - Optional: Decadron 4mg IV

    No relief in 15 minutes...

  - **C/I if risk for SAH
    - Phenergan 12.5mg IVP or Demerol 25mg
    - Toradol 30mg IV

MIGRAINE HEADACHES

- **Define**[268,269,270]
  - Two of four pain features (unilateral, pulsatile, moderate-severe intensity, symptoms impact daily activity) AND at least one of the following (nausea, photophobia/phonophobia). Often occur 1-5x/month lasting 4-72 hours at a time. F>M with + family history.
  - Often occur 1-5x/month lasting 4-72 hours at a time.
  - F>M with + family history.
- **Duration**
  - Episodic – fewer than 15 headache days per month
  - Chronic – at least 15 headache days per month
- **Types**
  - Migraine without aura (4-72 hours)
  - Migraine with aura (4-72 hours; visual changes last 15-20 minutes prior to HA)
    - Aura only occurs in 30% of patients
    - Typically characterized by any neurological event that can be a combination of visual, hemisensory, or language abnormalities, with each symptom developing over at least 5 minutes and lasting a maximum of 60 minutes.
  - Status migrainosus (>72 hours)
  - Migraine with Brainstem Aura (MBA)
    - Patients often present with basilar symptoms such as vertigo, dysarthria, tinnitus, diplopia, b/l visual sx, hypoacusis, ataxic gait, impaired consciousness.
  - Transformed
    - Initially episodic in duration but becomes more frequent and classified as chronic.
  - Retinal Migraines - spreading cortical depression that occurs in the retina. Fairly rare.
  - Abdominal Migraines - characterized by abdominal pain or vomiting as part of the headache syndrome. Symptoms predominate over the HA. Seen primarily in children and adolescents, although can manifest as cyclic abdominal pain and vomiting in adults.

NEUROLOGY

- o Hemiplegic Migraines - must have exam-confirmed motor weakness, as well as other aura (including dysphasia). Triptans are avoided in the management
- **Differential Diagnosis**
  - o Tension – does not have associated nausea and disability; not associated with activity, usually non pulsatile, bilateral and lasts from 30 minutes to 7 days. It is better described as vise-like that wraps around the head.
  - o Aneurysm
  - o GCA/PMR
  - o SAH
  - o Meningitis
  - o Glaucoma
  - o IIH
  - o TIA
  - o Intracranial neoplasia
- **Known Precipitants**
  - o Stress
  - o Foods
  - o Weather changes
  - o Smoke
  - o Hunger
  - o Fatigue
  - o Bright light sensitivity
  - o Menstruation - thought to be related to the sudden drop in estrogen levels
  - o Hormones
- **Evaluation/Work-up**
  - o Clinical diagnosis: physical exam is done to rule out secondary causes
    - Focal neurologic abnormality (consider mass)
    - Fever (consider inflammation, infection)
    - DBP>120 mmHg (consider malignant HTN)
    - Papilledema (consider pseudotumor; mass; meningitis)
    - Tender temporary arteries
    - Nuchal rigidity
  - o Imaging
    - Imaging is not appropriate for newly diagnosed migraine or tension-type headache with a normal neurologic exam or for chronic stable headache with no neurologic deficit.
    - In general imaging is only obtained if abnormal unexplained findings found on exam, or atypical features such as worsening with Valsalva, awaken from sleep due to HA, HA onset after age 50, aura lasting more than 1 hour, or progressively worsening.
    - Other imaging other than CT and MRI to consider include lumbar puncture, IOP, CT sinuses, MR angiogram
  - o Symptoms Suggestive of Secondary Headache
    - New onset headache in >50 YO
    - Headache lasting >72 hours
    - Visual/sensory/language sx lasting >1 hr.
    - Sudden onset with neurological symptoms
    - Abnormal neuro exam
    - Fever, systemic sx
  - o Concerning Symptoms
    - Change in quality of HA or frequency
    - Daily or continuous
    - Changes in mental status or personality

- Associated jaw pain (especially in older patient; consider GCA)
- New onset after 50 years old (consider neoplasm)
- **Consultation** - Referral is indicated if the headache is atypical, remains difficult to classify, or fails to respond to recommended management strategies
- **Pregnancy** – must rule out pre-eclampsia and pregnancy-induced HTN. Best preferred therapies are Mg OH and rest. Sumatriptan (nasal delivery system or nasal spray) for <9 days/month okay during pregnancy. For short term therapy, Tylenol and NSAIDs are best. Do not advise use of NSAIDs past 32 weeks. Preventive therapy has at least Category C rating. Best for now is beta blockers but should be tapered off the last few weeks of pregnancy.
    - During Lactation – sumatriptan and eletriptan are considered safe in the lowest effective dose.
- **Overuse Headache** – common in patients using OTC NSAIDs for 15 of the 30 days in a month with headaches occurring >10 days of the month. Consider use of Tylenol or Naproxen, these are less likely to cause overuse HA. In the acute setting, if needing to stop medication(s) immediately, steroid tapers have been used as well as gabapentin and hydroxyzine.
- **Treatment**
    - See table on next page
    - Menstruation related[271]
        - Remember women with aura cannot be on combined hormonal contraceptives (CHC) due to ↑ risk for stroke.
        - Common treatments include antihypertensives, anticonvulsants, and hormonal prophylaxis (i.e. transdermal estradiol gel 1.5mg applied 7 days starting on day 10 after ovulation and continued through the 2nd day of menstruation bleeding. Another option includes CHC throughout (skipping placebo period), ensuring at least **30** mcg of EE is prescribed. Overall goal is to prevent EE level from ↓ below 10mcg.

Hormonal Treatment Options for Menstrual Migraines		
Medication	Dose	Pearl
Continuous Formulation		
NuvaRing	Vaginal Ring	Women on the ring may notice ↑ sensitivity on week 4 and may require changing out the ring every 3 weeks as a result
Lybrel (Ashlyna)	20mcg EE+ 0.09 mg levonorgestrel once daily x 365d	
Extended Formulation		
LoSeasonique	20 mcg EE and 0.1 mg levonorgestrel for 84 d, followed by 7 d of 10 mcg EE	
Any 20-mcg EE CHC used in an extended manner	20 mcg EE used >2 mo without placebo	Add conjugated equine estrogens, 0.9 mg daily to achieve 30 mcg of EE
Any 30-mcg EE CHC used in an extended manner	30 mcg EE used >2 mo without placebo	
Monthly Formulation		
Lo Loestrin Fe 1/10	10 mcg EE and 1 mg norethindrone for 24d, f/b 10 mcg EE for 2d and then placebo for 2d	Ultralow doses may be a/w ↑ breakthrough bleeding, which may improve with time
Natazia	Gradually ↓ estradiol valerate dose from 3 to 2 to 1 mg ↑ dienogest dose from 2 to 3 mg	

Acute and chronic treatments for migraines in either inpatient or outpatient settings

Acute/Abortive

Contraindications of DHE and Triptans:
- Uncontrolled HTN, CAD, CVA, pregnant, coronary spasm
  - Causes vasoconstriction
  - Avoid concurrent use with SSRI (serotonin syndrome)

Inpatient / Clinic

- **Abortive ER Cocktail:**
  - Promethazine 25mg IM (caution with IV administration)
  - (or Reglan 10 mg IV or Chlorpromazine 0.1 mg/kg IV (to 25mg IV or IM) over 20 minutes, may repeat after 15 minutes to max of 37.5mg.
  - Pretreating with 5ml.kg of NS may prevent hypotensive effects)
  - +/-Dexamethasone 4mg
  - Toradol 15mg
  - Benadryl 50mg
- **Dihydroergotamine**
  - SQ/IM: 0.5-1mg (start with 0.33mg if first time) IM/SC/IV x1 & may be repeated in 1 hour.
  - Intranasal: 0.5mg (per actuation) q15m x2 (max 4 actuations/attack)

OR

- **Antiemetics**
  - Domperidone 10mg TID (or 60mg suppository)
  - Prochlorperazine 10mg IV, 25mg rectal, 3-6mg buccal
  - Promethazine 12.5-25mg IV (or 25mg rectal)
  - Chlorpromazine 10-25mg PO q4-6h / 12.5mg IM q30m *(also good for hiccups)*
  - Metoclopramide 10mg PO/IM/IV x1 (can give PO dose up to QID)
- **Analgesics/NSAIDs**
  - Ketorolac 60mg IM is very effective in severe cases[272]
  - Diclofenac (PO/IM) 50mg PO
  - Tylenol 325-1000mg PO q4-6h

Outpatient / Home

- **General Guidelines**
  - Triptan + NSAID
  - Triptan + Paracetamol + Anti-emetic
- **Mild (limit to <14d/month):**
  - ASA 600-900 mg PO Q 4 hours x2
  - Ibuprofen 400-800 mg PO Q 6 hours x2
  - Excedrin Migraine 2 tabs q3h (max 4 tabs/d)
  - Prodrin 1 tab q2-3h (max 3 doses)
  - Diclofenac 50mg dissolved q2-4h (max 150mg/d)
  - Ibuprofen 800mg q3h (max 2.4g)
  - Magnesium 400-500mg/d
- **Moderate:**
  - Consider DHE nasal spray as alternative.
  - Doxepin 10→25/50mg/d
  - Duloxetine 30-60mg/d

  or
  - Venlafaxine 75-200mg/d
- **Severe:**
  - Triptans
  - *Instruct patients to take up to 3x/week and alternate with NSAID; works within 2 hrs*
    - Sumatriptan 50-100 mg PO **q3h prn** (max 200mg) or nasal spray 40mg/d PLUS Aleve 440-500mg
    - Rizatriptan 10mg PO q4h prn (max 3 doses)

- Ketorolac 10mg PO q4-6h / 30mg IM or IV q6h / 60mg IM once
- Triptans
  - If patients have nausea and vomiting, use nasal formulation
  - If sx are rapidly progressing, use SQ or IN formulation; fast PO formulations are eletriptan, rizatriptan, and zolmitriptan
    - Sumatriptan 4 or 6mg SC (may repeat 6 mg SC in 1 hr. if not effective max 12mg/d). Other form is Sumatriptan PO 100mg at first visit (50mg if s/e noted) and 10mg IN
    - Rizatriptan 5-10mg (5mg if taking propranolol concurrently; 10mg if no beta blocker on board)
    - Eletriptan 40mg
    - Zolmitriptan 5mg nasal (first line tx for cluster)
    - Zolmitriptan 5mg PO (2.5mg if s/e)
    - Almotriptan 6.25mg-12.5mg PO (repeat 1x p̄ 2h)
- Zomig 2.5/5mg q3-4h prn (max 10mg/d) → nasal better for severe symptoms such as nausea/vomiting

Preventative
- Indicated if freq >2x/week or 4+ days/month or acute tx unsuccessful, prolonged auras >1hr, disabling nature of HA, interfere with daily routine.
- Consider tapering off therapy after 6-12 months of stability.
- Habits - Counsel patients on getting consistent, quality sleep and stress management with yoga or meditation.
- Dietary – missed or delayed meals are common trigger. Other triggers include caffeine, artificial sweeteners, additives (i.e. MSG)
- A common measure of success for migraine prevention is at least a 50% reduction in migraine attack frequency or days, which is the clinical trial end point recommended by the Clinical Trials Subcommittee of the International Headache Society
- Avoid OCP in patients with migraine with aura if possible.

Name	Great For	Side Effects
Depakote 250-500mg BID or Depakote ER 500-1000mg daily	Concurrent anxiety or mood stabilization	Nausea, fatigue, tremor, weight gain. Contraindicated in pregnancy!

Medication / Dosing	Notes / Side Effects
Frovatriptan 2.5mg BID	Best for **menstrual** related migraines. Best to start therapy 2 days before expected period and continue for total duration of 6 days
	Best for **menstrual** related migraines
Propranolol LA 80mg/d to max dose of 160-240mg/d	Anxiety, palpitations, **HTN**
Metoprolol succinate 100mg/d increased q1-2w to max of 200mg/d	
Timolol 5-30mg/d	Fatigue, reduced exercise tolerance, nausea, dizziness, insomnia, ED, and depression
Amitriptyline 10mg QHS ↑ by 10mg q1-2w to target dose of 20-40mg qhs	Parasthesias, depression
Fluoxetine 40mg/d	Insomnia, Anorexia, IBS, fibromyalgia
Gabapentin 300mg/d ↑ by 300mg q3-5d to target 1200-1500mg/d divided TID	drowsiness, weight gain, and dry mouth
Tizanidine 8mg TID	
Topiramate 25mg QHS ↑ by 25mg/d per week to target 100mg/daily divided BID or daily in ER formulations	Refractory migraine, aura, underweight, bipolar, depression, may ↓ effectiveness of OCP at doses ↑200mg
Magnesium Oxide 400-800mg/d (400mg BID)	Parasthesias, fatigue, anorexia, nausea, ↓concentration
Botox injections	Constipation
	>15 episodes/month (8 must be migraines) lasting 3 months duration with each HA ≥ 4 hrs/d
	Avoid s/e of other medications
Fremanezumab (single high dose of 675mg SQ quarterly or 3 monthly doses of 225mg SQ)	Patients on multiple medications (few drug-drug interactions noted)
	May work quicker than other preventive meds
Venlafaxine 37.5/d for 1 week then increase weekly by 37.5mg to target 150mg/d	Concurrent anxiety or depression
	Cardiovascular abnormalities (↑ risk if known history)
	No reversal strategy
	Beware in pts with HTN, h/o seizure disorder, and MAOI use within 14 days.
Open Label	
Pregabalin 150mg BID	Neuticeutical:
Zonisamide 100-400mg	Butterbur
Atenolol 50mg/d	Coenzyme-Q10 100mg TDS
Olanzapine 2.5-35mg/d	Riboflavin 400mg daily
	Mg 600mg/d

NEUROLOGY

PARKINSON'S DISEASE

- **Diagnosis**[273]
  o Clinical
  o Essential criterion is bradykinesia in combination with either resting tremor or rigidity
    - Supporting criteria: clear and marked improvement with dopaminergic tx
- **Clinical Features**[274,275]
  o <u>Tremor</u> – **resting** pill-rolling tremor @ 4-6hz; worse when ask patient to do mental calculations; gets worse with progression of disease
  o <u>Bradykinesia</u> – generalized slowness of movement; patient may state "I want to move; I just can't get my legs to move"; also seen as the 'shuffling gait'. Small handwriting.

Gait Type	Description
Parkinsonian	<ul><li>Patient will take small steps without raising feet</li><li>When stopping, patient appears to "freeze"</li></ul>
Senile Gait	<ul><li>"Walking on Ice"</li><li>Feet wide apart, knees and hips flexed</li><li>Walk as if they are expecting to fall</li></ul>
Spastic Paraparesis	<ul><li>Dragging of each leg with steps</li><li>No flexion of the knees</li><li>Due to circular leg movements (scissor gait)</li></ul>
Distal LMN disease	<ul><li>Steppage gait</li><li>Foot drop</li><li>Excessive elevation of legs during walking (toes touch floor before heals)</li></ul>

USMLEWorld

  o <u>Cogwheel Rigidity</u> – resistance of passive movement throughout wrist or elbow
  o <u>Postural instability</u> – ↑ tendency to fall; tested by standing behind patient and pulling their shoulders back – normal response is for pt to only have to take one step backward to get balanced whereas in PD patients may fall
  o Others
    - ↓eye blinking
    - blurred vision
    - dysphagia
    - kyphosis
    - fatigue
    - masked facies

Motor vs. Non-motor symptoms of PD	
Motor	Non-Motor
Tremor	Hyposmia
Rigidity	Depression, Anxiety, Apathy
Bradykinesia	Dementia, MCI
Postural instability	Urinary frequency, urgency
Gait disturbance (i.e. freezing)	Delayed gastric emptying
Altered blinking	Dysphagia
Micrographia	Postural orthostatic symptoms

- **Differential Diagnosis**
  o Tremors – general approach is to do the following in sequence:

1. Determine if the patient has a postural tremor (outstretched arms with palms facing straight ahead or facing down or towards each other)
2. See if there is a kinetic tremor (FTN, drawing a spiral, writing a sentence)
   - Intentional (approaching target during FTN)
3. Look for rest tremor
4. Assess for tremors in the head, jaw, chin, tongue, or voice

Differentiating Essential Tremor from Parkinson's Disease		
	Essential Tremor (ET)	Parkinson Disease (PD)
Onset of disease	Asymmetric arm involvement that is out of phase between each	Unilateral tremor, associated with stooped posture, shuffling gait, memory loss
Body affected by tremor	Postural, arms m/c then head, legs, larynx, trunk	Stooped posture, shuffling gait
Tremor characteristics	Kinetic tremor; associated with purposeful movement (i.e. utensils, writing, transferring water between cups, pouring drinks)	Tremor in arms at side @ rest
Latency period	Immediate	Longer (several seconds)

- **Causes** – r/o drug-induced (2/2 to exposure to anti-dopaminergics, anti-emetics, or neuroleptics), MSA (concurrent dysautonomia), PSP
- **Labs/Diagnostic**
  - Clinical impression
    - Bradykinesia + tremor or rigidity must be present
  - Response to DA
- **Dementia**
  - Memory difficulty, altered personality, difficulty multi-tasking
  - Lewy Body type is associated with visual hallucinations and altered cognition
- **Treatment**

Pharmacologic Management of Parkinson's Disease			
Generic name	Trade name	Starting dose	Maintenance dose
Dopamine Precursors			
Carbidopa/levodopa	Sinemet	25/100 mg TID *start ½ tab TID increase by ½ tab qweek to max 3 tabs/TID	25/250 mg TID-QID
Carbidopa/levodopa	Sinemet CR	25/100 mg TID	50/200 mg TID
Dopamine Agonists *(typically first line in <50YO, when added to precursors, decreases "off" time and manage dyskinesia)*			
Pramipexole	Mirapex	0.125 mg TID	1.5 mg TID
Ropinirole	Requip	0.25 mg TID	1.0 mg TID
Apomorphine	Apokyn	2 mg SC test dose	2 to 10 mg SC TID
Bromocriptine	Parlodel	2.5 mg daily	5 to 10 mg QID
COMT inhibitors *(commonly added to Sinemet to ↑duration of rx by 30m; reduces off time if combined with levodopa)*			
Entacapone	Comtan	200 mg with L-dopa	600 to 800 mg a day
Tolcapone	Tasmar	100 mg TID	100 to 200 mg TID
MAO-B inhibitors *(added to levodopa to reduce off time, moderate benefit in early disease)*			
Selegiline	Eldepryl	5 mg	5 mg qam
Anticholinergics			
Trihexyphenidyl	Artane	1 mg BID	2 mg BID-TID
Benztropine	Cogentin	0.5 mg BID	1 to 2 mg BID-TID
Other *(may help target tremor specifically, added after levodopa for dyskinesias)*			
Amantadine	Symmetrel	100 mg BID	100 mg BID-TID

  - Hallucinations/Delusions/Psychosis: consider pimavanserin

- Non-pharmacologic management
    - Deep Brain Stimulators (DBS) – for advanced disease; acts on STN, globus pallidus, or thalamus

SENSORY/MOTOR DEFICITS

- **History**
    - Definitive date of onset → immune, vasculitic, infectious, neoplastic
    - Stepwise progression → multiple mononeuropathies
    - Relapsing/Remitting → MS, intermittent exposure, CIDP
    - Positive symptoms (burning, tingling, shooting)→ think acquired
    - Loss of symptoms (feel lack of sensation, thick layers on top of skin) → think genetic/inherited
- **Large vs Small Fiber Neuropathies**
    - Large → proprioception, vibration; loss of reflexes, abnormal EMG, weakness
    - Small → pain, temperature
- **Localization**
    - Supratentorial (cerebral cortex and subcortical regions, including the basal ganglia, hypothalamus, and thalamus)
    - Posterior fossa (cerebellum, brainstem, and cranial nerves)
    - Spinal cord (including extramedullary, intramedullary, cauda equina, and conus medullaris lesions)
    - Peripheral
        - Peripheral are divided by the following:
            1. Pattern
                - Length-dependent* vs length independent vs multifocal
            2. Modality
                - Sensory* vs motor vs autonomic
        *most common
- **Differential Diagnosis**
    - Peripheral Neuropathy – toxic medication s/e (i.e. amiodarone, colchicine, hydralazine), vitamin b12 deficiency, hyperglycemia/type 2 diabetes, MGUS, hereditary (CMT), chemotherapy, amyloidosis
- **Diagnostic Testing**
    - 128 Hz tuning fork and monofilament >90% sensitivity for peripheral neuropathy
    - Ankle reflexes
    - Labs (peripheral neuropathy)
        - Highest yield: fasting glucose, monoclonal protein (immunofixation>SPEP), B12
            1. Consider adding MMA>homocysteine esp. in VB12 that are low-normal (200-500 mcg/mL)
        - Others to consider: CMP, ESR, TSH, Lyme, HIV, tissue-transglutaminase, Vitamin-E, Copper
    - Studies – EMG (helps define axonal vs demyelinating and severity)
    - Imaging
        - CT is a good starting point for TIA/Stroke for acute hemorrhage
        - MRI - far superior in hyperacute stages
- **UMN vs. LMN**
    - UMN damage occurs above the red nucleus resulting in a decorticate posture (with arms flexed and hands fisted)

- o LMN damage occurs below the red nucleus and above the vestibulospinal and reticulospinal tracts resulting in a decerebrate posture

Differentiating UMN vs. LMN disease		
	UMN	LMN
Location	Cerebral cortex	Brain stem, cranial nerves
Tone	↑	↓
Fasciculations	None	Present
Muscle	No atrophy, stiff	Atrophied, weak
Babinski	Present	Negative
Reflexes	Increased/Clonus	Decreased
Pattern of weakness	Pyramidal/regional	Distal/segmental
Hoffman	+	-
Spasticity	+	-

- **When to refer**
  - o Peripheral neuropathy
    - Acute or subacute onset
    - Progressive
    - Functionally limiting

SEIZURE

- **Defined**
  - o Epileptic seizure – transient occurrence of signs and/or symptoms due to abnormal excessive or synchronous neuronal activity in the brain
  - o Epilepsy – at least 2 unprovoked seizures on separate days, generally 24/h apart
  - o Status epilepticus – single seizure episode lasting 5+ minutes or 2 or more sequential seizures without full recovery of consciousness
- **Questions to ask**
  - o Current or new medications (i.e. Wellbutrin, tramadol)
  - o History of childhood/febrile seizures or even seizures as an adult
  - o Family history?
  - o History of head trauma (fx; TBI does not necessarily ↑ risk)
  - o Does the patient recall any part of the event?
  - o Any warning signs prior to event
  - o Any witnesses
  - o Incontinence, lateral tongue/cheek biting?
- **Admission Criteria**[276,277]
  - o First unprovoked non-recurrent seizure evaluation:
    - Clinically significant abnormality on neuroimaging or labs which require admission
    - Abnormality on neurologic exam/failure to return to baseline status
    - Patient does not have a responsible adult to stay with for 24hrs following discharge
    - Patient has not been given written instructions regarding driving and duty restrictions
  - o Second (or more) unprovoked recurrent seizure not on medication:
    - MRI Brain and/or EEG has not been performed
    - Abnormality on neuroimaging or labs which require admission
    - Abnormality on neurologic exam/failure to return to baseline status
    - Patient does not have a responsible adult to stay with for 24hrs following discharge
    - Patient has not been given written instructions regarding driving and duty restrictions

- AED therapy can be started in the ER (initiation of therapy alone does not require admission)
- If admitted neurology will consult in the inpatient setting
- **Etiology**
  - Toxic-Metabolic
    - Systemic illness- hypoglycemia, hyperglycemia, hypoxia, hypocalcemia, hyponatremia, hypomagnesemia, uremia, hepatic failure, TTP, Whipple's.
    - Drugs or toxins – cocaine, amphetamine, PCP, lead, TCAs, PCN
    - Withdrawal syndromes – EtOH, hypnotics
  - Acquired structural lesions
    - Infection – brain abscess, meningitis, encephalitis (HSV), AIDS, syphilis, post infectious encephalitis
    - Vascular – vasculitis (SLE), ischemic CVA, hemorrhagic CVA, central venous thrombosis, AVM
    - Trauma - SDH
    - Malignancy – primary, hamartomas
    - Other – temporal sclerosis, Alzheimer's, CJD, paraneoplastic d/o, limbic encephalitis, MS
    - Autoimmune – NMDA encephalitis
  - Familial
  - Genetic – tuberous sclerosis, NF, phenylketonuria
- Provoked – occurring within 7 days of acute brain insult secondary to:
  - Structural – head injury, NS intervention, stroke, CNS infection, malignancy
  - Metabolic/toxic – EtOH w/d, liver or kidney failure

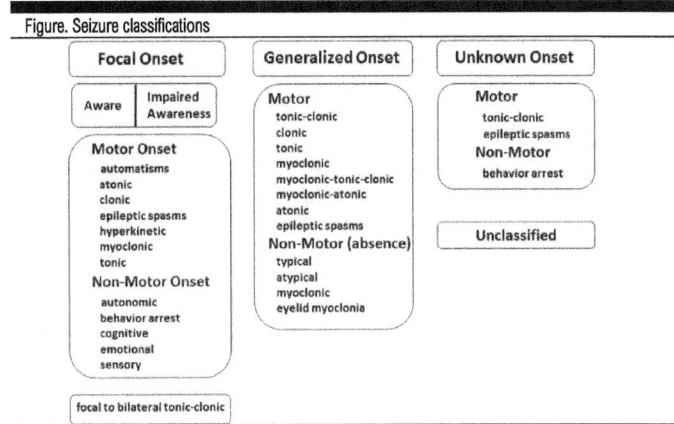

Figure. Seizure classifications

- **Types**
  - Acute
  - Symptomatic – occur in the setting of EtoH w/d, hypoglycemia, head trauma
  - Unprovoked – absence of provoking factors
- **Classification Scheme**
  Epileptic seizures are classified by whether or not the seizure is localized to 1 area of a lobe (focal) or is widespread, involving both cerebral hemispheres (generalized)
  - Focal (originates in a single focus; can become generalized; most commonly affecting the temporal lobe). Can be seen with meningitis or encephalitis, temporal lobe seizures

- *Simple* – no loss of consciousness; motor/sensory/ or autonomic phenomena are in the beginning; affect only single cortex region (face, limb), sweating, vomiting. May end in Todd's Paralysis which may be an indication of an underlying brain mass.
- *Complex* – partial seizures with impaired consciousness; also begin with an aura which then leads to loss of consciousness; characterized by coordinated involuntary muscle movements (automatism)
- Partial seizures with secondary generalization
  - Generalized
    - *Tonic clonic* – loss of consciousness without warning aura; patients will have stiffening and bilateral tonic-clonic activity is observed. Typically, metabolic or toxic cause, meningitis, or encephalitis.
    - *Absence* – m/c in childhood with rare occurrence in adolescence; brief LOC with eye blinking, rare loss of motor tone, immobile
      - Typical
      - Atypical
      - Absence with special features (myoclonic, eyelid myoclonia)
    - *Myoclonic* – single or repetitive jerks are observed; usually bilateral and involving face, trunk, UE, very brief lasting <1s with no post-ictal confusion
  - Focal – may or may not have impairment of consciousness or awareness; may have Todd's paralysis after event
  - Unknown
  - Status Epilepticus
    - Seizures prolonging for ≥ 30 minutes without spontaneous cease
- **Phases**
  - Tonic phase – contraction of limbs flexion then extension of the back and neck, tongue biting occurs with contraction of mastication muscles; may become cyanotic
  - Clonic phase – alternative contraction and relaxation for additional 30-60s ending with flaccid muscles, urinary incontinence can occur d/t effects on detrusor muscle
- **Clinical Symptoms**
  - Generalized seizures → think metabolic or toxic encephalopathy. HSV encephalitis,
  - Focal → nonketotic hyperglycemia, post hypoxic coma, meningitis, encephalitis, temporal lobe (auras present as nausea, GI complaints, visual or auditory hallucinations, déjà vu, olfactory sensation).
- **Diagnosis/Workup**
  - EEG
    - The EEG (routine) should be considered as part of the neuro diagnostic evaluation of the adult with an apparent unprovoked first seizure because it has a substantial yield (Level B)
    - Only 1/3 will be abnormal
    - Can help not only classify the type of seizure but also beneficial for surgical localization
  - Neuroimaging
    - Brain imaging using CT or MRI should be considered as part of the neurodiagnostic evaluation of adults presenting with an apparent unprovoked first seizure (Level B).
  - Labs
    - Blood glucose, RPR, UDS, CBC, and electrolyte panels (particularly sodium, mg, Ca), toxicology screening, LFTs
    - Prolactin is nonspecific!
  - Lumbar Puncture
    - Helpful in patients who are febrile, but there are insufficient data to support or refute recommending routine lumbar puncture (Level U).
- **Treatment/Prophylaxis (see table on next page)**

AED by seizure type

Seizure type	Presentation	First-line drugs	Adjuvant drugs	Drugs to avoid
Generalized tonic-clonic	Initial general muscle stiffening, jerking of limbs in rhythmic pattern	Carbamazepine Lamotrigine Oxcarbazepine Valproic acid	Lamotrigine Levetiracetam Valproic acid Topiramate	Gabapentin Phenytoin Vigabatrin
Tonic or atonic	Sudden and general stiffening of muscles for about a minute. Atonic is when you suddenly lose muscle tone	Valproic acid	Lamotrigine	Gabapentin Carbamazepine Oxcarbazepine Pregabalin
Absense	Seizure with arrest of current behavior	Lamotrigine Valproic Acid	Ethosuximide Lamotrigine Valproic acid	Carbamezepine Phenytoin
Focal	Seizure limited to one hemisphere, localized or widely distributed	Carbamezapine Lamotrigine Levetiracetam Oxcarbazepine Valproic acid	Carbamezapine Gabapentin Lamotrigine Topiramate	N/A
Myoclonic	Sudden and short jerking movements	Levetiracetam Valproic acid Topiramate	Levetiracetam Valproic Acid	Gabapentin Oxcarbazepine Phenytoin

- o Initiating AED reduces risk of recurrence by 35% within the first 2 years
- o Treatment Physiology
    - Benzodiazepines enhance neurotransmission of GABA at the GABAA receptor, increasing the frequency of chloride ion channel opening in response to GABA.
    - Valproate prolongs sodium channel inactivation, attenuates calcium mediated transient currents and augments GABA.
- o Treatment aimed at seizure freedom with no side effects
- o In women of child-bearing age, add folic acid 1mg/d (do not use pre-natal vitamin only)
    - If using contraception, avoid enzyme inducer medications such as Phenobarbital, phenytoin, carbamazepine, and primidone as they ↓ efficacy of OCP
    - Combined OCPs can ↓ lamotrigine levels by up to 50%
- o Anti-epileptic drug therapy (AED) often for those with ≥ 2 unprovoked seizures or a single seizure with high risk occupation or (i.e. bus driver) high risk for recurrence (abnormal EEG, abnormal MRI, nocturnal occurrence) or known structural abnormality (CT or MRI).
    - After first unprovoked seizure, however, consider pros and cons of starting AED
- **Status Epilepticus**
  - o *Defined* – continuous convulsive seizure ≥5 minutes or > 2 seizures w/o resolution of postictal encephalopathy
  - o *Orders*
    - Bedside glucose, serum glucose, ABG, U&E, Ca, FBC, ECG
    - Consider anticonvulsant levels, tox screen, LP, BCx, UCx, EEG, CT head, CO level
    - Pulse ox and continuous cardiac monitoring

Pharmacologic Management of Epilepsy

Drug	Doses	Loading / Initial Dose[1]	Maint. Dose[1]	Therapeutic Serum Levels	Pearl
Narrow spectrum for Focal Seizure (in order of selection)					
Lamotrigine (Lamictal) *First line for focal epilepsy; can be used in generalized seizure as well*	50, 100, 200 mg	25 mg twice a day then slowly increase[2]	200-500 mg/day in two doses[2]	3-15 g/mL*	Broad spectrum; good for concurrent mood d/o
Carbamazepine (Tegretol) *S/E include SJS esp. in Asian pop., not good to use with OCP*	200, 300 mg; XR: 100, 200, 400 mg	400mg divided 2-4 doses; increase q2-3w for max 2400mg	400-1,600 mg/day in 2-4 doses, or in 2 doses if XR form	4-12 mcg/mL	Narrow spectrum (used for focal onset seizure); good for concurrent migraine d/o, ↓Na, ↑LFT, ↑PR interval, ↓Na
Levetiracetam (Keppra) *S/E include aplastic anemia, ↓WBC, rash (SJS), S/E include GI upset*	250, 500, 750 mg	250-500 mg twice a day	1,000-3,000 mg/day in two doses	10-60 mcg/mL*	Broad spectrum. Good for women of childbearing age
Phenytoin (Dilantin) *S/E include gum hyperplasia, SJS, cerebellar atrophy* *Fosphenytoin is form for IM or IV use*	100 mg; 30, 50 mg also available	Oral loading: 15mg/kg TID over 9-12 hours; Intravenous loading: 15 mg/kg (not more than 50 mg/m)	300-400 mg/day in a single dose or divided doses	10-20 mcg/mL	Narrow spectrum (used for focal onset seizure)
Oxcarbazepine (Trileptal) *S/E include ↓Na, rash, ↑LFT*	150, 300, 600 mg	600mg BID	Increase by 300mg as tolerated q3d to max dose 1200mg (or as tolerated)	12-35 mcg/mL*	Narrow spectrum (used for focal onset seizure)
Phenobarbital (Luminal) *S/E include rash, SJS*	15, 30, 60, 100 mg	180 mg twice a day for 3 days or same as maintenance dose	90-180 mg/day in a single dose	15-40 mcg/mL	Broad spectrum
Lacosamide (Vimpat) *S/E include diplopia, dizziness, fatigue, HA, n/v, sedation*	10 mg/mL	100mg once or in 2 divided doses	Increase by 100mg q1-2w as tolerated (Max 600mg)	1-10 mcg/mL	May be affected when combined with sodium channel blockers†
Broad spectrum for Generalized, Focal, or Unknown-Type Seizure (in order of selection)					
Valproic acid (Depakote, Depakene) *First line for generalized epilepsy*	125, 250	15 mg/kg/d (500-1000mg) BID-TID and increase by 5-10mg/kg/d	-----	50-100 mcg/mL	Broad spectrum; good for concurrent mood and HA d/o; do DEXA scan if on

S/E include ↑LFTs, ↑NH3, ↑wt, ↓hair, SJS, osteoporosis, tremor		**every week as needed (max 60mg/kg/d; 3000-5000mg)**			for 3-5 years. **Avoid in pregnancy**
Lamotrigine(Lamictal) *First line for focal epilepsy; can be used in generalized seizure as well* *S/E include **SJS esp. in Asian pop.**, not good to use with OCP*	50, 100, 200 mg	Taking enzyme-inducing AED 25 mg twice a day then slowly increase by 50mg increments every 1-2 weeks as needed[2] Taking Valproate 25mg QOD with increases of 25-50mg every 2 weeks prn to max as noted to right	300-500 mg/day in two doses[2]	3-15 mcg/mL*	Broad spectrum; good for concurrent mood d/o
Topamax(Topiramate) *S/E include nephrolithiasis, metabolic acidosis, hyperthermia, AACG, dizziness*	25, 50, 100, 150, 200	25-50mg/d	Increase as tolerated by 50mg at weeks 2, 3 and 4 then from that point, increase by 100mg at weeks 5 and 6 (max 400mg/d)	5-20 mcg/mL	Weight loss can be used for migraine prophylaxis, diabetic neuropathy, bipolar disorder, EtOH dependence. Associated with teratogenicity.
Levetiracetam(Keppra) *S/E include GI upset*	250, 500, 750 mg	500-1000mg BID	Increase as tolerated every 2 weeks until response (max dose 4000mg)	10-60 mcg/mL*	Broad spectrum. Good for women of childbearing age

†Mediations that inhibit voltage-gated sodium channels include primidone, phenytoin, carbamazepine, valproic acid, lamotrigine, topiramate, oxcarbazepine, Zonisamide, rufinamide, lacosamide, and eslicarbazepine

Status epilepticus treatment[278]

Time	Phase	Treatment
0-5min	STABILIZATION PHASE	Stabilize patient via monitoring of O2 sat, ECG, establishing IV access Labs: CBC, CHEM7, AED, UDS, ABG, TOX screen 50cc D50W if finger glucose < 60mg/dl f/b Thiamine 200mg IV, Consider naloxone 0.4-2mg IV added to D5 if history suggests

5-20min	INITIAL THERAPY PHASE	**CONSIDER INTUBATION, EEG, AND ICU TRANSFER**
		• Consider intubation
		• Give thiamine 200mg IV and D50W 50cc
		
		FIRST GIVE….
		IV ACCESS: Lorazepam 2mg IV bolus (follow with sequential boluses every 5 minutes for total of 0.1mg/kg)
		NO IV ACCESS: Diazepam 20mg (or 0.2mg/kg) PR or Midazolam 10mg IN/IM (repeat after 10 min if necessary)
		THEN GIVE….
		• Fosphenytoin: Load 20 mg/kg PE* IV at max 150 mg/min. Keep on cardiac monitoring (goal therapeutic level: 22-25 μg/mL). Start maintenance 12-24h after load.
		   o May give an additional 5-10 PE/kg IV if no response
		   o Maintenance @ 5-7mg PE/kg/d divided q8h dosing
		Alternatives
		   o Valproate 20-30mg/kg IV over 15-20 min can be given if patient is allergic to phenytoin. Therapeutic level is 70-140. May give an additional 500 mg after 20 min. Maintenance rate at 15-20mg/kg/d given in 8-hour intervals with first maintenance dose started 6 hours after initial load.
		   o Levetiracetam 20-30mg/kg over 5-15min (maintenance dosing started 12h later at 500-1500mg BID)
		   o Dilantin 1,000 mg IV at <50 mg/min. May give an additional 500 mg IV if no response after 20 min. (Note: Do not give w/ glucose or dextrose due to precipitation.)
		   o Propofol 15mg/kg IV followed by 0.5-4 mg/kg/h
		• Levels should be checked >2 h after an IV load or >4 h after an IM load.

IV Access Available	No IV Access Available
Drip	Midazolam 10mg IN

Phase	Time	Treatment
SECOND THERAPY PHASE (refractory S.E.)	20-40min	Lorazepam 0.1mg/kg (@ 2mg/min; max 4mg) may repeat once Diazepam 0.15-0.2 mg/kg (max 10mg/dose) may repeat once IV phenobarbital 15mg/kg/dose x1 Diazepam 0.2-0.5mg/kg PR (max 20mg) over 5 minutes x1 Versed 5 mg IM if no IV access **Non-Drip** Lorazepam 2mg IV over 2min max 0.1-1.5mg/kg - IV Midazolam (load with 0.2mg/kg then infuse at 0.05-2 mg/kg/h)
THIRD THERAPY PHASE	40-60min	*Other Options* - IV propofol: Load 1-2 mg/kg; repeat 1-2 mg/kg boluses every 3-5 min until seizures stop, up to a maximum total loading dose of 10 mg/kg. Initial IV rate: 2 mg/kg/h. IV dose range: 1-15 mg/kg/h. If still having seizures, switch to midazolam, valproate, or pentobarbital. - IV Ketamine 5mg/kg/h - IV levetiracetam 60mg/kg max 4500mg/dose x 1 (47% recovered at 60m) - IV valproate: 40 mg/kg over ~10 min max 3000mg/dose x1 (46% recovered at 60m) - IV fosphenytoin 20mg phenytoin equivalents/kg IV max 1500mg PE/dose x 1 (45% recovered at 60m) - IV phenobarbital: 20 mg/kg @ 50-75 mg/min - IV pentobarbital: Load 5 mg/kg at up to 50 mg/min; repeat 5 mg/kg boluses until seizures stop. Initial IV rate: 1 mg/kg/h. IV dose range: 0.5-10 mg/kg/h; traditionally titrated to burst suppression on EEG but titrating to seizure suppression is reasonable as well. Therapeutic level: 30-45 mcg/mL. - Pt will need to be admitted to an intensive care unit. Begin EEG monitoring as soon as possible if patient does not rapidly awaken or if any continuous IV Rx is used. - Consider CT brain or MRI brain. Evaluate for & correct underlying causes.

*PE = phenytoin equivalents; 75mg of Fosphenytoin = 50mg of phenytoin

NEUROLOGY

- o When patient has stopped...
  - Phenytoin or Fosphenytoin (preferred) 20 mg/kg IV in 3 doses @ 50 mg/min (25 mg/min in cardiac pt) over 2 hours (any shorter you ↑ risk for cardiac rhythm disturbances). Again, can use valproic acid if allergies exist to above.
  - Ensure glucose and thiamine were already given
  - Consider EEG
  - Consider MRI, brain
  - Must give while on cardiac monitor (may prolong QRS)
    1. If either Phenytoin or Fosphenytoin ineffective then try Phenobarbital
  - Phenobarbital 20 mg/kg @ 100 mg/min
    1. May repeat up to 30 mg/kg
    2. May cause ↓BP and depressed respirations
- o Risk for seizure recurrence
  - +EEG
  - Abnormal brain imaging
  - Nocturnal seizure

UNRESPONSIVE PATIENT

- **Common Causes**
  - o Hypoglycemia
  - o CVA/subdural hematoma
  - o Postictal state
  - o Cardiovascular (↓BP, arrhythmia)
  - o Drug (narcotic, sedative, EtOH)
  - o Metabolic/respiratory encephalopathy
  - o CNS tumor/meningitis
- **Questions to Ask**
  - o Any recent narcotics, sedatives, falls? Hx of DM? *Think D50, Narcan*
  - o History of alcoholism? *Think thiamine*
  - o Any trauma? *Think CT head, c-spine precautions*
  - o History of depression? *Think overdose*
- **Exam**
  - o Vital signs
    - Clear the airway, stabilize c-spine if necessary
    - If inadequate ventilation with O2, use NRB
    - ↑RR → obstructed airway, aspiration, PNA, DKA
    - ↓RR → poisoning, ↑ICP
    - ↓HR → hypoxia, CHB, ↑ICP, digoxin
    - ↑HR → airway obstruction, pain, ↓volume, SVT, VT, AF
    - Rectal temp (coma common in T<86F)
  - o Physical Exam
    - Neuro Exam
      □ Measure GCS score
      □ Limb strength, muscle tone and reflexes, neck stiffness (except in neck injury).
      □ Lateralizing signs - facial or limb weakness, may be caused by a stroke, intracranial bleeding or preexisting problems
      □ Ocular nerve palsy or divergent squint with coma s/o Wernicke's encephalopathy
      □ Look for signs of seizure activity which may indicate non-convulsive status epilepticus.
- **Interventions**
  - o Make sure there is IV access.

- **Treatment**
  (airway→breathing→circulation)
  - Diagnostics
    - Consider ECG, CXR
    - CT head to r/o SAH, CVA, injury
  - Labs
    - Get a stat fingerstick, Chem 7, ABG, UDS
  - Medications
    - Coma cocktail:
      - Dextrose 1 amp
      - O2
      - **Naloxone**
        - Remember that Narcan may need to be repeated multiple times in patients with fentanyl overdose.
        - Titrate effect to RR of ≥12
          - Dosing:
            - *IV/IM/SQ*: Narcan 0.4mg (can do 0.2mg initially if patient is opiate naïve) repeated q2-3 minutes in escalating doses (0.9mg/2mg/4mg/10mg/15mg)
              - Apnea/cardiac arrest/very low RR patients: bag mask ventilation and start dose at 2mg (or 0.005-0.1 mg/kg q2-3m)
              - At 10-15mg, if no improvement, consider alternative causes
            - *Intranasal*: 2mg/4mg intranasal repeated q3-5 minutes until effect (1 spray in 1 nostril, new spray canister per attempt). Not as effective as IM form.[279]
            - *Drip*: often done in patients on methadone; use 2/3 of total effective dose of naloxone per hour (typically 0.25-6.25mg/hr) and provide ½ of that bolus dose about 15 minutes after starting the drip to prevent a drop in naloxone levels
    - Thiamine 100mg IV
    - Magnesium 1-2g IV in alcoholics
    - Ceftriaxone IV if meningitis suspected

STROKE

- **Evaluation**[280,281,282,283,284,285,286,287]
  - If any of these signs are present, the probability of a stroke is 72%[288]
    - Facial droop: Ask patient to smile; sign is present if one side does not move as well as the other
    - Arm drift: Ask patient to close eyes and hold arms out for 10 s; sign is present if one arm does not move or drifts downward
    - Abnormal speech: Sign is present if the patient slurs speech or uses wrong words
  - Obtain vitals including oxygen saturation. Keep patient on a continuous cardiac monitor and obtain frequent vital sign measurements and neurologic checks every 1-2 hours.
  - Blood glucose check: Keep BS <200 avoiding dextrose-containing solutions for the first 24 hours.
  - In young women presenting with stroke like symptoms and predominant headache consider cerebral venous thrombosis.
- **Types (*TOAST*)**
  - Cardioembolic, small vessel (lacunar), large vessel (carotid or intracranial), cryptogenic (no etiology identified), other (drug induced, carotid dissection)

- Ischemic (83%) – large vessel (ICA, basal ganglia, cerebellar), small vessel (i.e. lacunar), embolic, unknown
  - Lacunar (25%)
    1. Pure motor or pure sensory
    2. Face-arm or arm-leg syndromes
  - Atherothrombotic large vessel (20%)
  - Embolism (20-30%) – associated with higher risk of hemorrhagic transformation
  - Cryptogenic (30%)
- Hemorrhagic (17%)
  - Types
    1. ICH (59%) – HTN, amyloid, anticoagulants, tumors, avm, aneurysm, IVDA
    2. SAH (41%)
  - Risk factors on admission (3/4 = 99% spec for hemorrhage):
    1. Vomiting
    2. Headache
    3. Elevated WBC
    4. Decline in neurological status within 3 hours of admission
    5. Decreased LOC
- CVT[289]
  - Risk factors associated with thrombogenic states (pregnancy, hypercoagulable d/o, trauma, stasis, OCP)
  - Symptoms
    1. HA (diffuse, progresses in severity over weeks)
    2. Papilledema (d/t ↑ICP; consider in patients who present with sx c/w PTC/IIH)
    3. Neurological signs: hemiparesis, aphasia
- **Etiology**
  - AF (15-20%)
  - Anticoagulation (hemorrhagic type)
  - HTN
  - DM
  - Tobacco use
  - HLD
- **Examination**
  - History and Physical: focus on when symptoms began (i.e. when patient was last known to be symptom/deficit free as this will determine possible eligibility for thrombolytics), look for focal neurologic findings
    - Supinator
    - Spinatus (tests by external rotation)
    - Wrist flexors
    - Fingers
    - Psoas
    - Dorsiflexion (tests by heel walk)
  - Mimic: look for Bell's Palsy which presents with facial paralysis (upper **and** lower) along with often a change in taste perception and hearing. Treatment with steroids recommended.
- **Determining severity of stroke in acute setting**
  The NIHSS was developed to help physicians objectively determine the severity of an ischemic stroke. The higher the score, the larger the stroke likely to be found on imaging. Must be performed within 48 hours of presentation.
  - Based on NIHSS score
    - *Minor*: NIHSS score ≤ 3
    - *Moderate*: NIHSS score 15-24

NEUROLOGY

- *Severe*: NIHSS score ≥ 25
- *Severity*: NIH stroke scale recommended & document vitals and time
  o <u>Based on ABC/2 score</u> – see page 454

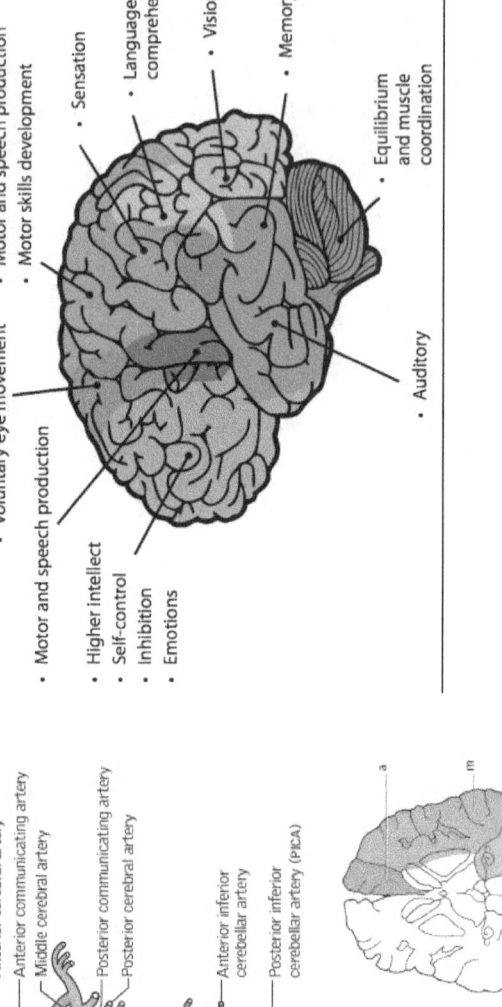

Figure. Arteries of the brain and associated distributions

Figure. Regions of the brain and associated functions

Clinical symptoms based on arterial involvement in stroke

Artery	Findings
Anterior Cerebral	Legs weaker than arms, frontal lobe signs (agitation, lack of motivation)
Middle Cerebral	Aphasia (if dominant side i.e. R sided weakness, then expect aphasia),
	Arms weaker than legs
	Contralateral hemiplegia and hemianopia
	Unilateral neglect (if R MCA affected)
Posterior Cerebral	Visual hemianopia
Basilar	Cortical blindness (blind with preserved pupillary reflexes)
	Same side (L or R) should be affected on each eye's field of vision
Vertebral	The most common clinical features included
	• vertigo (57%) (do HINTS exam)
	• unilateral facial paresthesia (46%)
	• cerebellar signs (33%)
	• lateral medullary signs (26%)
	• visual field defects (15%).
Brain Stem	Quadriplegia
	Hemiparesis
	Double vision
	Impaired swallowing → often require intubation
	Sensory loss across entire half of body

NEUROLOGY

- **Location**
  - Large vessel vs. small vessel (lacunes)
  - Large vessel: arm/face>leg or leg>arm/face with sensory **and** motor
    - 2/2 thrombosis of intracranial vessels or embolus from aortic arch, carotids
  - Small vessel: arm/leg/face equal with sensory **or** motor
    - 2/2 lipohyalinosis, HTN, DM2
    - Modify stroke RF's: LDL, BP, diabetes, smoking
- **History**
  - Sx c/w hemorrhagic include HA, meningismus, vomiting, coma
  - HA should make you consider hemorrhagic vs hemiplegic migraine if hx of migraine w/aura
  - Trauma → r/o SAH
  - Young patient → always consider CVT
- **Disposition location**
  - Ward/Tele – no risk for cerebellar involvement, no hemorrhage
  - PCU – concern for cerebellar involvement (and thus herniation)
- **Management**
  - Labs
    - ICU Panel → glucose level required prior to any TPA
    - Lipid panel (LDL goal <70 mg/dL)[290]
    - ECG
    - TROP
    - A1c
    - CBC
    - ESR/CRP if considering CVT
    - Hypercoagulable w/u if considering CVT
    - Coagulation panel
    - Oxygen saturation
    - Selected patients
      1. Toxicology screen
      2. Blood alcohol level
      3. Pregnancy test
      4. Arterial blood gas tests (if hypoxia is suspected)
  - Imaging
    - **CT**
      1. **NCCT scan within 20 minutes of arrival**
      2. **CTA should be obtained in patients presenting within 6-24 hours of symptoms with evidence of large vessel occlusion in the anterior circulation**
    - **MRI/DWI** of brain and MRA of brain and neck
      - In patients with AIS who awake with stroke symptoms or have unclear time of onset > 4.5 hours from last known well or at baseline state, MRI to identify diffusion-positive FLAIR-negative lesions can be useful for selecting those who can benefit from IV alteplase administration within 4.5 hours of stroke symptom recognition *(WAKE-UP)*
        - DW-MRI lesion must be smaller than 1/3 of the MCA territory and FLAIR shows no signal change.
    - TTE
      1. Aortic atherosclerotic plaque
      2. Left atrial enlargement
      3. Left ventricular hypertrophy
      4. ASD/PFO
    - Carotid US *(NACET)*

1. Patients with carotid artery stenosis should be tx with ASA, high-dose statin and referred to vascular surgery for endarterectomy if high grade lesion (70-99%) in the 1-2 weeks following hospitalization.
     - Patients that are candidates include those with TIA or ischemic stroke within the distribution of the affected vessel.
- ECG, CXR
- Consider CT angiogram to r/o aneurysmal source if hemorrhagic stroke noted
o Orders
    - Telemetry
    - NPO
    - Maintain oxygen $\geq$ 94%
    - Walk with assist
o Consults
    - **Swallow evaluation** - to reduce risk of aspiration and pneumonia, ALL patients with stroke should have swallowing evaluated
        o Nutrition should be given within 7 days of stroke
    - PT/OT
    - Neurology

Criteria for determining thrombolytic use (TPA) in Ischemic strokes

Inclusion criteria	Exclusion criteria
1. Age >18 years	1. NIH stroke scale 0-5 (nondisabling)
2. Clinical diagnosis of ischemic stroke with a defined onset of symptoms <3 hours from time TPA is to be started	2. INR>1.7
3. IV TPA may be helpful if given within 4.5 hours of recognition of symptoms with imaging confirming acute ischemic stroke, DW-MRI lesion is < 1/3 of the MCA territory, and FLAIR shows no signal change	3. PLT<100
	4. Seizure at onset or low glucose
	5. Recent surgery or hemorrhage
	6. ICH present
4. NIH stroke scale >5	7. Recent stroke or head trauma (in past 3 months)
5. CT scan shows no evidence of intracranial hemorrhage	8. Recent heparin use in past 48 hours
	9. SBP>185, DBP>110
	10. Hypoglycemic (<50)
	11. Recent surgery in past 3 months
	12. Some consider avoiding if NIHSS score of >22 due to ↑ risk for hemorrhagic conversion

BP in Ischemic Stroke[251]

No-TPA

First 48 hours goal:
- No thrombectomy: Systolic BP <220 mm Hg; diastolic BP <120 mm Hg with ↓ by 15-20% over 24h
- Thrombectomy planned: goals ≤185/110, then ≤180/105 during procedure and 24h after

***If blood pressure drops below 120/80; intravenous crystalloids should be given (assuming no evidence of CHF present) to maintain perfusion

Further Management:
All patients get ASA 325mg/d within 48 hours
Systolic BP >220 mm Hg or diastolic BP 121–140 mm Hg
1. Labetalol 10–20 mg IV over 1–2 min. May repeat or double every 10 min to a maximum dose

TPA

Indications:
0-3 hours: IV-TPA
3-6 hours: IV-TPA ** controversial
**TPA given within 4.5h of recognition of stroke sx can be considered
6-16 hours: mechanical embolectomy (ACA occlusion and meet DAWN or DEFUSE 3 criteria)
>8 hours: anticoagulation/antiplatelet

Pretreatment:
Glucose should be checked
SBP <185 or diastolic <110 (if you cannot meet this goal, do NOT start TPA)
- Labetalol 10-20mg IV over 1-2min may repeat 1x
- Nicardipine 5mg/h IV; titrate up by 2.5mg/h every 5-15min; max 15mg/h

of 300 mg
2. Nicardipine 5 mg/h IV infusion as initial dose; titrate to desired effect by increasing by 2.5 mg/h every 5 min to maximum of 15 mg/h (target 10%–15% reduction **in first 24 hours**)
3. Nitroprusside 0.5 microm/kg/min IV; titrate to goal

Diastolic BP >140 mm Hg
- Sodium nitroprusside 0.5 microm/kg per min IV with continuous BP monitoring (target 10%–15% reduction)
- Clevidipine 1-2mg/h IV; titrate by doubling dose q2-5min (max 21mg/h)
- Others: hydralazine, enalaprilat

During and After TPA:
- Blood Pressure Management
  o Goal <180/105 for first 24h
    Measure BP every 15 minutes for 2 hours → then every 30 minutes for 6 hours → then hourly for 16 hours
- Other Monitoring
  o If the patient develops severe headache, acute hypertension, nausea, or vomiting or has a worsening neurological examination, discontinue the infusion (if IV alteplase is being administered) and obtain emergency head CT scan.
  o Delay placement of nasogastric tubes, indwelling bladder catheters, or intraarterial pressure catheters if the patient can be safely managed without them
  o Obtain a follow-up CT or MRI scan at 24 h after IV alteplase before starting anticoagulants or antiplatelet agents

Further Management:
SBP 180-230 or DBP 105-120
- IV 10 mg labetalol over 1–2 min; may repeat or double labetalol q10min to a maximum dose of 300 mg or can start with the initial bolus dose of labetalol and then follow-up with a continuous labetalol infusion administered at a rate of 2–8 mg/min
- Nicardipine 5 mg/h IV infusion as initial dose, titrate by increasing 2.5 mg/h q 5 min to maximum of 15 mg/h.
- If the blood pressure is not controlled with above two, consider starting an infusion of sodium nitroprusside

DBP >140
- Nitroprusside 0.5 mc/kg/min IV infusion; titrate as desired

Intracranial Bleeding After TPA

1. Stop Alteplase
2. Obtain labs: CBC, Coags, T&C, Fibrinogen
3. NCCT stat
4. Consult neurology + heme/onc
5. Cryoprecipitate 10U IV over 10-30m with additional dose if fibrinogen <150 mg/dL
6. Tranexamic acid 1000 mg IV infused over 10 min OR ε-aminocaproic acid 4–5 g over 1 h, followed by 1 g IV until bleeding is controlled (peak onset in 3 h)
7. Monitor BP, ICP, CPP, MAP, temperature, and glucose

NEUROLOGY

Treatment of Acute Ischemic Stroke

Category	Intervention
Blood Pressure	See above depending on intervention given; in general, reduce BP by 15%. Consider restarting home medications if BP is >140/90 in the hospital.
Glucose	Insulin if BG>140-180 mg/dL; replace K if also giving insulin! Avoid BG<60 mg/dL
Antiplatelet[292]	• Do not give IV ASA within 90 minutes of tPA • Give ASA 325mg then 81mg/d within 24-48h of AIS, delay 24 hours if TPA given (*CAST*). Studied dose of ASA suggests 162-325mg however most will use 81mg/d. • Add Plavix (300mg for *CHANCE*, 600mg for *POINT*) load then 75mg/d) if minor CVA (NIHSS <3) or TIA within 24 hours of admission and continue for 21 days then stop (*CAPRIE, FASTER, CHANCE, POINT*) or continue combined for 90 days (*POINT*) but increased bleeding risk observed. CVA while on ASA • Clopidogrel 75mg monotherapy or ASA+dipyridamole 25/200mg are both better options than ASA alone. • Only do combination therapy of ASA+plavix for minor stroke or high-risk TIA • *Contraindications: ASA allergy, GIB, TPA* ○ *If allergy, consider Plavix alone* • Continue for 2 weeks then consider prolonged anticoagulation options
NOACs	Not currently recommended unless other indications exist
Oxygen[293]	Maintain >94%

Embolic?	1. Thrombolytics
	   • Dose: TPA (alteplase) 0.9 mg/kg (max 90mg; consider lower dose of 0.6 mg/kg in Asian population per *ENCHANTED* study) IV as 10% over 1 min, then 90% over 1 hr
	   • Indications: ischemic stroke (CT neg for hemorrhage) with neurological deficits with pt presentation **within 3-4.5 hrs** of sx onset and pt BP <185/110
	      ○ Exclusions: possible SAH, surgery in past 14d, head trauma or MI in past 3mo, GI bleed in past 21d, ANY hx of ICH, any active bleeding, INR>1.7, thrombocytopenia, hypoglycemic (<50)
	      ○ Considered: >80YO, any use of oral anticoagulant, NIH>25
	   • Monitoring
	      ○ Patient should be monitored carefully for signs of symptomatic ICH, which include changes in level of alertness, headaches, nausea, vomiting, and worsening neurologic examination findings.
	      ○ The blood pressure should be maintained below **180/105 mm Hg** after thrombolysis to prevent this complication
	      ○ Frequent vital sign checks and neurologic examinations are recommended for the first 24 hours.
	2. *Endovascular mechanical embolus removal*
	   MERCI reasonable option to extract intra-arterial thrombi
	3. *NOAC or Warfarin*– see page 453

HDL	Continue statin if already on one, poor indication to start if not on already (Level B) with goal LDL of < 70
Fever	Tylenol as needed to maintain temperature <38°C
Statin	High intensity; LDL goal <70[294]; see page 667
Anticoagulation	Use SCDs or prophylactic dose (Grade 1A). Chemical prophylaxis is often okay by HD#4 if imaging shows stability
tPA	0.9 mg/kg, maximum dose 90 mg over 60 minutes with initial 10% of dose given as bolus over 1 minute administered within 4.5 hours of stroke symptom recognition (*WAKE-UP*) Can be beneficial in patients with AIS who awake with stroke symptoms or have unclear time of onset >4.5 hours from last known well or at baseline state and who

have a DW-MRI lesion smaller than one-third of the MCA territory and no visible signal change on FLAIR

- **Treatment**
    - *Edema* - Decompressive surgery within 48 hours reduces mortality; restrict free water; correct hypoxemia, hypercarbia and hyperthermia. Elevated HOB>30degrees and avoid anti HTN agents that increase vasodilation
        1. Brief hyperventilation to a PCO2 of 30-34 for severe edema is reasonable as a bridge to more definitive treatment.
    - *Hemorrhagic conversion*
        1. Highest risk is in patients who undergo reperfusion therapy (i.e. Alteplase), ↑age, ↑glucose, prev. on antiplatelet therapy, on DAPT, triple therapy, CHF, ↑BP, prior ICH
        2. Patients will present with new neurologic symptoms
        3. Stat CT head without contrast
        4. Transfer patient to neuro ICU
    - *Increased ICP –*
        1. STAT mannitol
            - 100 g IV bolus, followed by 0.5-1 g/kg
            - Contraindications: low BP, anuria secondary to renal disease, serum osm > 340. Hold dose for Na > 160, serum osm > 340, or osm gap > 10.
        2. Hypertonic saline:
            - Goal sodium 145-155
            - 3% saline, 40-50 cc/h can go through peripheral IV for up to 12 h, then needs a central line.
            - Contraindications: Na > 160.
        3. Hyperventilation: For goal pCO2 30
  - Hemorrhagic strokes (ICH):

Physical symptoms based on site of ICH	
Site	Findings
Basal Ganglia	Hemiplegia
	Homonymous hemianopsia
	Gaze palsy
	Stupor, Coma
Cerebellum	Neck stiffness
	Facial weakness
	No hemiparesis
	Stupor / Coma
Thalamus	Hemiparesis
	Hemi-sensory loss
	Upgaze palsy
	Nonreactive miotic pupils
	Eyes deviate **toward** the hemiparesis
Cerebral Lobe	Associated with seizures
	Occipital lobe causes CTL homonymous hemi.
	Eyes deviate away from hemiparesis
Pons	**Pinpoint** reactive pupils
	Deep coma
	Paralysis

USMLEWorld

- Consult: neurology and neurosurgery
- Orders
    1. Activate the STROKE TEAM (call page operator)
    2. Q2-4 hour neuro checks.

3. For DVT prophylaxis, use intermittent pneumatic compression together with elastic stockings (can consider elevation to LMWH or UFH if patient non ambulatory after 4 days and no bleeding noted on CT)
4. PT, OT, speech therapy.
5. Passive full ROM exercises of paralyzed limbs should be started during the first 24 hours.
6. NPO if patient is at risk of aspiration.
- Blood Pressure
  1. Early intense SBP reduction best (*INTENSE*-2), keep SBP $\leq$140 with IV nicardipine, labetalol (any rapidly titratable medication) [295]
     - PO nicardipine studied at 60mg q4h x21d (*Cochrane review, 2010*)
     - The lower the better, however few studies have shown adverse effects with very low SBP (this was rare).
     - Concept is to ↓ risk for cerebral vasospasm
- On anticoagulation – reverse!
  1. Warfarin: rapid correction with FFP, 3 Factor PCC (20-40cc; contains Factors II, IX, and X)), rFVII (Factor VII not part of 3-F-PCC but if you do 4-F-PCC it is included) and/or IV Vitamin K (5-10mg) recommended
  2. DOAC: consider specific reversal agent
  3. ASA not indicated until 2-4 weeks after stroke onset if hematoma has resolved
- DVT prophylaxis
  1. LMWH can be restarted assuming 48-hour CT imaging shows no active bleeding
  2. Use compression, SCDs
- Glucose
  1. Should be monitored, manage hyper and hypoglycemia as needed with goal of (80-110 for FBG)
- ↑ICP
  1. Monitoring (CPP target: 50-70mmHg)
  2. Ventricular drainage (EVD) for hydrocephalus reasonable if ↓LOC (esp. GCS 8), severe mass effect
  3. STAT mannitol
     - 100 g IV bolus, followed by 0.5-1 g/kg
     - Contraindications: low BP, anuria secondary to renal disease, S_{OSM} > 340. Hold dose for Na > 160, S_{OSM} > 340, or osm gap > 10.
  4. Hypertonic saline:
     - Goal sodium 145-155
     - 3% saline, 40-50 cc/h can go through peripheral IV for up to 12 h, then needs a central line.
     - Contraindications: Na > 160.
  5. Hyperventilation: For goal pCO2 30
  6. Avoid corticosteroids
- **Subarachnoid Hemorrhage[296]**
  1. Etiology
     - M/c causes include rupture of aneurysm or AVM
     - Atypical: mycotic aneurysm
  2. Symptoms
     - Headache → LOC
     - Seizure activity (given risk, prophylactic anticonvulsants are often given)
  3. Examination
     - Fundoscopic exam reveals hemorrhage, dilated pupil

- ECG → look for T wave inversions d/t release of catecholamines 2/2 myocardial ischemia
4. Classification
    - *Hunt-Hess Grades*
        - Grade I: Mild headache with or without meningeal irritation
        - Grade II: Severe headache and a non-focal examination, with or without mydriasis
        - Grade III: Mild alteration in neurologic examination, including mental status
        - Grade IV: Obviously depressed level of consciousness or focal deficit
        - Grade V: Patient either posturing or comatose
5. Imaging
    - On CT-head, look for blood around the COW
        - Intraparenchymal – MCA, PCA
        - Interhemispheric/Intravascular – ACA
    - To identify location, CT angiograms are often ordered
6. LP – if CT negative with high suspicion, look for xanthochromia
7. Intubation
    - Often in HH Grades III-V
    - Target PaCO2 30-35, any lower and ↑ risk of vasospasm
8. Treatment
    - **Triple H Therapy**
        - *Hypertension*: goal CPP>70 or SBP 160-180 if clipped; 140-160 if unclipped; If vasospasm exists then goal is >130
            - ↓BP = labetalol
            - ↑BP = NE, phenylephrine
        - *Hemodilution*: goal HCT of 30-33% using albumin 5% 250cc q6h
        - *Hypervolemia*: goal CVP of 5-7 using NS @ 150cc/hr or 1/2NS if ↑Na
        - Mannitol (osmotic agent, ↓ICP by 50%, lasts 4 hours)
        - Consider prophylactic anticonvulsant
    - Statin therapy if LDL>100[297]
    - CCB
        - Nimodipine 60mg PO/NG q4h-q6h for 21 days
9. Monitoring
    - Neuro checks q1h
    - Pulse oximetry
    - EtCO2
    - UOP
    - Serum Na
10. Complications
    - Rebleed (peaks within 24 hours of event)
    - Hydrocephalus (peaks within 24 hours of event)
    - Hyponatremia (SIADH, cerebral salt wasting, within first week of event)
    - Vasospasm (worst is day 7-10; ↑risk with higher HH grade; prevention with nimodipine, tx with HHH)
        - HHH
            - Hemodilution (HCT 30-35%)
            - Hypertension (vasopressors phenylephrine, NE)
            - Hypervolemia (CVP>12)
- **Prevention of medical complications as an inpatient in stroke patients**[298]
    - IS use due to ↑ risk for PNA
    - VTE prophylaxis → as above; LMWH can be started if 48 hour imaging shows no active bleed

- Speech pathology c/s for risk of dysphagia
- Hyperglycemia management with SSI
- Titrate NC to >92% due to risk for hypoxia
- Ambulation/bed turns for bed sores
- Telemetry due to cardiac abnormalities (arrest, CHF, arrhythmias)
- PPI prophylaxis
- Evaluation for depression
- **Secondary Prevention of Strokes (All Types)**
  - Most important factors (based on INTERSTROKE case study) to control in the patient are:
    - Lifestyle (↑exercise, ↓smoking, ↓alcohol, ↓weight)
    - BP management (ACEi+thiazide) for optimal reduction of 10/5mmHg rather than ACE alone (PROGERSS trial)
      - PRoFESS did not show ARB>placebo
    - Cholesterol reduction (Simvastatin (40mg/day based on Heart Protection Study) or Atorvastatin 80mg (SPARCL) recommended if LDL>=100 **with goal of reducing to 70** (or overall reduction by 50%)
      - May be contraindicated if patient has hx of intracerebral hemorrhage
      - No utility in treating ↓HDL
    - Lifestyle factors
      - Consider screening for OSA
      - Recommend regular exercise
      - Weight control (Screen for obesity and consider dietary consultation as outpatient)
    - PFO do not require treatment unless history of DVT (CLOSURE 1 study)
    - Antiplatelet therapy (unless anticoagulation indicated)[299]:
      - **Non cardioembolic, minor stroke, high risk TIA, lacunar, or cryptogenic:**
        - Clopidogrel 75mg daily combined with ASA 81mg/d after initial loading dose of each
          - Only done in high risk TIA (see below) or minor stroke
            - Start therapy **within** 24 hours of stroke and continue together for 21 days then stop Plavix and continue ASA 81mg/d indefinitely.
          - Plavix failures may be due to CYP450 genetic abnormalities as liver modification is required to create active metabolite
          - More beneficial than ASA alone and lower bleeding risk Level 2; MATCH, CHANCE (sub-analysis) trial
          - Plavix>ASA if hx of PAD (Clopidogrel versus Aspirin in Patients at Risk of Ischemic Events (CAPRIE) study)
          - POINT and CHANCE trials suggested possible benefit of initial dual therapy with Plavix+ASA for 90 days or 21 days respectively and then continuation of Plavix indefinitely in patients with TIA and high ABCD2 score.
        - ASA 25mg+dipyridamole 200mg BID
          - More beneficial than ASA alone
          - Higher hemorrhage risk
        - ASA 75-100mg once daily
      - **Cardioembolic (atrial fibrillation):**
        - Higher risk for hemorrhagic transformation
        - Heparin not advised d/t ↑ risk of ICH
        - Agents approved: dabigatran, apixaban, rivaroxaban, edoxaban, and warfarin. Less rates of ICH compared to Warfarin.
        - **The optimal time to start (or re-initiate) these agents after an AIS in patients with AF remains uncertain.**

NEUROLOGY

- o ASA should be given until deciding which anticoagulation regimen to treat with
- o Understand for NOACs, trials below did not study patients receiving medication up to 1 year of ischemic stroke.
- o 1-3-6-12 rule (*ESC*)
  - TIA: initiate 1 day after acute event
  - Mild stroke (NIHSS score < 8): initiate 3 days after acute event
  - Moderate stroke (NIHSS score 8-16): evaluate hemorrhagic transformation at day 6, initiate 6 days after acute event
  - Severe stroke (NIHSS score > 16): evaluate hemorrhagic transformation at day 12, initiate 12 days after acute event
- Most start/re-start therapy 3-14 days of event but can delay >14d if ↑size (based on NIHSS score or calculated volume of infarct based on ABC/2 method). **ABC/2 method** is **A** (greatest diameter on axial view) **x B** (widest diameter 90 degrees to A) **x C** (# of slices that show stroke multiplied by slice thickness)
  - o Edoxaban (*ENGAGE AF-TIMI 48*) 60mg/d (consider 50% dose reduction if GFR<50)
  - o Dabigatran (*RE-LY*) 150mg BID (unless CrCl <30 cc/min) (Grade 2B)
  - o Apixaban (*ARISTOTLE*)
  - o Rivaroxiban (*ROCKET-AF, RELAXED, Triple AXEL*)
  - o Warfarin (*EAFT, RAF, VISTA*) Can use ASA as bridge (ACC, ESC, CSG) but defer to Neurology. Early therapy with heparin is class III recommendation and suggests harm.

  If patient does not desire anticoagulant then...
  - o ASA 81mg/d + Plavix (Grade 1B)
    - Start 24-48 hours after stroke (>24h if received tPA)
- **Carotid Stenosis** - best to treat with endarterectomy over stenting when occlusion >70% (NASCET trial)

TRANSIENT ISCHEMIC ATTACK

- **Definition**[300,301]
  - o Temporary neurologic deficit attributable to vascular ischemia, but not infarction. TIA symptoms last <24 hours and show no sign of infarction on MRI
  - o Vascular events (stroke and TIA) will be sudden and close to maximal in onset
    - Symptoms are usually focal in nature, should not be diffuse or scattered.
    - More diffuse symptomatology like confusion or not thinking straight is unlikely to be a TIA or stroke
  - o Compare to complex migraine with lack of associated HA or photophobia
- **High Risk to Progress to Stroke**
  - o High ABCD2 (see below)
  - o Recurrent symptoms in same vascular territory
  - o Ischemic findings on MRI
- **Indications for Hospitalization/Risk Determination:**
  - o Obtain ABCD2 score to determine **risk** of re-stroke in 7 days → score **≥3 warrants** admission if symptoms occurred within the past 72 hours
    - Age>60 (1pt)
    - BP>140/90 (1 pt)
    - Clinical features
    - **Unilateral** Weakness (2pt)

- **Abnormal speech**: Sign is present if the patient slurs speech or uses wrong words (1pt)
- Duration: 10-59m (1pt), >60m (2pt)
- DM2 (1pt)

Risk of CVA in 7 days: 6-7 (11.7%), 4-5 (5.9%), 0-3 (1.2%)
>>high is considered scores of 6-7

- If concurrent risk factors (AF, multiple TIAs, hypercoagulable state, symptoms > 1 hour, sx carotid artery disease >50%) or high ABCD2 score (>6)
- **Labs**
    - CBC
    - CMP
    - Lipid panel in AM
    - HgA1c
    - Consider RPR
- **Imaging**[302]
    - TTE (r/o ASD therefore consider bubble study)
    - Risk of recurrent stroke within 14 days of initial stroke is 8% (RF include ↑age, LAE, LVD, ↑CHADS2VASC, ↑size of ischemic stroke based on NIHSS score)
        - Consider reserving bubble study for patients younger than 60 years old.
            - The biggest correlation between PFO closure and reduction in stroke is in young patients with cryptogenic stroke
        - Difficult to implicate a PFO as the cause because PFOs are common (~1 in 4 people).
    - MRI brain without contrast
        - Look for acute ischemia on diffusion weighted imaging (DWI).
        - Use FLAIR or T2 to look for old injury or chronic infarcts.
        - Microvascular disease (or nonspecific white matter disease) on MRI suggests increased risk of future stroke.
        - Chronic embolic appearing infarcts should direct an evaluation for sources of emboli
    - CTA/MRA with contrast to evaluate anterior and posterior circulation
        - Carotid duplex US will not evaluate posterior circ
    - Telemetry monitoring with ECG qAM
- **Consults**
    - PT/OT evaluation
    - Speech pathology
    - Neurology
    - Consider outpatient event monitor (28 days) to r/o arrythmia in pts at high risk
- **Treatment**
    - Non-Cardioembolic TIA
        - First event: ASA 325mg (alternative is Plavix if ASA allergy) within 24 hours of event then 81mg/d with Plavix 75mg/d combination (if high risk TIA: defined as ABCD2 score of 6+) for 21 days then 81mg/d alone thereafter indefinitely.
            - If already on ASA
                - Considered failure
                - Start Plavix 75mg or Aggrenox
    - Cardioembolic TIA
    Concerning for underlying AF as the source
        - Start within 24 hours of admission
        - Long term oral anticoagulation with target INR of 2-3
        - If cannot tolerate above and nonvalvular AF (rheumatic disease, hemodynamically significant MS):

- ASA 325mg
- Plavix 75mg
- Concurrent STEMI/USA
  - Start ASA 325mg and Plavix 75mg
- **Prevention**
  - LDL goal ≤ 70 (*SPARCL*); all patients will benefit from statin regardless of LDL
  - BP goal <140/90
  - Fasting glucose goal of <126
  - All smokers should be counseled to quit
  - Lifestyle changes if BMI>25
  - Physical activity for 3-4x/week lasting at least 10 minutes
  - ↓Salt intake

VERTIGO

- **General**[303,304]
  - Sensation of motion (most often rotational) and is **not** the same as dizziness or lightheadedness
  - Vestibular dysfunction (asymmetry) caused by central or peripheral lesion (see table below)
  - 2/3 more common in women than men
- **Historical Questions**
  - Define: Patient will endorse the room spinning around them **not** feeling lightheaded
  - Time-course:
    - BPPV is suggestive of recurring vertigo lasting a few minutes or less
      - (1) a sensation that the surroundings or the patient were spinning
      - (2) dizziness occurring mostly with head movement
      - (3) duration of dizziness less than 3 minutes.
      Among patients who answered "yes" to all three questions, 80% received BPPV diagnoses. Among patients who answered "no" to any of these questions, 94% did not have BPPV.[305]
    - Vestibular migraine or TIA can be described as a single episode lasting minutes to hours
    - Vestibular neuritis and stroke are more prolonged episodes
  - Associated symptoms
    - Nausea/vomiting (non-specific)
    - Suggests central cause:
      - Focal neurologic deficits (dipoplia, dysarthria, dysphagia, numbness, weakness)
      - Headache, photophobia, visual auras
    - Suggests peripheral cause:
      - Deafness, tinnitus (Meniere's)
      - Recent viral infection (labyrinthitis, vestibular neuritis)
      - New medications (anticonvulsant, salicylates, ABx)
- **HINTS Exam**
  When the head impulse test is combined with an examination of nystagmus and a test for skew this is referred to as the HINTS (Head Impulse-Nystagmus-Test for Skew) test. The HINTS test may be more sensitive for the diagnosis of acute stroke than even MRI within the first 48 hours following symptom onset.
  - Nystagmus – have patient look at you; using a piece of paper, hold it to one side of their face (against cheek) and have them turn their eyes (not head) to look at the paper. Observe for nystagmus. Then put the paper on the other cheek and have them

look in the other direction and again observe for nystagmus. Worrisome finding is if the nystagmus (fast beat) occurs in different directions depending on what direction they look (if it's always fast beating to left, or right, it's considered unilateral and not worrisome).
- *Peripheral lesion* - horizontal direction (and torsional).
- *Central lesions* - in any direction but often vertical.

o Test of Skew - involves the examiner covering one eye and observing for a vertical shift in the eye when uncovered and then covering the opposite eye. Repeat for the opposite eye. Central lesions sometimes produce a slight skew deviation.

o Head Impulse Test – abnormal finding is good, suggestive of vestibular neuritis.
  1. Hold on to the patient's skull
  2. Have patient fixate on your nose
  3. Patient's muscles in the neck should be completely relaxed
  4. Move the head to the left and right slowly by about 15 degrees, the **briskly** to the center
  5. Look for a catch-up saccade
     - A normal response occurs when the eyes remain on the target.
       o A normal test on both sides with direction changing nystagmus or skew deviation is concerning for a central lesion
     - An abnormal response (see an abnormal long jump in the eyes to move to the nose when you briskly move the head to the center).
       o An abnormal head impulse test with unidirectional nystagmus and absent skew strongly suggests a peripheral lesion.

Evaluation of vertigo

		Peripheral Vertigo	Central Vertigo
Pathophysiology		Disorder of vestibular nerve (cn viii)	Disorder of brain stem or cerebellum
Severity		Intense	Less intense
Onset		Sudden	Slow
Pattern		Intermittent	Constant
Nausea and vomiting		Usually present	Usually absent
Exacerbated by position		Yes	No
Hearing abnormalities		Yes	No
Focal neurologic deficits		No	Yes
Fatigability of symptoms		Yes	No
HINTS EXAM	Nystagmus	Horizontal, direction fixed, beating away from the affected side (no matter the gaze, fast beating always in same 1 direction)	Vertical, torsional, horizontal; direction-changing on left/right gaze (fast beat **changes** depending on direction of gaze)
	Test of skew (alternating cover test)	No vertical nystagmus when uncovering either eye	Vertical nystagmus when uncovering either eye
	Head Impulse Test (HIT); looks for nerve problem	Unilateral **abnormality** with head movement toward affected side	Bilateral **normality** (no correction)
DDx		FB Cerumen impaction Acute otitis media BPPV Meniere's dz Vestibular neuronitis Trauma Motion sickness Neuroma Ototoxic Medications	Infection (i.e. encephalitis, meningitis) Vertebrobasilar Migraine Brainstem hemorrhage Infarction (cerebellum or VB system) Migraine Tumor MS Temp. lobe epilepsy

SOURCE: USMLEASY

- **Differential Diagnosis**

NEUROLOGY

- BPPV (dx with Dix-Hallpike Maneuver, episodic positionally induced vertigo)
  - Sudden onset, recurrent and brief (<1 min) associated with positional changes in head
  - No headache or diplopia should be present
  - Normal CN2-12 exam
  - Latency present with onset of nystagmus, lasts <1 minute, fatigable, and unidirectional (often horizontal)
- Vestibular neuritis (not induced with movement like BPPV)
- Labyrinthitis (may be associated with unilateral hearing loss, single acute event like VN)
- Migraine
- "Dizziness" with fatigue, consider POTS
- Severe VB12 deficiency
- Cerebellar stroke (associated sx include headache, instability, diplopia, wide based gait, ataxia, vomiting, nystagmus)
  - Look for immediate onset nystagmus, that lasts >1 minute, that is non-fatigable and vertical
- Multiple Sclerosis (d/t plaques at CN 8, vision changes (optic neuritis), look for hx suggestive of relapse/remittance, dx with MRI)
- Medication toxicity (i.e. phenytoin)
- Persistent postural-perceptual dizziness (PPPD) (functional d/o in patients with chronic symptoms (>3mo) despite appropriate therapy and no objective sx). Typically, preceded by vestibular event (BPPV, vestibular neuritis, trauma, migraine, major depression, anxiety, CVA.

Vestibular syndromes based on description

Description	Benign Cause	Concerning Cause
Acute, **continuous** dizziness lasting days, accompanied by nausea, vomiting, nystagmus, head motion intolerance, and gait unsteadiness that is **exacerbated** by movement	Vestibular Neuritis (dizziness only, may be d/t HSV; **m/c**) Labyrinthitis (dizziness+↓hearing or tinnitus)	Posterior circulation ischemic stroke (**cannot** be r/o with CT) MS Cerebellar hemorrhage
Episodic dizziness that occurs spontaneously, is not triggered, and usually last minutes to hours	Vestibular migraine Meniere's disease	TIA
Episodic dizziness brought on by a specific, obligate trigger (typically a change in head position or standing up), and usually lasting less than 1 min. **At baseline, no symptoms**	BPPV	Central paroxysmal pos. vertigo Orthostatic ↓BP 2/2 illness

- Check Orthostatic BP
  - Defined as a ↓ in SBP of ≥20 mmHg and DBP ≥10 mmHg within 5 minutes of standing.
  - Meclizine 25 PO TID (1/2-1-tab PO TID)
- **Treatment**

Vertigo treatment based on situation

Scenario	Class	Treatment
Vestibular nausea/motion sickness	Histamine ACh	Meclizine 25mg q6h Scopolamine 1ptch q3d Benadryl 25mg q6h

Migraine-associated *(consider Migraine with Brainstem Aura diagnosis)*	Dopamine	Metoclopramide 10mg q4h Promethazine 25mg q6h
Gastroenteritis	Dopamine Serotonin	Promethazine 25mg q6h Zofran 2mg PO
Pregnancy	Unknown	Ginger 250mg q6h Pyridoxine 25mg x 1 Zofran 2mg PO Methylprednisolone 40mg IV
PPPD	SSRI SNRI Vestibular Rehab	Any from prior classes are acceptable treatment options. Effects take minimum 8-12 weeks and tx should last minimum 1 year

Bibliography

[258] Cooper et al. Synopsis of the National Institute for Health and Clinical Excellence Guideline for Management of Transient Loss of Consciousness. Ann Intern Med. 2011;155:543-549

[259] Brignole et al. European Heart Journal, Volume 39, Issue 21, 1 June 2018.

[260] Michele Brignole, Angel Moya, Frederik J de Lange, Jean-Claude Deharo, Perry M Elliott, Alessandra Fanciulli, Artur Fedorowski, Raffaello Furlan, Rose Anne Kenny, Alfonso Martín, Vincent Probst, Matthew J Reed, Ciara P Rice, Richard Sutton, Andrea Ungar, J Gert van Dijk, ESC Scientific Document Group; 2018 ESC Guidelines for the diagnosis and management of syncope, European Heart Journal, , ehy037

[261] Matuszak JM, McVige J, McPherson J, Willer B, Leddy J. A Practical Concussion Physical Examination Toolbox: Evidence-Based Physical Examination for Concussion. Sports Health. 2016;8:260-269.

[262] Matuszak JM, McVige J, McPherson J, Willer B, Leddy J. A Practical Concussion Physical Examination Toolbox: Evidence-Based Physical Examination for Concussion. Sports Health. 2016;8:260-269.

[263] Stillman et al. "Concussion: Evaluation and management." Cleveland Clinic Journal of Medicine. 2017 August;84(8):623-630.

[264] Berry et al. Return-to-Play After Concussion: Clinical Guidelines for Young Athletes. JAOA. 2019.

[265] Watto, M. (2018, November 5). #123 Sleep Apnea Pearls and Pitfalls [Audio blog post]. Retrieved November 5, 2018, from https://thecurbsiders.com/podcast/123-sleep-apnea-pearls-and-pitfalls

[266] Sinclair et al. Prac Neurol. 2015.

[267] Clinical Policy: Critical Issues in the Evaluation and Management of Adult Patients Presenting to the Emergency Department With Acute Headache: Approved by the ACEP Board of Directors June 26, 2019 Clinical Policy Endorsed by the Emergency Nurses Association (July 31, 2019). Ann Emerg Med. 2019 Oct;74(4):e41-e74. doi: 10.1016/j.annemergmed.2019.07.009.

[268] Robbins et al. "Migraine Treatment From A to Z." Practical Pain Management. April 2012.

[269] Charles, Andrew. "Migraine." NEJM. 2017: 377; 553-561.

[270] Watto, M. (n.d.). #122 Headaches Advanced Class: Migraines, medication overuse, and more! [Audio blog post]. Retrieved from https://thecurbsiders.com/podcast/122-headaches-advanced-class

[271] Faubion et al. "Migraine Throughout the Female Reproductive Life Cycle." Mayo Clin Proc. 2018;93(5):639-645.

[272] Taggart et al. "Ketorolac in the treatment of acute migraine: a systematic review." Headache. 2013 Feb;53(2):277-87.

[273] Balestrino, R., & Schapira, A. H. V. (2019). Parkinson Disease. European Journal of Neurology. doi:10.1111/ene.14108.

[274] Chou, Kelvin et al. "Diagnosis of Parkinson disease. " UpToDate 20JUL2012

[275] DeLong MR, Luncos JL. Parkinson's disease and other movement disorders. In: Kasper DL, Fauci AS, Longo DL, et al, eds. Harrison's Principles of Internal Medicine. Vol 2. 16th ed. New York: McGraw-Hill. 2005:2406–2418.

[276] Wills AJ, Stevens DL. Epilepsy in the accident and emergency department. Br J Hosp Med 1994;52:42–5. Morrison AD, McAlpine CH. The management of first seizures in adults in a district general hospital. Scot Med J 1997;42:73–5. Pellegrino TR. An emergency department approach to first-time seizures. Emerg Med Clin North Am 1994;12:925–39.

[277] Greenberg DA, Aminoff MJ, Simon RP. Chapter 12. Seizures & Syncope. In: Greenberg DA, Aminoff MJ, Simon RP, eds. Clinical Neurology. 8th ed. New York: McGraw-Hill; 2012.

[278] Kapur et al. Randomized Trial of Three Anticonvulsant Medications for Status Epilepticus. NEJM. 2019.

[279] Dietze et al. JAMA Netw Open. 2019.

[280] Adapted from Status Epilepticus/Stroke 2/22/01 by Dr. Steve Lee and Stroke 2006 by Nereses Sanossian, MD

[281] Rob's Pearls

[282] Go S, Worman DJ. Chapter 161. Stroke, Transient Ischemic Attack, and Cervical Artery Dissection. In: Tintinalli JE, Stapczynski JS, Cline DM, Ma OJ, Cydulka RK, Meckler GD, eds. Tintinalli's Emergency Medicine: A Comprehensive Study Guide. 7th ed. New York: McGraw-Hill; 2011

[283] Badruddin A, Gorelick PB. Antiplatelet therapy for prevention of recurrent stroke. Curr Treat Options Neurol. 2009 Nov;11(6):452-9. PMID: 20848331 [PubMed]

[284] Adams et al. "Guidelines for the Early Management of Adults With Ischemic Stroke : A Guideline From the American Heart Association/American Stroke Association Stroke Council, Clinical Cardiology Council, Cardiovascular Radiology and Intervention Council, and the Atherosclerotic Peripheral Vascular Disease and Quality of Care Outcomes in Research Interdisciplinary Working Groups: The American Academy of Neurology affirms the value of this guideline as an educational tool for neurologists." Stroke. 2007;38:1655-1711

[285] Goldstein, Larry B. Blood Pressure Management in Patients With Acute Ischemic Stroke. Hypertension. 2004;43:137-141

[286] Powers et al. "2018 Guidelines for the Early Management of Patients With Acute Ischemic Stroke: A Guideline for Healthcare Professionals From the American Heart Association/American Stroke Association." Stroke; a Journal of Cerebral Circulation 2018 January 24.

[287] Oxford Handbook of Clinical Medicine (10th Edition)

[288] Circulation 2005;112:IV-111–IV-120

[289] Saposnik et al. "AHA/ASA Scientific Statement. Diagnosis and Management of Cerebral Venous Thrombosis" Stroke. 2011; 42: 1158-1192

[290] Amarenco et al. A Comparison of Two LDL Cholesterol Targets after Ischemic Stroke. N Engl J Med 2020; 382:9-19.

[291] Cumbler E, Glasheen J. "Management of Blood Pressure after Acute Ischemic Stroke: An Evidenced-Base Guide for the Hospitalist." Journal of Hospital Medicine 2007;2: 261–267.

[292] Prasad K, Siemieniuk R, Hao Q, et al. Dual antiplatelet therapy with aspirin and clopidogrel for acute high risk transient ischaemic attack and minor ischaemic stroke: a clinical practice guideline [published online Decembre 18, 2018]. BMJ.

[293] Siemieniuk RAC, Chu DK, Kim LH, et al. Oxygen therapy for acutely ill medical patients: a clinical practice guideline. BMJ. 2018;363:k4169. PMID: 30355567 doi:10.1136/bmj.k4169

[294] Amarenco P et al. A comparison of two LDL cholesterol targets after ischemic stroke. N Engl J Med 2019 Nov 18; [e-pub].

[295] Morgenstern LB, Hemphill JC 3rd, Anderson C, et al; American Heart Association Stroke Council and Council on Cardiovascular Nursing. Guidelines for the management of spontaneous intracerebral hemorrhage: a guideline for healthcare professionals from the American Heart Association/American Stroke Association. Stroke. 2010 Sep;41(9): 2108-29.

[296] Neligan, Patrick. Subarachnoid Hemorrhage. CCMTutorials.com

[297] McGirt et al. "Risk of cerebral vasospasm after subarachnoid hemorrhage reduced by statin therapy: a multivariate analysis of an institutional experience." Journal of Neurosurgery. November 2006. Vol. 105 (5) 671-674.

[298] Kumar et al. "Medical complications after stroke." Lancet Neurology. 2010: 9. 105-108.

[299] Lansberg et al. "Antithrombotic and thrombolytic therapy for ischemic stroke, Ninth Edition" Chest. 2012: 141(2).

[300] Johnston et al. "National Stroke Association Guidelines for the Management of TIAs." Ann Neurol 2006. Vol 60 (301-313).

[301] Giles M, Rothwell P. Transient ischaemic attack: clinical relevance, risk prediction and urgency of secondary prevention. Current Opinion in Neurology. 2009, 22:46–53

[302] Chutinet et al. White matter disease as a biomarker for long-term cerebrovascular disease and dementia. Curr Treat Options Cardiovasc Med. 2014 Mar; 16(3): 292.

[303] Stanton M, Freeman AM. Vertigo. [Updated 2018 Oct 27]. In: StatPearls [Internet]. Treasure Island (FL): StatPearls Publishing; 2019 Jan-. Available from: https://www.ncbi.nlm.nih.gov/books/NBK482356/

[304] Gurley et al. "Acute Dizziness." Semin Neurol. 2019 Feb;39(1):27-40. doi: 10.1055/s-0038-1676857.

[305] Kim H-J et al. Questionnaire-based diagnosis of benign paroxysmal positional vertigo. Neurology 2020 Mar 3; 94:e942

PULMONOLOGY/ CRITICAL CARE

Section Editors: Ricki Kumar DO, Drew Van Boening DO

Cough	462
Dyspnea	463
Interpretation of PFT's	465
Asthma	472
COPD	480
Interstitial Lung Diseases	490
Hypoxia	494
Supplemental Oxygen	495
Pleural Effusion	496
Solitary Pulmonary Nodule	499
Pulmonary Hypertension	501
Obstructive Sleep Apnea	502
Hemodynamic Monitoring in the ICU	503
Intubation	504
Extubation Criteria	516
Ventilator Review	517
ARDS	523
Anaphylaxis	525
Shock	526

PULMONOLOGY/CRITICAL CARE

COUGH

- **Definitions**[306,307]
    - Acute – less than 21 days (3 weeks)
    - Chronic - cough persisting for longer than 8 weeks
- **Causes**
    - Acute – likely viral upper respiratory illness (consider infectious cause)
    - Chronic – up to 50% of cases will be multifactorial; smoking (COPD), medication side effect (i.e. ACE inhibitors), upper airway cough syndrome (UACS; postnasal drip), airway bronchospasm (asthma ~ 10% of cases), GERD
        - **UACS** – most often caused by allergic rhinitis, non-allergic rhinitis/vasomotor, rhinitis medicamentosa, infection (chronic bacterial sinusitis), allergic fungal sinusitis, deviated septum.
        - **Asthma** – routine testing using PFTs with methacholine challenge; can mimic non-asthmatic eosinophilic bronchitis except the PFTs are normal but bronchoscopy and lavage will reveal elevated eosinophil counts.
        - **Cough hypersensitivity syndrome** – symptoms suggestive of pharyngeal/laryngeal hypersensitivity, such as throat tickling, irritation or blockage, and dysphonia. Cough is often triggered by low levels of thermal, mechanical, or chemical exposure. Pts develop cough in response to stimuli/ concentrations, that wouldn't otherwise elicit cough.
        - **GERD** – Reflux triggers cough due to the effect of acid on the proximal part of the esophagus. Look for other symptoms of acid reflux (e.g. heartburn) but understand that they may be absent (silent reflux) in as many as 75% of cases of a reflux-induced cough. Esophageal PH monitoring may confirm the presence of silent reflux, although anti-reflux therapy does not always resolve a cough.
        - **Neurogenic** – unexplained cough in excess of 8 weeks with normal diagnostic testing (i.e. CXR, pH monitor).
- **Diagnosis**[308,309]
    - Predominance of cough
        - Duration (less than 3 weeks, 3 to 8 weeks, more than 8 weeks)
        - Productive or nonproductive of sputum
    - Can be accompanied by other respiratory and constitutional symptoms
    - Physical exam suggesting pneumonia:
        - Heart rate >100 beats per minute
        - Respiratory rate >24 breaths per minute
        - Temperature >100.4F (38C)
        - Lung findings suggest a consolidation process
- **Diagnostic Testing**
    - CXR (to r/o PNA) if
        - Dyspnea or blood/rust colored sputum
        - Pulse>100
        - RR>24
        - T>100F
        - Focal consolidation on lung exam
    - CT Chest if patient is smoker or suspecting chronic lung disease
    - CT Sinus if suspecting UACS
    - PFTs
    - pH monitor
    - Procalcitonin (PCT)
    - Sputum (for eosinophil count) if suspecting asthma or NAEB
- **Treatment**

- o Acute
  - At least 90% of acute bronchitis episodes are viral → antibiotics not routinely recommended (per AAFP, evidence rating A)
    - Consider PCT to aid in consideration of bacterial origin
    - Viral Bronchitis/Supportive
      - Robitussin AC 10/100/5ml 1 tsp (5ml) PO Q 4-6 hours prn cough
      - Benzonatate (Tessalon Pearls) 100 mg PO Q 8 hours prn cough
      - Dextromethorphan 15-30 mg PO 4 times daily
      - Most effective: Codeine Phosphate 10-30 mg Q 4-6 hours
      - Diphenhydramine HCl 25 mg Q 4-6 hours
  - Over-the-counter medications are recommended as first-line treatment for acute cough
    - Consider using dextromethorphan, guaifenesin, or honey to manage acute bronchitis symptoms (per AAFP, evidence rating B)
      - Three placebo-controlled trials show that dextromethorphan, 30 mg, decreased the cough count by 19% to 36% compared with placebo
      - One study comparing benzonatate, guaifenesin, and placebo showed significant improvement with the combination of benzonatate and guaifenesin, but not with either agent alone.
    - RCT showed that in comparison to placebo, no benefit from NSAID in decreasing severity or duration of cough in patients with acute bronchitis.
- o Chronic
  - First generation antihistamine (Benadryl) + decongestant or as alternative: second generation antihistamine (Claritin) + nasal corticosteroids. If no response to this, then trial asthma treatment with inhaled corticosteroids. If still no response, then high-dose PPI (i.e. 40mg daily or BID).
    - UACS – first generation anti-H1; intranasal steroids, ipratropium
    - Asthma – PFTs
    - GERD – PPI, pH monitor
    - Neurogenic - May have paradoxical vocal cord movements. Consider treatment with voice rehabilitation or speech pathology. Can consider pharmacologic therapy with Gabapentin, Pregabalin, or Amitriptyline however data regarding their efficacy is sparse. High dose tramadol (50mg TID) has been used by laryngologists (start at 25mg QHS then increase to BID; after coughing has stopped, wean off).
  - In patients with evidence of bronchial hyper responsiveness, consider treatment with
    - Albuterol for 1 to 2 weeks (per AAFP, evidence rating B)
    - Robitussin in those with cough for 2 to 3 weeks
    - Tylenol prn
    - Smoking cessation
    - Education: cough likely to last 3 weeks or more

DYSPNEA

- **Definition**[310] - subjective experience of breathing discomfort that consists of qualitatively distinct sensations that vary in intensity[311]
- **Qualities**
  - o Work/effort/exertion: often due to cardiorespiratory disease, likely due to underlying respiratory muscle issue
  - o Chest tightness: due to constriction of the airways, consider asthma and COPD in differential

PULMONOLOGY/CRITICAL CARE

- o Unsatisfied inspiration: or air hunger, often in patients with respiratory dz at the end of exercising
- **History**
  - o Look for fever, cough, chest pain
  - o Rapid onset dyspnea in the absence of other clinical findings are concerning for:
    - PTX – CP, ↑HR, think trauma, thin young males, or those with h/o lung dz
    - PE – see page 340
    - ↑LVEDP – can result from a myocardial infarction leading to ↑LVEDP, CHF. Look for ↑HR, ↓BP, JVD, HJR, S3, LE edema.
  - o Wheezing → think acute bronchitis, asthma, foreign body, vocal cord dysfunction
  - o Cough+fever → pulmonary infection, myocarditis, pericarditis, septic emboli
  - o Dyspnea as a single symptom☐ anemia, methemoglobinemia and carbon monoxide (esp. if other family members affected), chronic PE (only dx with VQ scan)
  - o Dizziness + syncope → VHD, HOCM, anxiety, ↑RR, anemia
  - o Hemoptysis → lung CA, PE, bronchiectasis, TB
  - o Hoarseness → disease of the glottis, laryngeal nerve palsy
- **Differential Diagnosis**
  Too vast to list all, however, below are the most common to consider

Differential diagnosis of dyspnea	
Acute	**Chronic**
Head/Neck	
- Angioedema - Anaphylaxis - Pharyngitis - VCD - Foreign body - Trauma	- Laryngeal tumor - VCD - Tumor compressing the upper airways - Tracheal stenosis - Goiter
Chest Wall	
- Rib fx - Flail chest - Pneumomediastinum - COPD exacerbation - Asthma *(pg 472)* - PE *(pg 340)* - PTX - Pleural effusion - PNA - ARF - Lung contusion/trauma - Hemorrhage - Lung CA	- Bronchial asthma - Bronchiectasis - Bronchiolitis - COPD - Emphysema - CTED - ILD - Sarcoidosis - Bronchiolitis obliterans - CF
Cardiac	
- ACS - AECHF - Pulmonary edema - High-output failure - Cardiomyopathy - VHD - Pericardial tamponade	- Arrhythmia - Pericarditis (constrictive, restrictive) - Pericardial effusion/tamponade - CHD - CHF - VHD
CNS	
- Stroke - Neuromuscular dz	- ALS - Polymyositis
Other	

- Poisoning
- Sepsis
- Anemia
- TBI
- ARF
- ↑RR
- Anxiety
- Pregnancy
- Kyphoscoliosis
- Obesity
- Abdominal wall hernia
- Medications (BB, NSAIDs)

- **Clinical Exam**[312]
  o VS and pulse oximetry (SaO2>96% correspond to PO2 >70 mmHg)
  o Visual inspection may reveal e/o:
    - obstructive airway disease (pursed-lip breathing, use of accessory respiratory muscles, barrel-shaped chest)
    - pneumothorax (asymmetric excursion)
    - metabolic acidosis (Kussmaul respirations).
  o Patients with impending upper airway obstruction (e.g., epiglottitis, foreign body) or severe asthma exacerbation sometimes assume a tripod position.
  o Focal wheezing is c/f a foreign body or other bronchial obstruction.
  o Absent breath sounds in one area of the exam s/o PTX.
  o An ↑P2 is a sign of pHTN and PE
  o Pursed-lip breathing is suggestive of COPD (mechanism increases PEEP/airway resistance)
- **Diagnostics**[313]
  o CXR (with PCT if concern for pulm infxn)
    - Look for pulm venous redistribution, effusions, interstitial changes, hyperinflation, infiltrates, enlargement of the pulm arteries, cardiac chamber enlargement, and valve calcification.
    - Upper zone redistribution of pulm blood flow may be seen in COPD because of destruction of vessels in the lower lung fields.
  o ABG lactic acid
  o Labs: pro-BNP (may be caused by AF, RV strain, pHTN, ARDS), CBC (r/o anemia), CMP (calculate if gap present), TSH, glucose
  o PFTs with DLCO
  o ECG
  o Advanced
    - TTE
    - VQ scan (r/o CTED)
    - Bronchoscopy (r/o VCD, obstruction)
    - Chest CT or MRI
    - Stress testing

INTERPRETATION OF PFT'S

Contributor: Eric Crawley, M.D.[314,315,316,317]

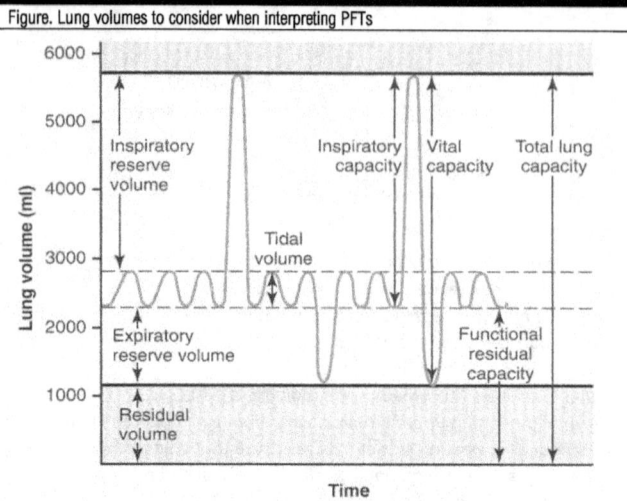

Figure. Lung volumes to consider when interpreting PFTs

- **Background**
  o Tool used to diagnose and manage respiratory, or suspected respiratory, problems
  o Gold standard for diagnosis of obstructive lung disease (NLHEP, NHLBI, WHO)
  o Used for the diagnosis of lung disease (detect presence thereof)
  o Helps to quantify the extent of disease if present and can be utilized to measure the benefit of therapy administered
- **Types**
  o <u>Spirometry</u> – includes measurement of exhaled or inhaled air during forced maneuvers
  o <u>Diffusion capacity</u> – measures diffusion of CO, can help evaluate parenchyma, see DLCO below
  o <u>Lung volumes</u> – obtains total lung volumes to include TLC, RV, etc.
- **Definitions**
  o <u>FVC</u> – Forced vital capacity; the total volume of air that can be exhaled during a maximal forced expiration effort. Will be displayed graphically as to the right. It's important to ensure that a full 6 seconds is seen of effort with an obvious plateau with no early termination/cut-off. Healthy people can exhale the FVC in 4-6 seconds, with COPD patients, you will see this extended to 15+ seconds.
    ▪ Ideally the FVC value is within 150cc of the VC
    ▪ Often in healthy patients this will be quite close to the VC if not equal
    ▪ In obstructive and restrictive disease, we will see this value decreased (mucus plug, bronchial narrowing, CF, asthma, PF, MG, GBS)
  o <u>FEV1</u> – Forced expiratory volume in one second; the volume of air exhaled in the first second under force after a maximal inhalation. Represented on the graph to the bottom right.
  o <u>FEV1/ FVC ratio</u> – the percentage of the FVC expired in one second.
  o <u>FEF25-75%</u> – Forced expiratory flow over the middle one half of the FVC; the average flow from the point at which 25 percent of the FVC has been exhaled to the point at which 75 percent of the FVC has been exhaled. This is rarely used but used if the FEV1/FVC was questionable, you can use this to confirm evidence of obstructive disease if it is also low.
  o <u>MVV</u> – Maximal voluntary ventilation; measure of how rapidly and deeply someone breaths in and out; decreased in patients with poor test performance or NM disease

- o Flow volume loop - provides important clues about the quality, acceptability, and reproducibility of the maneuver, which is determined by national standards and controlled by each individual laboratory.
- o BDR[318] – stands for bronchodilator response, or reversibility, increase of 12% and 200 ml in FEV1 or FVC over the baseline value; does not necessarily distinguish asthma from COPD (for which methacholine challenge may help).
- **Lung volumes**
  - o ERV—Expiratory reserve volume; the maximal volume of air exhaled from end expiration.
  - o IRV—Inspiratory reserve volume; the maximal volume of air inhaled from end inspiration.
  - o RV—Residual volume; the volume of air remaining in the lungs after a maximal exhalation. Increase in RV associated with air trapping.
  - o V_T—Tidal volume; the volume of air inhaled or exhaled during each respiratory cycle.
  - o Lung capacities
  - o FRC—Functional residual capacity; the volume of air in the lungs at resting end expiration.
  - o IC—Inspiratory capacity; the maximal volume of air that can be inhaled from the resting expiratory level.
  - o TLC—Total lung capacity; the volume of air in the lungs at maximal inflation (TLC=IC+FRC); increase in TLC associated with hyperinflation
  - o VC—Vital capacity; the largest volume measured on complete exhalation after full inspiration (but not forced)
    - Conditions associated with decreased VC:
      - ▫ Lung cancer, pulm edema, PNA, surgical tissue resection, OLD, PTX, pregnancy (limited movement of diaphragm), tumors, scleroderma and kyphoscoliosis due to limited chest wall movement)
  - o DLCO - diffusing capacity of the lung for carbon monoxide. This measurement represents the adequacy of the surface area for gas exchange and can be used along with spirometry and lung volumes to understand the patient's underlying physiology and generate a differential diagnosis. Normal spirometry and isolated low DLCO can be seen with pHTN and anemia. With concurrent obstructive pattern, suggestive of emphysema. With concurrent restrictive pattern, suggestive of pulmonary fibrosis.
    - *Low DLCO:* post-exercise, standing, valsalva, ILD, anemia, medications, emphysema
    - *High DLCO:* polycythemia, obesity, asthma, chronic bronchitis, pregnancy, pulmonary hemorrhage
- **Normal Values**
  - o Pulmonary Normal value (95 percent function test confidence interval)
  - o FEV1 80% to 120%
  - o FVC 80% to 120%
  - o Absolute FEV1 / FVC Within 5% of the predicted ratio
  - o TLC 80% to 120%
  - o FRC 75% to 120%
  - o RV 75% to 120%
  - o DLCO > 60% to < 120%
- **Others Not Commonly Used**
  - o Peak Expiratory Flow (aka Peak Flow) is the maximum flow during an FVC, measuring large airway function. Normal being 100-850 cc/min, used often with asthmatics, and patients with MG.
    - Have patients monitor their own function; they should know what their "normal" is, along with their personal best.

PULMONOLOGY/CRITICAL CARE

- For asthmatics specifically, this can determine the likelihood of an exacerbation by the % reduction in peak flow from their personal best (<80% is worrisome)
  o Reports will have the following information:
    - Actual – what the patient performed
    - Predicted – what the patient should be able to perform based on epidemiology
    - % Predicted – actual/predicted
    - Flow Volume Loop (FVL), exhibited below:

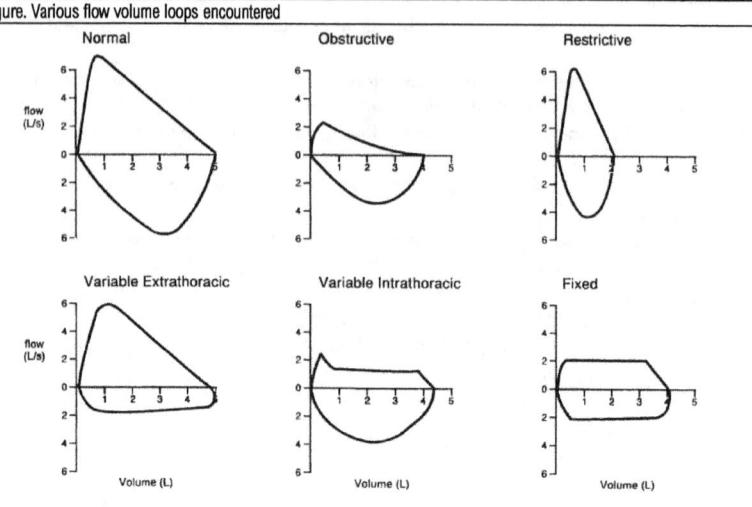

Figure. Various flow volume loops encountered

- **Interpretation**
  o Ensure the following are present:
    - Volume/time curve reaches a plateau lasting at least 6 seconds
    - Results are reproducible: on at least two attempts, the values were within 0.2L
      ▫ Flow-volume loop show no evidence of abnormalities

Step by Step Evaluation of PFTs	
Step	Evaluation
STEP 1	**Look at the flow volume loop:** • Look for scooped or scalloped appearance c/w COPD • Narrow loops are c/w restrictive disease • Inspiratory flows are disproportionately reduced from lesions in the upper/extrathoracic airway • Expiratory flows are disproportionately reduced from lesions in the lower/intrathoracic airway (trachea, main stem) • Restrictions in both inspiratory and expiratory suggest a fixed lesion
STEP 2	**Look at FEV1:FVC ratio to see if there is an obvious obstructive or restrictive defect:**

Obstructive	Restrictive	Mixed
FEV1/FVC < 70%	FEV1/FVC nml	FEV1/FVC <70%
FVC nml or ↑	FVC ↑	FVC↓

- GOLD: <70% ← the expert consensus criteria to use for patients >65 years
- ATS: Less than the LLN ← the expert consensus criteria to use for patients <65 years

	• *Anything* less than the predicted lower limit of normal (<70%)→obstructive pattern
STEP 3	**Look at FVC**
	• If it is reduced in the presence of a reduced FEV1/FVC then mixed pattern present, this is because most patients with a restrictive defect have a low FVC
	• If reduced in the presence of a normal FEV1/FVC then restrictive pattern present
	• Officially use the LLN to determine if FVC is reduced, but the below can help categorize the severity:
	Look at FEV1
	• *Officially use the LLN to determine if FVC is reduced, but the below can help categorize the severity:*
	• *Only of benefit if there was an obstructive process going on in step 1*
	• *If FEV1 is disproportionally reduced relative to FVC, then might be a mixed picture*
STEP 4	**Confirm Restrictive Pattern→Defect**
	• If pattern above is consistent with restrictive pattern, then obtain full volumes along with DLCO (↓DLCo, ↓TLC compared to LLN, ↓RV compared to LLN)
STEP 5	**Assess Severity**
	• Determine severity obstruction based on the percentage of FEV1 predicted
	o FEV1>70% predicted: mild.
	o FEV1 60-69% predicted: moderate obstruction.
	o FEV1 50-59% predicted: moderate severe obstruction.
	o FEV1 35-49% predicted: severe obstruction.
	o FEV1 <35% predicted: very severe obstruction.
STEP 6	**Reversibility after bronchodilator (bronchodilator response)**
	• Ensure patients have not taken their medication at least 4 hours prior to testing in lab
	• If obstructive defect, determine reversibility based on the increase in FEV1 and/or FVC after bronchodilator challenge
	o 12% **and** 200cc in either FEV1 **or** FVC
	• For mixed pattern, full reversibility to the LLN of the FVC suggests pure obstruction
	o If it doesn't reverse to the LLN, it confirms restrictive disease
STEP 7	**Bronchoprovocation**
	• If PFT is normal (FEV1>70%) but you still suspect disease (i.e. EIB, allergen-induced) then perform testing with methacholine challenge, exercise testing, or mannitol inhalation.
	o Methacholine: 20% reduction in FEV1 is diagnostic
	o Exercise: 10% or more reduction in FEV1 or FVC is diagnostic if it occurs over two time points (i.e. 1/3/5/10/15/20/30/45 min)
	• If FEV1/FVC was normal but FEV1<70% go ahead and give them albuterol as trial

Figure. Interpretation of pulmonary function tests in flow-chart format

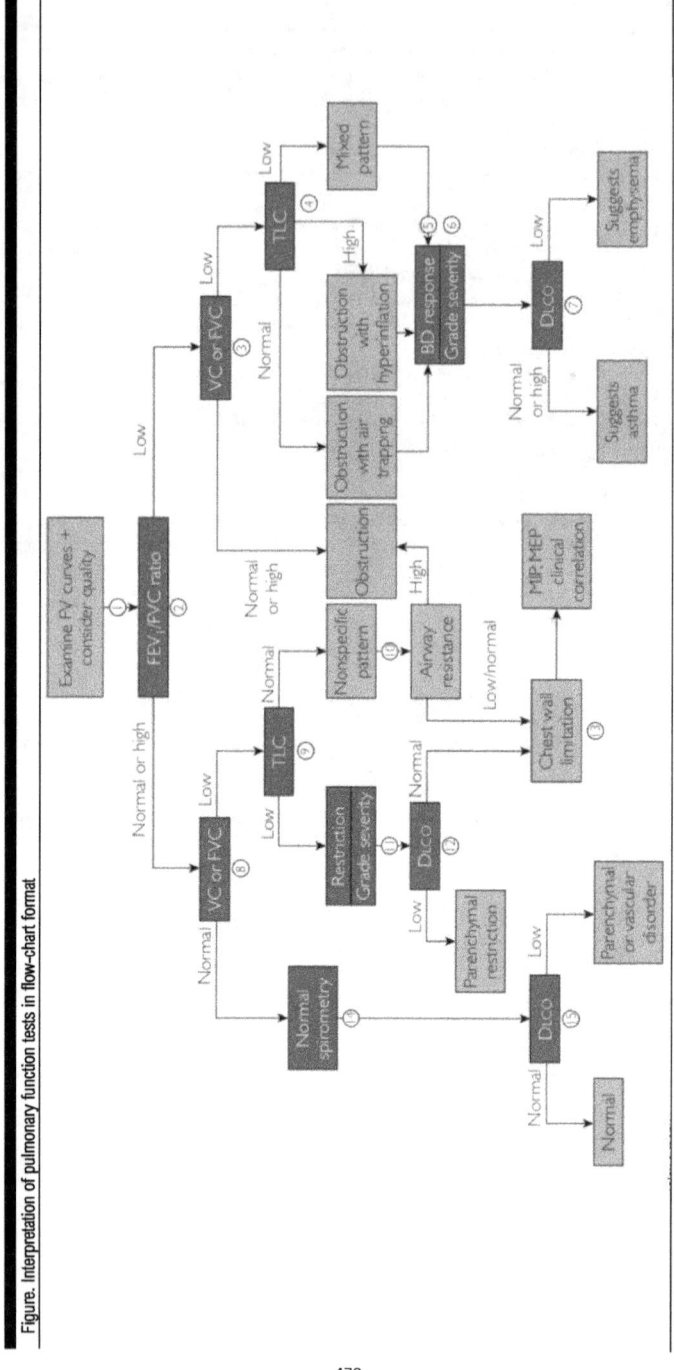

- Lung volumes
    - *Obstructive pattern:*
        - ↑TLC (hyperinflation)
        - ↑RV (gas trapping)
        - If you suspect a defect but don't see it on initial testing (i.e. asthma, EIB, allergen-induced), consider bronchoprovocation testing with methacholine challenge
    - *Restrictive pattern:*
        - ↓FVC
        - ↓TLC
        - Severity:
            - Mild: TLC or FVC 65 - 80% predicted
            - Moderate: TLC or FVC 50 -65% predicted
            - Severe: TLC or FVC < 50% predicted
        - ↓RV
        - Diffusion Capacity (DLCO2) (Parenchymal Process)
            - ↓DLCO2 + normal spirometry: early ILD, pHTN, pulmonary vascular disease, anemia, early emphysema.
            - ↓DLCO2 + obstruction: emphysema, bronchiolitis obliterans, cystic fibrosis, bronchiectasis
            - ↓DLCO2 + restriction: ILD, hypersensitivity pneumonitis, drug toxicity, CHF.
            - ↑DLCO2: polycythemia, pulmonary hemorrhage, asthma, intracardiac shunt
    - *Mixed pattern:*
        - ↓FEV1/FVC and ↓FVC and the severity is monitored by the FEV1 specifically
        - These are more difficult to interpret:
            - With the reduced ratio and reduced FVC specifically, if the bronchodilator leads to improvement (remember 12% and 200cc) then it's suggestive of a pure obstructive defect → COPD. If there is no response to bronchodilator, then get full pulmonary testing to evaluate for evidence of restrictive defect (i.e. TLC, RV reduced)
- **Differential**
    - Obstructive
        - α1-antitrypsin deficiency
        - Asthma
        - Bronchiectasis
        - Bronchiolitis obliterans
        - Chronic obstructive pulmonary disease
        - Cystic fibrosis
        - Silicosis (early)
    - Restrictive
        - Chest wall
            - Ankylosing spondylitis
            - Kyphosis
            - Morbid obesity
            - Scoliosis
            - Drugs (adverse reaction)
                - Amiodarone
                - Methotrexate
                - Nitrofurantoin
        - Interstitial lung disease
            - Asbestosis
            - Berylliosis
            - Eosinophilic pneumonia
            - Hypersensitivity pneumonitis
            - Idiopathic pulmonary fibrosis
            - Sarcoidosis
            - Silicosis (late)
        - Neuromuscular disorders
            - Amyotrophic lateral sclerosis
            - Guillain-Barré syndrome
            - Muscular dystrophy
            - Myasthenia gravis
- **Summary**
    - FEV1, FVC, TLC and DLCO are pretty much the major variables to know

- An obstructive defect is indicted by a low FEV1/FVC ratio which overall is defined as < 70%
- Reversible obstruction (i.e. asthma) is evaluated by post bronchodilator response (12% or 200cc improvement)
- Suspect a restrictive lung disease in patients with a normal FEV1/FVC ratio but the FVC itself is <80%. DLCO is best to obtain at this point to r/o IPF or other diffusion defects

ASTHMA

- **Background**[319,320]
  - Family history
  - Allergies (seasonal or NSAIDs/ASA)
  - Sx more prominent in AM vs PM (PM more s/o dx)
  - F>M; AA>Caucasian
- **Definition** – chronic inflammatory disorder of the airways triggered by various sensitizing stimuli resulting in reversible airflow obstruction.
- **Types**
  - Type 2 – irritant asthma (painting, bleach, cold)
    - Most common form; peaking in the 2nd decade
    - Atopic (extrinsic)
    - Commonly associated with positive family history
    - Look for IgE+ to specific antigens such as dust, pollen, dander, mold
    - Common concurrent conditions: AERD, ABPA, chronic rhinosinusitis, nasal polyposis, atopic dermatitis
    - Treatment is commonly with immunomodulators
  - Non-Type 2 – allergen induced (dust, mold)
    - IgE mediated via IL-4 associated with mast cells and eosinophils
    - Blood eosinophils >150
    - Sputum eosinophils >2%
    - FeNO > 20 ppb
    - Less common; associated with later age of onset
    - Non-atopic (intrinsic)
    - Triggers are not really allergy related but more with exercise, cold exposure, smoke, viruses, fumes, medications
    - Treatment is with bronchial thermoplasty
- Exacerbating Factors[321]
  - Anxiety→VCD
  - Systemic or Eosinophilic inflammation
  - OSA
  - Depression
  - Not taking inhaler correctly
- **Endotypes**
  - Eosinophilic – early onset, allergic IL-4, IL-13 mediated. Late onset, IL-5
  - Exercise Induced – mast cell associated; often leads to late onset obesity-related asthma. IL-9.
  - Obesity – leukotriene associated; patients will respond best to Singulair
- **Classification**
  - See table on next page

Classification of Asthma

Type	Symptoms	Treatment req	Spirometry	Treatment
Intermittent	Sx ≤2 days/week, PM awakenings ≤2 times per month No interference with normal activity	SABA use ≤2 days/week	Normal FEV1 b/w exacerbations	SABA
Mild persistent	Sx >2 days/week but not daily, PM awakenings 3-4 times per month Minor limitations in normal activity	SABA use >2 days/week but not daily	Normal FEV1 b/w exacerbations	SABA +/- LABA/LAMA+ICS (low dose) PRN LABA+ICS (budesonide+fomoterol) equal to PRN SABA *cannot give LABA alone* *consider adding leukotriene inhibitor, theophylline or cromolyn sodium
Moderate persistent	Daily symptoms, PM awakenings ≥ 1x/week but not nightly Some limitation in normal activity	Daily use of SABA	FEV1 (predicted) 60-80% FEV1/FVC 75-80%	SABA+ICS (high/medium dose) +LABA/LAMA+leukotriene inhibitor Add tiotropium
Severe persistent	Sx throughout the day, PM awakenings often 7 times per week Extremely limited normal activity, and	SABA use several times a day	FEV1 (predicted) <60% FEV1/FVC <75%	Low dose oral Steroid + ICS+LABA+LAMA Consider referring for add-on treatment (i.e. tiotropium, biologics) Consider bronchial thermoplasty if non-allergic Triple therapy with LABA+LAMA+ICS has not been found to be beneficial

- **Exam**
  - Nasal polyps (consider AERD)
  - Nasal mucosal bogginess
  - Sinus tenderness
  - Wheezing (expiratory)
- **Diagnosis**
  - Look for the typical pattern of symptoms with the correct objective data on PFTs and appropriate response to therapy (beta agonists).
    - Symptoms - Combination of consistent symptoms (i.e. cough, chest tightness, wheezing, SOB) with documented reversible airway obstruction (on PFTs or home peak-flow)
- **Diagnostics**
  - Pulmonary Function Testing
    - Reversible obstruction on PFTs showing FEV1/FVC < 70% with reversibility of 12% AND 200cc in FEV1 OR FVC with administration of SABA.
      - If PFT's are "normal" and no reversibility noted, proceed with methacholine challenge (drop in 20% of FEV1; 80% SN, 96% SP) to test bronchial hyperactivity
      - If ratio is normal, but reversibility is still present, diagnosis is still made
  - Labs - *be aware that FeNO, RAST, and serum eosinophils affected by concurrent OCS use*
    - CBC with serum eosinophils (>150 diagnostic)
    - Anti-IgE level (repeat up to 3 times if initial negative as it can be falsely negative with concurrent steroid use)
    - FeNO – look for >20 ppb; levels are often high due to ↑ eosinophils; can be used for long term monitoring
    - Immunoglobulin levels (severe; step 5)
    - RAST (IgE specific)
    - Fungal precipitants
    - Skin allergy testing
  - Other Diagnostics
    - CXR +/- HRCT
- **Treatment**
  - Treat to symptom control, not based on severity "levels"
    - Goal is for patient to have no limitations on physical activity, no nighttime awakenings, normal lung function, and 2x/week or less of daytime sx.
  - In pregnant patients, keep SaO2>95%
  - Pharmacologic Options
    - **Never provide LABA monotherapy without concurrent ICS treatment**
    - *Direct Bronchodilators*
      - B2 agonists –
        - Short acting: albuterol, levalbuterol, metaproterenol, pirbuterol
        - Long acting: salmeterol, vilanterol
      - Anti-cholinergics
        - Short acting: Ipratropium bromide
        - Long acting: Tiotropium bromide, glycopyrronium, aclidinium
      - Methylxanthines – aminophylline, theophylline, daliresp (PDE-4 inhibitor)
      - Adrenergic agonists - epinephrine
    - *Anti-inflammatory medications*
      - Corticosteroids (inhaled, PO, IV, IM): Fluticasone, prednisone, beclomethasone
    - *Mast cell stabilizers* – cromolyn sodium, nedocromil
    - *Leukotriene Antagonists* – zileuton, montelukast. Work best in obese patients.
    - *Immunomodulators/Biologics* – for patients with severe asthma only
      - Prior to starting

- Confirm the diagnosis via lab testing of IgE, sputum EOS, etc.
- Perform baseline phenotyping to understand if the patient has type 2 asthma
- Assess inhaler technique, adherence, contributing factors, and manage comorbidities
- Identify appropriate biologic based on patient characteristics (see table below)
- Re-assess patient every 4 months while on therapy

Biologics in Severe Asthma				
Agent	Target	Eosinophils	FeNO	Clinical/Factors
Dupilumab	IL-4	150/mcl		Steroid-dependent asthma, moderate to severe asthma
Mepolizumab	IL-5	150/mcl or 3% sputum eos		Steroid-dependent asthma, severe asthma
Resilizumab	IL-5	400/mcl or 3% sputum eos		Severe asthma; requires IV infusion, no improvement on steroid req'd
Benralizumab	IL-5 receptor	300/mcl or 2% sputum eos	50 ppb	Steroid-dependent asthma; moderate to severe asthma
Omalizumab	IgE	300/mcl	19.5 ppb	IgE 30-700; weight-based

- Should be started by Pulmonology; commonly used with severe allergic type asthma that is refractory to traditional therapy
- Options based on laboratory results:
  - Elevated serum eosinophils
    - **> 150** – Mepolizumab 100mg SQ q4w at home
    - **> 300** – Benralizumab 30mg SQ q4w x3 then q8w at infusion center
    - **> 400** – Resilizumab 3mg/kg IV over 20-50min
  - IgE – omalizumab weight-based dosing, given in hospital, q2w or q4w
  - FeNO > 50 - Benralizumab 30mg SQ q4w x3 then q8w at infusion center
- Patients should be re-assessed every 4 months on biologic therapy with FEV1, ACT, FeNO, serum eosinophils, and ask if they have required any oral steroids.

o Non-Pharmacologic
- Nonpharmacologic includes removal of allergens, patient education on how to use inhaler, physical training, smoking cessation, weight loss (if applicable).
- Bronchial thermoplasty is an option in non-allergic asthma in patients with severe asthma; in allergic asthma patients 40% reduction in symptoms seen

o Pregnancy
- Inhaled beta-agonists safe (SABA, LABA), cromolyn sodium, PO and IV steroids
- Leukotriene inhibitors should be avoided if possible

Long-term control medications for asthma

Medication	Dosage Form	Adult Dose	Comments
Systemic Corticosteroids			
Methylprednisolone	2, 4, 6, 8, 16, 32 mg tablets	7.5-60 mg daily in a single dose in AM or every other day as needed for control	Administer single dose in AM either daily or on alternate days (alternate-day therapy may produce less adrenal suppression).
Prednisolone	5 mg tablets, 5 mg/5 mL, 15 mg/5 mL	Short course "burst": to achieve control, 40-60 mg per day as single or 2 divided doses for 3-10 days	Short courses or "bursts" are effective for establishing control when initiating therapy or during a period of gradual deterioration.
Prednisone	1, 2.5, 5, 10, 20, 50 mg tablets; 5 mg/mL, 5 mg/mL		
Inhaled Long-Acting β₂-Agonists			
Salmeterol	DPI 50 mcg/blister	1 blister every 12 hors	Decreased duration of protection against EIB may occur with regular use.
Combined Medication			
Fluticasone/Salmeterol	DPI 100 mcg/50 mcg 250 mcg/50 mcg, or 500 mcg/50 mcg HFA 45 mcg/21 mcg 115 mcg/21 mcg 230 mcg/21 mcg	1 inhalation twice daily; dose depends on severity of asthma	100/50 DPI or 45/21 HFA for patient not controlled on low- to medium-dose inhaled corticosteroids 250/50 DPI or 115/21 HFA for patients not controlled on medium- to high-dose inhaled corticosteroids
Budesonide/Formoterol	HFA MDI 80 mcg/4.5 mcg 160 mcg/4.5 mcg	2 inhalations twice daily; dose depends on severity of asthma Shown to be equal in benefit to prn SABA in mild-persistent asthma d/t fast onset of action of fomoterol[322]	80/4.5 for asthma not controlled on low- to medium-dose inhaled corticosteroids 160/4.5 for asthma not controlled on medium- to high-dose inhaled corticosteroids

	Low Dose	Medium Dose	High-Dose
Inhaled Steroids			
Beclomethasone dipropionate (CFC)*	200–500	>500–1000	>1000
Beclomethasone dipropionate (HFA)	100–200	>200–400	>400

Budesonide (DPI)	200–400	>400–800
Fluticasone propionate (HFA)	100–250	>250–500
Mometasone furoate	110–220	>220–440
Triamcinolone acetonide	400–1000	>1000–2000
Leukotriene Modifiers		
Montelukast	10mg	One tablet daily
Zafirlukast	20mg	One tablet BID
Zileuton	600mg	Two tablets BID within 1 hour of meals

- **Refractory Asthma**
  - Represents a subgroup of patients (<5%) with high medication requirements to maintain good disease control or those with persistent symptoms despite high medication use
  - Most asthma patients can be controlled with use of beta-agonists and low dose anti-inflammatory agents
  - Assess inhaler technique
  - Encompasses asthma patients known to have 'severe' asthma or 'steroid-dependent' asthma
  - Severe asthma defined as steroid dependence with FEV1 < 50% predicted
  - Clinical Presentation
    - Widely varying peak flows
    - Copious phlegm production
    - Chronic airflow limitation
    - Rapidly progressive loss of lung function
  - 2 major, 7 minor criteria

Criteria for Diagnosis	
Major	Minor
Treatment with continuous or near continuous (>50%/year) oral steroids	Requirement for daily treatment with a controller medication in addition to inhaled steroids (i.e. LABA, montelukast, theophylline)
Requirement for treatment with high-dose inhaled steroids	Asthma symptoms requiring SABA use on daily or near daily basis
	Persistent airway obstruction (FEV1<80%)
	One or more urgent care visits/year
	3+ oral steroid bursts/year
	Prompt deterioration with <25% reduction in oral or inhaled steroid dose
	Near fatal asthma event in the past

  - **Evaluation**
    - Confirm reversible airflow limitation and quantify severity
      - FEV1, peak flow, and flow–volume loop before and after bronchodilator treatment
      - Total lung capacity and residual volume
      - Diffusion capacity (in adults—usually not indicated in children)
    - Consider other diagnoses
      - AF
      - COPD
      - Depression
      - Anxiety
      - Rhinosinusitis
      - GERD
      - VAD
      - OSA
    - Investigate concomitant diseases
      - Allergen skin tests
      - CT sinus
      - 24-hour pH for GERD
      - Environmental/occupational exposures
        - Smoking
        - Viral Infections

- Occupational agents (wood, birds, coal) → allergies
- **Therapy**
  - Controller Therapy – initial therapies include inhaled GA's, LABA with combination of 2+ controller agents
    - Oral Steroids – given in patients with frequent daytime or nocturnal sx, recent deterioration, or FEV1<60% of predicted for 2-3 weeks
    - Inhaled GAS – with increases to up to 1600-2000/day
    - LABA
    - Theophylline – not used as much, for rare cases
    - Anti-leukotriene agent – Zileuton, montelukast, and zafirlukast
      - Anti-IgE therapy – omalizumab (check IgE level), often takes 12 weeks minimum before response
  - Spirometry
    - Obtain in all patients with consideration for diagnosis of Asthma
    - Perform Asthma Control Test (ACT) questionnaire with each clinic visit
    - Repeat after symptoms are under control on pharmacologic therapy to obtain true baseline
    - After this, repeat q1-2y or after episodes of poor control

Asthma Exacerbation
- Causes
  - Infection (viral vs bacterial)
  - Exposure (pollen, ozone, cold air, humidity, smoke)
  - Non-adherence to tx
- Clinical Exam
  - ↑HR, ↑RR, ↓SaO2, dyspnea, hyperresonance, ↓breath sounds
- Labs
  - CBC
  - CMP
  - TROP
  - Procalcitonin (reduces initiation of antibiotic treatment in the ED without adverse outcomes)
  - Sputum Cx
  - ABG
  - Peak flows
- Imaging: CXR
- Categorization
  - Mild/Moderate (M)
    - Talks in phrases, not agitated, able to lie down
    - Normal RR, Pulse 100-120; O2 90-95%, PEF>50% predicted/or best
  - Severe (S)
    - Talks in words, agitated, must sit up
    - RR>30/m, Pulse>120, O2<90%, PEF<50%
- Acute Management
  - See table below
  - O2 to keep PaO2>92%
  - Bronchodilator
    - Neb treatment (albuterol 2.5 5.0mg NEB q6h +q1h prn + ipratropium 0.5mg NEB q6h)
  - Steroids (IV = PO)
    - IV: methylprednisolone 1mg/kg or appx 80mg IV q8h x5-10d
    - PO: prednisone 30-45mg daily x5-10d
  - Consider MgSO4 1.2 or 2g as a single IV infusion over 15-30m in refractory cases

PULMONOLOGY/CRITICAL CARE

- Hospital Admission Criteria
  - PaO2<90% on supplemental oxygen
  - FEV1 <2.1L and PEF < 300 L/min

Asthma treatment options based on severity of attack

Cat	Treatment	Dosage
M/S	Oxygen	Maintain SpO2>92%
M/S	Albuterol	2.5 mg by nebulization q20min or 4–6 puffs by MDI w/spacer q20min
S	Epinephrine	0.3 mL of a 1:1000 solution subcutaneously every 20 minutes x 3. Terbutaline is favored in pregnancy when parenteral therapy is indicated. Use with caution in patients > age 40 and in the presence of cardiac disease
M/S	Ipratropium bromide	0.5 mg combined with albuterol by nebulization every 20 minutes or 4–6 puffs by MDI with spacer combined with albuterol every 20 minutes
S	Methylprednisolone	60 mg IV every 6 hours or prednisone PO 40 mg Q6H
S	Magnesium sulfate	2 g IV over 20 minutes, repeat in 20 minutes if clinically indicated (total 4 g unless hypomagnesemia)
M/S	Theophylline	5 mg/kg IV over 30 minutes loading dose in patients not on theophylline, followed by 0.4 mg/kg per hour IV maintenance dose. Watch for drug interactions and disease states that alter clearance. Follow serum levels
M/S	montelukast	10 mg PO (the chewable formulation may have quicker onset of action)
S	Heliox	80:20 or 70:30 helium:oxygen mix by tight-fitting, nonrebreathing face mask. Higher helium concentrations are needed for maximal effect

COPD

The following is for chronic, outpatient management. For acute exacerbations, see page 488

- **Pathophysiology**[323,324,325,326]
  - Hallmark is sudden and marked imbalance between respiratory load and capacity.
  - The inciting event is a flare up in inflammation in the airways that leads to increased airway edema, bronchospasm, and increased sputum production.
  - All these lead to an increase in the elastic and resistive loads and worsening of airflow resistance, with consequent increase in the labor of breathing.
  - Patients respond with rapid, shallow, ineffective breaths
  - There is increased dead space breathing, leading to further deterioration in alveolar ventilation.
  - Severe airflow resistance leads to dynamic hyperinflation, which results in a flattening of the diaphragm that further increases the work of breathing.
- **Symptoms (assessed via mMRC scale or the COPD assessment test [CAT])**
  *Those **bolded** below are suggestive of an acute exacerbation when present*
  - **SOB**
  - Chest tightness
  - **Change in sputum purulence**
  - **Change in sputum volume**
  - Cough
  - Confusion
  - ↑HR

- o ↑RR
- o Wheezing
- o Fatigue
- o Fever
- o Malaise
- **Diagnosis**
    - o Symptoms of SOB+chronic cough+sputum with appropriate risk factors (i.e. tobacco, occupational exposure, pollution)
    - o Spirometry results (post bronchodilator FEV1/FVC < 70%)
        - Severity based on FEV1 (see table on page 483)
- **Etiology**
    - o Medication noncompliance
    - o Exposure (tobacco, allergies, air pollution)
    - o CHF
    - o Infection
    - o PE
    - o PTX
- **Classification (see following Table)**
  GOLD classification based on airflow limitation (FEV1). Symptom burden determines what group (A-D) they belong to which helps therapeutic management.
  + Grade airflow limitation/severity based on GOLD
  + Assess symptoms and risk of exacerbation (apply ABCD tool)
  = *Example: FEV1/FVC <0.7; GOLD grade 2; group A*
- **Assessment of Symptoms**[327]
    - o COPD Assessment Tool (CAT) (reviews current symptoms and control)
    - o Modified Medical Research Council dyspnea scale (predicts severity and future *mortality* risk)
    - o Use ABCD status to assign combined assessment based on symptoms

ABCD Assessment Tool		
History of Exacerbations	Symptom Score	GOLD group
No hospitalizations	Low	A
And <2 exacerbations	High	B
Hospitalization	Low	C
Or ≥2 exacerbations	High	D

Low=mMRC 0-1/CAT<10
High=mMRC ≥2/CAT≥10

- **Labs**
    - o CBC
    - o Blood eosinophil count
        - Biomarker to guide **ICS** use
            - □ EOS<100 cells/mcL or <2% → ICS will have minimal benefit
            - □ EOS>100 cells/mcL or >2% → ICS to have ↑ benefit
        - Can be used to monitor risk for exacerbations
        - Higher levels = pts more likely to have beneficial response with the addition of ICS (*COPENHAGEN GENERAL POPULATION STUDY*).
    - o BMP, Mg, Phosphorus
    - o Alpha-1-antitrypsin deficiency once after initial diagnosis is confirmed of COPD
    - o 12 lead ECG
    - o Procalcitonin (in acute exacerbations, reduces initiation of Abx treatment in the ED)
    - o BNP (r/o CHF)
    - o Troponin

- ABG (O2, CO2)
  - ↓O2 = CPAP
  - ↑CO2 = BiPAP
  - Mechanical ventilation for pH<7.36, CO2>45mm
  - Repeat 30-60min after providing O2
  - BNP (to rule out underlying HF)
- **Diagnostics**
  - Spirometry
  - CT Imaging – helps define phenotypes (pink puffers, or emphysematous, associated with loss of mesenchymal tissue) vs the (blue bloaters, or chronic bronchitis patients, associated with airway luminal narrowing and wall thickening manifesting as a chronic cough, phlegm production, or discoloration.
- **Treatment**
  - Goals: ↓COPD sx, ↑exercise tolerance, ↓progression, ↓mortality
  - Approach
    - *Mild COPD (FEV1/FVC≥80%; GOLD 1)* - reasonable to start with one bronchodilator (LABA or SABA); beyond SABA, can use either LABA or LAMA
    - *Moderate/severe COPD* - dual bronchodilator therapy with LABA+LAMA combinations are helpful
      - *ICS are rarely used but when necessary are added to single bronchodilator therapy (moderate disease) before going to dual bronchodilators **or** if patients are not responding to LABA+LAMA combinations then add ICS **or** patients have ↑serum eosinophils **or** have asthma like symptoms.*

GOLD Criteria

Class/Symptoms	Group	Risk	PFTs	Assessment	Treatment
I (mild)	A	Low (<1 exacerbation & no hospitalizations/year)	FEV1 ≥ 80% predicted	mMRC ≤ 1 CAT <10	SABA -or- SAMA
II (moderate)	B		FEV1 50-79%	mMRC ≥ 2 CAT ≥ 10	SABA + LAMA +/- LABA (LAMA preferred per UPLIFT) *If further exacerbations...* Combine LAMA+LABA (SPARK) *Or* *Try the other long acting bronchodilator alone*
III (severe)	C	High (≥ 2 exacerbations or ≥1 hospitalization/year)	FEV1 30-49%	mMRC ≤ 1 CAT <10	SABA + LAMA -or- LABA *If further exacerbations...* LAMA+LABA (SPARK) (indacaterol/glycopyrronium) -or- LABA+ICS (FLAME) if eos ≥ 300/uL/>2%, h/o asthma, allergies, rhinitis
IV (very severe)	D		FEV1 ≤ 30% or FEV1 <50% + chronic resp failure	mMRC ≥ 2 CAT ≥ 10	SABA + LAMA+LABA+ICS (advised if 1+ hospitalizations for AECOPD, or 2 exacerb/year) (LABA+ICS preferred in patients with asthma component or ↑blood eosinophils >2%; ≥ 300/uL) +/- Azithromycin (hospitalized) -or- Roflumilast (chronic bronchitis)

GOLD Criteria

Class/Symptoms	Group	Risk	PFTs	Assessment	Treatment
					If further exacerbations... - Add ICS (triple therapy, *IMPACT*) - Long term O2 if hypoxemic (PaO2 $\leq$ 55% or SpO2 $\leq$ 88%) - Consider lung reduction surgery - Consider roflumilast if FEV1 <50%+chronic bronchitis - Consider stopping ICS if no improvement while on it (patient with low eosinophil count and rare exacerbation history) - Consider macrolide (in former smokers)

- o Short acting bronchodilators scheduled
  - Include beta-agonists and anticholinergic bronchodilators via neb or MDI
  - Patients with severe dyspnea may benefit from nebulizer due to poor inhalation technique and can later be transitioned to MDI
- **Inhaler Technique**
  - o MDI (Metered Dose Inhaler)
    Examples include flovent, azmacort, beclovent, vanceril, budesonide, aerobid
    - Instructions
      1. Must shake before use for about 5 seconds with the cap on, drug is in a suspension
      2. Take the cap off and hold upright
      3. Breath out completely
      4. While pressing the inhaler, slowly breath in and as deep as possible
      5. Hold breath for about 10 seconds
    - Can use spacer if patient has problems with coordinating breaths or has arthritis
  - o DPI (Dry Powder Inhaler)
    Examples include breezhaler, diskus, ellipta, spiromax
    - Medication is in a loose powder form
    - Easier to use
    - Activated by the breath, no timing required like with MDIs
  - o Soft Mist Liquid Inhaler
    Examples include spiriva respimat, olodaterol, stiolto
    - Think of this as a combination between an MDI and a nebulizer
    - Less of the medication gets stuck in the upper airway and no propellant is present
  - o Nebulizer
    - Allows for a large dose of medication without any required coordination
    - Problem is they are not portable and take a while to set up

Management of step-up therapy	
If on	Then
LAMA or LABA	Switch to combination LAMA+LABA
	If EOS$\geq$300 -or- $\leq$100 but 1 hospitalization or s/o asthma then ICS+LABA
ICS+LABA	Add LAMA or stop ICS and do LAMA+LABA
LAMA+LABA	Add ICS if EOS $\geq$100
	Add roflumilast if EOS <100
	Consider starting azithromycin
LAMA+LABA+ICS	Stop ICS
	Consider adding roflumilast if FEV<50
	Consider starting azithromycin

- o LABA/LAMA combinations (moderate/severe disease) (*FLAME*)
  - These combinations improve lung function compared to placebo and have a greater impact on patient reported outcomes compared to monotherapies.
  - LABA/LAMA improves symptoms and health status in COPD patients, is more effective than long-acting bronchodilator monotherapy for preventing exacerbations and decreases exacerbations to a greater extent than ICS/LABA combination.
  - **Options**
    - **Indacaterol+glycopyrronium** 27.5/15.6 & 110/50 *(FLAME, LANTERN)*
    - Formoterol+aclidinium 12/400
    - Formoterol+glycopyrronium 9.6/14.4

- Vilanterol+umeclidinium 25/62.5
- Tiotropium+olodaterol
- Triple Therapy (LAMA+LABA/ICS) shows improved lung function but evidence is scarce *(IMPACT)*
  - Patients had higher incident of PNA but ↑QOL, FEV1 and ↓exacerbations, mortality
  - *IMPACT, FULFIL* - Fluticasone furoate 100mcg+umeclidinium 62.5mg+vilanterol 25mcg (DPI)
  - *TRILOGY, TRINITY, TRIBUTE* - Beclomethasone+formoterol+glycopyrronium (MDI)
- +/- Antibiotics (↑sputum production, frequency)
  - Goal is to improve airflow and decrease hyperinflation of lungs
  - Provided in the acute setting
  - May benefit patients with mild exacerbations and **purulent** sputum
  - Levofloxacin 500mg PO daily x 3-10 days vs. 750mg PO daily for 7 days
  - Doxycycline 100mg PO BID x 3-10 days
  - Amoxicillin-clavulanate 875 mg, Tab, PO, q12h
  - Prophylactic Use:
    - Azithromycin (250 mg/day or 500 mg 3x/week) or erythromycin (500 mg two times per day) for 1 year reduces the risk of exacerbations in patients prone to exacerbations (>2 per year).
      - No effect on mortality
      - Use ↓ exacerbation rate in **former smokers only** in patients who have frequent exacerbations despite optimal maintenance inhaler therapy
        - Associated with an ↑ incidence of bacterial resistance and impaired hearing tests.
        - Pulse moxifloxacin therapy in patients with chronic bronchitis and frequent exacerbations does not reduce exacerbation rate.
- Beta Agonists
  - Duoneb 2ml Q 6 hours with Q 4 hours prn SOB/Wheezing
  - Xopenex (Levalbuterol) 1.25/3ml neb Q 4-6 hour prn SOB/wheezing (hold for tachycardia)
  - Neb: Albuterol 2.5 mg & Atrovent 0.5 mg in 3 cc NS q 4 hours
    or
  - MDI: 4-8 puffs (90 mcg per puff) with a spacer q1-4 hour as needed
- Anticholinergics *(UPLIFT)*
  - Nebulizer
  - Ipratropium (Atrovent) 0.5mg (500mcg) by neb q4h daily (or PRN SOB wheezing), or desaturation
    vs
    Ipratropium/Albuterol (Duoneb) by neb every 4 hours PRN SOB, wheezing
  - MDI
  - Spiriva (Tiotropium) 18mcg 2 puffs by MDI q4h PRN
- Systemic Glucocorticoids
  - Associated with greater FEV1, ↓hospitalization relapse, and improved oxygenation
  - No associated mortality benefits
  - Caution in patients with concurrent DM
  - No efficacy difference in PO vs. IV; 10 day course no better than 5 day course
    - PO: prednisone 40mg daily for **5 days** (*GOLD 2017*)
      or prednisolone 30mg daily x 7-14 days (*NICE 2016*)
    - IV: Methylprednisolone 60-125mg IV Q6H (PO equiv to IV; *GOLD 2017*)
- Oxygen Therapy
  - Does not provide mortality benefit nor decreased hospitalization benefit

- Mortality benefit @ PaO2 ≤ 55 mmHg or SaO2 ≤ 88% (goal PaO2 60-70; SaO2 of 88-92%
- Indicated in any of the following:
  - PaO2 ≤ 7.3 kPa or SaO2 ≤ 88% +/- hypercapnia confirmed 2x over a 3-week period
  - PaO2 of 7.3–8.0 kPa or SaO2 of 88%, with evidence of pHTN, peripheral edema suggesting CHF, or polycythemia.
- Patients should be re-evaluated after 60 to 90 days to determine if the treatment is still indicated and effective
- Stepwise oxygen requirement progression
  - NC→Simple Mask→VM
  - BiPAP is best if hypoxia and hypercapnia above baseline; IPAP 8-12; EPAP 3-5 with changes to IPAP to alleviate dyspnea
- Inhaled Steroids
  NOT recommended in the acute setting
  - Use guided by blood EOS level (>2% or sputum >300 cells/mcL)
  - Used per GOLD for categories C + D (higher risk patients)
  - Work best in patients with ↑ serum eosinophils (>2%; ≥300 cells/mcl in *SUNSET* and >400 cells/mcl with 2+ exacerbations in *WISDOM*), not responding to LABA+LAMA or have asthma like symptoms. If patients have a low EOS count (<300), you may actually ↑ exacerbations if you use ICS. (*WISDOM*)
  - ICS ↑ risk for pneumonia
  - Understand risks of w/d if stopping this medication class (*SUNSET, WISDOM*)
  - Options
    - Advair (Fluticasone/salmeterol) 250/50 daily vs. BID
    - Flovent (Fluticasone) 110mcg 2 puffs BID
  - If patient is already on and want to switch to LABA/LAMA, no increased risk of exacerbations seen with w/d of medication (*WISDOM*)
- Mucolytics
  - Options: erdosteine 600mg/d, N-acetylcysteine, carbocysteine
  - Studied only in those **not** taking ICS
  - High dose (1200mg/d) for long term may lead to ↓ exacerbations[328]
  - Weak recommendation to use NAC in moderate to severe COPD (not recommended for acute exacerbations)[329]
- Roflumilast
  - Consider in:
    - GOLD Stage D and if FEV1<50% in patients with chronic bronchitis
    - Adding on if already on LAMA+LABA and low Eos count (<100)
    - Adding on if already on triple therapy (LAMA+LABA+ICS) and not improving (stop ICS, replace with roflumilast)
  - Improved lung function and reduced exacerbations in participants with frequent exacerbations and hospitalization history
  - **Best to be added in patients on fixed-dose LABA+ICS**
  - Cannot be used concurrently with theophylline
  - Not to be used in acute setting
- **Routine Management**
  - Measure FEV1 annually
  - Assess symptoms at each visit
  - Assess inhaler technique
- **Preventive/Secondary Management**
  - Smoking cessation is key
  - Influenza and pneumococcal vaccinations are important in ↓ risk for lower respiratory tract infections

PULMONOLOGY/CRITICAL CARE

- o Pulmonary rehabilitation to increase exercise tolerance and decrease dependence on supplemental oxygen
- o Long-volume reduction surgery (primarily in those with upper long predominant disease)
- o Long term oxygen improves survival in patients with low resting oxygenation level
- o **Air Travel**[330]
  - When planes travel >8000ft, normal oxygenation drops to 89-94% in healthy passengers
  - Patients with severe COPD may not be able to compensate and may develop lightheadedness, chest pain, neurological sequelae in the extremities, palpitations, and dyspnea
  - The following patients should be tested:

Indications for oxygen management with COPD with air travel (flying)	
Resting Pulse Ox	Management
>95%	No testing required
92-95%	Testing if RF such as previous dyspnea during air travel, cannot walk to 50m w/o respiratory distress, mod/severe pulm HTN, FEV<50% are present → hypoxia altitude simulation test
≤92%	Supplement with oxygen without testing
On home O2	Increase flow to 1-2L/min from baseline

Figure. Determining O2 requirements during air travel in patients with COPD

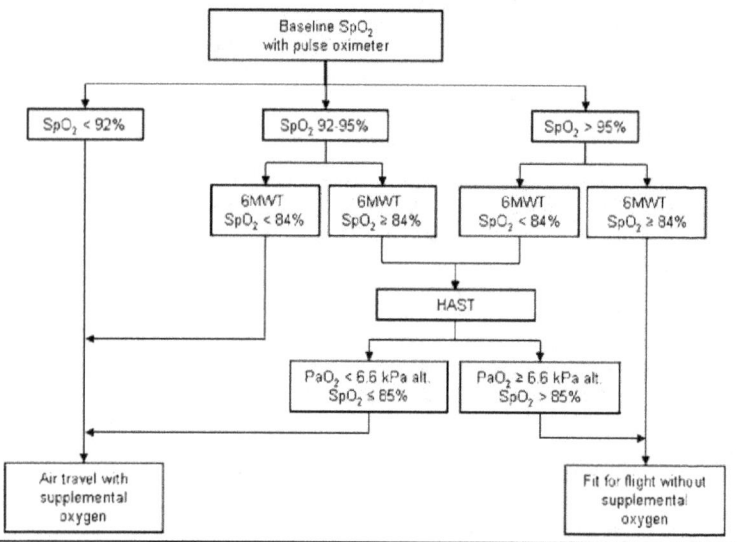

- **COPD Exacerbation**[331,332]
  - Defined - AECOPD is an event characterized by an acute or subacute change in one of 3 cardinal symptoms: (1) a patient's baseline dyspnea (particularly with exertion), and/or (2-3) sputum production (volume [more phlegm or unexpectedly less], purulence) over 2 to 3 days, enough to warrant concern and a call for advice and help with a change in treatment and management
  - General Facts

- Approximately 50% are due to viral infections
- Treat for 5 days duration
- Precipitated by m/c respiratory tract infections, aspiration, pollution, allergens, PE, poor adherence.
- SABA+/-SAMA, are recommended as the initial bronchodilators to treat an acute exacerbation.
- Maintenance therapy with LABA or LAMA should be initiated as soon as possible before hospital discharge.
- Systemic corticosteroids improve lung function (FEV1), oxygenation and shorten recovery time and hospitalization duration.
    - **5-day course** is just as good as 14-day course (*REDUCE*)
- ABx, when indicated, shorten recovery time, and reduce the risk of early relapse or treatment failure, and hospitalization duration.
    - S. pneumoniae, H influenzae, M. catarrhalis are important targets during AECOPD.
    - Remember the possibility for Pseudomonas species to cause AECOPDs in more severely affected patients and when patients do not experience clinical improvement after 2 days of treatment.
  - Non-invasive mechanical ventilation should be the first mode of ventilation used to treat acute respiratory failure.
  - Exacerbations associated with an increase in sputum or blood eosinophils may be more responsive to systemic steroids
  - Symptoms usually last between 7 to 10 days during an exacerbation,
  - Acid-Base

Acid-base correction			
Condition	△ in PCO2	△ in HCO3	pH
Acute	Every ↑10	↑1	↓.1
Chronic	Every ↑10	↑4	↓.015
Acute on Chronic	Every ↑10	↑1	↓.1

  - <u>Oxygen</u> to target saturation of 90 to 92% and PaO2 of 60-65 mmHg with gradual increases in FiO2 by 4-7% (from 24-28%).
    - Venturi masks are preferred means of O2 delivery because they permit a precise delivered fraction of inspired oxygen (FiO2) such as 24, 28, 31, 35, 40, or 60 percent.
    - Nasal cannula can provide flow rates up to 6 L per minute with an associated FiO2 of approximately 40 percent
  - <u>Imaging</u> – CXR to r/o PNA, PTX, or aspiration
  - <u>Diagnostics</u> – ECG to r/o cardiac source, ABG
  - <u>Labs</u> – CBC, BNP, BMP

Treatment for COPD exacerbation	
Therapy	Dose
SABA	
DuoNeb	2cc q4h
Xopenex	1.25/3ml neb Q6h
Ipratropium (AC)	500 mcg via neb q6h → transition to 2 puffs via MDI q4h prn
Steroids	
Solu Medrol	125 mg-200mg IV now (admit) then 80 mg IV Q 6-8 hours
Prednisone	40mg/d = 5 days (no benefit to prolonged 7-14 day course)
Oxygen	

PULMONOLOGY/CRITICAL CARE

Oxygen Therapy:	If SaO2 <88% or PaO2 <7 kPa with goal 88-92%
Antibiotics	
Augmentin	875 mg BID or 500mg TID x5d
Amoxicillin	500mg TID PO x3-14d
Azithromycin	500mg/d x3d
Doxycycline	100mg BID x3-14d
Clarithromycin XL	1g/d (or 500mg BID) x7d
Levofloxacin	500mg daily x5d
Moxifloxacin	400mg/d x5d
Mucolytics	
NAC	600mg BID

- Treatment
    - **Beta Agonists**
        - Goal is to use combination SABA and SAAC
            - Albuterol 5mg via neb q4h prn→ transition to MDI 4-8puffs q1-4h prn
            - Ipratropium (AC) 500 micrograms via nebulizer q6h prn → transition to 2 puffs via MDI q4h prn
            - Others
                - Xopenex (SABA) 1.25/3ml neb Q 6-hour prn SOB/wheezing
                - DuoNeb 2ml Q 4 hours with Q 2 hours prn SOB/Wheezing
    - **Oxygen Therapy**: if SaO2 <88% or PaO2 <7 kPa with goal 88-92%
    - **Solumedrol** 125 mg-200mg IV now (admit) then 80 mg IV Q 6-8 hours OR Solu Medrol **40mg** IV Q 24 hours
        - Duration of Prednisone 40mg/d = 5 days (no benefit to prolonged 7-14 day course) (*REDUCE*)
    - **Antibiotics**
        - No single ABx proven superior over others
        - Typical duration: 5-7 days
        - Cover *S.pneumoniae, H.influenzae, M.catarrhalis*
        - See specific dosage above
        - IV route ↓ tx failure for those in ICU
    - **Physiotherapy**: aids in sputum expulsion
    - **Mucolytics/Anti-Inflammation**: more data needed, however smaller studies have suggested that 600mg BID may be beneficial in acute exacerbations (↓PaCO2, ↑expectoration, ↓C-RP) through antioxidant actions as well as breaking down disulfide which has mucolytic activity.
    - **Non-Invasive PPV** - Consider if patient does not improve with above interventions or if ↑RR, ↓pH or ↑PaCO2 suggestive of impending failure
    - **Intubation**: Consider if not improving to NIPPV or pH <7.26 and PaCO2 ↑

INTERSTITIAL LUNG DISEASES

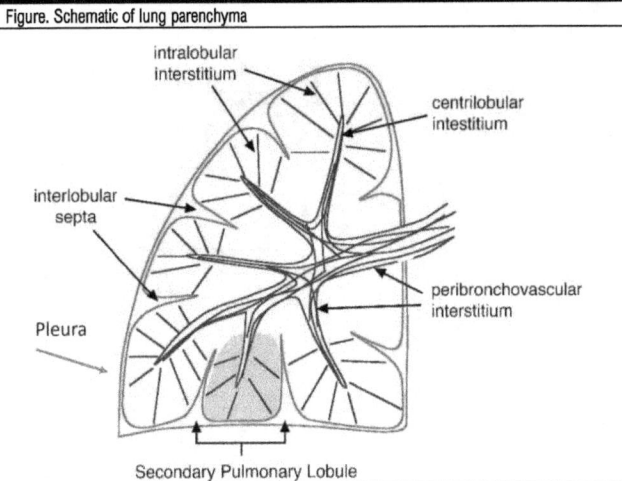
Figure. Schematic of lung parenchyma

- **Defined** - Interstitial lung disease is a term encompassing a diverse range of lung conditions that primarily affect the lung interstitium. ILD should be considered in any person presenting with breathlessness or cough along with abnormal chest radiology or lung function testing.[333,334,335]
- **Symptoms/Exam**
    - Progressive dyspnea
    - Tachypnea
    - Orthopnea
    - Chest discomfort
    - Fatigue
    - Nonproductive cough
    - Inspiratory crackles
    - Digital clubbing
- **Labs/Imaging**
    - Labs
        - ESR/CRP
        - Autoimmune workup
            - ANCAS: C-ANCA, p-ANCA, anti-MRO, anti-PR3
            - RA: Anti-CCP with RF
            - SLE/MCTD/Sjogren's: ANA, ds-DNA, smith, SS-A, SS-B, RNP
            - Sclerosis: SCL-70, centromere
            - Myositis: JO1, CPK, aldolase
    - Imaging/Diagnostics
        - CXR (reticulonodular pattern)
        - HRCT (honeycombing, GGO, mosaicism, see tables below)
        - PFTs (restrictive defect, ↓DLCO, ↓TLV)
        - Bronchoscopy
        - Consider TTE to evaluate for pHTN
- **Classification**

Figure. Classification of ILD

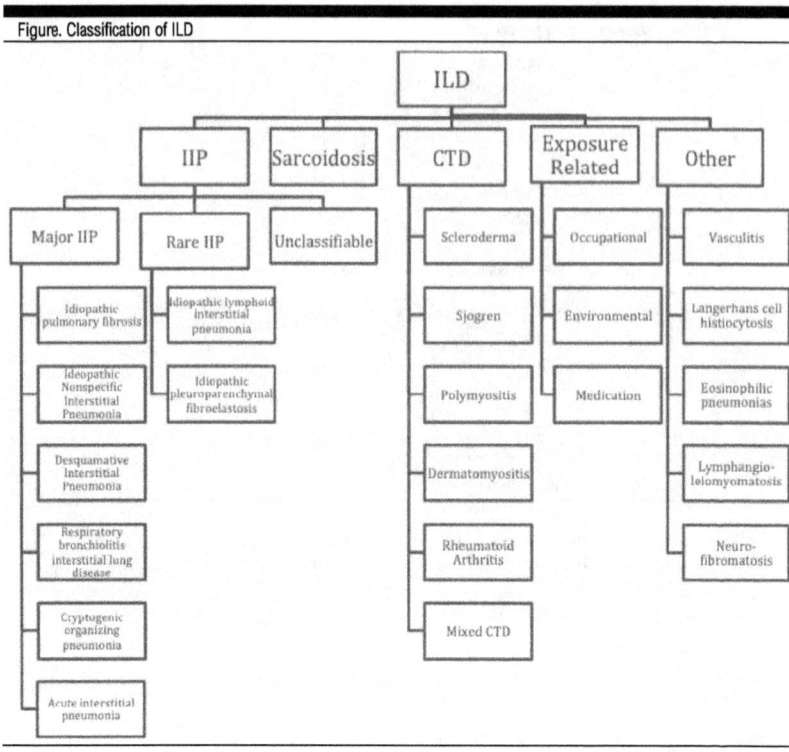

- **Differential Diagnosis**

Differential Diagnosis: subdividing groups of ILD	
Inflammation/fibrosis	**Granulomatous reaction**
<ul><li>Inflammation/Fibrosis<ul><li>Exposure: asbestosis, radiation, coal, metals</li><li>Medication-induced<ul><li>Amiodarone</li><li>Cyclophosphamide</li><li>MTX</li><li>Nitrofurantoin</li></ul></li><li>Smoking-related</li><li>Environmental: birds, hay, mold</li><li>Unknown<ul><li>IIP (NSIP, COP, DSIP, AIP, LIP)<ul><li>DIP = smoking</li><li>NSIP/IPF = chronic fibrosis</li><li>COP/AIP = acute/subacute IIP</li></ul></li><li>IPF</li><li>CTD (RA, scleroderma, SLE, AS, Sjogren's, myositis)</li><li>Eosinophilic pneumonias</li><li>Amyloidosis</li><li>Inherited: TS, LAM neurofibromatosis, PBC</li></ul></li></ul></li></ul>	<ul><li>Granulomatous<ul><li>HSP</li><li>Occupation related dusts (silica, beryllium)</li><li>Sarcoidosis</li><li>Wegener's</li><li>Churg-Strauss</li></ul></li></ul>

- Others (LAM, eosinophilic, Langerhans)
- Pulmonary hemorrhages
- Pulmonary alveolar proteinosis

Distinguishing features of most common ILD groups

Group	History	CT findings	Serologies	Treatments
Smoking	H/o tobacco use, biomass exposure	GGO, emphysema, mosaic	DIP, normal a/i labs	Smoking cessation Remove exposure
HSP	Exposure to organic antigens (avian, mold, farming)	GGO, mosaic, upper lobe fibrosis, centrilobular nodules	Multinucleated giant cells on histology, normal a/i w/u	Remove exposure Anti-inflammatory therapy required
CTD	Constitutional sx Arthralgias Raynaud's	GGO, reticular opacities, fibrosis, consolidation, peripheral sparing	Histology s/o UIP, NSIP, OP, consider a/i w/u	Immunosuppressive therapy with steroids
Medications	Offending rx use	GGO, reticular opacities, consolidation, nodules	Histology shows UIP, NSIP, OP with normal a/i w/u	Stop rx
IPF	M>F, 60-70 YO Past tobacco use Dust exposure	Peripheral and basilar fibrosis with honeycombing	UIP on histology, normal a/i w/u	Antifibrotic therapy, lung transplant evaluation

Diseases associated with Reticulation Pattern on CT

Traction & Honeycombing	Variable traction & honeycombing	Without traction & honeycombing
Lower zone predominant with some upper lobe reticulation	Features not c/w UIP (not lower zone) and are homogenous appearance & septal thickening	Interlobular septal thickening with 2/2 lobules; variable GGO
UIP	Fibrotic interstitial lung disease	Interstitial pulmonary edema
IPF	Indeterminant UIP	Lymphangitic carcinomatosis
UIO	Fibrotic NSIP	Septal amyloidosis
Asbestosis	Fibrotic HP	
RA	Organizing PNA	
	Chronic gastric aspiration	

Differentials based on lung pattern involvement on CT

Decreased lung density	Heterogeneous/Incr lung density
Diffuse low attenuation	*Heterogenous/Mosaic pattern*
-Bronchiolitis obliterans	-Post viral bronchiolitis
-Toxic fume inhalation	-Subacute HP
-Lung transplant recipient	-CTEPH
-Drug toxicity	-PVHTN
-Idiopathic	
Focal areas of attenuation	*Diffuse GGO*
-Centrilobular emphysema	-Crazy Paving consider → subacute diffuse alveolar damage, cellular NSIP, subacute pulm hem, alveolar proteinosis
-LAM	
-Tuberous sclerosis	

PULMONOLOGY/CRITICAL CARE

    -Amyloidosis   -GGO without intralobular lines → interstitial pulm
    -Cystic lung diseases   edema, acute pulm hem, acute lung injury, infxn

- **Diagnosis**
  - Lung biopsy is often required for dx, however BAL and classic imaging findings may suffice
  - Major criteria
    - Exclusion of known causes of ILD
    - Abnormal lung function (restriction and impaired gas exchange)
    - Hypoxia (rest or exercise)
    - Bibasilar reticular abnormalities with minimal ground glass opacities on HRCT
    - Transbronchial lung biopsy or bronchoalveolar lavage (BAL) showing no features to support an alternative diagnosis
  - Minor criteria
    - \>50 years YO
    - Insidious onset of otherwise unexplained dyspnea on exertion
    - Duration of illness >3 months
    - Bi-basal inspiratory crackles
- **Management/Treatment**
  - Acute Respiratory Failure
    - Causes: CHF, arrythmia (check electrolytes), ACS, PNA, sepsis, ILD exacerbation (steroids), PE (anticoag, lytics), anemia (transfuse, address cause), acid/base disturbance
  - Pulmonary rehabilitation
  - Smoking cessation
  - Consider supplemental oxygen if SpO2<88%
  - Treat GERD if present
  - Screen for depression
  - IPF – no therapy proven to ↑survival, consider prednisone, prednisolone, azathioprine, NAC. Consider lung transplantation evaluation.
  - Sarcoidosis – tx indicated in progressive dz, prednisolone 0.5mg/kg for 1 month weaning to maintenance dose for up to 6-24 months
  - CTD – often requires steroids as above, tapering to 10mg/d. Can consider cyclophosphamide.

HYPOXIA

- **Physiology**[336,337]
  - The arterial pH is the main respiratory drive as it is affected by CO2 and is monitored by <u>peripheral</u> (carotid body; PNS/CNS effects) and <u>central</u> (brainstem; monitor H+ levels) chemoreceptors
  - Linear relationship exists between MV (TVxRR) and CO2; this is why with intubated patients these are the variables you monitor to alter CO2 levels
    - ↑CO2 leads to ↓consciousness, ↑CBF (aka ICP, which is why you hyperventilate pts with suspected ↑ICP), decreased myocardial contractility
  - MV is not as closely correlated with PaO2 when PaO2 levels drop below 60. This is the theory behind COPD patients and their ultimate respiratory drive as their PaO2 is often low due to a chronic elevated PaCO2 therefore their senses are 'blunted' to any abnormal levels due to chronically being in this state, as a result they rely on hypoxia instead to drive respirations.
- **Classifications**
  - Mild - PaO2/FIO2 > 200 mmHg

        - Moderate - PaO2/FIO2 100-200 mmHg
        - Severe - PaO2/FIO2 < 100 mmHg
- **A-a gradient**
    - $PAO_2 - PaO_2$ (Alveolar oxygen - capillary oxygen)
    - PAO_2 is calculated and PaO_2 is obtained from blood gas
    - $PAO_2 = 150 - (1.25 \times PACO_2)$
    - Normal gradient 5-20, anything > 20 is abnormal
    - Only causes below that ↑A-a gradient are diffusion defect, V/Q, hypoventilation, Low FiO2, and true shunt
        - Shunt will not improve with supplemental oxygen, require PEEP
        - V/Q mismatch WILL improve with oxygen
- **Five major causes include:**
    - ↓RR / Low alveolar PO2 – low oxygen delivered from lungs into HGB therefore low O2 available to tissues; caused by depressed RAS, respiratory muscle injury, spinal cord injury, NMJ disease (MG), kyphoscoliosis. Anemia can also be considered (1g HGB = 1.34-1.39 ml O2)
    - Diffusion impairment - seen in conditions such as pulmonary fibrosis, interstitial/alveolar edema
    - V/Q mismatch – large areas of lung that are under perfused
        - Major cause of hypercapnia in COPD patients due to emphysema which makes it more difficult to remove CO2 from the lungs due to ↑dead space
        - COPD patients compensate for the ↑ dead space by ↑MV (RR primarily) to try and blow off CO2
    - Shunt – R→L shunt seen with atelectasis, PNA, ARDS, CHF
    - ↓FIO2 – high altitudes

Causes of hypoxia						
Classification	PA_{O2}	Pa_{O2}	Ca_{O2}	P_{O2}	C_{O2}	Increased FI_{O2} Helpful?
↓RR	Low	Low	Low	Low	Low	Yes
Diffusion impairment	N	Low	Low	Low	Low	Yes
Right-to-left shunts	N	Low	Low	Low	Low	No
V/Q mismatch	N	Low	Low	Low	Low	Yes

- **Treatment**
    - Patients with moderate to severe ARDS respond best to prone positioning and NMBD
- **Outcome**
    - Calculate the oxygenation index (see Formulas below)

SUPPLEMENTAL OXYGEN

- Nearly all oxygen is carried to the tissues by hemoglobin (Hb). Each gram/dl of Hb carries 1·3 ml oxygen when fully saturated. A negligible amount is dissolved in plasma. The oxygen content of blood can therefore be calculated:

$$\text{Hb (g/dl)} \times \text{oxygen saturation of Hb} \times 1\cdot3 \text{ and} \times 10 \text{ to convert to litres}$$

- In a 70 kg man a normal HGB is 14 g/dl, normal saturation is above 95% and normal co is 5 liters per minute. Oxygen delivery is therefore: 14 × 0·95 × 1·3 × 10 × 5 = 864·5 ml o2 per minute.

- Low flow devices deliver oxygen at less than the inspiratory flow rate, for example nasal cannula and simple face masks (including masks with a reservoir bag). Although they are low flow, they can deliver a high concentration of oxygen. The oxygen concentration is variable.
    - Nasal canula: fio2 ≈ 21% + (3 x LPM) (maximum 40%)
        - Are commonly used because they are convenient and comfortable. They deliver 2-4 liters per minute of 100% oxygen in addition to the air a person is breathing. Thus, nasal cannula
        - Deliver a variable concentration of oxygen depending on how the patient is breathing → the person breathing slowly
        - Receives a large proportion of oxygen whilst the person breathing quickly receives much less.
    - Simple face mask = up to an fio2 of 50%
        - Deliver up to 50% oxygen when set to 15 liters per minute. Like nasal cannula, the concentration is variable depending on the fit of the mask and how the patient is breathing.
    - Venturi face mask = based on color-coded adaptor, up to an FiO2 of 50%
        - High flow devices deliver oxygen at above the inspiratory flow rate, such as venturi masks. Although they are high flow, a low concentration of oxygen may be delivered. The oxygen concentration is fixed.
    - Nonrebreather face mask = always at an FiO2 of ~60%
- **Diagnoses that satisfy Medicare requirement for home oxygen therapy**
  Diagnosis/ICD-10
    - COPD (J44.9) – *failed SABA, LABA, steroids*
        - Chronic Bronchitis (J42)
        - Emphysema (J43.9)
    - Cystic Fibrosis (E84, E84.9) – *failed mucolytics, inhaled ABx*
    - Bronchiectasis – *failed ABx, steroids, bronchodilators*
    - Pulmonary Hypertension (I27) – *on anticoagulation, drug therapies to dilate arteries, diuretics*
    - Lung Cancer – *on chemotherapy, radiation, etc.*

PLEURAL EFFUSION

- **Causes**[338,339]
    - HF
    - Bacterial pneumonia
    - PE
    - Malignancy
    - Viral infection
    - Cardiac surgery
    - Pancreatitis
- **Types**
    - Uncomplicated – sterile (think CHF)
    - Complicated – due to infection or inflammation from a concurrent infection; also referred to as empyema when due to infection. Diagnosis can be suggested by clinical symptoms but only confirmed on pleural fluid analysis (see below).
- **Thoracentesis**
    - Purpose/Indications: Diagnostic and therapeutic
        - Required when concern for complicated effusion present (parapneumonic)
        - Emergently indicated in patients with respiratory distress or cardiac decompensation as it may improve respiratory status
    - Indications (c/f complicated parapneumonic effusion):

- Effusion on decubitus chest XR is >10mm (with or without loculations, thickened pleura or encompassing more than ½ of the hemithorax)
    - Chest tube should be considered if + gram stain, pH<7.2, or glucose <60
  o Can help diagnose: malignancy, empyema (pus and + gram stain), TB, fungal infections, hemothorax, etc.
    - Malignant effusions may require therapeutic if initial diagnostic performed
- **Characterization**
Done via the Light's Criteria Rule through comparison of serum and pleural protein and LDH

> **Lights Criteria**[340]
> - If at least one of the three is present the fluid is considered an exudate:
>   o Pleural:Serum Protein ratio is > 0.5
>   o Pleural:Serum LDH ratio is > 0.6
>   o Pleural LDH value in total is > 2/3 upper limit of normal LDH for the lab's normal LDH
> - Light's Criteria can falsely diagnose up to 20% of transudative effusions as exudative.
>   o An example of this is patients receiving diuresis will lose fluid component from the effusion increasing the concentration of pleural fluid protein and LDH → appears exudative
> - If Light's Criteria results in exudative, but clinically you suspect it should be transudative, use the <u>Modified Light's Criteria</u>. Considered exudative is one is present:
>   o Serum albumn - pleural albumin ≤ 1.2g/dL
>   o Pleural cholesterol > 45mg/dL

Transudative vs Exudative Pleural Effusion		
Variable	Transudative	Exudative
Concept	Physiologically due to an imbalance of oncotic pressures in the chest (↓albumin) resulting in the shift of fluid from peritoneal/retroperitoneal/etc. spaces	Physiologic basis is behind concept that inflammation of the lung and pleura leads to increased capillary and pleural membrane permeability allowing for increased movement of fluid.
Labs	pH 7.4-7.55 + normal glucose + few WBCs (<1000)	pH < 7.3 + low glucose ▫ pH of 7.3 or below itself is an indication for thoracostomy
Differential	▫ CHF ▫ Cirrhosis ▫ Nephrotic syndrome ▫ Peritoneal dialysis (within 48hrs of starting dialysis) ▫ Urinothorax (in presence of obstructive uropathy)	▫ Infection (PNA, abscesses, hepatitis, TB) ▫ Malignancy ▫ Inflammation (pancreatitis, uremia, ARDS) ▫ PE (can be either) ▫ Sarcoidosis ▫ Esophageal perforation (↑amylase)

- **Fluid Analysis**

PULMONOLOGY/CRITICAL CARE

Pleural Fluid Analysis: Appearance

Color	Suspected Diagnosis
Yellow	Transudates
Blood	Malignancy/Trauma/PE
White	Chylothorax, cholesterol effusion, empyema → centrifuge and see below
Brown	Long standing bloody effusion
Black	Aspergillosis
Green	Biliothorax

Pleural Fluid Analysis: Consistency

Type	Suspected Diagnosis
Clear supernatant above white cells	Empyema (if malodorous, consider anaerobic source)
Viscous	Mesothelioma
Debris	Rheumatoid pleurisy
Turbid	Chylous fluid v. inflammation

- **Imaging**
  - On a standard upright CXR:
    - 75–100 mL of pleural fluid must accumulate in the posterior costophrenic sulcus to be visible on the lateral view
    - 175–200 mL must be present in the lateral costophrenic sulcus to be visible on the frontal view
  - Chest CT scans may identify as little as 10 mL of fluid
- **Procedure Pearls**
  - Needle entry should occur <u>at least</u> 1 intercostal space below the top of the effusion aimed at the posterior hemithorax line and <u>not below</u> the 9th rib
  - Never leave the catheter hub open to the atmosphere → may cause PTX
  - Stop cock points towards side of closure
- **Labs to order**
  - <u>Cell Count</u> – levels >50k suggestive of parapneumonic effusion, empyema
  - <u>pH</u> – normal level is 7.60, if pH < 7.30 this suggests exudative (bacteria produce H+; less efflux of H+ in other exudative processes); 7.4-7.55 is more transudative
  - <u>Protein</u> – should be low in transudative source UNLESS patient is s/p Lasix administration
  - <u>LDH</u> – highly specific in differentiating transudative vs. exudative as elevated LDH in the pleural fluid is suggestive of exudative process (often empyema) as lysis of PMN ↑ LDH levels
  - <u>Glucose</u> – used to help differentiate type of exudative effusion (low levels are less likely infectious); can be seen with rheumatoid causes
  - Cytology
  - Culture
  - Gram Stain
  - Additional: amylase (esophageal perf; pancreatitis), TG (↑ in chylothorax), cholesterol (↑ in exudative), AFB stain/culture, ADA (suspected TB source)
- **Treatment**
  - Antibiotics
    - Can be used for uncomplicated parapneumonic effusions (free-flowing, non-loculated)
    - Treat for anaerobic infection:
      - Clindamycin
      - Amoxicillin-Clavulanic Acid

- Ampicillin-Sulbactam
- Piperacillin-Tazobactam
- Treat until there is resolution of the fluid on plain films (2-4 weeks)
  - Intrapleural tPA DNAse (dornase alfa)
    - Indicated for loculated pleural effusions due to bacterial PNA and trying to avoid surgical intervention (*MIST-2*)
  - Thoracostomy
    - AKA: Chest tube drainage
    - Mostly indicated in:
      - Complicated parapneumonic effusions (loculation present)
        - Severe exudative effusions, pH <7.3 + glucose < 60
      - Empyema (+GS or culture and frank pus)
    - May require additional treatment: thoracoscopy with adhesion lysis and decortication
    - CT are continued until drainage falls below 50 mL/day AND the cavity has closed

SOLITARY PULMONARY NODULE

- **Defined**[341,342,343]
  - <3cm (>3cm is considered mass)
  - Round opacity
  - Surrounded by pulmonary parenchyma
  - Without regional LN
- **Differential Diagnosis**
  - Nonspecific granuloma
  - Hamartoma
  - Infectious granuloma (i.e. aspergillosis, cocci, crypto, histo)
  - Malignancy (i.e. adeno, small cell, mets, squamous)
- **Pearls**
  - Solid nodules <6mm in low risk patients do not require further w/u
  - Solid nodules between 6-8mm should have repeat CT imaging
  - Solid nodules >8mm should have f/u CT imaging (+PET) sooner (3 months)

Radiologic features suggestive of benign vs. Malignant nodule		
Feature	Benign	Malignant
Size	<5mm	>10mm
Border	Smooth	Irregular or spiculated
Density	Dense, solid	Nonsolid or "ground-glass"
Calcification	Typically, a benign feature, especially in "concentric," "central," "popcorn-like," or "homogeneous" patterns	noncalcified, or "eccentric" calcification
Doubling time	<1mo; more than 1 year	1mo-1year

- **Assessment**[187]
  - Radiographic Appearance
    - Size (8mm→8-30mm→>30mm)
    - Appearance (ground glass vs mixed vs solid)
    - Density (fat, hamartoma)
    - Borders (spiculated vs smooth)
    - Location (upper lobe vs middle lobe)
    - Stability (over time)
  - Clinical Risk Factors

- Age
- Smoking history
- H/o malignancy
- *Categorizing risk*:
  - Low risk – minimal or absent history of smoking and other known risk factors
  - High risk – History of smoking or other known risk factors
  - Calculators (Gurney, Mayo, Herder)
- **Screening for SPN with low-dose CT**
  - Asymptomatic smokers ages 55 to 77 years who have smoked 30 pack-years or more and continue to smoke
  - Former smokers ages 55 to 77 years who have smoked 30 pack-years or more and quit within the past 15 years
  - If patient considered high risk of having/developing lung cancer based on clinical risk prediction calculators then still do CT regardless of above criteria

SPN Evaluation			
	Low cancer risk	Intermediate Cancer risk	High cancer risk
Diameter of nodule (cm)	<0.8	0.8-3.0	≥3.0
Age (years)	<40	40-60	>60
Smoking Cessation?	Never Quit > 15 years ago	Current (<20/d) Quit 5-15 years ago	Current (>20/d) <5
Nodule characteristics	Smooth	Scalloped	Spiculated Corona radiata
PET	Low or no activity	Weak or moderate activity	Intense hypermetabolic
Cancer risk	<5%	5-65%	>65%

Fleischner Society Guidelines (2017)			
Size	# of nodules	Low cancer risk	High cancer risk
<6mm	Single	No routine f/u	Optional CT @ 12mo
	Multiple	No routine f/u	Optional CT @ 12mo
6-8mm	Single	CT @ 6-12 mo then consider @ 18-24	CT @ 6-12 mo then @ 18-24
	Multiple	CT @ 3-6 mo then consider @ 18-24	CT @ 3-6 mo then @ 18-24
>8mm	Single	Consider CT @ 3 mo, PET/CT, or biopsy	
	Multiple	CT @ 3-6 mo then consider CT @ 18-24 mo	CT @ 3-6 mo then CT @ 18-24 mo

- **Intervention**
  - *Use the Fleischner Society Guidelines (above)*
  - Intervention depends on combination of risk factors and pre-test probability of malignancy based on radiographic appearance
    - High Risk - Surgical excision
    - Intermediate Risk
      - <1cm nodule
        - Serial CT scans
      - >1cm nodule
        - FDG-PET scan
          - Hot – excise
          - Cold- serial CT scans
    - Low Risk
      - <6mm, solid, noncalcified, age<35 → serial CT scans (see Fleischner Report Criteria) **not required** unless patient is high risk. If high risk, CT remains

optional. CT should be considered though in patients with spiculated margins on the nodule, and/or a nodule in the upper lobe.
- For patients with solid SPNs that have been stable on serial CT over a two year period, or with subsolid SPNs that have been stable over a five year period, no further diagnostic testing req' d.

PULMONARY HYPERTENSION

- **Defined** – high blood pressure in the pulmonary arteries causing increased pressure on the right heart → right heart remodeling → hemodynamic compromise. Can be caused by several conditions.
- **WHO Classification**:
  - Class 1 (*intrinsic pulm artery*): idiopathic, systemic sclerosis, connective tissue disease, drug/toxin induced, familial HIV, congenital heart conditions (shunts), sickle cell, schistosomiasis, portal HTN, genetic (BMPR2 mutation)
  - Class 2 (*heart*): L sided heart failure
  - Class 3 (*lungs*): COPD, ILD, fibrosis, hypoxemia, sleep apnea
  - Class 4: CTEPH
  - Class 5 (*other*): polycythemia vera, sarcoidosis, vasculitis, glycogen storage diseases, kidney disease, essential thrombocythemia, external compression of pulm arteries by tumor
- **Clinical Symptoms**
  - Dyspnea +/- with exertion *(most common presenting Sx)*
  - Fatigue
  - Lower extremity swelling
  - Chest pain
  - Palpitations
  - Dizziness, syncope
  - Bluish discoloration of lips
- **Risk factors:**
  - Obesity
  - Sleep apnea
  - Age (elevated pulm HTN in older patients; however, idiopathic PAH more common in younger patients)
  - Family history
  - Clotting disorder
  - Drug use
  - Arrhythmias
  - Pregnancy
- **Examination**
  - ↑ JVP
  - Peripheral edema, cyanosis
  - TV regurg murmur
  - RV heave/parasternal lift (palpable)
- **Diagnosis**
  - Echocardiogram -- will show elevated PASP or RVSP (surrogate marker for PASP)
  - Right heart cath -- confirmatory test, mean pulm artery pressure >25mmHg
    - Mild: 25-40mmHg
    - Moderate: 41-55mmHg
    - Severe: >55mmHg
- **Treatment**
  - For WHO Class 2-5, treat underlying cause

- For WHO Class 1 → different classes
  - CCBs: amlodipine (only if vasoreactive on right heart cath)
  - PDE-5 inhibitors: sildenafil, tadalafil
  - Endothelin receptor antagonists: Bosentan, Ambrisentan, Macitentan
  - Prostacyclin analogue: Epoprostenol, Treprostinil, Iloprost
  - Prostacyclin IP receptor agonist: Selexipag
  - cGMP stimulators: Riociguat
- For symptomatic pulm HTN with cor pulmonale (right heart failure) → diurese, treat hypoxemia, treat concomitant conditions (COPD exacerbation), HF exacerbation, hypercarbia with BiPAP, etc.)

OBSTRUCTIVE SLEEP APNEA

- **Defined**[344] – cessation of breathing caused by repetitive, episodic collapse of the pharyngeal airway due to an obstruction or airway resistance
  - Central sleep apnea is not the same as OSA, it is respiratory drive cessation due to dysfunction in central respiratory network
- **Screening**[345,346]
  - In patients who are dissatisfied with their sleep quality should undergo a questionnaire (STOP-BANG or Epworth)
  - Consider screening also in those with high risk occupations like bus drivers, truck drivers, surgeons, etc.
- **Clinical Symptoms / Risk Factors**
  - Daytime fatigue
  - Obesity
  - Family history of OSA
  - CHF
  - Stroke
  - AFib
  - Resistant HTN
  - Morning headaches
  - Snoring
  - Apneic episodes
  - Prior diagnosis of hypothyroidism
  - Concurrent metabolic syndrome is often found
- **Examination**
  - Obesity
  - Neck circumference (>16" women; >17" men)
  - Mallampati 3 or 4
  - Macroglossia
  - Tonsillar hypertrophy
- **Red Flags**
  - Excessive daytime fatigue
  - Morning headaches
  - Neck circumference of greater than or equal to 17 inches in males and 16 inches in females
  - Polycythemia
- **Pursuing sleep study**
  - STOP BANG ≥ 3
  - Epworth > 8 (however some studies recommend 10)
- **Diagnosis**
  - Home sleep testing (HST) – noninferior to traditional lab testing

- In-lab sleep study – best for patients with significant cardiovascular disease, chronic opiate use, h/o stroke, h/o insomnia, neuromuscular disorders among others.
- In patients already on CPAP therapy, a CPAP titration study may be warranted if there has been a significant change in body habitus, has been several years since last sleep study or develops clinical symptoms despite being on therapy
- **Severity/Grading (AHI)**
    - Apnea-Hypopnea Index (AHI) - number of times a patient has an episode of complete apnea (stops breathing for 10 or more seconds) + episodes of hypopnea (the definition of which varies) / hour.
        - < 5 – normal
        - 5-14 is - mild OSA
        - 15-29 - moderate OSA
        - 30+ - severe OSA
    - The number of times oxygen a patient's oxygen saturation drops from baseline by 4% or more / hour, or Oxygen Desaturation Index (ODI) and time spent with oxygen less than 90% (T90) are better markers for determining severity
- **Treatment**
    - Mild OSA may not require treatment if patients do not have excessive daytime sleepiness
    - Other levels can be treated with positional therapy with sleep position trainer or tennis ball technique (best for mild positional OSA), autoPAP, BiPAP (in patients with high pressure requirements), a mouth appliance (best for mild-moderate apnea and patients who are resistant to CPAP), nasal surgery (anatomic nasal obstruction preventing PAP use), and bariatric surgery.[347]

HEMODYNAMIC MONITORING IN THE ICU

Hemodynamic variables[348,349]

Item	Acronym	Normal	Interpretation
Evaluation of Volume Status			
Stroke volume variation (Pulse Contour Analysis)	SVV	<10%-15%	Best for patients with combined septic and cardiogenic shock. For ventilated patients, SVV is highly sensitive and specific for **preload responsiveness**. More variation may be indicative of **low volume** status, atrial or ventricular arrhythmia, IABP, ECMO, massive PE. Remember **the correlation between SVV and Frank-Starling Curve.**
Stroke volume index	SVI	35-45	Similar as above
Central Venous Pressure	CVP	8-12	A measurement of **cardiac preload** by looking at the pressure within the thoracic veins. It may be low in low volume states and elevated in either high volume states or RV dysfunction. Patients with atrial fibrillation or dissociation will have altered waveform.
Passive Leg-Raising Test[350]	PLR	<10%	Lift the legs at a 45-degree angle with the patient supine which can result in appx 150cc of blood return; used to predict responsiveness to cardiac output by providing an endogenous **fluid challenge** by monitoring CO after 60-90s. Increase in

Evaluation of Cardiac Function

			SV of >10% indicates patient is pre-load responsive.
Cardiac Index	CI	2.5-4.5	Assessment of cardiac output based on the patient's BMI. Basically, this will tell you how well the heart is pumping. Dobutamine and other inotropes will help increase CI.
Cardiac Output	CO	3-7 L/m	Affected by arrhythmias and ↑HR
Pulmonary Capillary Wedge Pressure	PCWP	2-12 mmHg	An indirect measurement of R atrial pressure and thus, when elevated, can point towards ventricular dysfunction. Most acruately measured with PA cather (i.e. Swan-Ganz) to directly measure LV filling pressure.

Other

Central Venous Oxygen	ScvO2	≥70	Used as a marker of balance between systemic oxygen supply and demand obtained through a VBG from a central line. May require vasopressors +/- transfusions to improve.
Mean Arterial Pressure	MAP	≥65	Invasively measured through arterial line (most preferred); non-invasively estimated through blood pressure cuff (1/3SP + 2/3DP). Should have good dicrotic notch. If overdamped, think soft tubing or bubbles in line. If underdamped, think long stiff tubing or too large of catheter. Increase in variability of measurements in those who are hypovolemic or in atrial fibrillation.
Systemic Vascular Resistance	SVR	900-1200 dyn/s/cm²	

INTUBATION

- **Indications for intubation**[2]
    - Respiratory rate > 35-40 for extended period (minutes can count in a severely debilitated patient.
    - pCO2 > 60 in patient who does not chronically retain CO2
    - pO2 < 50-55 despite therapy and high FiO2 in patient without chronically low values
    - Gross respiratory distress, especially if it is apparent that patient is tiring or too weak to continue arduous respiration for much longer
    - Signs/symptoms of acute respiratory failure:
        - Resp rate > 35
        - Tachycardia
        - PaCO2 > 55 (acute)
    - Cyanosis
    - Change in mental status
    - PaCO2 < 70 on supplemental O2

    Be sure that patient is not a DO NOT INTUBATE before initiating process. Call anesthesia to place the tube and consult pulmonary for ventilator management.

    NOTE: Most people get into trouble by thinking about intubation too late, rather than too early. Don't intubate without calling your resident -- unless it's too late to wait!

- **Intubate if:**
  - Response to tx is inadequate.
  - Airway obstructed or unstable.
  - Work of breathing becomes overwhelming w/ other organ system failure.
  - Inability to protect airway (decreased LOC with no gag/cough).
  - Severe metabolic acidosis with respiratory distress

Sedation / Induction medications used in the intubation of a patient

Drug	MOA	Dose	Onset	Duration	Elimination	Positive Considerations	Negative Considerations
Etomidate		0.1-0.2 mg/kg (usual dose ~20 mg IV)	10-15 seconds	4-10 minutes		• **First line sedative for rapid sequence intubation (RSI).** • Rapid onset • Short duration • No ↓BP, lowers ICP	• tendency to induce vomiting (use with paralytic) • C/I in adrenal insufficiency
Midazolam (Versed)	GABAergic	0.05-0.1 mg/kg over 1-2min	2-5 min	2-4h	Liver	• Good when used in combination with fentanyl • CV stability (no bradycardia, little ↓BP) • Low cost • Anti-convulsant properties	• Risk of ICU delirium (benzos) • Accumulation • Active metabolite • Use lower dose in elderly • High risk for respiratory depression • Daily awakenings and scheduled dose taper can minimize accumulation
Lorazepam (Ativan)	GABAergic	1-15 mg/hr	5-20 min	4-6h	Liver	• Effective sedation	• Accumulation (long T1/2) • Consider only using boluses • Propylene glycol toxicity at high doses
Propofol (Diprivan)	GABAergic	15-50 mcg/kg/m RSI dose is 0.5 mg/kg, sedative dose is 1 mg/kg	30-90s	3-10m	Liver	• Effective sedation • No risk of accumulation • Easily titratable with no need to bolus • Fast recovery, so good for patients in whom neuro exam must be checked frequently (can turn off and check neuro exam in ~10 minutes)	• ↓BP • ↑TRIG due to lipid emulsion • Check TRIG 48 hrs. after use • Propofol related infusion syndrome (PRIS) rare but associated with ST elevation, acidosis, electrolyte imbalance, rhabdo, CV collapse • Expensive,

Sedation / Induction medications used in the intubation of a patient

Drug	MOA	Dose	Onset	Duration	Elimination	Positive Considerations	Negative Considerations
Dexmedetomidine (Precedex)	Alpha-2 agonist	IV 1 mcg/kg loading dose (over 10 min) f/b 0.5-2 mcg/kg/h continuous infusion. Use 0.5 mcg/kg for geriatric patients	15-30m	20-30m	Liver	• Unique sedative profile (can remain arousable) • ↓ICU delirium • Opioid sparing • No respiratory suppression	• Most common adverse events include bradycardia and ↓BP • Avoid if patient on paralytic/NMBA • Avoid in hemodynamic shock • High cost • Some data to suggest use in benzo-refractory delirium tremens • Depresses myocardial contractility
Thiopental	Barbiturate	3-5 mg/kg SE: 15-20 mg/kg IV loading dose over 10-15m	<30 seconds	5-10m	Mostly liver	• Great for RSI in neuro patients (high ICP, CVA, **status epilepticus**). • Rapid onset, ultra-short acting.	• <u>Disadvantages</u>: **not routinely used**, causes ↓BP—reduce dose or use alternative sedative. • Monitor K levels. • Contraindications: severe ↓BP.
Ketamine	Dissociative anesthetic	General Anesthesia: 0.5-1.0 mg/kg IV Further boluses: 10-20mg IV	45-60s	10-20m		• Good option for patients with reactive airway disease or who are hypovolemic, hemorrhaging, or in shock	• ↑HR and ↑BP • ↑Intraocular pressure • Not recommended in hypertensive patients • Caution in those with CVD

Sedation / Induction medications used in the intubation of a patient

Pain medications used in the intubation of a patient

Drug	MOA	Dose	Equianalgesic Dose	Onset	Duration	Elimination	Positive Considerations	Negative Considerations
Fentanyl (DOC for continuous analgesia)	Opioid	25-300 mcg/h	100mcg	1-2m	1-2h	Liver	<ul><li>Short DOA</li><li>Eliminated 1-2h after infusion is D/C</li><li>Low risk of accumulation</li></ul>	<ul><li>Very potent</li><li>Dosing error risk</li><li>Respiratory suppression</li><li>Constipation/Ileus</li><li>Fentanyl induced Rigidity (rare, a/w large bolus doses)</li></ul> Contraindications: increased ICP, end stage liver disease, severe respiratory depression (not yet intubated)
Morphine	Opioid	2-30 mg/h	10mg	2-8m	2-6h	Liver	<ul><li>Most clinicians are familiar with dosing</li><li>Longer duration of action allows for bolus dosing without continuous infusion</li><li>Avoid in CKD</li></ul>	<ul><li>Histamine release</li><li>Flushing</li><li>↓BP</li><li>Constipation/Ileus</li></ul>

Sedation / Induction medications used in the intubation of a patient

Drug	MOA	Dose	Onset	Duration	Elimination	Positive Considerations	Negative Considerations
Hydromorphone (Dilaudid)	Opioid	0.5-10 mg/h 3.5mg	2-8m	2-4h	Liver	• Longer DOA allows bolus dosing without continuous infusion • **Can be used in renal dysfunction** • No or less histamine release	• Less histamine release • Constipation/Ileus

Rapid Sequence Intubation Step by Step

	Class	Medication	Time to Effect	Miscellaneous Information

1	Preparation	• Monitors, laryngoscope, fiberoptic, crico kit, ETT/stylet/syringe, all medications, suction, IV, rescue devices, fluids hanging, pressors if possible, place CXR order
		• LEMON for difficult airway
		  ○ Look, Evaluate (3-3-2 rule), Mallampati, Obstruction evidence, Neck mobility
		  ○ Risk
		    ▪ Mallampati Score (1→4; easy→hard)
		    ▪ Thyromental distance (more = better)
		    ▪ ROM
		    ▪ Size of neck
		    ▪ Size of open mouth
		    ▪ Neck instability (RA, Down's, OA)
		  ○ Sniff
		    ▪ Put pillow rolls under shoulder
		• Preoxygenation with 100% O2
		  ○ 100% O2 for 5 minutes OR 2-6 Full Vital Capacity breaths of 100% O2
		  ○ Denitrogenizes alveoli to allow much longer time before desaturation occurs		

2	Pain medication	Fentanyl 2-10mcg/kg		
3	Premedication	Atropine 0.5-1 mg IV	1-2min	Antisialagogue Inhibits bradycardic response to hypoxia
		Glycopyrrolate 0.005-0.01 mg/kg	1-2min	Antisialagogue Inhibits bradycardic response to hypoxia
4	Induction/Sedative	Etomidate 0.3mg/kg	15-45 sec	Good for ↓BP patients; ↓cortisol (avoid in sepsis)
		Versed 0.3mg/kg	30-60 sec	
		Propofol 1-2mg/kg	15-45 sec	Can ↓BP, good for status epilepticus patients Good for patients with bronchospasm, can ↓BP, no analgesic properties
		Ketamine 1-2mcg/kg	30 sec	Arrythmia, increases secretions; elev BP, elev HR
		Fentanyl 2-5mcg/kg	1-3min	May lower BP, minimal histamine release
5	Paralytic	Succinylcholine 1-1.5 mg/kg	30s-1min	Depolarizing. Typically, first line due to short onset; lasts 6-10 m. ↑K, ↓HR, GBS, ↑muscle fasciculations, ↑IOP, avoid in burn/crush pts, denervation syndromes, severe infection

	Rocuronium 0.6-1.2 mg/kg	45s-1min	Nondepolarizing, rapid onset, used with succinylcholine c/I. Lasts 37-72min.
	Vecuronium 0.1-0.2 mg/kg	2-3m	Higher doses mean quicker onset and longer duration
6	Confirmation	Check placement with end-tidal CO2, t/c NGT, OGT, CXR (ETT should be just below head of clavicles)	

Initial ventilator settings

Calculate predicted body weight (PBW)

Male = 50 + 2.3 [height (inches) - 60] **OR**
50 + 0.91 [height (cm) - 152.4]

Female = 45.5 + 2.3 [height (inches) - 60] **OR**
45.5 + 0.91 [height (cm) - 152.4]

Set mode to volume assist-control
Set initial tidal volume to 8 mL/kg PBW
Reduce tidal volume to 7 and then to 6 mL/kg over 1 to 3 hours
Set initial ventilator rate ≤35 breaths/min to match baseline minute ventilation
Subsequent tidal volume adjustment
Plateau pressure (Pplat) goal ≤30 cm H_2O
Check inspiratory plateau pressure with 0.5 second inspiratory pause at least every four hours and after each change in PEEP or tidal volume.
If Pplat >30 cm H_2O, decrease tidal volume in 1 mL/kg PBW steps to 5 or if necessary, to 4 mL/kg PBW.
If Pplat <25 cm H_2O and tidal volume <6 mL/kg, increase tidal volume by 1 mL/kg PBW until Pplat >25 cm H_2O or tidal volume = 6 mL/kg.
If breath stacking (auto PEEP) or severe dyspnea occurs, tidal volume may be increased to 7 or 8 mL/kg PBW if Pplat remains ≤30 cm H_2O.

Arterial oxygenation and PEEP
Oxygenation goal PaO_2 55 to 80 mmHg or SpO_2: 88 to 95 percent
Use these FiO_2/PEEP combinations to achieve oxygenation goal:

FiO_2	0.3	0.4	0.5	0.6	0.7	0.8	0.9	1.0
PEEP	5	5 to 8	8 to 10	10	10 to 14	14	14 to 18	18 to 24

PEEP should be applied starting with the minimum value for a given FiO_2.

Intubation/Medications

Induction	RSI	Maintenance
Etomidate	30mg	N/A
Ketamine	150mg	50mg/hr
Paralytic		
Succinylcholine	100mg	N/A
Rocuronium	150mg	N/A
Pain		
Fentanyl	50mcg	50mcg/hr

Vent Settings

- Mode: AC
- Rate = 12
- VT = 500cc (6cc/kg; ARDSNet Protocol)
- I:E ratio: 1:2 or 1:3
- FiO2 = 1.0 (wean down rapidly to < 60% to avoid oxygen toxicity).
- PS (pressure support) = 5-10 (5cm H20 needed to overcome resistance of endotracheal tube).
- IFR: 80cc
- PEEP (positive end-expiratory pressure) = 0-15 (start low; cautious use in asthmatics and COPD patients as "auto PEEP" occurs often).

Neuromuscular Blockade Agents[351,352]

	Agent	Onset of Action	Duration of Action	Recommended Bolus Dose	Infusion Rate
Short-Acting	Mivacurium	2min	17min	150 mcg/kg	1-15 mcg/kg/min
	Rocuronium	0.7-1min	30-60min	0.6-1.2 mg/kg	10-40 mcg/kg/min
	Succinylcholine	0.5-1min	5-10min	1-2 mg/kg	2.5 mg/min
Intermediate-Acting	Atracurium	2	30 min	0.5 mg/kg	5 mcg/kg/min
	Cisatracurium	2	30 min	100-200 mcg/kg	1-5 mcg/kg/min
	Pancuronium	2-3	60-90min	0.05-0.1 mg/kg	0.05-1 mg/kg q2 prn
	Vecuronium	1.5	30-60min	0.08-0.1 mg/kg	0.1-0.2 mg/kg q2 prn
Long-Acting	Doxacurium	6	80 min	50 mcg/kg	N/A
	Pipecuronium	3-5	70-120 min	50-100 mcg/kg	N/A

Figure. View of different support modes on ventilator[353]

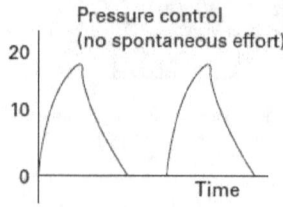
Pressure control (no spontaneous effort)

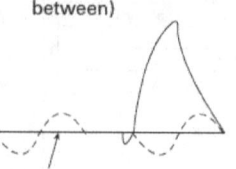
SIMV (spontaneous breaths in between)

Patient's spontaneous breath

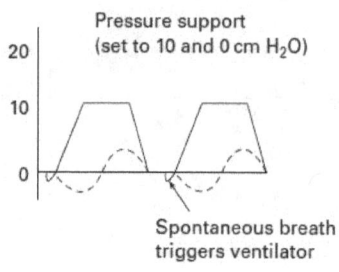
Pressure support (set to 10 and 0 cm H$_2$O)

Spontaneous breath triggers ventilator

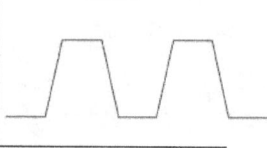
BiPAP

Inspiratory and expiratory times can be adjusted (e.g. longer time allowed for expiration in wheeze)

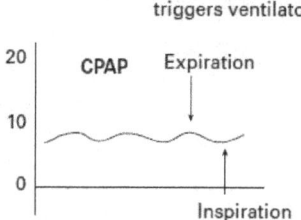
CPAP Expiration

Inspiration

Figure. Example timeline for RSI

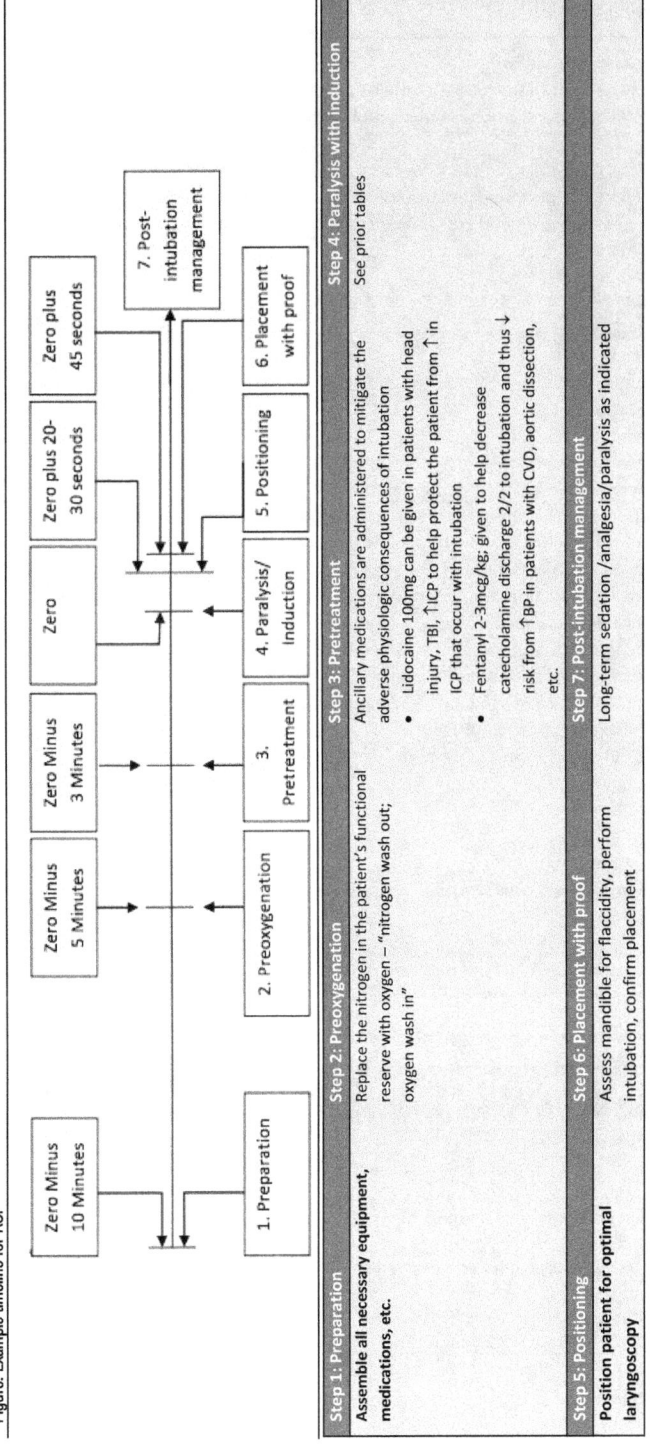

PULMONOLOGY/CRITICAL CARE

- **Rapid Sequence Intubation**
  Used in anyone at risk for aspiration. Major difference is that there is no bag-mask ventilation following induction, as this could introduce air into the GI track causing vomiting.

  1) Be prepared to perform surgical airway in event airway control is lost
  2) Ensure suction is on and you can delivery PP ventilation
  3) Equipment:
     - Laryngoscope
     - Blade
     - NPA/OPA
     - Suction
     - Bougie
     - Glideslope
     - Fiberoptic
     - LMA
  4) Preoxygenate to 100% O2 for 5 minutes
  5) The application of pressure to the cricoid cartilage (to close esophagus and ↓ aspiration) is no longer recommended for use in the ER setting. It has not been tested for appropriateness in pre-hospital care.
  6) **Administer induction drug** (etomidate 0.3 mg/kg or 20mg)
     ****Depresses adrenal function*
  7) **Administer pain drug** (fentanyl 0.3mcg/kg)
  8) **Administer paralyzing drug**: 1-2mg/kg succinylcholine IV (or 100mg)
     Avoid if ↑K, crush injuries, burns, CRF, neuromuscular disease
  9) After relaxation, start intubation
  10) Inflate cuff and confirm placement
      - Auscultation
      - B/L chest rise
      - CO2
      - O2 waves on monitor
      - Release cricoid pressure
  11) Ventilate
  12) CXR
     ETT should be 3-7cm from the carina (Remember 357 magnum) often just below the clavicles. Insertion depth of ETT from corner of mouth of 21cm for women, 23cm for men

EXTUBATION CRITERIA

Required Criteria
1. The cause of the respiratory failure has improved.
2. Tidal volume > 5cc/kg
3. Respirations spontaneous and >8/min
4. NIF of -10 to -15
5. Patient showing purposeful movement
6. Temperature of 35 C or greater
7. Hemodynamic stability
8. PaO2 ≥ 60 on FiO2 40, Pco2 ≤ 55 mmHg

- **Weaning Predictors**

- o   Rapid shallow breathing index — the ratio of respiratory frequency to tidal volume (f/VT). It is the most extensively studied and commonly used weaning predictor. Aim for RSBI <105 breaths/min/L
- o   Minute ventilation: aim for 5-6L/min
- **Good Parameters for Successful Extubation**
  - o   FiO2 < 0.5 *with* PEEP ≤ 5 cmH2O
  - o   PaO2 > 70 mmHg ** lower values may be appropriate in SpO2 > 90% chronically hypoxemic patients
  - o   RR < 30 *with* PS ≤ 5cmH2O
  - o   pH > 7.2
  - o   No respiratory distress
  - o   Patient able to obey commands
  - o   Patient able to protect airway and cough
  - o   Patient able to cope with amount of secretions
  - o   Reason for intubation resolved
- **Bedside Equipment**
  - o   Oxygen source
  - o   Suction
  - o   Oral/Nasal airways
  - o   Face masks
  - o   Endotracheal tubes
  - o   LMA
  - o   Pulse ox
  - o   Cardiac Monitors
  - o   CO2 detectors
  - o   Ambu bags
- **Risk Factors**
  - o   ICU patient
  - o   Age > 70 or < 24 months
  - o   Hemoglobin <10 mg/dL
  - o   Longer duration of mechanical ventilation
  - o   Medical or surgical airway condition
  - o   Frequent pulmonary toilet
  - o   Loss of airway protective reflexes
- **Post Extubation**
  - o   NIPPV for 24 hours if high risk of being reintubated, or to nasal cannula if stable

VENTILATOR REVIEW

- **Overview**
  - o   Vocabulary:
    - **Presentation:**
      MODE/TV/RATE/PEEP/FIO2 WITH PEAK **, PLATEAU *, PULLING TV OF ****
    - *Pressure support* – pressure that augments a spontaneous breath
      1. "10 over 5" or "10/5" – (pressure support) above (PEEP). The assigned pressure support, which is above and beyond the continuous PEEP, for spontaneous breaths.
    - *PEEP* – positive end expiratory pressure. Pressure that is maintained at the end of expiration to prevent alveolar collapse. This in effect increases compliance, and thus oxygenation.
    - *I:E ratio* – the inspiratory time to expiratory time ratio. Normal is 3:1.
  - o   Pressures

PULMONOLOGY/CRITICAL CARE

- *Peak* – PIP - marker of upper airway pressures (trachea/bronchi); equals the sum of the resistive pressure (flow x resistance) and the plateau pressure. Dynamic pressures that measure the resistance to flow of air. Ideally maintained < 35 cm H20. Differential: bronchospasm, mucus plug, biting ET tube.
- *Plateau* – Pplat - marker of alveolar trauma; pressure maintained during inspiratory hold maneuver. Static pressure that gives an estimate of lung compliance. Ideally maintained < 30 cm H20. Differential: PTX, Pulm Edema, PNA, Atelectasis, R mainstem intubation
- Static = (Peak – Plateau). A measure of resistance in the circuit.
- Minute Ventilation (total volume ventilated in 1 minute)
- Elevated Pressure Alarm
   1. Management for ↑ pressure – disconnect patient from ventilator and bag with 100% O2, if patient is difficult to bag consider suctioning ETT (if not, then likely d/t bronchospasm or asynchrony and can re-connect to vent), look for tracheal obstruction, PTX, RMS intubation, bronchospasm. Treat with bronchodilators, steroids, and pull back ETT.
   o Modes of ventilation
   - **Volume-based ventilation:**
      1. Assist-Control.
         - "assist" – refers to assisting a spontaneous breath
         - "control" –refers to a fully controlled breath without spontaneous effort
         - Delivers set volume of air upon patient initiated breath
         - Controls breath at predetermined frequency and tidal volume (TV) if patient breath not initiated
         - On AC rate 12 with TV 700, patient will receive 12 ventilator delivered breaths/minute, each with a volume of 700 cc. If the patient initiates a breath on his/her own, the vent will also deliver volume of 700 cc. Tachypnea in this mode may cause respiratory alkalosis.
      2. SIMV – intermittent mandatory ventilation
         - "mandatory" – refers to assigned rate of full mandatory breaths
         - All other breaths are spontaneous or assisted with pressure support
         - "synchronized" – refers to synchronization of mandatory breaths with pt's diaphragm
         - Intermittently supplies mandatory frequency of breaths at predetermined volume or pressure that is synchronized with patient breathing efforts
         - Commonly used in conjunction with PSV during weaning process
         - On SIMV rate 12 with TV 700, patient will receive at least 12 breaths/min, each with volume of 700cc. If patient initiates > 12 breaths/min, the vent provides no support during those breaths unless pressure support is added. This mode prevents over-ventilation in patients with rapid respiratory rates; however, SIMV requires more respiratory muscle work than AC.
   - **Pressure-based ventilation:**
      1. Pressure Control
         - Set the PEEP and initial rate. Then adjust inspiratory pressure to obtain desired tidal volume.
            o Watch for patient agitation (sedate), tachypnea (sedate), and auto-PEEP (reduce set respiratory rate, ↓inspiratory time, ↑expiratory time, use bronchodilators+inhalted steroids; see Figure below).
         - Volumes will vary.
         - Flow rate will vary.

Figure. Appearance of flow volume in normal patient vs. patient with auto-PEEP

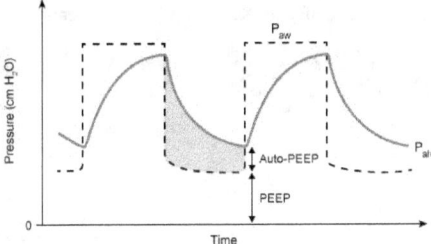

2. Pressure Support
    - Augments spontaneous breathing. Helps overcome tubing.
    - Supports patient breathing by delivering air at **predetermined pressure**
    - Adjunctive positive end-expiratory pressure (PEEP): **constant pressure** applied to maintain functional residual capacity & aid gas exchange
    - PRVC – pressure regulated volume control
    - Adjusts I:E time and other factors to accomplish a rate with volume minimums and pressure maximums.
3. Bi-Level[354]
    - Concept of alternating between two different pressures of CPAP
    - Pressure controlled, not respiratory rate dependent, allows for spontaneous breathing
    - Variables: P_{high}, P_{low}, T_{high}, T_{low}
    - **Good if low PaO2 and maxed on FiO2 and PEEP, allows for higher PaO2/FiO2 ratio**
    - Indications: ARDS, CHF
    - Contraindications: COPD, barotrauma
    - Settings:
        o Start with the "respiratory rate": 60/RR gives you your cycle time. Example RR 15 gives cycle time of 4 seconds
        o Set T1 and T2: Example I:E ratio 4:1 results in T1 of 3.2 seconds and T2 of 0.8 seconds
        o Set P1 and P2: Set P2 at the PEEP set on previous mode of ventilation. Set P1 to appropriate TV
    - Pearls
        o ↑O2 - ↑P1 or ↑T1
        o ↓CO2 - ↑T2 or ↓P2
- **Noninvasive ventilation:**
    1. CPAP – continuous positive airway pressure
        - Vent maintains constant positive pressure during entire respiratory cycle. This is equivalent to setting PEEP to the desired CPAP level and setting pressure support to zero.
        - Tight fitting mask, only temporary, can't eat
        - Stents open alveoli with continuous pressure. No rate, no volume.
        - Indications: OSA, COPD, **hypoxemia** but not hypercapnia
    2. BiPAP – bidirectional positive airway pressure
        - Tight fitting mask, only temporary, can't eat
        - IPAP – inspiratory positive airway pressure (ventilation)
        - EPAP – expiratory positive airway pressure (oxygenation)
        - Can set rate (not that helpful)

- In BiPAP "10/5", the IPAP is 10, the EPAP is 5. In SIMV "10/5", the IPAP is 15, the EPAP is 5.
- Best for COPD or CHF with CO2 retention (**hypercapnia**)

Characteristics of non-invasive ventilation		
	CPAP[355,356]	BiPAP
Set Variables	CPAP, FiO2	IPAP, EPAP, RR[set], FiO2
Dep. Variables	TV, RR	TV
End-Trigger Trigger	N/A	Patient determines
Notes	= to EPAP (on BiPAP) and cont. PEEP	IPAP=inspiratory positive airway pressure (i.e. PS; effects CO2). EPAP=expiratory positive airway pressure (i.e. PEEP; effects O2). Caution if pressure >=15 → can lead to ↓BP
Initial Settings	CPAP = 5-15 cmH2O	IPAP = 8-10; EPAP = 3-4 Mode: spontaneous ↑EPAP 1-2cm with IPAP constant for ratio 1:2.5
Populations Indications	COPD (acute exacerbation) Acute Cardiogenic PE Hypoxemia but <u>not</u> exhausted Weaning off ventilator	Acute Cardiogenic PE (CHF) Hypercapnia (retained CO2)
Modifications		Continued hypercapnia = ↑IPAP in 1-3cm interv.
Contraindications	• Cardiac/Resp arrest • Acidosis (pH<7.10) • ARDS • Organ failure • Cannot protect airway • Cannot clear secretions • Recent facial surgery • Upper airway obstruction	

- **Generic Initial vent settings**
  - Mode: AC or SIMV.
  - Rate = 12 (lower rate in COPD/asthma).
  - VT = 6cc/kg (ARDSNet Protocol)
  - I:E ratio: no less than 1:2; up to 1:4.
  - FiO2 = 1.0 (wean down rapidly to < 60% to avoid oxygen toxicity).
  - PS (pressure support) = 5-10 (5cm H20 needed to overcome resistance of endotracheal tube).
  - PEEP (positive end-expiratory pressure) = 0-15 (start low; cautious use in asthmatics and COPD patients as "auto PEEP" occurs often).
    - **Auto-PEEP**
      1. Check w/ expiratory pause
      2. ↓MV (↓TV, ↓RR)
      3. Provide long expiratory phase (I:E ratio)
      4. ↓air flow resistance with use of bronchodilators and steroids
      5. Providing external PEEP may be beneficial
- **Tweaking the Vent**
  - ↑/↓ vent rate → ↑/↓ CO2 and ↑/↓ pH.
  - ↑/↓ FIO2 → ↑/↓ PaO2 (adjust FiO2 in increments of 10-20%).
  - Adding PEEP can increase PaO2 (then you can FiO2).
  - **Low pO2**: ↑FiO2, ↑PEEP (to recruit more alveoli).
  - **High pCO2**: ↑TV or ↑RR (suction, bronchodilators), check for auto-PEEP

Recheck ABG 30 min after change

Figure. Titrating the vent based on ABG

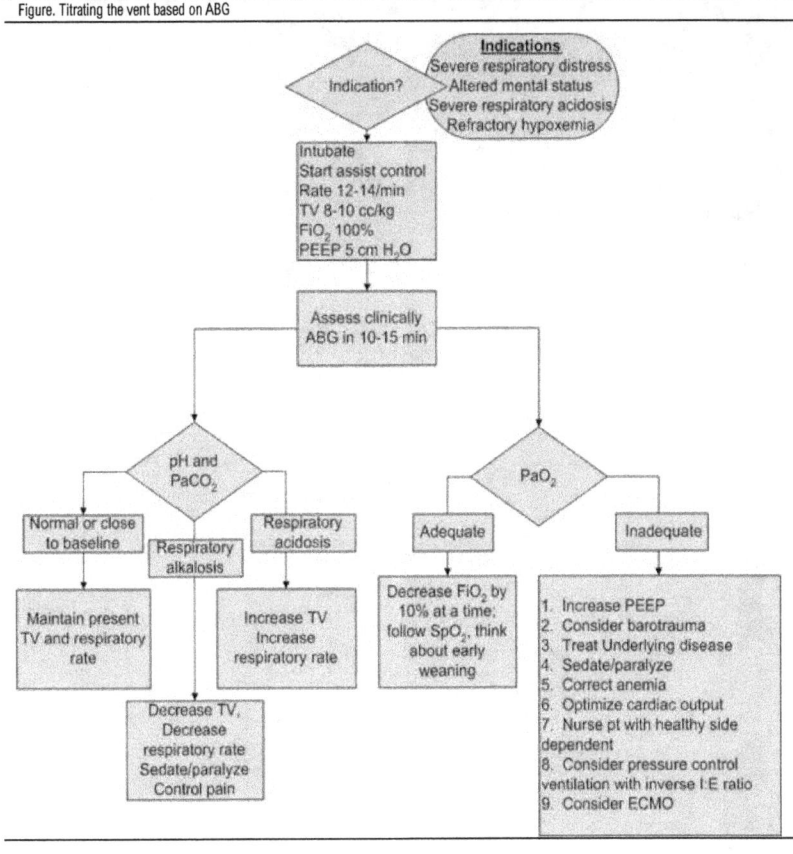

Common Vent Settings by Condition

Condition	Mode	RR	TV (ml/kg)	FIO2	PEEP	Add'tl vent issues	Pearls
Airway protection	AC SIMV PS	10-14	8-10		5	Peak flow 60 L/min	Maintain on MV until upper airway issues resolved. Patients with hepatic encephalopathy are prone to develop a respiratory alkalosis, so TV may need to be reduced
Asthma exacerbation (see page 472)	AC	8-12 (low)	6-8		0-5	High peak flows Allow adeq. Exp time	Permissive hypercarbia Higher peak airway press. Monitor for auto-PEEP Do **not** attempt to get normal ABG
COPD exacerbation	AC	8-12 (low)	6-8	Wean to SpO2 to 92%	0-5	High peak flows Allow adeq. Exp time	Monitor auto-PEEP Avoid posthypercapnic alkalosis Permissive hypercarbia Extubate to NIPPV
Hypoxemic respiratory failure with pneumonia or pulmonary edema	AC	High rates (16-24) due to high V_E requirements	6-8		5-10	High V_E requirements	Manage secretions
ARDS	AC PS APRV	High often up to 30	6		5-15	I:E of 1:1 or 1.5:1, allow permissive hypercarbia to pH of 7.20	Consider neb nitrous oxide Monitor for barotrauma Often require heavy sedation Avoid neuromuscular blockade
Postoperative respiratory failure	AC	10-16	8-10		5	Verify placement of all lines and tubes	Wait out the clearance of sedatives and paralytics Prone to hypoventilate after extubation Watch for atelectasis

PULMONOLOGY/CRITICAL CARE

Weaning parameters[357]	
Method of Assessment	Value
Vital capacity	10 mL/kg
Tidal volume	> 4 mL/kg
Minute ventilation	<15L
Respiratory rate	< 30 breath/min
Dynamic compliance	> 22 mL/cm H2O
Static compliance	> 33 mL/cm H2O
PaO2/FiO2 ratio	> 0.35
Negative inspiratory force (NIF)	20-30 cm H2O
Dead space to tidal volume ratio	0.6
Rapid shallow breathing index (RSBI)	< 105 breaths/min/L
Crop index	> 13 mL/breath/min
Pressors	Not present

- **When to attempt weaning (PS mode)**
  - PaO2/FiO2 ratio > 150
  - Patient can take spontaneous breaths if vent resp-rate reduced
- **Weaning Modes**
  - Preferred method: spontaneous breathing trial (30-120 minutes), T-piece or CPAP x 1-2 hours, check Tobin Index.
  - Decrease SIMV rate (2-4 breaths/min Q12h) ® decrease PS ® T-piece trials.
  - PS wean by decreasing PS until patient on CPAP (i.e., IPAP=PEEP)
  - During weaning, follow ABG, RR, HR and BP to determine when extubation is appropriate.
- **Failure to Wean**
  - F Fluid overload - diuresis if indicated.
  - An Airway resistance - check endotracheal tube; is it obstructed or too small?
  - I Infection - treat as indicated.
  - L Lying down, bad V/Q mismatch - elevate head of bed.
  - T Thyroid, toxicity of drugs - check TFT's, check med list.
  - O Oxygen - increase FiO2 as patient is taken off ventilator.
  - W Wheezing - treat with nebs.
  - E Electrolytes, eating - correct K/Mg/PO4/Ca; provide adequate nutrition.
  - An Anti-inflammatory needed? Consider steroids in asthma/COPD.
  - N Neuromuscular disease, neuro status compromised - think of myasthenia gravis, ALS, steroid/paralytic
  neuropathy, etc.; assure that patient is in fact awake and alert.

ARDS

- **Pearls**
  - ↓Mortality noted with lung-protective ventilation alone (↓V_T and pulm pressures), whereas use of systemic steroids, ↑PEEP (increases oxygenation), prone ventilation, and ECMO have had mixed results.[358]
- **Clinical**[359]
  - Dyspnea, cyanosis, and diffuse crackles not explained by cardiac process often in 6-72 hrs of event
  - Respiratory distress further shown by tachypnea, tachycardia, and diaphoresis
  - Causes
    - Direct Insult to Lung: PNA, aspiration, pulmonary contusion, vasculitis, drowning, DAH
    - Indirect Insult to Lung: sepsis, acute pancreatitis, massive blood transfusions (TRALI), trauma, drug overdose, severe burns

PULMONOLOGY/CRITICAL CARE

Berlin Criteria for ARDS

Item	Defined
Timing	Within 1 week of a known clinical insult or new or worsening respiratory symptoms
ALI	• Mild: 200 mm Hg < PaO2/FIO2 ≤ 300 mm Hg with PEEP or CPAP ≥5 cm H2O • Moderate: 100 mm Hg < PaO2/FIO2 ≤ 200 mm Hg • Severe: PaO2/FIO2 ≤ 100 mm Hg
Oxygenation	• Mild: PEEP or CPAP ≥5 cm H2O • Moderate-severe: PEEP ≥5 cm H2O
Chest Imaging	Bilateral opacities—not fully explained by effusions, lobar or lung collapse, or nodules
PAWP	Respiratory failure not fully explained by cardiac failure or fluid Overload (nml TTE, pro-BNP<300)

- **Severity Calculator**
  - Based off the CESAR study, patients with severe ARDS should be referred to an ECMO center. The severity can be determined by the Murray calculator found <http://cesar.lshtm.ac.uk/murrayscorecalculator.htm>
  - Variables include:
    - Ratio of arterial oxygen tension to the fraction of inspired oxygen (PaO2/FiO2)
    - Positive end-expiratory pressure (PEEP)
    - Lung compliance (V_T/(PIP-PEEP))
    - Chest radiograph quadrants with infiltrates (normal = 0; 1 per quadrant)
- **Treatment**
  - Cornerstone of therapy is mechanical ventilation to reduce ventilation induced lung injury → this can increase the systemic inflammatory response leading to the development of MOSF (multi-organ system failure). This is done through the **lung protective strategy of ventilation** by aiming for low tidal volumes (TV) and low inspiratory pressures.
    - Target TV should be at 0.6cc/kg (up to 0.8cc/kg) of <u>ideal body weight</u> with a maximum plateau pressure (P_{PL}) of 30[360]
    - Consider higher PEEP in moderate and severe ARDS
- **Adjunctive Therapies**
  - <u>Reduced tidal volume</u> - to protect the lungs may lead to hypercapnia and respiratory acidosis. Extracorporeal CO2 removal has not been found to be helpful.
  - <u>Prone ventilation</u> - should be initiated. It encourages homogenous lung ventilation to help distribute the mechanical forces in the lung. Benefits were seen in those with PaO2/FiO2 ratio ≤ 150 mmHg when performed for at least 16 hours/d.
  - <u>Nitric Oxide</u> - did not show mortality benefit
  - <u>Nutritional support</u>: improved survival and oxygenation when using low carb high fat enteral formulas
  - <u>Corticosteroids</u>: not helpful
  - <u>ECMO</u>: not promising (*CESAR*)
  - <u>Neuromuscular blockade</u>: controversial but promising; may ↓ barotrauma. Often utilized if PaO2/FiO2 ratio ≤ 150 mmHg.[361]
  - <u>Fluid-conservative</u>: When giving Lasix for diuresis, if total protein <6, consider co-administration of albumin[362] Does not improve survival.
- **Complications to Expect**
  - Barotrauma – due to PEEP on damaged lung tissue; prevented by keeping **plateau pressure** < 30. See page 517 for information on ventilator management and peak vs. plateau pressures.
  - Delirium – often treated with sedation and NM blockade

- o Infection – often VAP
- o DVT (lack of mobility; see page 340)
- o GI bleed (stress ulcers)

ANAPHYLAXIS

- **Defined** - acute, potentially lethal, multisystem (2+) syndrome resulting from the sudden release of mast cell and basophil-derived mediators into the circulation due to hypersensitivity to an exposed allergen (type 1 immunologic reaction)
- **General**[363,364,365]
  - o Most cases are immunoglobulin E (IgE)–mediated; non IgE mediated are termed *anaphylactoid*.
  - o Antibodies exposed to a particular allergen attach to mast cells and basophils, resulting in their activation and degranulation.
  - o A variety of chemical mediators are released including histamine, heparin, tryptase, kallikrein, platelet-activating factor, bradykinin, tumor necrosis factor, nitrous oxide, and several types of interleukins.[5]
- **Most common causes**
  - o <u>Drugs</u> – ABx, ASA, NSAID, monoclonal ABs
  - o <u>Foods</u> – shellfish, soy, wheat, milk, nuts
  - o <u>Other</u> – insects, mold, hymenoptera sting, iodine/contrast
- **Presentation**
  - o Urticaria, generalized pruritis, flushing +/- edema of the mucous membranes +/- respiratory distress and hemodynamic collapse
    - Signs and symptoms usually develop within five to 30 minutes (50% of fatal reactions) of exposure to the offending allergen but may not develop for several hours.
  - o A biphasic reaction is a <u>second</u> acute anaphylactic reaction occurring <u>hours</u> after the first response and without further exposure to the allergen.
- **Labs**
  Treatment should not depend on awaiting lab results
  - o Plasma histamine within 1 hour of symptoms but rarely performed
  - o Tryptase levels 15 min to 3 hours after symptom onset
  - o Skin testing should occur within 4-6 weeks of severe reaction to avoid false negative refractory period[366]
- **Diagnosis** – clinical
  - o <u>Criteria</u> (SN 95%, SP 71%)
    - Acute onset (min to h) with involvement of skin/mucosa/both (e.g. hives, prurits, flushing as mentioned above) and at least one of the following: respiratory compromise, dyspnea, wheeze/bronchospasm, stridor, hypoxia)
      -and/or-
      Reduced BP or associated end organ dysfunction (hypotension, syncope, incontinence)
    - Two or more of the following (min to h) after exposure to likely allergen:
      - skin mucosal tissue involvement (gen hives, itch/flush, swollen lips/tongue/uvula)
      - respiratory compromise (dyspnea, wheeze/bronchospasm, stridor, hypoxia)
      - reduced BP or associated sx (hypotension, collapse, syncope, incontinence)
      - persistent GI symptoms (crampy abd pain, vomiting)
    - Reduced BP after exposure (SBP less than 90 mmHg or >30% decrease from baseline)
- **Treatment**

- First Line
  - Epinephrine 1:1000 0.01 ml/kg to max 0.5 ml IM (normotensive)
    - Usual initial dose is 0.3-0.5 ml IM/SC; Repeat every 5-15 minutes as necessary.
    - Give 0.1-0.2 ml of total dose at site of antigenic exposure
    - 1 cc of 1:1000 epinephrine is 1 mg
    - Epinephrine 1 mg IM may be repeated every 3-5 minutes up to a maximum of 3 mg.
  - Epinephrine IV if hypotensive or respiratory failure
    - 0.3 mg & if no improvement continuous drip at 1-4 mcg/min of 1:10,000 dilution
- Second / Third line
  - H1- and H2- antihistamines for symptoms; glucocorticoids to prevent biphasic/protracted episodes
    - Pepcid: 20mg IVPB or Zantac 50 mg IV over 5 min
    - Diphenhydramine 50 mg IV/IM/PO q2h (max 400mg)
  - Supine with legs elevated
  - 100% O2 NRB
  - Albuterol 2.5 mg nebulized
  - Fluid bolus of 1-2L 0.9NS to maintain urine output and BP (pts often ↓BP).
  - What is the allergy? Discontinue medication if found to be the cause
  - Racemic Epinephrine neb 0.5 cc in 2.5 ml NS to temporize airway management
  - Solu-Medrol 125-250 mg IV q6h or repeat w/ 50mg/d vs 1-2mg/kg/d x 48 hours
    - Or Prednisone 60 mg PO
  - If on beta blocker → Glucagon 3.5-5mg IV x1 (0.5 mg peds) with prn infusion 1-5 mg/hr
    - Useful in refractory cases, especially in pts on β-Blockers

SHOCK

- **Defined** - Inadequate tissue perfusion and oxygenation 2/2 circulatory failure. Use qSOFA for triage purposes.
- **Pathophysiology**
  - Remember CO = SV x HR and this is ultimately determined by preload, afterload, and contractility
  - Preload determined by volume status and venous capacitance. ↓venous return leads to decreased muscle stretch, leading to ↓frank-starling stretch, and thus less contractility. Increased afterload itself is separate and associated with vascular resistance towards the forward flow of blood
  - In shock, early compensation seen as peripheral vasoconstriction to preserve flow to vital organs (kidney, brain, and heart) → seen as resting tachycardia
  - Inadequately perfused tissues do not get adequate oxygen and are deprived of completing normal aerobic metabolism thus the cells shift to anaerobic metabolism producing lactic acid → metabolic acidosis.
- **Assessment**
  1. Start with ABCs
  2. Establish IV access; 2 large bore vs CVC
  3. Monitor MAP (target 65-70mmHg), UOP, and telemetry
  4. Evaluate for evidence of end organ damage
  5. Determine etiology and type of shock
  6. Maintain perfusion via IV hydration vs. blood transfusion
- **Clinical symptoms**

- SIRS (≥2 of the following: T>100.4F or <96.8F, HR>90, RR>20, WBC>12k or <4k or >10% bands)
    -or-
    Use qSOFA (≥2 of the following: RR≥22, ΔMS, SBP≤110 mmHg
    - Sepsis: life threatening organ dysfunction (SOFA Δ ≥2) in the setting of SIRS with suspected or confirmed infectious source
- ↑RR
- ↓skin circulation

Types of Shock

Types	CVP or RA (Preload)	PA	PCWP	CO (Pump fxn)	SVR	MAP
Hypovolemic	↓	↓	↓	↓	↑	↓
Cardiogenic	↑↓	↑	↑	↓	↑	↓
Massive PE	↑	↑	↓/↔	↓	↑	↓
Acute LV Failure	↔	↑	↑	↓	↑/↔	↓/↔
Early Sepsis	↓	↓	↓	↑	↓	↓/↔

- **Types**
    - Hypovolemic
        - Most common type, 2/2 acute blood loss, severe DKA, GI loss
        - See page 125 for vasopressor support options
        - EBL:
            - Class I - < 15% blood volume loss (750cc); tx with crystalloid
            - Class II – 15-30% blood volume loss (750-1500cc); treat with crystalloid
            - Class III – 30-40% blood volume loss (1500-2000cc); treat with crystalloid and blood
            - Class IV - >40% BVL (>2000cc); treat with crystalloid and blood
    - Cardiogenic
        - 2/2 myocardial dysfunction from blunt injury → tamponade, ACS, valvular, mechanical complications of MI, arrhythmias, drugs.
        - Cardiology consult for cardiac cath vs mechanical circulatory support device
        - Obtain ECG to detect injury patterns
        - Get new echo or look at prior TTE
        - R/O tamponade with FAST
        - Pressors: dobutamine + dopamine +/- IABP
    - Septic[367]
        - See page 121
        - Due to infection leading to tachycardia, and cutaneous vasoconstriction
        - Look for warm, pink skin due to peripheral vasodilation
        - Start empiric antibiotics within 1 hour of recognition of severe sepsis or shock
            - Broad spectrum gram-positive (MRSA) and gram-negative coverage +/- anaerobes
        - Infectious work-up (i.e. 2x blood cultures, urine culture, +/- procalcitonin)
    - Obstructive
        - 2/2 obstructed blood flow into or exiting the heart
        - ex: PE, pericardial tamponade, tension PTX
        - treat underlying cause
    - Neurogenic
        - Hypotension due to loss of sympathetic tone ⦿ hypovolemia/hypotension w/o tachycardia
        - Often, like hemorrhagic shock, see no response to fluid resuscitation

Bibliography

[306] Andreas Achilleos, Evidence-based Evaluation and Management of Chronic Cough, Medical Clinics of North America, Volume 100, Issue 5, September 2016, Pages 1033-1045, ISSN 0025-7125, http://dx.doi.org/10.1016/j.mcna.2016.04.008.
[307] Alhajjaj MS, Bhimji SS. Cough, Chronic. [Updated 2017 Feb 10]. In: StatPearls [Internet]. Treasure Island (FL): StatPearls Publishing; 2018 Jan-. Available from: https://www.ncbi.nlm.nih.gov/books/NBK430791/
[308] Davids, Susan. "The Respiratory System." Conn's Current Therapy 2013.
[309] Kinkade S, Long NA. "Acute Bronchitis." Am Fam Physician. 2016 Oct 1;94(7):560-565.
[310] Gillespie et al. Mayo Clinic Proceedings, 1994.
[311] Berliner D, Schneider N, Welte T, Bauersachs J. The Differential Diagnosis of Dyspnea. Dtsch Arztebl Int. 2016;113(49):834-845.
[312] Wang et al. JAMA. 2005.
[313] Maisel. NEJM. 2002.
[314] Barreirotin et al. An Approach to Interpreting Spirometry. Am Fam Physician 2004;69:1107-14
[315] John A Gjevre, MD FRCPC, Thomas S Hurst, MVetSc FCCP, Regina M Taylor-Gjevre, MD MSc FRCPC, and Donald W Cockroft, MD FRCP. The American Thoracic Society's spirometric criteria alone is inadequate in asthma diagnosis. Can Respir J. 2006 Nov-Dec; 13(8): 433-437.
[316] Dempsey TM et al. "Pulmonary Function Tests for the Generalist: A Brief Review." Mayo Clinic Proceedings, Volume 93, Issue 6, 763 - 771.
[317] Sabatine et al. Pocket Medicine. 2016.
[318] Chhabra SK. Lung India. 2013.
[319] Latifi et al. "Is spirometry necessary to diagnose and control asthma?" Cleveland Clinic Journal of Medicine. 2017 August;84(8):597-599.
[320] Lazarus et al. NEJM 2010. | Calhoun et al. Chest. 2003. | GINA guidelines | Martinez et al. Lancet, 2013. | Bel et al. N Engl J Med 2013. | Fanta, Christopher. NEJM. 2009. | Papi et al. The Lancet. 2018.
[321] Wark, Peter AB. Contemporary Concise Review. 2020.
[322] Bateman ED et al. As-needed budesonide–formoterol versus maintenance budesonide in mild asthma. N Engl J Med 2018 May 17; 378:1877. (https://doi.org/10.1056/NEJMoa1715275)
[323] Evensen AE. "Management of COPD exacerbations." Am Fam Physician. 2010 Mar 1;81(5):607-13.
[324] Vogelmeier et al. "Global Strategy for the Diagnosis, Management, and Prevention of Chronic Obstructive Lung Disease 2017 Report: GOLD Executive Summary." European Respiratory Journal Mar 2017, 49 (3) 1700214
[325] Craddock et al. "ACUTE EXACERBATIONS OF COPD: AVOIDING DANGER AND DEATH." Consultant. 2016;56(8):740-745.
[326] Khilnani et al. "Noninvasive ventilation in patients with chronic obstructive airway disease." International Journal of COPD. 2008: 3(3).
[327] Zwolak Z, Rohlfing J. Pulmonary. In: David JA. eds. CURRENT Practice Guidelines in Inpatient Medicine 2018–2019 New York, NY: McGraw-Hill.
[328] Shen et al. COPD (2014).
[329] Banerjee S, McCormack A. Acetylcysteine for Patients Requiring Secretion Clearance: A Review of Guidelines [Internet]. Ottawa (ON): Canadian Agency for Drugs and Technologies in Health; 2019 Jul 3.
[330] Edvardsen et al. "Air travel and chronic obstructive pulmonary disease: a new algorithm for pre-flight evaluation." Thorax 2012;67:964–969.
[331] Pavord et al. Int J Chron Obstruct Pulmon Dis. 2016.
[332] Crisafulli et al. Multidiscip Respir Med. 2018.
[333] Ward et al. Australian Family Physician. 2010.
[334] Kalchiem-Dekel et al. Journal of Clinical Medicine. 2018.
[335] Vahdatpour, C. A., Darnell, M. L., & Palevsky, H. I. (2019). Acute respiratory failure in interstitial lung disease complicated by pulmonary hypertension. Respiratory Medicine, 105825. doi:10.1016/j.rmed.2019.105825
[336] West JB. Compr Physiol. 2011
[337] Sarkar et al. Lung India. 2017.
[338] Chesnutt MS, Chesnutt MC, Prendergast TJ, Tavan ET, Tavan ET. Chapter 9. Pulmonary Disorders. In: McPhee SJ, Papadakis MA, Rabow MW, eds. CURRENT Medical Diagnosis & Treatment 2012. New York: McGraw-Hill; 2012.
[339] Strange, Charlie et al. "Parapneumonic effusion and empyema in adults." In: UpToDate, Basow, DS (Ed), UpToDate, Waltham, MA, 2012.
[340] Hamal AB, Yogi KN, Bam N, Das SK, Karn R. Pleural fluid cholesterol in differentiating exudative and transudative pleural effusion. Pulm Med. 2013;2013:135036. doi:10.1155/2013/135036
[341] Ost et al. N Engl J Med 2003.
[342] McWilliams et al. N Engl J Med 2013.
[343] Gould et al. JAMA. 2001.
[344] Ramirez JM, Garcia AJ 3rd, Anderson TM, et al. Central and peripheral factors contributing to obstructive sleep apneas. Respir Physiol Neurobiol. 2013;189(2):344–353. doi:10.1016/j.resp.2013.06.004
[345] Watto, M. (2018, November 5). #123 Sleep Apnea Pearls and Pitfalls [Audio blog post]. Retrieved November 5, 2018, from https://thecurbsiders.com/podcast/123-sleep-apnea-pearls-and-pitfalls
[346] Balachandran JS, Patel SR. Obstructive Sleep Apnea. Ann Intern Med. ;161:ITC1. doi: 10.7326/0003-4819-161-9-201411040-01005
[347] Eijsvogel MM, Ubbink R, Dekker J, et al. Sleep position trainer versus tennis ball technique in positional obstructive sleep apnea syndrome. J Clin Sleep Med. 2015;11(2):139–147. Published 2015 Jan 15. doi:10.5664/jcsm.4460
[348] Marino, Paul L. The Little ICU Book Of Facts And Formulas. Philadelphia : Wolter Kluwer Health/Lippincott Williams & Wilkins, 2009.
[349] Fundamental Critical Care Support Course
[350] Farahnak Assadi. Int J Prev Med. 2017.
[351] Case Approach Resident Guide to IM (UH Case Medical Center) 2015-2016.

[352] Case Approach Resident Guide to IM (UH Case Medical Center) 2015-2016.
[353] Case Approach Resident Guide to IM (UH Case Medical Center) 2015-2016.
[354] Dettbarn, Kyle MD. "Bi-Level Ventilation/APRV." http://www.wsrconline.org/read/Bi-Level%20Ventilation.pdf
[355] Peter JV, Moran JL, Phillips-Hughes J, et al. Effect of non-invasive positive pressure ventilation (NIPPV) on mortality in patients with acute cardiogenic pulmonary oedema: a meta-analysis. *Lancet.* 2006;367:1155-63.
[356] Kirkland, Lisa. "Noninvasive positive-pressure ventilation." ACP Hospitalist. September. 2010.
[357] Tobin MJ. Advances in mechanical ventilation. N Engl J Med 2001; 344:1986-96.
[358] Matthay et al. "Acute respiratory distress syndrome." Nature Reviews. Disease Primers 2019 March 14, 5 (1): 18.
[359] Fan et al. "Acute Respiratory Distress Syndrome Advances in Diagnosis and Treatment." JAMA. 2018;319(7):698-710.
[360] Ventilation with lower tidal volumes as compared with traditional tidal volumes for acute lung injury and the acute respiratory distress syndrome. The Acute Respiratory Distress Syndrome Network. N Engl J Med. 2000 May 4;342(18):1301-8. PubMed PMID: 10793162
[361] Parhar et al. J Thorac Dis. 2019.
[362] Martin et al. "A randomized, controlled trial of furosemide with or without albumin in hypoproteinemic patients with acute lung injury." Critical Care Medicine. 2005. 33(8).
[363] Gomella L.G., Haist S.A. (2007). Chapter 21. Common Medical Emergencies. In L.G. Gomella, S.A. Haist (Eds), *Clinician's Pocket Reference: The Scut Monkey*, 11e. Retrieved May 5, 2012
[364] Arnold JJ, Williams PM. "Anaphylaxis: recognition and management." Am Fam Physician. 2011 Nov 15;84(10):1111-8.
[365] Rowe BH, Grunau B. Allergy and Anaphylaxis. In: Tintinalli JE, Ma O, Yealy DM, Meckler GD, Stapczynski J, Cline DM, Thomas SH. eds. Tintinalli's Emergency Medicine: A Comprehensive Study Guide, 9e New York, NY: McGraw-Hill
[366] Hellmann DB, Imboden Jr. JB. Immediate Hypersensitivity. In: Papadakis MA, McPhee SJ, Rabow MW. eds. Current Medical Diagnosis and Treatment 2020 New York, NY: McGraw-Hill
[367] Dellinger et al. "Surviving Sepsis Campaign: International Guidelines for Management of Severe Sepsis and Septic Shock: 2012" CCJM. February 2013 • Volume 41 • Number 2

NEPHROLOGY

Acid Base Physiology 531
Acute Kidney Injury 536
Chronic Kidney Disease 543
Polyuria 547
Glomerular Disease 551
Nephrolithiasis 553

ACID BASE PHYSIOLOGY

STEP 1: Gather the necessary data (electrolytes and an ABG) Make sure the HCO3 from the electrolyte panel and ABG are within 2 (if not the results are uninterpretable) **Understand the Normals** PaO2: 80-100mmHg PaCO2: 35-45mmHg HCO3: 22-28mEq/L SaO2: 95-100% SvO2: 60-80%	pH | CO2 | HCO3
STEP 2: Look at the pH If pH > 7.4, then pt is alkalemic (proceed to step 3a) If pH < 7.4, the pt is acidemic (proceed to step 3b)	Patient has primary: Acidosis / Alkalosis
STEP 3: Determine the primary etiology 3a Alkalemia ↑HCO3 = Metabolic alkalosis (go to step 5) 　　　　　　　↓pCO2 = Respiratory alkalosis (go to step 4a) 3b Acidosis ↓HCO3 = Metabolic acidosis (go to step 5) 　　　　　　　↑pCO2 = Respiratory acidosis (go to step 4b)	Primary process is: Respiratory / Metabolic

Respiratory Disorders

STEP 4: If primary respiratory disorder, determine whether acute or chronic

Respiratory Acidosis		Respiratory Alkalosis		Respiratory process: Acute / Chronic / Unknown
For each ↑ PCO2 of 10 above 40		For each ↓ PCO2 of 10 above 40		
Acute	**Chronic**	**Acute**	**Chronic**	
HCO3 ↑ 1 mEq	HCO3 ↑ 4-5 mEq	HCO3 ↓ 2 mEq	HCO3 ↓ 4-5 mEq	
pH ↓ 0.08	pH ↓ 0.03	pH ↑ 0.07	pH ↑ 0.02	

All

STEP 5: Calculate the anion gap. 5a If ↓alb or PO4 then normal gap calculated as: 　　AG = (albumin x 2.5) + (0.5)(PO4) 5b Na − (HCO3 + Cl) = _____ 　　　　If > 12 (or 3xalbumin) then pt has an anion gap 　　　　metabolic acidosis (proceed to step 5b) 　　　　If <12, skip to Step 6b 5c Calculate the excess anion gap 　　　　Calculated anion gap + 12 (or 3xalbumin) =	Anion gap? Yes / No Excess gap: _____

NEPHROLOGY

Metabolic Acidosis

STEP 6: Identify concomitant disorders.

6a Calculate the corrected HCO3. You must understand that this step essentially compares the decrease in measured HCO3 to the expected decrease in HCO3 based on the degree of anion gap.

Measured HCO3 + excess anion gap = _____
  *If the corrected HCO3 is >30, then the patient has a concomitant metabolic alkalosis (more HCO3 than expected for the degree of gap acidosis).

  *If the corrected HCO3 is <23, then the patient has a concomitant NAGMA (less HCO3 than expected for the degree of gap). See page 534 for more on this.

Metabolic alkalosis present:

yes / no

NAGMA present:

yes / no

6b Calculate the expected pCO2. Winter's formula shows what the pCO2 should be for the level of acidosis present (omit if primary disorder is respiratory).

Winter's formula = expected pCO2 = 1.5(HCO3) +8 +/- 2
pCO2 = (1.5)(_____) + 8 +/- 2
  *If the actual pCO2 > calculated pCO2 then pt has concomitant respiratory acidosis
  *If the actual pCO2 < calculated pCO2 then pt has concomitant respiratory alkalosis

Respiratory disorder present:

yes / no

Metabolic Acidosis	Metabolic Alkalosis
For each ↓ HCO3 of 1 mEq...	For each ↑ HCO3 of 1 mEq...
PCO2 ↓ 1.25 mmHg	PCO2 ↑ 0.75 mmHg
Formula	Formula
$Pa_{co2} = [HCO_3^-] + 15$	$Pa_{co2} = [HCO_3^-] + 15$
pCO2 = 1.5 x [HCO3] + 8 ± 2	pCO2 = 0.7 x [HCO3] + 20 ± 5

STEP 7: Figure out what's causing the problem(s)

AGMA	NAGMA	ACUTE RESP ACIDOSIS	METABOLIC ALKALOSIS	RESPIRATORY ALKALOSIS
"MUDPILERS"	"HARDUPS"	Anything that causes hypoventilation	"CLEVER PD"	"CHAMPS" Anything that causes hypervent.
Methanol	↑0.9NS fluids	CNS depression Airway obstruction	Vomiting (↓U$_{Cl}$)	CNS dz
Uremia	Hyperalimentation	PNA	Diuretics	Hypoxia
DKA/	Acetazolamide	PE	Hypokalemia	Anxiety
EtOH/	RTA	Hemo/PTX	Hyperaldosterone	Mech ventilation
starvation	Diarrhea	Myopathy	Licorice	Progesterone
Paraldehyde	Uretero-pelvic shunt	Chronic resp acid. Is caused by COPD and restrictive lung dz	Conn's	Salicylates/ sepsis
INH	Post-hypocapnia		Cushing's Bartter's	
Lactic acid	Spironolactone		Hypercalcemia	
EtOH/ ethylene glycol	Normal saline		Refeeding	
Rhabdo/renal fail.			Post-hypercapnia	
Salicylates			Laxative abuse	

STEP 8: Fix it!

Figure. Flow chart interpretation of ABG

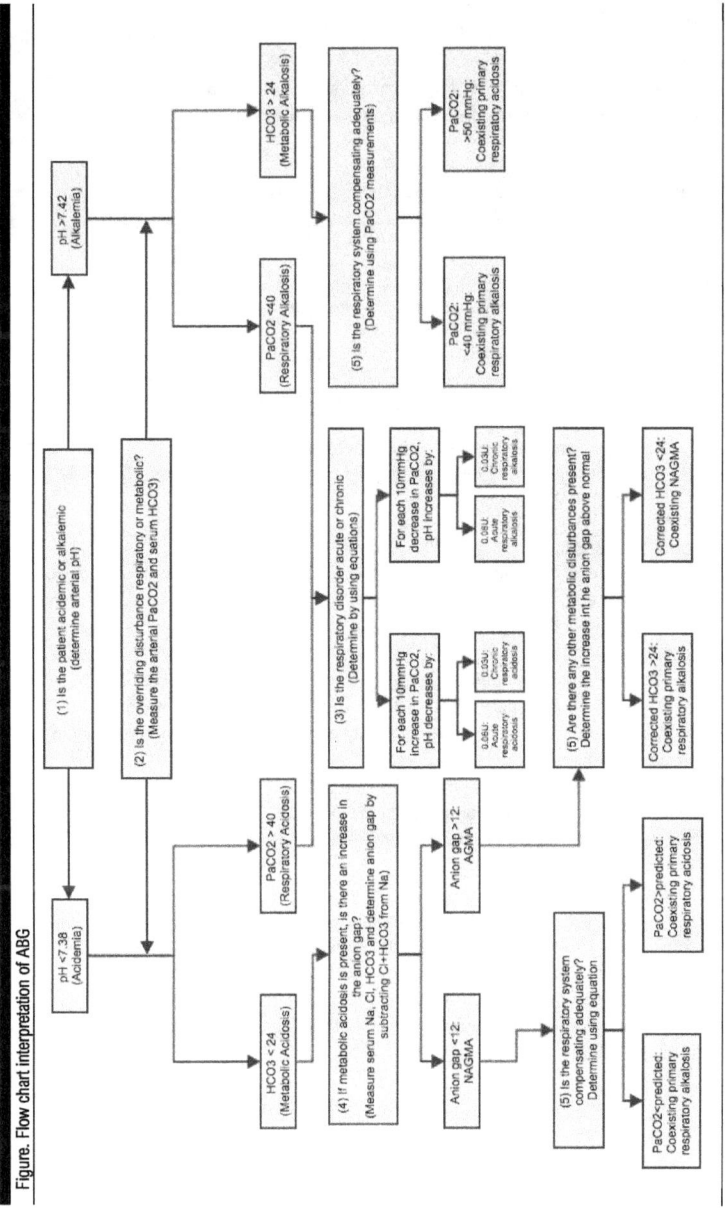

NEPHROLOGY

- **More on Delta Gap**
  - If there is an AG, determine whether this alone accounts for the change in HCO3. Calculate the gap-gap: (delta-gap) = patient's anion gap – 12 (normal anion gap).
  - Compensate for low albumin (for every 1 g/dl decrease from normal, increase AG by 2.5 mmol/L)
  - Add this to the measured HCO3. If the result is >30, then an additional metabolic alkalosis exists. If the result is <23, then an additional non-gap metabolic acidosis is present
  - Osmolar
    Done when considering concurrent toxic alcohols as cause
    - (2xNa)+(Bun/3)+Gluc/18
    - (+): methanol, ethanol, ethylene glycol
    - (0) or (-): other causes
  - Urine AG
    Calculated for NAGMA to determine urinary vs gastrointestinal cause
    - Urinary Na + Urinary K - Urinary Cl
      1. The urinary anion gap can help to differentiate between GIT and renal causes of a NAG metabolic acidosis.
      2. In general, ↑Cl excretion (suggestive of ↑NH3 excretion) seen with GI cause and causes a <u>negative</u> UAG
         - + gap: failure of kidneys to excrete NH4+ and retain HCO3 → RTA1 or RTA4
         - - gap: appropriate increased renal NH4+ excretion (GI loss, dilutional, exogenous acid)
- **Differentials of Acidosis/Alkalosis**
  - Respiratory alkalosis
    - CNS disorders, hypoxia, pulmonary receptor stimulation (asthma, pneumonia, pulmonary edema, PE), anxiety, drugs (ASA, Theo), liver failure, sepsis, recovery phase of met acidosis
  - Respiratory acidosis
    - Respiratory center inhibition (opiates, myxedema, o2 in co2 retainer), neuromuscular disorder (Guillain–Barré, myasthenia gravis, botulism, hypokalemia), chest wall disorder, airway obstruction, acute and chronic lung disease
  - Metabolic alkalosis
    - Saline/chloride–responsive (urine Cl– <20 mEq/L): GI; due to low volume state vomiting, diarrhea, ng drainage, diuretics, post–hypercapnic, cystic fibrosis, villous adenoma
    - Saline/chloride–resistant (urine Cl– >20 mEq/L): ↑BP think primary aldosteronism, secondary aldosteronism (CHF, cirrhosis & ascites, Cushing's, Bartter's), if ↓BP think congenital adrenal hyperplasia, Liddle's, licorice
    - Miscellaneous: poorly resorbed anion (PCN, carbenicillin), refeeding alkalosis, administration of alkali (e.g. antacids, overshoot from rx of acidosis, massive transfusions with citrate anticoagulant, milk alkali)
  - Metabolic acidosis
    - **Gap**
      - Are ketones present?
        - Yes → diabetic ketoacidosis/starvation/EtOH ketoacidosis
        - No →
          - There is an unmeasured anion
          - Measure the serum osmolarity and compare to calculated osmolarity
            - Increased – methanol, ethylene glycol
            - Normal – uremia, paraldehyde, INH, iron toxicity, lactic acidosis, rhabdomyolysis / renal (ESRD - uremic), salicylates
    - **Non-gap**

- Common causes: low albumin (cirrhosis, CKD), multiple myeloma, ↑Mg, ↑Ca, lithium, bromide
- Clinically, the major distinction is between: renal and extrarenal (usually GI) causes.
  - Renal: RTA, either proximal, distal, or due to hypoaldosteronism
  - GI: diarrhea, surgical drains, fistulas, cholestyramine
  - To differentiate, calculate the urine anion gap as below [368]

	$U_{AG} = (NA+K)-Cl$
- UAG	(i.e. -30) – appropriate renal response → NH3 is in the urine which is appropriate → suggests GI loss of bicarbonate (e.g. diarrhea) with renal continuing to be able to acidify urine. However, if proximal RTA (type 2) can be negative as well.
+ UAG	(i.e. +25) – suggests impaired renal distal acidification (i.e. renal tubular acidosis because kidney cannot excrete h).

- o **Renal**
  - Renal tubular acidosis: NAGMA, ↑Cl, normal GFR
  - Failure of the kidney to reabsorb, synthesize or stow H+ ions in NH3

Evaluation of RTA Causes			
	Type I	Type II	Type IV
Location	Distal	Proximal	Distal
Inability to...	H+ secretion	Reabsorb HCO₃ at proximal tubule	Produce NH₃
Urine pH	>6	<5.5	<5.5
Urine K+	↓↓↓	↓	↑↑↑
Serum K	↓	↓	↑
HCO3	↓↓↓	↓↓	>17
UAG	Positive	Negative at baseline Positive during tx	Positive
Associated with	TMP-SMX Autoimmune dz Hypercalcemia Nephrolithiasis	Osteomalacia Multiple myeloma Nephrotoxic mediations	Spironolactone ACEi/ARB Diabetic nephropathy Heparin AIDS Hypertensive nephro Hyperaldosteronism

- Type I RTA:
  - *Location*: proximal tubule (re-absorption of HCO3 problem)
  - *Causes:* drugs (ampho), chronic pyelonephritis, obstructive uropathy, nephrocalcinosis, autoimmune (SLE, Sjogren's, thyroiditis, cryoglobulinemia, chronic active hepatitis, PBC), amyloidosis, myeloma
  - ↓K
  - Positive UAG (alkalotic urine noted with attempt to acidify urine with NH3Cl via PO administration)
- Type II RTA:
  - *Location*: cortical collecting tubule, distal (synthesizing problem)
  - *Causes*: Primary (hereditary), MM, amyloidosis, Sjogren's, PNH, acetazolamide, hyperglobulinemia, heavy metals (Pb, Cd, Hg, Cu, others), Wilson's, ↑PTH
  - ↑HCO3 with ↑Fractional excretion of HCO3
  - ↓K
  - Negative UAG
- Type IV RTA: inadequate aldo activity, leads to ↑K causing acidosis

- Causes:
    i. Low aldo levels with normal/increased renin levels: Addison's dz, isolated decreased aldo synthesis a/w heparin or LMWH, ACEi, ARB, critically ill patients
    ii. Low aldo levels with low renin levels: DM (most common), NSAIDS, HIV
    iii. Aldo antagonists: Aldactone, TMP, pentamidine, amiloride
    iv. DM patients with Type IV are sensitive to ACE inhibitors (↑K)
    v. Miscellaneous: obstructive uropathy, sickle cell disease, amyloidosis, AIN
  - **Non-Renal**
    - Bicarb wasting: Gi: diarrhea, ileus, fistula, villous adenoma
    - Urinary tract diversions: ureterosigmoidostomy, ileal conduit
    - Administration of chloride-containing acid: NH4Cl, HCl, TPN, cholestyramine
    - Normal saline
    - Spironolactone
    - Topiramate
    - Post hypercapnia (transient)
  - Low Anion Gap
    - As above, ensure you are correcting for ↓albumin and ↓PO$_4$
    - Causes include: ↑Cl d/t ↑TG, ↓albumin, ↓PO4, ↓IgA, ↑K, ↑Ca, ↑Mg, ↑Lithium
- **Treatment**
  - In general, severe acidosis (pH < 7.10) warrants the IV administration of 50–100 mEq of NaHCO3, over 30–45 min, during the initial 1–2 h of therapy.
  - A reasonable approach is to infuse enough NaHCO3 to raise the arterial pH to no more than 7.2 over 30–40 min.
  - It is essential to monitor plasma electrolytes during therapy, because the [K+] may decline as pH rises. The goal is to increase the [HCO3−] to 10 mEq/l and the pH to 7.20, not to increase these values to normal.
  - Chronic Metabolic Acidosis
    - Seen with CKD
    - If HCO3 is 19-21 mEq/L on 2 consecutive measurements or ≤18 on one measurement, then consider treating
      - 19-21 mEq/L: start NaHCO3 650mg BID (≈15 mEq HCO3)
      - ≤18 mEq/L: start NaHCO3 1300mg BID (≈30 mEq HCO3)
      - In either scenario above, **goal is to titrate to 1950mg BID (max TID) to target a HCO3 of 24-26 mEq/L**
    - Alternatives to NaHCO3 tablet
      - NaHCO3 powder: 1/8 teaspoon = 600mg
      - Sodium Citrate: 500mg/334mg per 5cc
        - Less GI sx with no K
        - Do not use in patients with liver dz
      - K-citrate: 540mg (≈ 5 mEq of HCO3); 1080mg (≈10 mEq of HCO3)
        - More potent than NaHCO3
        - May ↑K
        - Dissolve in water before consumption

ACUTE KIDNEY INJURY

- Definition/Risk stratification
  - KDIGO consensus

- ↑SCr ≥ 0.3 mg per deciliter within 48 hours (>24 hours is sustained; over 48 hours is abrupt)
- ↑SCr ≥ 1.5x baseline within 7 days
- A urine volume of less than 0.5 ml per kilogram of body weight per hour for 6 hours
- **Etiology**
  - Occurs in about 10-25% of hospitalized patients → ATN is most common cause from ischemic or nephrotoxic injury
  - In hospital mortality of 23-80%

Diagnostic comparisons of common causes of AKI					
	Pre-Renal	Post-Renal	ATN	AGN	AIN
BUN/SCr	>20:1	>20:1	<20:1	>20:1	<20:1
U_{Na}	<20	Varies	>40	<20	<20 (acute) >40 (days)
U_{Osm}	>500	<400	<400	>400	Variable
FE_{Na}	<1	Varies	>2	<1	<1 (acute) >1 (days)
FE_{Urea}	<35%	Varies	>35%		
Urine sediment	Benign Hyaline cast	Normal RBCs WBCs Crystals	Muddy brown casts RT epithelial cells Granular casts	Dysmorphic RBCs RBC casts	WBCs WBC casts +/- eos +Hansel stain

- **Risks**
  - Hyperkalemia
  - Metabolic acidosis (loss of bicarb)

Comparing AKI, AKD, and CKD			
	AKI	AKD	CKD
Duration	2-7 days	≤ 3 months	> 3 months
Functional Criteria	↑ in SCr by ≥50% in 7 days -or- ↑ in SCr by ≥0.3 mg/dL within 2 days -or- Oliguria for ≥ 6h	AKI -or- GFR <60 -or- ↓ in GFR by ≥35%x baseline GFR -or- ↑ in SCr by ≥50%x baseline	GFR<60
Structural criteria	Not defined	Marker of kidney damage (albuminuria, hematuria, or pyuria is m/c)	Marker of kidney damage for >3 months (albuminuria, is m/c)
Examples	Prerenal Intrinsic Postrenal	AGN Nephrotic syndrome Pyelonephritis	T2DM Hypertension

AKI = acute kidney injury   AKD = acute kidney disease   CKD = chronic kidney disease

- **Staging**

  The worse the stage, the worse the prognosis for the patient

NEPHROLOGY

Acute Kidney Injury Staging		
Stage	SCr	UOP
1	1.5-1.9x baseline within 1 week or ≥ 0.3 mg/dl ↑ within 48 hours	<0.5 cc/kg/h for 6-12h
2	2.0-2.9x baseline	<0.5 cc/kg/h ≥ 12h
3	3.0x baseline	<0.3 cc/kg/h ≥ 24h or anuria ≥ 12 h

- **Classification**
  - Prerenal (↓volume)
  - Intrinsic (AGN, AIN, ATN)
  - Postrenal (obstruction)

Lab associations with renal injury			
	Prerenal	Intrinsic	Postrenal
Labs	Urine Osmolality >500 U_{Na} <20 Urine/Plasma Cr >40 FE_{Na} <1 FE_{Urea} <35	Urine Osmolality <400 U_{Na} >40 Urine/Plasma Cr <20 FE_{Na} >2 FE_{Urea} >35	± nondysmorphic RBCs FE_{Na} variable
Urine Sediment	Normal; occasional hyaline cast or fine granular cast	Renal tubular epithelial cells; granular and muddy brown casts	Bland
DDx	Ischemia Toxins Hypotension	AIN AGN ATN SIADH ATN	BPH Prostate CA Nephrolithiasis Anticholinergics Neurog. bladder

- **Determine cause**
  - Labs
    - General
      - **Urinalysis**
      - Random urine electrolytes (will help for FENa)
      - Urine creatinine (will help for FENa)
      - Urine microscopy (↑casts/sediment suggestive of AIN)
      - CBC
    - *Others to consider if overt failure*
      - Glomerulonephritis/Vasculitis
        - ANCA (C-ANCA seen with Wegener's)
        - ANA
        - Anti-GBM
        - Anti-dsDNA, ANA (SLE)
        - ENA
        - IgG, IgA
        - Cryoglobulins
        - Hepatitis B, C
        - HIV
        - Renal bx
        - C3, C4 (low levels may be s/o SLE)
        - Anti-SPO (UA: Coca-Cola color)
      - Malignancy:
        - Urine cytology
        - Light chains

- SPEP and UPEP
- Interstitial Nephritis
  - Eosinophils
  - Urine eosinophils
  - Renal bx
- TTP/HUS
  - LDH
  - Haptoglobin
  - PLT
  - Reticulocytes
  - Bilirubin
- FENa is the most accurate screening test to differentiate between prerenal disease and acute tubular necrosis.
  - Not beneficial if patient has received Lasix or IV contrast recently! If this is the case, get a FEUrea and look for a value <35% which indicates pre-renal etiology.

$$FE_{UREA} = UREA \times S_{Cr} / BUN \times U_{Cr} \times 100$$

  - The urine sodium concentration is usually above 40 mEq/l in intrinsic or post renal causes, and below 20 mEq/l in prerenal conditions. However, since the urinary sodium concentration is influenced by the urine output, there is substantial overlap due in part to variations in the urine volume.

$$FE_{NA} = U_{Na} \times S_{Cr} / S_{NA} \times U_{Cr} \times 100$$

  - A value below 1 percent suggests prerenal disease, where the reabsorption of almost all the filtered sodium represents an appropriate response to decreased renal perfusion; in comparison, a value between 1 and 2 percent may be seen with either disorder, while a value above 2 percent usually indicates ATN.
- UA with electrolytes
  - Pre-renal is suspicious on UA if you see high spec grav, low pH, hyaline casts, low urinary Na
  - Intra-renal is suspicious on UA if you see low spec grav with muddy brown casts, normal or elevated urinary Na >40 (urinary Na often elevated with ATN and SIADH due to lack of ability to reabsorb Na)

NEPHROLOGY

Urinary findings and associated renal disease	
Urinary pattern	Renal disease
Hematuria with red cell casts (>3 RBC on microscopy), dysmorphic red cells, heavy proteinuria, or lipiduria	Glomerular disease or vasculitis
Multiple granular and epithelial cell casts with free epithelial cells	Acute tubular necrosis in a patient with acute renal failure
White cell and granular or waxy casts and no or mild proteinuria	Tubular or interstitial disease or urinary tract obstruction
Hematuria and pyuria with no or variable casts (excluding red cell casts)	May be observed in acute interstitial nephritis, glomerular disease, vasculitis, obstruction, and renal infarction
Epithelial Cells	Normal
Renal tubular cells	Acute tubular injury
Non-dysmorphic red cells	Non-glomerular bleeding from anywhere in the urinary tract
Hyaline casts	Any type of renal disease
Leukocytes	Inflammation in urinary tract

- **Complications**
  - ↑K, ↑volume, acidosis, anemia, ↓immune response, myopathy, pleural effusion
- **Imaging**
  - Renal ultrasound
  - MAG3 scan – when considering post obstructive
  - Renal biopsy
    - Major indications include
      - Isolated glomerular hematuria with proteinuria
      - Nephrotic syndrome
      - Acute nephritic syndrome
      - Unexplained acute or rapidly progressive renal failure
    - Contraindications include:
      - Uncorrectable bleeding diathesis
      - Small kidneys which are generally indicative of chronic irreversible disease
      - Severe hypertension, which cannot be controlled with antihypertensive medications
      - Multiple, bilateral cysts or a renal tumor
      - Hydronephrosis
      - Active renal or perirenal infection
      - An uncooperative patient
- **Treatment**

  Remove the offending agent, improve hemodynamics, make non-oliguric, fix electrolytes, and avoid nephrotoxins. Assess for indications for urgent dialysis (↑volume, uremia, electrolyte disorders, drug toxicity)
  - Pre-renal – isotonic fluids
  - Intrinsic
    - *Etiology*
      - Nephrotoxin
        - Contrast induced nephropathy – fluids are best. Give 1cc/kg/hr of 0.9NaCl 6 hours prior to procedure and continue for 6 hours after. If short notice, can use 3cc/kg/hr for 1 hour prior to procedure, and then decrease to 1cc/kg/hr for 6 hours post.
      - Ischemia from vasoconstriction
      - Obstruction
    - *Phases*
      - Initiation – acute drop in GFR and increase in SCr

- ▫ Maintenance – sustained low GFR with continued elevation of SCr for 1-2 weeks
- ▫ Recovery – tubular function restored leading to polyuria with ↓SCr
- CRRT – clears solutes that are not being filed through process of diffusion and convection. Main disadvantage is risk of ↓BP (less so with CRRT than intermittent hemodialysis)
    1. *Indications* - ↑K, metabolic acidosis, anuria, diuretic resistant volume overload, uremia
    2. *Flow* – 20-25aa/kg/hr
    3. *Anticoagulation* – citrate is recommended, if cannot be used, then UFH or LMWH

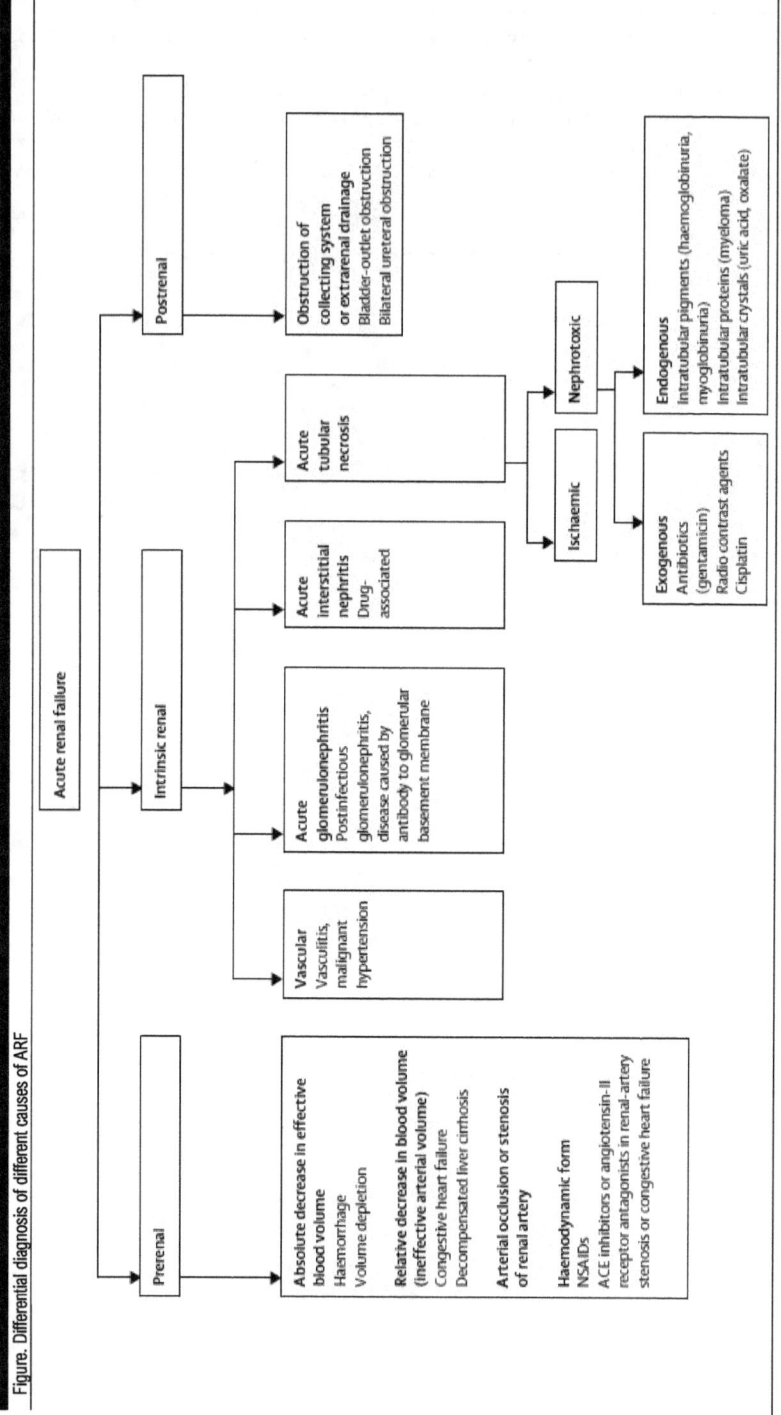

Figure. Differential diagnosis of different causes of ARF

CHRONIC KIDNEY DISEASE

- **Definition (any of the following)** [369,370]
    - Kidney damage for 3 or more months based on findings of abnormal structure (imaging studies) or abnormal function (microalbuminuria is 30-300mg, hematuria, electrolyte issues)
    - GFR < 60 mL per minute per 1.73 m2 for ≥3 months with or without evidence of kidney damage

CKD Stages		
Stage	Damage	GFR
1	Kidney Damage	GFR≥90 mL/min
2	Kidney Damage	GFR 60-89 mL/min
3	Moderate	GFR 30-59 mL/min
4	Severe	GFR 15-29 mL/min
5	Failure	GFR<15 mL/min

KDIGO classification				Persistent albuminuria Categories		
				Normal to mildly ↑	Moderately ↑	Severely ↑
				<30 mg/g	30-300 mg/g	>300 mg/g
GFR Category	1	Normal	>90	1 if CKD	1	2
	2	Mildly decreased	60-89	1 if CKD	1	2
	3a	Mild-moderate decreased	45-59	1	2	3
	3b	Moderate to severe decreased	30-44	2	3	3
	4	Severely decreased	15-29	3	3	4+
	5	Kidney failure	<15	4+	4+	4+

- **Screening**
    - In general, anyone at higher risk of chronic kidney disease should be screened for it. This group includes US minorities and patients with hypertension, cardiovascular disease, and diabetes mellitus, among others. Screening includes an assessment of estimated GFR and urinalysis for proteinuria or hematuria.
    - SCr
        - Factors that alter SCr without changing GFR
            - Muscle mass
            - Dietary protein intake
            - Exercise
            - Cimetidine
            - Fibrates
            - Methyldopa
        - The serum creatinine concentration is directly dependent on muscle mass, which varies with sex (women tend to have less muscle mass as a percent of body weight than men), age (muscle mass decreases with age), and race (African Americans have a higher serum creatinine level for the same GFR than other Americans). Thus, there is no "normal" value for serum creatinine that applies to all patients.
        - Proteinuria on UA → if +1 then obtain...
            - Protein/SCr ratio: >200 should prompt nephrology referral
            - Albumin/SCr ratio: <30 nml, 30-300 is microalbuminuria, >300 is macroalbuminuria

- Repeat yearly for progression

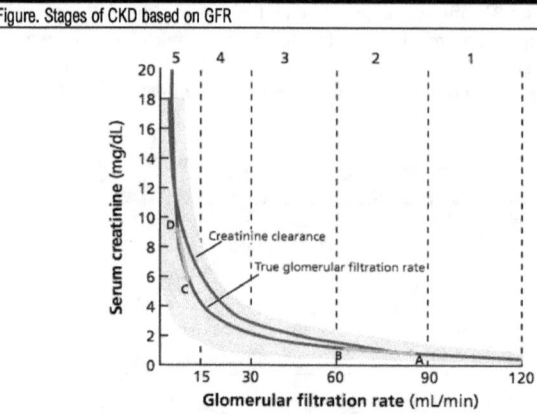

Figure. Stages of CKD based on GFR

- **Etiologies**
  - DM (45%)
  - HTN (29%)
  - Glomerulonephritis (presence of dysmorphic RBCs) (5.5%)
  - C3/C4, anti-ASO, HIV, HepB, HCV, RPR
  - ANA, ANCA
  - SPEP/UPEP if age > 40
  - Interstitial nephritis (presence of WBC casts d/t medication s/e, fever, rash)
  - Ischemia/Hypovolemia (presence of hyaline casts (test for FENa, eosinophilia)
  - Chronic UTI
  - Malignancy
  - Tobacco use
  - RVD (doppler US)
  - Vasculitis (C3, C4, ANA, ANCA; HBsAg, HCV, cryoglobulins, ESR, RF, SS–A, SS–B, HIV)
- **Labs**
  - CMP (W/ Albumin)
  - Albumin/SCr ratio (>300 = nephrotic range, 30-300 = microalbuminuria)
  - Protein/SCr ratio (>200 = proteinuria)
  - CBC (eval for normocytic anemia)
  - Vitamin D / PTH
  - UA
  - A1c and Lipid panel (eval. for risk factors)
  - Other possible screening tests:
    - SPEP/UPEP
    - Serum and urine free light chains
    - ANA, ds-DNA
    - C3/C4 (if concerned for glomerulonephritis based on presence of dysmorphic RBCs)
    - ANCA
    - Anti-GBM
    - HIV
    - Hepatitis B and C

- Kidney biopsy
- **Imaging**
  - Renal US (eval. for hydronephrosis, medical renal disease)
- **Complications**
  - HTN, anemia, secondary hyperparathyroidism, renal osteodystrophy, sleep disturbances, infections, malnutrition, electrolyte imbalances, platelet dysfunction/bleeding, pseudogout, gout, metabolic calcification, sexual dysfunction
- **Treatment/Management**
  - Hypertension
    - Goal in adults is:
      - <130/80 mm Hg if urine albumin excretion is ≥30 mg/24 hr; with ACEi or ARB
      - <140/90 mm Hg if urine albumin excretion is <30 mg/24 hr
  - Anemia (goal HGB 11-12; transferrin sat > 20%, ferritin <200)[371]
    - Iron Deficiency
      - Supplementation, particularly with IV iron, enhances erythropoiesis and raises HGB levels in CKD patients with anemia.
      - ↑risk for ↓BP but ↓GI s/e which is higher in oral iron supplementation (constipation)
      - In ESRD
        - The only accurate way of diagnosing IDA in an anemic dialysis patient is to administer a therapeutic trial of iron and document a rise in the hematocrit.
        - Should be checked q1-3m
        - Goal ferritin: 200-500; transferrin saturation >20%
      - See page 305 for full details
    - EPO
      - Anemia in ESRD characterized by a reduced ability to produce EPO, the hormone involved in proliferation and maturation of red blood cells in the bone marrow
      - Initiated if Hgb<11, stop when Hgb>12 despite iron replacement
        - The usual starting dose is 80-120 U/kg/week in divided doses.
        - When HCT ↑ above 36 g/dl, it is best to give low maintenance doses of EPO (e.g. 1000 or 2,000 U) once or twice weekly, rather than stopping the drug
      - After administration of EPO, there is ↑RBC production for 5-7 hours during which large amounts of iron must be available for RBC production
  - Acidosis
    - Goal is HCo3 23-28
    - See page 536 for more
  - Electrolyte targets (mostly in ESRD)
    - Normalize Calcium (corrected): 8.4-9.5 mg/dL
    - Normalize Phosphate **toward** normal range but no benefit in stage 3a and 4 (3.5-5.5 mg/dL)
      - Restrict dietary phosphorus to 900mg/d
      - If remains high, test calcium level:
        - Calcium <9.5→ treat with calcium carbonate or calcium acetate
        - Calcium >9.5→ treat with sevelamer or lanthanum
    - Lower salt intake to <2g/d unless contraindicated
    - Normalize PTH: 150-300 pg/mL
      - Correct vitamin D deficiencies and normalize Ca^{2+} and Phos
      - If despite above treatments, PTH is >300 pg/mL, test phosphorus level
        - Phosphorus <5.5 mg/dL
          - And serum calcium <9.5
            - Treat with vitamin D
          - And serum calcium >9.5

- - - Treat with cinacalcet (only in ESRD)
  - Phosphorus >5.5 mg/dL
    - Treat with cinacalcet (only in ESRD)
  - Tertiary hyperparathyroidism
    - Result of chronically elevated PTH, leads to ↑Ca levels and parathyroid hyperplasia with ↑PTH that will not respond to phosphate binders and calcitriol therapy
    - Requires parathyroidectomy
  - Protein - restriction to 0.8 g/kg/day is recommended in CKD G4 to G5.
    - CKD at risk of progression should avoid dietary protein >1.3 g/kg/day to avoid accelerating progression
- **Referral Indications**
  - Nonurgent if GFR<60; more urgent with decreasing GFR

Monitoring for complications of CKD[372]			
Complication	Testing	Frequency	Other
Anemia	HGB	No anemia: • Stages 1-2: when clinically indicated • Stage 3: 1x per year • Stages 4-5: 2x/year With anemia: • Stages 3-5: q3m	R/O IDA, B12 deficiency, folate deficiency, bleed. Supplementation and EPO use as described above.
Bone disorder	Ca PO4 PTH 25-OH Vit D	Calcium/phosphate: • Stage 3: q 6-12 months • Stage 4: q 3-6 months • Stage 5: q 1-3 months Parathyroid hormone: • Stage 3: baseline, then prn • Stage 4: q 6-12 months • Stage 5: q 3-6 months Vitamin D: • Stages 3-5: baseline, then prn	Consider phosphate-lowering therapy (e.g., calcium acetate, sevelamer, iron-based binders) and vitamin D supplementation
Hyperkalemia	K	Baseline, then prn	Advise low K diet and correct elevated glucose. K-binders may be necessary.
Metabolic Acidosis	HCO3	Baseline, then prn	PO HCO3 supplementation for HCO3 < 22 mmol/L
CVD	Lipid	Baseline, then prn	Low- to moderate-dose statin therapy for ≥50 years with CKD Statin therapy for patients aged 18-49 years with CKD and coronary artery disease, diabetes, prior ischemic stroke, or high risk of myocardial infarction or cardiovascular death

POLYURIA

- **Clinical Symptoms**[373]
    - Orthostatic hypotension
    - Polydipsia
    - Nocturia
    - ↓fluid intake
    - Ask about history of lithium use
    - PMHx of bipolar disorder
    - ↑HR, dry mucous membranes, ↓skin turgor
- **Differential**
    - <u>Volume Depleted</u>
        - Diabetes Insipidus (excess water loss by the kidney due to deficiency of ADH or renal resistance to ADH. Can be acquired due to medications, protein malnutrition, or metabolic abnormalities. Congenital causes of rarer.
            - Central (family history, head trauma)→ appropriate increase in urine osmolality after AVP challenge
            - Nephrogenic (chronic renal disease, ↑ca 2/2 malignancy such as MM, lithium, gentamycin) → no increase in urine osmolality after AVP challenge
        - Diuretic induced
            - Osmotic
            - Medication s/e
    - <u>Euvolemic</u> → primary polydipsia (h/o psychiatric disease; likely if water deprivation leads to increase in Urine osmolality of 1000-1200)
- **Labs**
    - Serum and urine osmolarity
        - Expect ↑serum Na (>143) and ↑serum osmolality (>295)
    - Urine sodium
    - Serum sodium
    - 24-hour urine
    - UPEP
    - SPEP
- **Testing**
1. <u>Confirm</u> hypotonic polyuria on 24 hour urine volume and osmolality
    - 24-hour urine volume is typically ≥3L in patients with DI
    - Urine osmolality is typically <300 mOsm/kg
2. Consider obtaining plasma vasopressin level (↑in nephrogenic DI) and plasma copeptin level (↑in nephrogenic DI)
3. If ↑Na and serum ↑osmolality → unlikely PP; perform vasopressin challenge test (good test for differentiating nephrogenic from central DI)
    - <u>Water deprivation testing / Vasopressin challenge test</u>
    To be done after vasopressin challenge test in patients with ↑Na (≥143) and ↑serum osmolality (≥295). Otherwise, perform before vasopressin challenge test in patients with normal Na and osmolality
        - Measure urine osmolality
        - Administer exogenous dose of ADH
        - Repeat urine osmolality measurement to evaluate response to ADH
4. If Na and serum osmolality are normal though, perform water deprivation testing **then** do to vasopressin challenge test

Water deprivation testing (WDT) Protocol: varies by hospital, typically avoid alcohol, caffeine and tobacco 24 hours prior to test. STOP testing if body weight ↓ by 3-5%,

significant orthostatic BP changes noted, urine osmolality plateaus (defined as <10% change over 3 consecutive measurements), urine osmolality normalizes (>750 mOsm/kg), plasma osmolality >295-300, or serum sodium is above 143. The following labs should be obtained during test: plasma arginine vasopressin level at baseline; monitor body weight, BP, HR, serum sodium, plasma osmolality, urine osmolality, and urine volume **hourly** during water deprivation.
- If total daily urine volume is <3L in testing above, start testing at midnight
- If total daily urine volume is >3L in testing above, start testing 2 hours before test
    - Interpretation
        - Little increase or no increase in urine osmolality (remaining below 300 mOsm/kg) during water deprivation → complete diabetes insipidus
        - Small increase in urine osmolality (increase to about 400-500 mOsm/kg) during water deprivation → partial diabetes insipidus or primary polydipsia
        - Increase in serum osmolality and urine osmolality → healthy response

Vasopressin challenge testing
Patient must be in a hyperosmolar state; if not, perform WDT above
- **Protocol**: varies by hospital, Administer arginine vasopressin (AVP) 5U or DDAVP 1-2 mcg SQ or IM. Check urine osmolality q30min for 2-4hours. If no change in urine osmolality, likely nephrogenic DI. If increase in urine osmolality by >50%, likely central DI. See table below.

Differentiating polyuria states: AVP stimulation test evaluation				
Condition	Uosm Max dehydration	Uosm Max after AVP	% change	Uosm Increase
Normal	1068±69	979±79	-9±3	<9%
Psychogenic polydipsia	738±53	780±73	-5±2	<9%
Partial central DI	438±34	549±28	28±5	>9%<50%
Complete central DI	168±13	445±52	183±41	**>50%**
Nephrogenic DI	124	174	42	**<50%**

- **Treatment/Management**
    - Ensure adequate water intake to prevent dehydration
    - Stop lithium if patient taking; consider starting amiloride
    - Low Na diet (<500mg/d)
    - Nephrology and endocrinology consultation

Figure. Algorithm for the differential diagnosis of polyuria

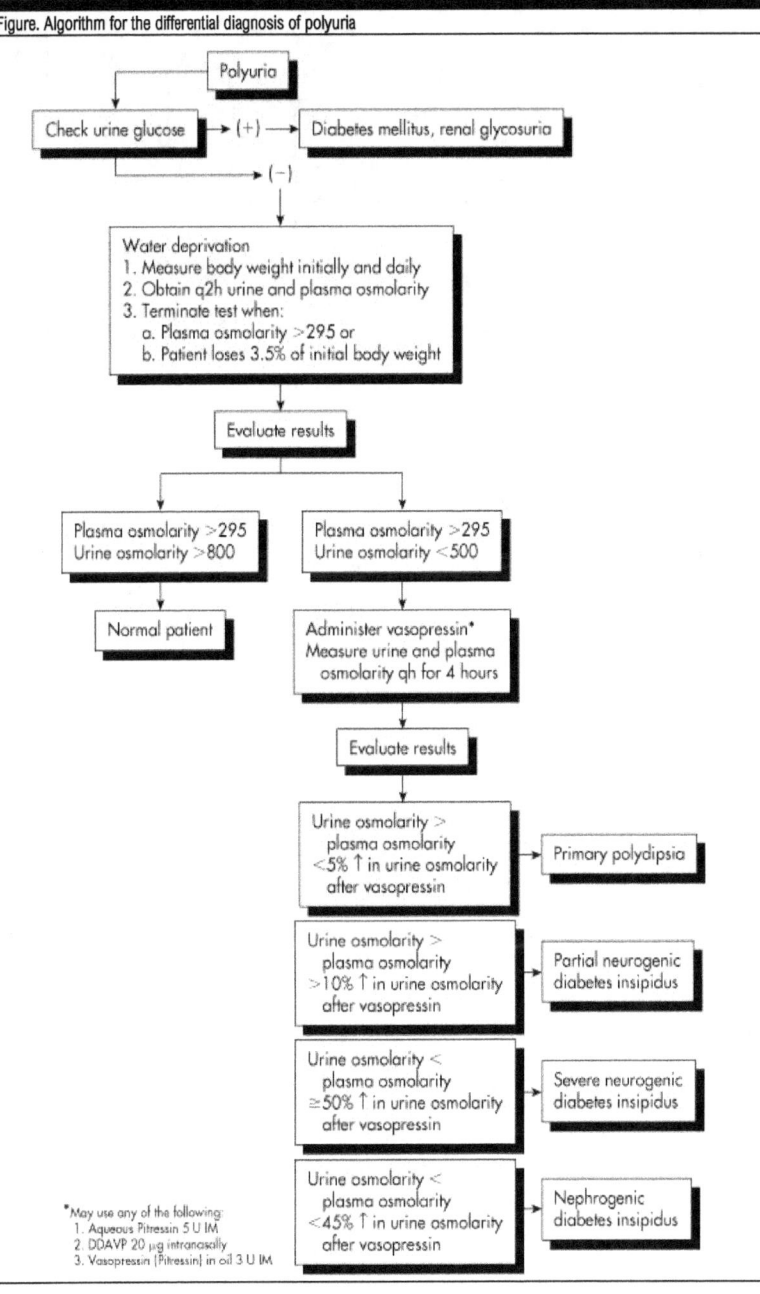

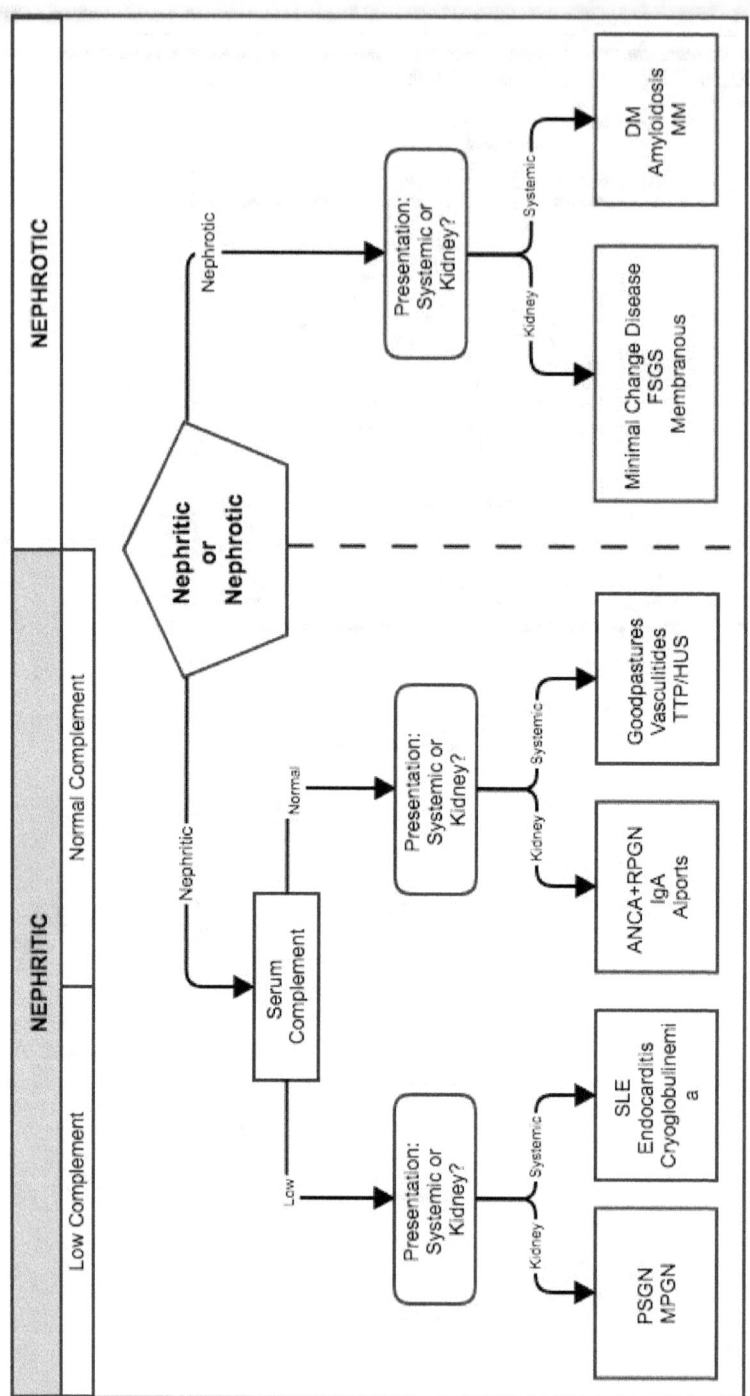

GLOMERULAR DISEASE

- **Background**
    - Account for majority of acute and chronic kidney disease
    - Due to both immunologic, infectious, and metabolic causes
    - This section will focus on Glomerulonephritis
- **Types**[374]
    (see chart on prior page)
    - Nephritic
        - *Features*
            - HTN
            - Hematuria
            - Oliguria
        - *Examples*
            - MGN
            - MPGN
            - IgA nephropathy (triggered by URI, associated with HSP; >50% → ESRD)
            - Anti-GBM disease
            - PSGN – associated with URI or skin infection. AS)+, back pain w/hematuria.
            - HSP
            - SLE
            - Wegener's
            - Orthostatic proteinuria (young adults) → dx with split 24-hour urine protein collection
    - Nephrotic
        - *Features*
            - Massive proteinuria (>3g)
            - ↓albumin
            - edema
            - hyperlipidemia
        - *Examples*
            - Primary Causes
                - Membranous (most common overall, Hepatitis B, cancer)
                - FSGS (African Americans, HIV, Heroin, chronic HTN)
                - Minimal change disease (most common in children; 25% of adult cases)
                - Membranoproliferative Glomerulonephritis (MPGN)
            - Secondary Causes
                - Tumor (lymphoma) → MN
                - Heroin (FSGS)
                - Infection (HepB, C)
                - Systemic
                - Lupus
                - Amyloidosis
                - Sarcoidosis
                - DM
                - Hepatitis B, C (B=MN, C=MPGN)
                - AIDS
                - Syphilis (MN)

NEPHROLOGY

Lab findings in nephritic vs. nephrotic range proteinuria	
Nephrotic	Nephritic
Bland without casts	Active sediment (casts, RBCs, dysmorphic)
Severe proteinuria (Spot prot/creat ratio >3.5 mg/dl or albumin/creatinine ratio >300 mg/dL)	Sterile pyuria
	Spot prot/creat ratio <3
Lipiduria	
Associated hypoalbuminurea, hyperlipidemia	
Edema	

Differential of glomerulonephritis based on complement levels	
Low complement	Normal compliment
PSGN (↓C3)	Positive ANCA
Endocarditis	MPA (+P-ANCA/MPO, no lung granulomas)
SLE (↓CH50, ↓C3/4, +ANA +anti-SM +anti-dsDNA)	GPA (+C-ANCA/PR3, saddle-nose, pulm nodules)
Cryoglobulinemia (+HepC commonly)	EGPA (asthma, atrophy, ↓eosinophils)
MPGN (+HepC commonly, ↑monoclonal proteins)	Renal limited ANCA
	Negative ANCA
	Goodpasture's (hemoptysis common)
	Anti-GBM renal dz
	Immune Complex
	HSP/IgA vasculitis (palpable purpura, age<20)
	IgA nephropathy (gross hematuria post URI)

- **Poor prognostic indicators**
  - Severe proteinuria
  - Hypertension
  - Elevated SCr at presentation
  - Male gender
- **Exam**
  - Hypertension seen with nephritic
  - Hematuria associated with nephritis
  - Check for flank pain
- **Labs**
  - C3, ANCA, Hepatitis C, Hepatitis B, anti-GM
  - ABG to determine pH
  - UA
    - Presence of hematuria is often always seen with glomerulone**phritis** whereas it is rarely seen with nephrotic syndrome.
    - Nephritis is associated with more active sediment (RBC/WBC/Glomerular casts).
    - Presence of heavy proteinuria (4+ which equals album of 1000 mg/dl) and lipiduria is classic of nephrotic syndrome.
    - WBC casts associated with tubulointerstitial disease
  - Measure a spot urine Prot/SCr ratio from first morning void
    - Normal is <0.2 g/dL
    - Ratio >3.5g = nephrotic range
  - Glomerulonephritis
    - Anti-SPO (r/o PSGN)
    - ANA/anti-DNA (r/o SLE)
    - C3/C4/CH50 (r/o PSGN and MPGN)
    - ANCA (r/o Wegener's)
    - IgA level (HSP, IgA nephropathy)
    - Anti-GBM antibody

- o Nephrotic Syndrome
    - Hypoalbuminurea (<3 g/dl)
    - Hyperlipidemia
    - APOL-1 gene in FSGS
- **Biopsy**
    - o Determines diagnosis, amount of injury, and future
- **Medications/Management**
    - o Consult nephrology → bx +/- cytotoxic therapy w/ high dose steroids
    - o Control blood pressure to <130/80
    - o Consider starting ACEi
    - o Fish oil supplements may delay ESRD
    - o PSGN→treat underlying infection (PCN)
    - o Consider medications to control elevated PO4 (Renvela 1-2 tabs TID), low HCO3 (Bicitra 30cc/TID if NAGMA; HCO3 drip (D5W+150mEQ) if low pH)

NEPHROLITHIASIS

- **Causes**[375]
    - o Genetics – familial hypocalcemic hypocalciuria, homocystinuria, xanthine
    - o Low water intake
    - o RTA type 1
    - o Hyperuricemia
    - o M>F in 2:1 ratio
    - o UTIs (staghorn calculi)
    - o Hyperparathyroidism
- **Diagnosis**
    - o Labs
        - SCr, Uric Acid, Ionized Calcium, Na, K, Cl, PTH, CBC, CRP, Coagulation Panel (for future surgery)
        - UA (red cells, white cells, nitrite, pH, volume, spec grav)
        - Urine calcium, oxalate, uric acid, citrate, Mg
        - Urine culture and microscopy
        - **Multiple Episode Patient**
            1. 24hr urine collection for oxalate, calcium, citrate, sodium, and uric acid
            2. Serum Mg, PO4
            3. 24hr cysteine level
            4. PTH and VIT D
    - o Imaging
        - CT renal without contrast
        - US used to detect dilatation of ureters (upper) and stones at UVJ – imaging of choice if pregnant
    - o Stone analysis
        - Calcium oxalate stones occur in 2 forms
            1. dehydrated calcium oxalate crystals - pyramidal (squares with X's) and fragile
            2. monohydrated calcium oxalate crystals - modular and very hard
        - Uric acid stones - yellow, smooth surface, very hard, occur in acidic environment
        - Phosphate stones (apatite) - whitish powder (appears as micro-bubbles if in contact with hydrochloric acid), occur in alkaline environment
        - Calcium phosphate stones - may appear as brushite, occur in acidic environment
        - Phosphor-ammonium-magnesium stones (struvite) - whitish, prismatic crystals, occur in alkaline environment, usually with infection

NEPHROLOGY

Kidney Stone Make-up

Stone	Metabolic Abnormality	Clinical Setting	Urine Findings	Treatment
Calcium oxalate	↑calciuria	Hyperparathyroidism Immobilization ↑vitamin d Cushing Genetic	Envelope-shape	HCTZ 50mg/d Chlorthalidone 25-50mg/d
	Hyperoxaluria	Increased oxalate uptake IBD High dietary VitC		Pyridoxine 25-50mg/d
Calcium phosphate	Hypocitraturia Hypercalciuria High urine pH (>7)	Similar to calcium oxalate Distal RTA		K-citrate 30-60 U/d
Struvite	High urinary ammonium and Bicarb levels	UTI w/ urease splitting organisms	Staghorn calculi Coffin-lid crystals	Acetohydroxamic acid (10-15 mg/kg/day)
Uric Acid	Low urine pH (<5.5) Hyperuricosuria	Metabolic syndrome Insulin resistance T2DM	Rhomboid crystals Radiolucent Stone	Allopurinol 100-300mg/d K-citrate 30-60U/d
Cystine	Cystinuria	Genetics	Hexagonal green/yellow Large branched calculi	α-Mercaptopropionylglycine (400-1,200 mg/day) or D-penicillamine (1,000-2,000 mg/day)

- **Treatment**
  - Urology Consultation – recommended in the following situations
    - Stones ≥ 10mm
    - AKI
    - Sepsis
    - Complete ureteral obstruction
    - Uncontrolled pain
    - Nausea
  - Fluids
  - Pain control
    - NSAID – ketorolac, diclofenac, indomethacin, Toradol IM injection all remain the first line treatment options
    - Morphine (hydromorphone, pentazocine, tramadol) 3mg prn q2h
      +
      Dilaudid 0.2mg q2h
    - Antispasmodics – metamizole sodium
  - Facilitate passage (for stones >5mm)
    - Alfuzosin 10mg/d, tamsulosin 0.4mg/d
    - Nifedipine
  - Ureteral stone
    - Upper < 1cm – ESWL
    - Upper > 1cm/resistant to ESWL/any stone >2cm – percutaneous nephrolithotomy
    - Distal < 1cm – ESWL
    - Distal > 1cm – Ureterorenoscopy
  - Kidney
    - < 2cm – ESWL
    - > 2cm – percutaneous nephrolithotomy
- **Prevention**
  - Pain: diclofenac sodium 100-150 mg/day for 3-10 days

- >2.5L water/day
- ↓ salt & protein diet
- ↑dietary calcium intake
- ↑fruits/veggies
- Thiazide diuretics unless calcium stone composition

Bibliography

[368] Batlle et al. "The use of the urinary anion gap in the diagnosis of hyperchloremic metabolic acidosis." N Engl J Med. 1988 Mar 10;318(10):594-9.

[369] Simon, James. Interpreting the estimated glomerular filtration rate in primary care: Benefits and pitfalls." CCJM. 78(3). March, 2011.

[370] Frank J. Domino, MD, Jeremy Golding, MD, FAAFP, Mark B. Stephens, MD, Robert A. Baldor MD, FAAFP, eds. 2020. 5-Minute Clinical Consult - 28th Ed. Philadelphia, PA. Lippincott Williams & Wilkins Health. ISBN-10: 1-9751-3641-1, ISBN-13: 978-1-9751-3641-3. eISBN-10: 1-9751-3642-X, eISBN-13: 978-1-9751-3642-0. STAT!Ref Online Electronic Medical Library. https://online.statref.com/document/qs-2WY0RvmfAd-z5NvpQJN!!. 10/10/2019 9:32:07 PM CDT (UTC -05:00).

[371] KDOQI Clinical Practice Guideline and Clinical Practice Recommendations for anemia in chronic kidney disease: 2007 update of hemoglobin target. Am J Kidney Dis 2007; 50: 471–530.

[372] Chen et al. Chronic Kidney Disease Diagnosis and Management A Review. JAMA. 2019;322(13):1294-1304

[373] Fenske W, Allolio B. Clinical review: Current state and future perspectives in the diagnosis of diabetes insipidus: a clinical review. J Clin Endocrinol Metab. 2012 Oct;97(10):3426-37

[374] http://medicine.ucsf.edu/education/resed/Chiefs_cover_sheets/nephrotic.pdf

[375] Gottlieb M, Long B, Koyfman A. "The evaluation and management of urolithiasis in the emergency department: A review of the literature." Am J Emerg Med. 2018 Jan 5. pii: S0735-6757(18)30003-2.

OTOLARYNGOLOGY

Allergic Rhinitis 557
Rhinosinusitis 559
Pharyngitis 560
Epistaxis 564
Hearing Loss 565

ALLERGIC RHINITIS

- **Diagnosis**[376]
  Diagnosis is made through clinical and physical exam; can confirm with allergy testing (skin or IgE)
    - Intermittent: <4 days a week or less than 4 weeks
    - Persistent: >4 days week and for more than 4 weeks
    - Mild: none of the following are present: sleep disturbance; impairment of daily activities, leisure, and/or sport; impairment of school or work; troublesome symptoms.
    - Moderate to severe: one or more of the following symptoms are present: sleep disturbance; impairment of daily activities, leisure, and/or sport; impairment of school or work, troublesome symptoms.
- **Causes**
    - Allergic rhinitis is most common cause
    - Non-allergic rhinitis
    - Congestion
    - PND
    - Rhinorrhea
    - Vasomotor
    - Gustatory - common causes being smoking, perfume, car exhaust, medications, hormone changes, idiopathic.
    - Drug-induced rhinitis (recent use of afrin, NSAIDs, ACEi)
    - Nasal polyps
    - Adenoid hypertrophy
- **Exam**
    - Sneezing
    - Nasal itching
    - Rhinorrhea
    - Nasal congestion
    - Pruritis
- **Management/Treatment**

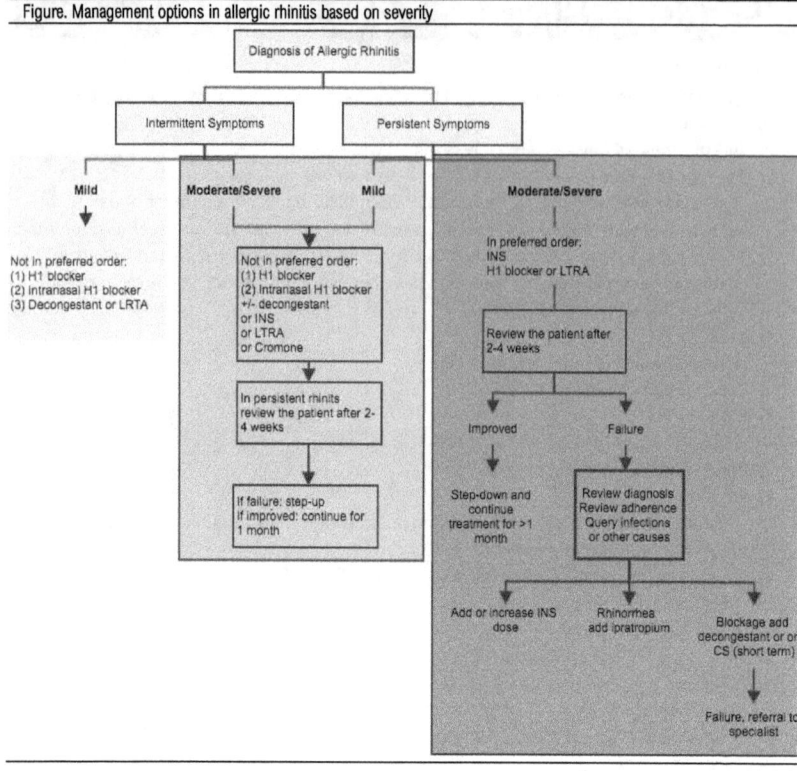

Figure. Management options in allergic rhinitis based on severity

- o Intranasal Corticosteroid (recommend 5 days on, 2 days off)
    - Treat nasal congestion and ocular symptoms
    - The combination with a second-generation antihistamine intranasal preparation has also been found to be effective
    - Rhinocort Aqua (good for pregnancy)
    - Flonase 2 sprays each nostril daily
    - Nasarel 2 sprays each nostril BID
    - Nasacort 1-2 sprays each nostril daily
    - Triamcinolone Acetate
    - Azelastine 137mcg/spray 1-2 sprays per nostril BID
    - Olopatadine 665mcg/spray 2 sprays per nostril BID
- o Oral Antihistamines
    Treat sneezing, purities, and rhinorrhea
    - Allegra 60mg/BID or 180mg/d *(180mg preferred dosing)*
    - Claritin 10mg/d or 5mg/*BID (best dose is 20mg but may be sedating)*
    - Clarinex 5mg/d *(best dose is 20mg but may be sedating)*
    - Zyrtec 5-10mg *(best dose is 20mg but may be sedating)*
- o Decongestants
    - Afrin 2 sprays into each nostril BID for < 3 days
    - Phenylephrine
    - Pseudoephedrine
- o Intranasal Antihistamines
    - Azelastine 0.15% 2 sprays/BID

- o Combination Therapy
  - Dymista (Azelastine+Fluticasone)
- o Acute
  - Afrin BID x 3 days
  - NEILmed saline rinse
  - ipratropium nasal spray 0.03% 2 sprays each nostril BID-TID
- o Chronic
  - Flonase (most effective)

RHINOSINUSITIS

- **Types**[377,378]
  - o Acute rhinosinusitis: Sudden onset, m/c involving maxillary sinus, lasting less than 6 weeks with complete resolution. Most commonly due to viruses and is usually self-limiting (only 1/3 due to bacteria).
  - o Subacute rhinosinusitis: A continuum of acute rhinosinusitis but less than 12 weeks.
  - o Recurrent acute rhinosinusitis: Four or more episodes of acute, lasting at least 7 days each, in any 1-year period.
  - o Chronic – presence of at least two of the following cardinal symptoms for at least 12 consecutive weeks:
    - Nasal obstruction
    - Nasal drainage
    - Facial pain/pressure
    - Hyposmia/anosmia
    -And-
    - Objective evidence on PE (mucopurulent d/c, edema, polyps in the middle of the meatus or XR/sinus
- **Symptoms** - nasal discharge, cough, congestion, headache, fever, facial pain
- **Diagnosis**
  - o The best predictors of bacterial infection were:
    - Purulent secretions from the nose
    - Halitosis
    - Pain in the teeth
    - Altered sense of smell
    - Purulent secretions in the posterior pharynx or postnasal region
- **Imaging** – CT or XR not advised in the acute setting
- **Treatment**
  - o Acute Rhinosinusitis
    - ABx indicated for:
      - Symptoms >10 days
      - Facial pain > 3 days +/- purulent discharge
      - Worsening symptoms after initial improvement
      - Temp>102.2F
    - Treatment (if no improvement in >7 days)
      - *Mild Disease:*
        - Amoxicillin 500mg q8h x5-10d or 875mg BID x5-10d
        - Augmentin 500/125 q8h x5-10d or 875/125 BID x5-10d recommended
        - *High S.pneumonia risk due to child at daycare:*
        - Amoxicillin 1g Q8H x5-10d or 1g QID x5-10d
      - *Mod/Severe Disease/Treatment Failure*
        - Augmentin XR 2g/125 BID x10d
        - PCN Allergy:

- Levaquin 500mg/d x10-14d
- Doxycycline 200mg/d x5-10d
- Chronic Rhinosinusitis
  - Treatment consists of medical mgmt. and endoscopic sinus surgery if meds are not successful
  - Options
    - Isotonic nasal saline rinse/irrigation (low pressure high volume 240cc)
    - Topical intranasal corticosteroids (i.e. Flonase) injected laterally away from septum while leaning forward
    - Anti-histamines (Claritin, Allegra, Zyrtec)
      - Can lead to impaired drainage.
      - They are only of benefit in early allergic sinusitis
    - Ipratropium 2 sprays of the 0.06% solution in each nostril 4 times daily
    - Decongestants: oxymetolazone 2-3 sprays each nostril BID (no more than 3d), pseudoephedrine 60mg q4-6h, nasal saline rinse, guaifenesin, Flonase (intranasal steroids), Afrin
    - Zinc 25mg/d
    - Humidification

PHARYNGITIS

- Cause[379]
  - Non-infectious (smoking, workplace inhalation exposure to chemicals, foreign body, GERD, allergic rhinitis
  - Viral vs. Bacterial
    - Viruses
      - Viral causes are most common (rhinovirus)
      - Others (adenovirus, HSV, Coxsackie)
    - Atypical (Mycoplasma, Chlamydophila pneumoniae
    - Remember prodrome of early HIV can present as pharyngitis/mono like symptoms (look for patients that participate in high risk sexual activity, IVDA)
      - R/o with HIV RNA testing or p24 antigen in serum
    - Bacterial
      - Bacterial m/c caused by GAS (pyogenes) → remember can lead to RF and PSGN

Pharyngitis Etiologies

Cause	Statistics	Facts/Findings
Strep	5-15% of cause	Group A Sudden onset sore throat Tonsillar exudates Fever No Cough Risk of progression to scarlet fever Group C/G Similar symptoms to GAS but negative rapid strep screen
EBV	Most Common (viral)	Can lead to infectious mono Malaise/Headache Low grade fever Prolonged course Rarely has exudates Severe pharyngotonsillar inflammation, which can be obstructive and require intensive anti-inflammatory treatment. Tonsillar exudates in 50% of cases. Inflammation of cervical lymph nodes. Takingantibiotics can result in a maculopapular rash on the trunk and extremities
CMV	Less common than EBV	Prolonged fever Less likely to have LAD Mild if any pharyngitis
HIV	Less Common	Mucosal ulcerations Febrile Pharyngeal edema WITHOUT exudates
Fusobacterium necrophorum	Less Common	Suspect in patients with negative RADT and not improving Cause in severe cases of Lemierre's syndrome

Figure. Evaluation of acute pharyngitis

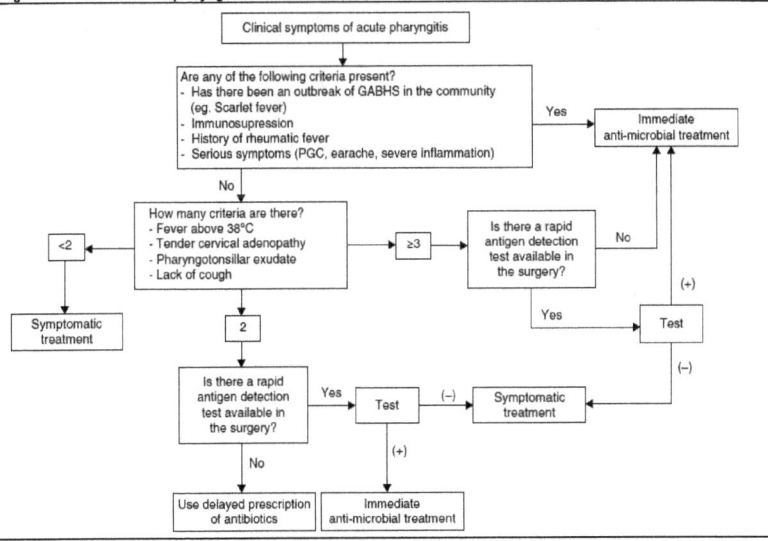

- **Signs/Symptoms**
  - <u>Bacterial</u>
    - Sore throat

- Fever
- Headache
- N/V/abdominal pain
- Cervical adenitis
  - Viral
    - Conjunctivitis
    - Cough
    - Diarrhea
    - Hoarseness
    - Rash
    - Presentation in winter
- **Serious Symptoms**
  - Stridor
  - Drooling
  - Respiratory Distress
  - Recent travel
  - Cases lasting over 2 weeks with poor outcome
  - Suspicion of lingual pharyngitis with obstruction
  - Concern for Lemierre's Syndrome – thrombophlebitis of the internal jugular vein (worsening sx with chills, fever, pain, and ipsilateral cervical swelling at the angle of the jaw and along the SCM and stiff neck)
- **Evaluation (Scoring System)**
  - Centor criteria (GABHS)
    - Fever (subjective or measured >100.5° F): 1 point
    - Absence of cough: 1 point
    - Tender anterior cervical lymphadenopathy: 1 point
    - Tonsillar exudates: 1 point
    - **Analysis**
      - 0-1 points: low risk therefore does not require treatment; probability 2.5-10%
      - 2-3 points: assess for GAS with rapid strep testing (RADT) without reflex culture for negative tests; probability 10-35%
      - 4+ points: empirical treatment; probability 39-57%
  - McIsaac criteria (modified Centor)
    - Fever (subjective or measured >100.5° F): 1 point
    - Absence of cough: 1 point
    - Tender anterior cervical lymphadenopathy: 1 point
    - Tonsillar exudates: 1 point
    - Age
      - 3–14 years: 1 point
      - 15–44 years: 0 point
      - 45 years or older: –1 point
    - **Analysis**
      - 0-1 points: low risk therefore does not require treatment
      - 2-3 points: assess for GAS with rapid strep testing (RADT) without reflex culture for negative tests
      - 4+ points: empirical treatment
- **Complications**
  - Epiglottitis
  - Peritonsillar abscess
  - Cervical lymphadenitis
  - Sinusitis
  - Mastoiditis
  - ARF

- o PSGN
- **Diagnostic Testing**
  - o RADT (if CENTOR 3+) but do not get reflex culture if negative
- **Treatment**
  - o Self-limited illness: viral pharyngitis resolves in 3-7 days
  - o If ABx are indicated, resolution noted within 24-48 hours of initiation
  - o Supportive therapy
    - <u>Analgesics</u>
      - □ NSAIDS to ↓ fever and pain
      - □ Tylenol 325mg for pain
    - <u>Nasal congestion</u>
      - □ Combination antihistamine+decongestant is best (i.e. Claritin+Sudafed)
        - Acute – Afrin BID x 3 days, NEILmed saline rinse, sodium cromoglycate dry powder (20mg/INH) q2h
        - Chronic – Flonase, sinus rinse, Sudafed IR 60mg q4-6h or ER 120mg q12h / 240mg daily
    - <u>Cough</u> (see page **Error! Bookmark not defined.** for more details)
      - □ 1tsp honey TID
      - □ Tessalon Pearls (best for nighttime cough due to reflux)
      - □ Robitussin (guaifenesin with codeine)
      - □ Mucinex
    - <u>Sneezing/Rhinorrhea</u>
      - □ ipratropium nasal spray 0.03% 2 sprays each nostril BID-TID
    - <u>Sore Throat</u>
      - □ 1tsp honey TID
      - □ Chloraseptic Spray 1 spray PO Q 2-hour prn sore throat
        - Leave in place x 15 sec then spit
      - □ Benzoate 100-200mg prn TID max 600 mg/day
      - □ Guaifenasin+Codeine
        - Capsule: G (200mg) and C (9mg) q4h max 12cap/24hr
        - Liquid: 15mL q4-6h max 45ml/day
        - Tablet G (400 mg) and C (10-20 mg): One tablet q4-6h (maximum: 6 tablets/24 hours)
      - □ Hurricane Spray
      - □ Benmalid (diphenhydramine/Maalox/lidocaine viscous) suspension 30ml swish and swallow Q2H prn.

Antibiotic Treatment		
Antibiotic	Dose	Duration
Penicillin V	250 mg QID or 500 mg BID	5 days
	1.2M I.U. /oral/12h	8-10 days
	**5 day duration only studied at 250mg dose*	
Penicillin G	1.2M I.U. I.M	1 dose
Amoxicillin	500mg BID	8-10 days
Cefadroxil	500mg BID	8-10 days
Recurrence		
Clindamycin	300mg Q8H	10 days
Augmentin	500mg/125mg Q8H	10 days

EPISTAXIS

- **Background**[380]
  - Nasal bleeds are either anterior, posterior, or a combination of the two.
  - About 5% of nasal bleeding originates in the posterior nasal cavity. Such bleeds are more commonly associated with atherosclerotic disease and hypertension.
- **Cause**
  - Digital trauma, a deviated septum, dry air exposure, rhinosinusitis, neoplasia, or chemical irritants such as inhaled corticosteroids or chronic nasal cannula oxygen use.
  - Systemic factors that increase the risk of bleeding include chronic renal insufficiency, alcoholism, hypertension, vascular malformations such as hereditary hemorrhagic telangiectasia, or any kind of coagulopathy, including warfarin administration, von Willebrand's disease, or hemophilia.
- **History**
  - Ask about prior or recurrent epistaxis, duration and severity of the current episode, and laterality.
  - Ask specifically about nonsteroidal anti-inflammatory drugs, warfarin, heparin, or aspirin use. Alcohol or cocaine abuse, trauma, prior head and neck procedures, and a personal and family history of coagulopathy should be assessed.
- **Tools**
  - Create an epistaxis kit containing nasal speculum, bonyet forceps, headlamp, suction catheter, cotton pledgets, 0.05% oxymetolazone an 4% lidocaine solutions, silver nitrate (AgNO3) swabs, petroleum jelly
- **Diagnosis/Testing**
  - The division between anterior and posterior bleeding is often based on the ability to visualize the site of bleeding with a light source and a nasal speculum.
  - Generally, the diagnosis of posterior hemorrhage is only made once measures to control anterior bleeding have failed.
  - Clinical features suggestive of a posterior source include elderly patients with either inherited or acquired coagulopathy, a significant amount of hemorrhage visible in the posterior nasopharynx, hemorrhage from bilateral nares, or epistaxis uncontrolled with either anterior rhinoscopy or an anterior pack.
    - Posterior, bilateral, or large-volume epistaxis should be triaged immediately to a specialist in a critical care setting.
  - Laboratory evaluation or other ancillary studies are not required unless management of comorbid illness requires it, or the hemorrhage is poorly controlled. In the latter case, collect blood for CBC, type and crossmatch, and coagulation studies if coagulopathy is suspected.
- **Treatment**
  - Anterior Bleed
    - Direct Nasal Pressure
    - Instill a topical vasoconstrictor such as oxymetazoline or phenylephrine.
    - The patient should lean forward in the "sniffing" position and pinch the soft nares between the thumb and the middle finger for a full 10 to 15 minutes, breathing through the mouth.
      - If the patient is uncooperative, fashion a hands-free pressure device made from two tongue depressors that are taped together between halfway and two thirds of the way up the depressors. Place the device on the nose and leave it undisturbed for 10 to 15 minutes. These initial measures are often enough to achieve hemostasis and facilitate further examination by anterior rhinoscopy.
  - Chemical Cauterization

- If two attempts at direct pressure have failed, chemical cauterization with silver nitrate is the next appropriate step for mild bleeding.
- Before cautery, anesthetize the nasal mucosa using three cotton pledgets soaked in a 1:1 mixture of 0.05% oxymetazoline and 4% lidocaine solution.
  - Do not attempt chemical cautery unless the bleeding vessel is visualized. Electrical cautery should be left to the otolaryngologist due to the risk of septal perforation.
- After visualizing the (anterior) bleeding site, silver nitrate sticks may be judiciously placed just proximal to the bleeding source on the anterior nasal septum. Silver nitrate requires a relatively bloodless field, as the chemical reaction leading to precipitation of silver metal and tissue coagulation cannot proceed in the setting of amative hemorrhage due to washout of substrate. Once a relatively bloodless field is achieved, gently and briefly (a few seconds) apply silver nitrate directly to the bleeding site. Chemical cautery should never be attempted on both sides of the nasal septum. Subsequent attempts on the same side of the nasal septum should be separated by 4 to 6 weeks to avoid perforation.
  - Iced Lavage
    1. If neither vasoconstrictors nor direct external pressure stops the bleeding, try an iced normal saline lavage of each nostril, with the patient leaning forward. This may help decrease or stop the bleeding and allow better assessment of bleeding sites.
    2. Have the patient seated during both the examination and the therapeutic procedures; this will lower his or her blood pressure.
  - Packing
    - Lubricating a vaginal tampon and slipping it into the nose can make an improvised "prepackaged" anterior pack.
      - As with anything else inserted into or through the nose, insert the tampon straight back along the floor of the nose.
      - May need to start oral antibiotics

HEARING LOSS

- **Overview**[381]
  - Sudden hearing loss is defined as a rapid onset, occurring over a 72-hour period, of a subjective sensation of hearing impairment in one or both ears.
  - Approximately 1 in 8 individuals aged 12 years or older in the United States have a bilateral hearing loss, and 1 in 5 have a unilateral hearing loss.1
  - Disorders anywhere along the auditory pathway from the external auditory canal to the central nervous system may result in diminished hearing.
  - Patients presenting with sudden sensorineural hearing loss (SSNHL), however, demand a more urgent and vigilant approach
- **Evaluation**
  - In a patient with auditory complaints, the goals in the evaluation are to determine:
    (1) the nature of the hearing impairment (conductive or sensorineural)
    (2) the severity of the impairment (mild, moderate, severe, profound)
    (3) the anatomy of the impairment (external ear, middle ear, inner ear, or central auditory pathway pathology)
    (4) the etiology
  - Onset
    - **Sudden**
      - A sudden onset of unilateral hearing loss, with or without tinnitus
      - May represent an inner ear viral infection or a vascular accident

- Patients with unilateral hearing loss (sensory or conductive) usually complain of reduced hearing, poor sound localization, and difficulty hearing clearly with background noise.
- **Gradual**
  - Gradual progression in a hearing deficit is common with otosclerosis, noise-induced hearing loss, vestibular schwannoma, or Meniere disease.
  - People with small vestibular schwannomas typically present with any or all the following conditions: asymmetric hearing impairment, tinnitus, and imbalance (although rarely vertigo).
  - Cranial neuropathy, especially of the trigeminal or facial nerve, may accompany larger tumors.
  - In addition to hearing loss, Meniere disease or endolymphatic hydrops may be associated with episodic vertigo, tinnitus, and aural fullness.
  - Hearing loss with otorrhea is most likely due to chronic otitis media or cholesteatoma.

Source of Hearing Loss Based on Weber / Rinne Testing			
Type	Rinne	Weber	DDx
Conductive	Bone>air	Localized to affected ear	Cerumen
			Otitis Media
			Otitis Externa
			Otosclerosis
			TM rupture
			Cholesteatoma
Sensorineural	Air>bone	Localizes to unaffected ear	Meniere
			Acoustic Neuroma
			Presbycusis
			Ototoxic Rx
Normal	Air=bone	No localization	N/a

- **Testing**
  - CT head not advised for presumptive SSNHL
    - Should undergo MRI or auditory brainstem response (ABR) to evaluate for retro cochlear pathology
  - Audiometry advised within 14 days of onset for SSNHL
  - Weber/Rinne - The combined information from the Weber and Rinne tests permits a tentative conclusion as to whether a conductive or sensorineural hearing loss is present. However, these tests are associated with significant false-positive and -negative responses and therefore should be used only as screening tools and not as a definitive evaluation of auditory function.
    - **Weber**
      - The Weber tuning fork test may be performed with a 256- or 512-Hz fork.
      - The stem of a vibrating tuning fork is placed on the head in the midline
      - The patient is asked whether the tone is heard in both ears or in one ear better than in the other.
        - With a unilateral conductive hearing loss, the tone localizes to the affected ear.
        - With a unilateral sensorineural hearing loss, the tone is perceived in the unaffected ear (the ear that is not localized to)
    - **Rinne**
      - Sensitive in detecting conductive hearing losses.
      - A Rinne test compares the ability to hear by air conduction with the ability to hear by bone conduction.

- Place vibrating tuning fork (256 or 512 Hz) over the mastoid bone of one ear, then move the tuning fork to the entrance of the ear canal (not touching the ear)
- The sound should be heard well via air conduction (at the entrance to the ear canal).
- If the sound is heard better by bone conduction, then there is a CHL in that ear.
- Repeat for the other ear

- **Types**
  - Sensorineural hearing loss
    - Decrease in hearing of 30 dB or greater across at least 3 consecutive frequencies
    - Etiology in up to 90% of cases remains elusive.
    - 10% or so of cases have been associated with neoplastic, autoimmune, infectious, circulatory, coagulation, and demyelinating disorders
    - **Weber/Rinne**
      - Weber tuning fork test lateralizes to the unaffected side
      - Rinne tuning fork test demonstrates air conduction greater than bone conduction
    - Speech discrimination testing less than 90% correct.
    - **Differential**
      - Age-related (presbycusis) - symmetric, high-frequency hearing loss that eventually progresses to involve all frequencies. The hearing loss is associated with a significant loss in clarity.
      - Alport
      - Otitis Media
      - Labyrinthitis
      - S/e of medication (i.e. aminoglycosides)
      - Head trauma
      - MS
      - Vestibular schwannoma
- **Treatment**
  - Sudden onset
    - Hydrocortisone (1mg/kg/d max 60mg/d x 7-14d f/b taper for same time period with repeat audiogram after)
    - Hyperbaric O2
    - If no response to above after 2-6 weeks, consider intratympanic steroid
  - Conductive hearing loss
    - Results from dysfunction of the external or middle ear.
    - There are four mechanisms, each resulting in impairment of the passage of sound vibrations to the inner ear:
      (1) Obstruction (e.g., cerumen impaction)
      (2) Mass loading (e.g., middle ear effusion)
      (3) Stiffness effect (e.g., otosclerosis)
      (4) Discontinuity (e.g., ossicular disruption).
    - Conductive losses in adults are most commonly due to cerumen impaction or transient eustachian tube dysfunction associated with upper respiratory tract infection.
    - Persistent conductive losses usually result from chronic ear infection, trauma, or otosclerosis. Conductive hearing loss is often correctable with medical or surgical therapy—or in some cases both.

Bibliography

[376] Sur et al. "Treatment of Allergic Rhinitis." Am Fam Physician. 2015;92(11):985-992.
[377] Battisti AS, Pangia J. Sinusitis. [Updated 2018 Jan 29]. In: StatPearls [Internet]. Treasure Island (FL): StatPearls Publishing; 2018 Jan-. Available from: https://www.ncbi.nlm.nih.gov/books/NBK470383/
[378] Ebell et al. "Accuracy of Signs and Symptoms for the Diagnosis of Acute Rhinosinusitis and Acute Bacterial Rhinosinusitis." Ann Fam Med March/April 2019 vol. 17 no. 2 164-172.
[379] Cots JM, Alós JI, Bárcena M, Boleda X, Ca͞nada JL, Gómez N, et al. Recomendaciones para el manejo de la faringoamigdalitis aguda del adulto. Acta Otorrinolaringol Esp. 2015;66:159---170.
[380] McGinnis HD. Nose and Sinuses. In: Tintinalli JE, Stapczynski J, Ma O, Yealy DM, Meckler GD, Cline DM. eds. *Tintinalli's Emergency Medicine: A Comprehensive Study Guide, 8e* New York, NY: McGraw-Hill; 2016. http://accessmedicine.mhmedical.com/content.aspx?bookid=1658&sectionid=109387197. Accessed November 26, 2017
[381] Chandrasekhar SS, Tsai Do BS, Schwartz SR, Bontempo LJ, Faucett EA, Finestone SA, et al. Clinical Practice Guideline: Sudden Hearing Loss (Update). Otolaryngol Head Neck Surg. 2019 Aug. 161 (1_suppl):S1-S45. https://journals.sagepub.com/doi/full/10.1177/0194599819859885#_i16

RHEUMATOLOGY

Gout	570
Approach to Joint Pain	573
Monoarthritis	574
Polyarticular Arthritis	575
Common Rheumatologic Labs	578

GOUT

- **Defined** - deposition of monosodium urate monohydrate (MSU) in synovial fluid and other tissues[382]
- **Background**[383,384]
  - Along with pseudogout, one of the most common crystal-induced arthropathies
  - Uric acid (UA) produced is the product of purine metabolism; 2/3rd derived from cellular turnover of nucleic acids and remaining is from dietary intake.
  - Longstanding gout will ultimately lead to polyarticular attacks
- **Symptoms**: sudden onset pain, warm and erythematous joint, often one joint but can become polyarticular, resolves spontaneously in days to weeks. Patients may have systemic symptoms of fever, chills, ↑WBC but often resolved spontaneously in a few days if untreated.
  - Joints affected often are 1st MTP (*podagra*), ankle, or knee
  - Postmenoupasual women may present differently with initial attacks, often involving the finger joints that are already affected by OA.
  - Soft tissue can also be involved manifesting as acute bursitis, periarthrritis, and gouty panniculitis
- **Risk Factors**
  - Older age, males, red meat consumption, shellfish, EtOH, ASA, loop diuretics, HTN, IV contrast
  - Hereditary undersecretion of uric acid
  - Proinflammatory states such as surgery, ACS can provoke aute gouty attacks due to volume and pH changes
- **Classification/Diagnosis**
  - Use web-based calculator: http://goutclassificationcalculator.auckland.ac.nz
    - Score $\geq$ 8 classifies an individual as having gout
  - At least 1 episode of swelling, pain (recurrent; developing over 24h and resolving in $\leq$ 14d back to baseline), erythema, or tenderness (can't bear touch or pressure, weight) in a peripheral joint/bursa either:
    - With documented presence of MSU crystals in that joint
    - Documented tophi
    - Anatomic involvement: ankle, mid-foot, first MTP
- **Diagnostics**
  - Synovial fluid aspiration of affected joint can help with diagnosis (+MSU) however NOT required as above
  - Urate deposition on XR/CT/MRI or double-contour sign on US
- **Labs**
  - Check LFTs if on allopurinol
  - Synovial fluid with 2k-100k WBC
  - Crystals during joint aspiration (needle shape, negative birefringent, **monosodium urate**)
  - Uric Acid level (may be normal during acute flare) but monitored monthly (or q6-12m) during prevention therapy titration
    - Highly suggestive if $\geq$10; goal after treatment is <6
  - HLA-B*5801 – consider testing in certain Asian ethnic groups who may have predisposition to allopurinol hypersensitivity.
- **Treatment**
  - <u>Acute Gouty Arthritis</u>
    - The acute phase is self-limited (1-2 weeks)
    - Primary treatments for acute gout attacks have NSAIDs, corticosteroids (intraarticular), colchicine.

- Never initiate ULT during an acute flare
- Monotherapy for mild-moderate pain and/or 1 joint involved
- Combination therapy for severe pain/polyarticular/large joints
  - Colchicine + NSAID
  - Oral corticosteroids + colchicine
  - Intra-articular steroids + (colchicine or NSAIDs)
    - Steroids: 9cc Marcaine + 1cc of 80mg methylprednisolone for large joint with 20g needle

Acute Gout Treatment Options

Treatment	Indications	Dose	C/I	S/E
NSAID	First line	Indomethacin 50mg-75mg PO TID and continued 48h after attack to ↓relapse Naproxen 750mg initial then 250mg TID x7d[385] Ibuprofen 800mg TID Diclofenac 75mg PO BID	PUD CKD CHF	GIB AKI Edema Sodium retention
Colchicine	NSAID intolerance	1-1.2mg PO f/b 0.5-0.6mg 1 hour later (dose not to exceed 1.8mg/d) on day 1 (or 0.6mg TID on day 1), then continue with 0.6mg BID on subsequent days until 48h past resolution of flare (alternate is 0.6mg TID x4d)[385] 0.5-0.6 mg/d if GFR 30-60 mL/min 0.5–0.6 mg every 2 or 3 days if GFR 15-30 mL/min. C/I if GFR <10	CKD	Diarrhea Abdominal pain Neuromyopathy
Intraarticular Steroids	1-2 inflamed joints NSAID/colchicine contraindications or intolerance	Methylprednisolone 20-80mg (80mg for large joints) Triamcinolone 10mg with Lidocaine and Marcaine	Drug rxn Inject up to 3x/year	No major systemic s/e
Systemic Steroids	>2 joints involved NSAID/colchicine intolerance	Prednisone 0.5mg/kg daily for 5-10d without taper -or- 40mg/d until resolution of sx (typically 1-3d) then 14d taper Prednisolone 30-40mg/d x3-5d	Drug rxn	Rebound attacks ↑BP ↑Glucose Fluid retention

C/I = contraindications

- Chronic/Tophaceous Gout
  - Per ACR guidelnes

- ULT indicated for:
  - ≥Stage 2 CKD
  - ≥ 2 acute attacks per year
  - History of (uric acid) nephrolithiasis
  - Presence of tophi
    - Solid chaulky white masses of uric acid surrounded by inflammatory cells and fibrous tissue. Can be deforming; interfereing with function and bony erosions
    - Tophi in joints, cartilage, bone, and auricular or other cutaneous tissues form after about 10 years of uncontrolled gout.
- Check uric acid levels every 3-6 mo (until goal reached, then q6m); goal is to maintain UA at ≤6 for 6-12 months to truly ↓ risk for flares
  - If UA level is ≥11 then monitor RFP routinely as patient is high risk for nephrolithiasis
- Pharmacotherapy
  - Goal UA level is ≤6 if no tophi present or 5 in the presence of tophi
    - **Anti-inflammatory** prophylaxis <u>must be co-administered</u> when starting ULT. Give for at least 3 months <u>after</u> achieving goal UA (extend to 6 months if tophi present)
    - Options include NSAIDs or colchicine (prednisone last resort if cannot tolerate other options).
      - Colchicine 0.6mg PO BID (use 0.6mg PO daily if ↓GFR)
  - Do not **start** chronic therapy during acute attack

	Chronic Gout Treatment Options (Urate Lowering Therapy)			
	Treatment	Indications	Dose	Comments
Xanthine Oxidase Inhibitor (XOI)	Allopurinol	First line	100 mg/day x 2w then 200mg daily x 2w; titrate to goal decrease in UA by 1mg/dL/wk with typical doses of 300-800mg/d until target UA reached (≤6) If CKD Stage 4, start at 50mg/d then ↑to 100mg/d @ 2 weeks then 200mg/d @ 4 weeks and 300mg/d @ 6 weeks	May ↓ progression to CKD, patients with underlying renal disease should be considered for early Allopurinol administration (CKD Stage II). May be associated with DRESS, but uncommon
	Febuxostat	Alternative 1st line	40-80mg/d	Potential association with ↑ cardiovascular morbidity. Equally or more efficacious than Allopurnol. Does not require dose adjustment in mild to moderate CKD. FDA blackbox warning re: CV death and all-cause mortality
Uricosuric Agent	Probenecid	2nd line	500mg BID	C/I if GFR<50. Less effective than XOI but when combined with XOI may be more effective. Appropriate for pts w/ ↓ renal UA secretion. May help reverse tophaceous changes over time. Higher risk for nephrolithiasis. Must remain well hydrated

Uricase	Pegloticase	2nd line	8 mg IV infusion every 2 weeks; optimum duration has not been established	Patients cannot be on any PO urate-lowering therapy. Requires q2w infusion; decreases serum urate to nearly 0. Indicated for patietns with severe recurrent or tophaceous gout. 30-50% develop antibodies to the drug within a month → may become ineffective and ↑ liklihood of infusion reactions.

Figure. Treatment of chronic gout

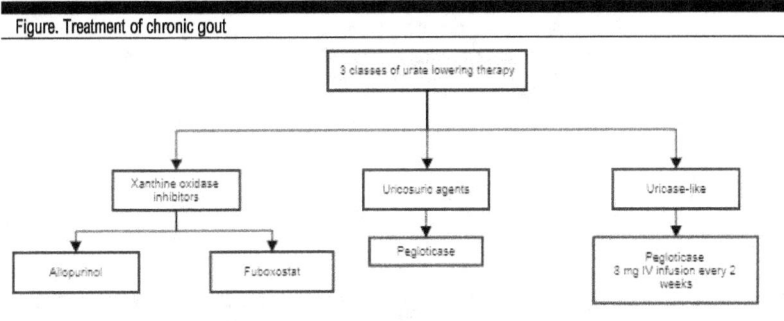

- **Referral**
    - If unable to bring serum uric acid levels to goal, ongoing clinical symptoms despite your best efforts, need for multiple medications to control gout, and the presence of joint deformities or tophaceous disease.

APPROACH TO JOINT PAIN

1. **Articular vs periarticular**
    - Articular
        - *Structures* - synovium, synovial fluid, articular cartilage, intraarticular ligaments, joint capsule.
        - *Symptoms* - deep or diffuse pain, pain or limited range of motion on active and passive movement, and swelling (caused by synovial proliferation, effusion, or bony enlargement), crepitation, instability, "locking," or deformity.
    - Periarticular
        - *Structures* - extraarticular ligaments, tendons, bursae, muscle, fascia, bone, nerve, and skin. Nonarticular disorders are painful on active, but not passive (or assisted), range of motion.
        - *Pain* - point or focal tenderness in regions adjacent to articular structures, are elicited with a specific movement or position, and have physical findings remote from the joint capsule. Rarely demonstrate swelling, crepitus, instability, or deformity of the joint itself.
2. **Inflammatory vs noninflammatory**
    - Inflammatory
        - *Differential* - infectious, crystal-induced (gout, pseudogout), immune-related (RA, SLE), reactive (RF, reactive arthritis), or idiopathic.
        - *Symptoms* - four cardinal signs of inflammation (erythema, warmth, pain, or swelling), systemic symptoms (fatigue, fever, rash, weight loss), or ↑ESR or C-RP, ↑PLT, ACD, or ↓albumin). Prolonged stiffness (>1hr)
    - Noninflammatory

- *Differential* - elated to trauma (rotator cuff tear), repetitive use (bursitis, tendinitis), degeneration (OA).
- *Symptoms* - intermittent stiffness that is shorter in duration (<1hr) and exacerbated by activity. Pain without synovial swelling or warmth, absence of inflammatory or systemic features, sx improve with activity/motion, and normal negative laboratory investigations.

Exam findings with joint pain presentation					
	Articular			Periarticular	
	OA	Inflamm	Arthralgia	Bursitis	Myofascial
Swelling	Varies	+	-	+	-
Erythema	-	Varies	-	+	-
Warmth	-	+	-	+	-
Tenderness	Joint line	+	Varies	Periarticular	+
ROM	Limited	Limited	Full	Full	Full
Pain w/ AROM/PROM	Both	Both	Both	AROM>PROM	Both
Acute onset	-	+	n/a	+	-

Pocket Medicine 6th Edition

MONOARTHRITIS

- **Etiology**[386]
    - Infection
        - Septic: RF include prosthesis, recent surgery, RA, overlying infection). Organisms include MRSA, GBS, Lyme disease, Gonorrhea (suspect if other joints previously affected) is the most common cause!
            - Consider in patients with prosthetic hip/knee, overlying skin infection, age>80, DM
        - Crystal (mc causes include monosodium urate, calcium pyrophosphate)
    - Trauma (fractures, ligament tears) → hemarthrosis
    - Osteonecrosis (chronic steroid use, alcoholism)
    - OA
    - Crystal Induced
        - Gout
        - Pseudogout
    - Reactive Arthritis
- **Presentation**
    - Isolated swollen joint(s)
    - Hot/warm to touch
- **Assessment**
    - Synovial Fluid Analysis
    - Clarity and color (clear = non inflammatory; yellow = inflammatory; red = traumatic vs hemarthrosis)
    - Viscosity = ↓ with inflammatory etiology
- **Labs**
    - Cell count
    - Differential
    - Suspect infection:
    - Gram stain
    - Culture
    - Crystal analysis
    - Cell Count

- **Assessment**

Synovial fluid analysis					
	Normal	Non-inflammatory	Inflammatory	Septic	Hemorrhagic
Class	N/a	1	II	III	IV
Appearance	Clear	Clear/yellow	Clear/opaque, yellow	Opaque	Red, Opaque
WBC	<200	<2000	2000-50,000 (may be up to 100,000)	>50,000 (or 100k)	N/A
PMN	<25%	<25%	≥50%	≥75%	
Cx	-	-	-	+	
Crystals	-	-	+ in gout		-
DDx	N/a	OA Trauma AVN Chondromalacia Hypothyroidism Amyloid	Gout (causes high range of WBC) RA SLE Stills Dermatomyositis Vasculitis	Septic Arth Gonococcal Mycobacterium	Trauma TB Neoplasia Coagulopathy Charcot arthro
X-ray	N/a	Osteophytes Joint spc narrow Subchondral scl	Periart osteop Erosions Asx joint spc narrow	Joint destruction edema	

POLYARTICULAR ARTHRITIS

- **Clinical/Evaluation**[387]
    - Determine chronicity (acute vs. chronic)
        - *Acute* – hours to two weeks
        - *Chronic* - >2 weeks
    - Duration, Triggers
        - Intermittent or Constant
    - Symmetric vs Asymmetric
    - Number of joints involved
        - *Pauciarticular* – 2 to 4 joints (i.e. spondyloarthropathies such as psoriatic, inflammatory, ankylosing, reactive)
        - *Polyarticular* – 5+ joints (i.e. RA)
    - Types of Joints Involved (see table below)
        - Spine, SI, hips, shoulder, knees – can be seen with OA, spondyloarthropathies
        - First digit – consider gout
        - Smaller joints (wrists, fingers, toes) – consider RA, SLE
    - Rule Out
        - Should rule out other causes of "joint" pain → depression, fibromyalgia, hypothyroidism, bursitis, metabolic factors (Ca), neuromuscular disease
- **Differential/Types**
    - Inflammatory – suggestive in patients with joint swelling, erythema, morning stiffness >1hr, symmetric, pain at rest, ↑C-RP, ↑ESR
        - Rheumatoid arthritis
        - Infectious arthritis (i.e. septic, Lyme)
        - Ankylosing spondylitis
        - Reactive arthritis
        - Psoriatic Arthritis
    - Non-Inflammatory – worse with weight bearing, asymmetric, morning stiffness for <1 hr., no pain rest, pain ↓ with activity, nml C-RP and ESR
        - Osteoarthritis (most often involves weight bearing joints such as the spine, hips, and knees along with distal finger joints such as the DIP)

- Crystal-Associated
  - Gout
  - Calcium pyrophosphate arthropathy
- Immune-Mediated
  - SLE
- **Labs**
  - ANA
  - ESR
  - C-RP
  - RF and anti-CCP
  - Uric acid
  - Hepatitis B, C, parvovirus
  - Synovial fluid aspiration (see page 575 for evaluation of aspirate)
  - Crystal analysis
- **Imaging**
  - Plain films – evaluate for erosive disease, calcium deposition, fractures, pencil-in-cup
- **Treatment/Management**
  - Treatment is based on ultimate diagnosis as above, this is beyond the scope of this book to list all individual treatment modalities

Joint involvement pattern and suggested diagnoses

Characteristic	Autoimmune / CTD			Spondyloarthropathies				Infectious		Crystal		Other
	RA	SLE	Vasculitis	AS	PA	RA	IBD	Bacterial	Viral	Gout	CPPD	OA
Symmetry												
>symmetric	x	x							x			
>asymmetric	x		x	x	x	x	x	x		x	x	x
Inflammatory	x	x										
Noninflammatory									x			x
Number												
>pauciarticular	x			x	x	x	x	x		x	x	x
>polyarticular	x	x	x				x		x			
Joints												
>Spine	x			x	x	x	x	x				x
>SI	x			x	x	x	x					x
Joints/Small												
>Wrist	x	x	x					x	x		x	x
>Carpo											x	x
>Metacarpoph	x	x	x		x				x			
>PIP	x	x			x				x			
>DIP	x			x	x	x			x			x
>Ankle	x				x	x	x		x	x		x
>Metatarsoph	x				x	x				x		x
Joints/Medium												
>Shoulders	x	x			x	x	x	x			x	
>Elbows	x	x			x	x	x	x				x
>Hips/Knees	x		x	x	x	x	x				x	x

COMMON RHEUMATOLOGIC LABS

- **Common Generic Rheumatologic Labs**
  - CBC, CMP, CK, UA
  - RF
  - ANA
  - Cryoglobulins
  - HBV (HBsAg with PAN)
  - HCV (Cryoglobulinemia, PAN)
  - CH50, C3, C4
  - HSV, HIV, CMV (r/o vasculitis)
  - Parvovirus IgM (GPA, PAN)
  - C-ANCA (PR3; GPA or MPA)
  - P-ANCA (MPO; MPA and CSS)
  - BCx (rules out SBE)
  - SPEP, UPEP (rule out MM)
- **Inflammatory Arthritis**
  - Rheumatoid Arthritis
    - ESR (normals: male = age/2; female = age+10/2)
    - C-RP (normals: male = age/50; female = age / 50 + 0.6)
    - RF (frequency of false positives ↑ with age; incidence of disease ↑ with ↑ titer)
    - CCP (can be diagnostic in RF negative dz, better predictor of erosive dz)
    - 1433 (presence is associated with worse dz)
- **ANA**
  - Seen in 5-30% of normal individuals

Significance of ANA Pattern			
Pattern	Nature of Antigens	Antibody	Associated Dz
Homogenous/diffuse	Histone (H1, H2a)	Histone dsDNA ssDNA	SLE, DIL, RA
Rim/Peripheral/Shaggy	Double or single stranded DNA	dsDNA	SLE
Speckled	Proteins A-G, snRNAs, U1-6	ENA-RNP & Smith SS-A, SS-B	SLE, MCTD, Sjogrens, RA, SSc, UCTD, EBV
Centromere	Kinetochore	Centromere	CREST Raynaud MCTD
Nucleolar	nRNA	Jo-1	Myositis Raynaud SSc SLE
Cytoplasmic	N/a	N/a	Dermatomyositis Polymyositis Inflamm. Myopathy SLE Sjogrens

Autoantibodies and Autoimmune diseases

Antibody	SLE	MCTD	Diff Sclerosis	Limited Sclerosis	Sjogren's	RA	Inflamm Myop
ANA	>95%	>95%	70-90%	60-90%	>70%	40-50%	100%
Anti-dsDNA	60%	Ø	Ø	Ø	Rare	Rare	Ø
Anti-Smith	30%	Ø	Ø	Ø	Ø	Ø	Ø
Anti-RNP	30%	>95%	Comm	Ø	Rare	Rare	10-20%
Anti-Centromere	Rare	Rare	10-15%	60-90%	Ø	Ø	Ø
Anti-Ro (SSA)	30%	Rare	Rare	Ø	70%	10-15%	Ø
Anti-La (SSB)	15%	Rare	Rare	Ø	60%	Rare	Ø
Anti-nucleolar	Occ	Ø	Comm	Ø	Occ	Rare	Ø
Anti-SCL-70	Rare	Ø	10-20%	Ø	Ø	Ø	Ø
Anti-Jo-1	Ø	Ø	Ø	Ø	Ø	Ø	20%
Anti-Histone	24-95%	Occ	Occ	Occ	Occ	20%	Ø
DDx	FUO, ILD, Pleuro-pericarditis, AKI, Neuropathy	Pulm HTN, ILD, pleuro-pericarditis	Diffuse: ILD, scleroderma renal crises	Limited: Pulm HTN	Neuropathy, AKI, Pleuro-pericarditis, ILD	Neuropathy, LD	FUO

- **Myopathies**
  - Commonly will have +ANA and +anti-cytoplasmic Ab (synthetase and anti-SRP)
- **Vasculitis**
  - Differential
    - *Large* – Takayasu, GCA
    - *Medium* – Kawasaki, PAN, Central Angiitis
    - *Small* –
      - Immune complex (Hypersensitivity, cryoglobulinemic, HSP)
      - Pauci Immune (GPA, microscopic polyangiitis, Churg-Strauss)
  - Labs
    - Systemic Inflammation
      - CBC
      - ESR
      - C-RP
      - ↓Albumin
    - Organ involvement
      - SCr, UA
      - LFT
      - CK
      - Occult blood
      - CXR
      - Brain MRI/MRA
      - Abdominal CTA

Bibliography

[382] Neogi T, Jansen TLTA, Dalbeth N, et al 2015 Gout classification criteria: an American College of Rheumatology/European League Against Rheumatism collaborative initiativeAnnals of the Rheumatic Diseases 2015;74:1789-1798.

[383] El-Zawawy et al. "Managing gout: How is it different in patients with chronic kidney disease?" CCJM. 77(12). 12/2010.

[384] Burns et al. " Latest evidence on gout management: what the clinician needs to know." Ther Adv Chronic Dis. 2012 Nov; 3(6): 271–286.

[385] Roddy E et al. Open-label randomised pragmatic trial (CONTACT) comparing naproxen and low-dose colchicine for the treatment of gout flares in primary care. Ann Rheum Dis 2020 Feb; 79:276.

[386] Siva et al. "Diagnosing acute monoarthritis in adults: a practical approach for the family physician." Am Fam Physician. 2003 Jul 1;68(1):83-90.

[387] Pujalte, George et al. Am Fam Physician. 2015.

PSYCHIATRY

Capacity	582
Delirium	582
Insomnia	587
Sedation of the Violent Patient	589
Depression	590
Alcoholic Patient	599
PTSD	601
Anxiety Disorder	602

CAPACITY

- **General**
  - Made by physician, not a lawyer or judge, often by neuropsychologist or forensic psychologist. You can consider getting specialists involved if, after performing the ACE below, you feel the patient is **incapable** of consenting to a procedure.[388]
  - (1) Capacity is imbedded in informed consent, one of a **triad** of factors that also includes: (2) disclosure and (3) voluntariness.
    - Capacity – consists of four criteria, to have capacity, patients must demonstrate the following:
      - Understand their situation and care options
      - Have appreciation of how information presented applies to their situation
      - Have reasoning consistent with their goals, preferences and values
      - Have ability to communicate a choice
      - Evaluation of capacity can be done with the ACE bedside test by answering yes or no to the following questions:

      Is the patient...
      1. Able to understand medical problem
      2. Able to understand proposed treatment
      3. Able to understand alternative to proposed treatment (if any)
      4. Able to understand option of refusing proposed treatment (including withholding or withdrawing treatment)
      5. Able to appreciate reasonably foreseeable consequences of accepting proposed treatment
      6. Able to appreciate reasonably foreseeable consequences of refusing proposed treatment (including withholding or withdrawing proposed treatment)
      7a. The person's decision is affected by depression
      7b. The person's decision is affected by delusions/psychosis
    - Disclosure - discussing the risks and benefits of available tests and treatments, including of declining care.
    - Voluntariness - the patient's decision isn't being forced or coerced by others.
  - All three—capacity, disclosure, voluntariness—must be present to meet ethical and legal muster
- **2 point test**
  1. Understands procedure action
  2. Understands consequences of decision—they say it out to you
     - Level of capacity increases the higher the risk of the procedure, i.e. demented patient doesn't need much capacity to agree to IV Fluids but does require higher level of capacity to agree to open heart surgery.

DELIRIUM

- **Definition**[389]
  - Disturbance of consciousness with ↓ ability to focus or maintain attention
  - No pre-existing or established dementia
  - Occurs over short period of time (hours/days) and fluctuates, sometimes lasting for months
  - Ultimately caused by a medical condition or substance intoxication
- **Types**
  - Hyperactive – restlessness, rapid mood changes, hallucinations, will not cooperate with medical care. RASS +1 to +4.
  - Hypoactive – inattention, reduced activity, drowsiness. RASS -1 to -4

- o Mixed – combination of above; patients may switch back and forth between the two
- **Risk Factors**
  - o Underlying dementia, hx of stroke, or Parkinson's disease
  - o Post-operative
  - o age >70, comorbidities, male, dementia, history of alcohol use, malnutrition, polypharmacy
  - o Admission risk factors
    - Infection, dehydration, severe pain, fracture, heart failure, abnormal blood pressure
- **Presentation**
  - o Disturbed Consciousness – inability to focus or maintain attention; "mother just isn't acting right."; patient may appear more lethargic, or if undergoing withdrawal will be hypervigilant
  - o Change in Cognition - ↓memory, disoriented (confirm A&O' s); perceptual disturbances (see objects or shadows in room); hallucinations
  - o Look for initial daytime fatigue, sleep disturbances which will then erupt into full on delirium
- **Causes**
  - o Highest causes are seen in the hospital (ICU, ER)
  - o Fluid and electrolyte disturbances (dehydration, hyponatremia/hypernatremia)
  - o Infections (silent UTI, respiratory tract, skin and soft-tissue, meningitis)
  - o Drug toxicity (Opioids, sedatives, anti-psychotics, NSAIDs; Withdrawal from EtOH or Benzodiazepines, use of Antihistamines)
  - o Metabolic disorders (hypoglycemia, hypercalcemia, uremia, liver failure, TSH)
  - o Low perfusion states (shock, heart failure)
  - o Immobility (restraints)
  - o Malnutrition
  - o Seizure (frontal or temporal region→causes behavioral changes such as sudden agitation, apathy, w/d)
  - o CVA (dominant hemisphere will cause confused state; alert but cannot name objects, repeat words, or follow commands); catatonic/hypoactive seen with basilar artery occlusion
  - o Organ failure (liver, renal)
  - o Pregnancy
    - Consider trauma, delirium, ICH, coagulopathy, ↓PLT, amniotic and venous thromboembolism, drug w/d. Consider eclampsia in those 20w-6w post-partum.
- **Stepwise evaluation[390]**
  - o Initial evaluation
    - History with special attention to medications (including over-the-counter and herbals)
    - Short onset of symptoms
    - Inability to focus when asking questions during initial examination
    - Tangential and disorganized speech
    - General physical examination and neurologic examination
    - Nonrhythmic, asynchronous muscle jerking (metabolic abnormality)
    - Flapping motion of outstretched hands (hepatic encephalopathy)
    - Nystagmus, ataxia (consider Wernicke's)
    - Complete blood count
    - Electrolyte panel including sodium, calcium, magnesium, phosphorus
    - Liver function tests, including albumin
    - Renal function tests

Common symptoms in delirium	
Feature	Assessment
Acute onset and fluctuating course	Usually obtained from a family member or nurse and shown by positive responses to the following questions: "Is there evidence of an acute change in mental status from the patient's baseline?". "Did the abnormal behavior fluctuate during the day, that is, tend to come and go, or increase and decrease in severity?"
Inattention	Shown by a positive response to the following: "Did the patient have difficulty focusing attention, for example, being easily distractible or having difficulty keeping track of what was being said?"
Disorganized thinking	Shown by a positive response to the following: "Was the patient's thinking disorganized or incoherent, such as rambling or irrelevant conversation, unclear or illogical flow of ideas, or unpredictable switching from subject to subject?"
Altered level of consciousness	Shown by any answer other than "alert" to the following: "Overall, how would you rate this patient's level of consciousness?" Normal = alert Hyper alert = vigilant Drowsy, arousable = lethargic Difficult to arouse = stupor Unarousable = coma

** The diagnosis of delirium requires the presence of features 1 AND 2 plus either 3 OR 4.

- First-tier further evaluation guided by initial evaluation
    - Systemic infection screen
        - Urinalysis and culture
        - Chest radiograph
        - Blood cultures
    - Electrocardiogram
    - Arterial blood gas
    - Serum and/or urine toxicology screen (perform earlier in young persons)
    - Brain imaging with MRI with diffusion and gadolinium (preferred) or CT
    - Suspected CNS infection: lumbar puncture after brain imaging
    - Suspected seizure-related etiology: electroencephalogram (G) (if high suspicion, should be performed immediately)
    - Tools
        - AWOL (**A:** Age is 80 years or older; **W:** Inability to spell "world" backwards; **O:** Not oriented to name, city, county, state, hospital, and floor; **L:** Nursing illness severity assessment moderately to severely ill
        - MOCA
        - CAM
- Second-tier further evaluation
    - Vitamin levels: B12, folate, thiamine
    - Endocrinologic laboratories: thyroid-stimulating hormone (TSH) and free t_4; cortisol
    - Serum ammonia
    - Sedimentation rate
    - Autoimmune serologies: antinuclear antibodies (ANA), complement levels; p-ANCA, c-ANCA
    - Infectious serologies: rapid plasmin reagin (RPR); fungal and viral serologies if high suspicion; HIV antibody
    - Lumbar puncture (if not already performed)

- Brain MRI with and without gadolinium (if not already performed)
- EEG (r/o Non-convulsive Status Epilepticus; look for nystagmus and anisocoria on exam; MRI may show frontal/parietal atrophy)
- **Diagnostics**
    - Labs
        - Electrolyte panel (ICU panel)
        - CBC
        - UA
        - Urine culture
        - LFTs (if history of cirrhosis)
        - TSH/FT4
        - Drug levels if appropriate (digoxin in AM assuming dose given in PM, lithium)
        - ABG (respiratory alkalosis is early sign of sepsis) helpful in hypoactive state
        - LP (older patients; suspecting bacterial meningitis)
    - Testing
        - EEG - indications in patient with AMS include suspected seizure (postictal state) or metabolic encephalopathy; AMS often associated with generalized slowing of normal 8- to 13-Hz α rhythm; they may have 6- to 7-Hz β activity or δ waves; triphasic waves with frontal predominance signature of hepatic or uremic encephalopathy; continuous spike-and-wave activity means NCSE; treatment often leads to rapid recovery
    - Imaging
        - CXR
        - CT head (if no cause is identified)
- **Treatment**
    - **Treat underlying cause**
        - **Current evidence does not support routine use of haloperidol or second-generation antipsychotics to treat delirium in adult inpatients.**
    - Behavior: sitters, family, reorientation, bed rails, minimize restraints

Medications for agitation based on demographic[391]		
Context	RX	Dosage
Severe violence	Droperidol	0.625-5mg IM/IV
	Midazolam	2.5-5mg IM/IV
	Haldol PLUS	2mg PO/IV
	Lorazepam	0.5mg IM/IV
	Generally, want to avoid benzodiazepines, but in conjunction with haloperidol can be useful. Haldol can be given 0.5-2.5mg IV prn (TID for example) then 1-2mg IV QHS short term with a quick taper.	
Undifferentiated	Lorazepam	2-4mg IM/IV
	Midazolam	2.5-5mg IM/IV
	Haldol PLUS	2mg IM/IV
	Lorazepam	2mg IM/IV
Known psych	Haldol	2-5mg IM/IV
	Droperidol	2.5-5mg IM/IV
	Haldol PLUS	5mg IM/IV
	Lorazepam	2mg IM/IV
Intoxication	Lorazepam	2-4mg IM/IV
	Midazolam	2.5-5mg IM/IV
Cooperative	Olanzapine	5-10mg IM/SL/or PO
	Ziprasidone	20mg IM
	Lorazepam	2-4mg IM/IV
	Risperidone	0.25mg PO

PSYCHIATRY

Elderly (all anti-psychotics are black-box)	Oxazepam	10mg BID-TID; ↑ to total 30-45mg/d
	Buspirone	5mg BID; ↑ by 5mg q2-3d up to 20-30/d
	Haldol AND Ativan	0.5mg to 2mg IM & 1 mg Q 8 hours prn; hold if BP<100/60
	Haldol	1mg po/IV Q30min prn
	Quetiapine	12.5mg PO (elderly dose) daily
		25-100mg PO (all other ages; divided BID)
		(Good for hyperactive; helps sedate)
	Olanzapine	2.5mg
Alternative	Divalproex sodium	500–1500 mg/d
	Carbamazepine	300–600 mg/d
	Olanzapine	2.5mg IM/PO
Sun downing (give at 1500)	Olanzapine	2.5mg – 5mg IM/PO (up to 10 mg po daily)
	Quetiapine	12.5mg po prn (elderly) up to BID
		25-100mg PO prn (other ages)
		if no response in 6h then give additional 12.5 mg p.o. May ↑ dose by 25 mg q2 days
	Risperidone	0.5mg po BID (max 2mg q12h)
		May be ↑ x 1 mg q 2 days. Max dose is 6 mg in 24 hours
Pregnancy[392]		**Recommended**: First generation antipsychotics safe (i.e. haloperidol, perphenazine) and have sedative and ↓BP effects
		Others
		Diphenhydramine 25-50mg PO, IV or IM q1-4h (max 300mg/d)
		-Onset: 15-30m PO, rapid if IM or IV
		-S/E: sedation, anticholinergic effects
		Haloperidol 2-10mg PO, IV or IM (max 20mg/d)
		-Onset: 15-30m PO, 20-30m if IM or IV
		-S/E: EPS, dystonia, sedation, NMS, anticholinergic
		Olanzapine 5-10mg PO or IM (max 30mg/d)
		-Onset: 15m-4h PO, 15-30m if IM
		-S/E: sedation, orthostatic, EPS
		Ziprasidone 20mg IM (max 40mg/d)
		-Onset: 15-30m
		-S/E: sedation, orthostatic, EPS, HA, nausea
		Lorazepam 0.5-2mg PO, IV, or IM
		-Onset: 15-30m PO, rapid if IM or IV
		-S/E: sedation, ↓RR

** *Risperdal or Haldol*: Caution if prolonged QT

1. Try having a 1:1 sitter in the room, move pt to room by nursing station, and/or decrease noise/light
2. Agitation in elderly may be first manifestation of an illness: new infection, MI, dyspnea/hypoxia, CVA, pain, etc.
3. Consider adding Cogentin to ↓ risk of EPS
4. Check vitals, Pulse Ox, Na/K, glucose, Fever, meds, sources of infection (UA, CXR)
5. Check ECG (esp. if post-operative patient)
6. Treatment
   - Agitation in context of non-acute psychosis
     - Risperidone (Risperdal) 0.25–1.5 mg/d
     - Olanzapine (Zyprexa, Zydis) 2.5–10mg/d
     - Quetiapine (Seroquel) 12.5–200 mg/d
     - Aripiprazole (Abilify) 2.5–12.5 mg/d
   - Acute in context of acute psychosis:

- Haloperidol (Haldol) 0.5–2 mg/d
  - Agitation in context of depression
    - SSRI, e.g., citalopram (Celexa) 10–30 mg/d
- **Delirium prophylaxis** [393]
  - General
    - When a consult is placed for altered mental status, it is important to determine the affected domain that has changed from the patient's normal state. Changes can include alterations in consciousness, attention, behavior, cognition, language, speech, and praxis and can reflect varying degrees of cerebral dysfunction.
  - Orientation: accurately assess baseline, provide orientation clues, perception aids (hearing aids, glasses), regulate sleep-wake cycle, active involvement of family/caregivers
  - Minimize iatrogenesis: stop inappropriate/unnecessary medications, minimize urinary catheters, minimize restraints
  - Housekeeping measures: oxygen delivery, hydration, monitor electrolytes/glucose
  - Prophylaxis: bowel regimen, nutrition, early mobilization, pain control
  - Red Flag: an isolated alteration in speech, language, behavior, or praxis should suggest an underlying neurologic or psychiatric substrate in the early evaluation for delirium

Compare and Contrast Delirium and Dementia	
Delirium	Dementia
Onset: over hours to days	Onset: over months to years
Disturbance of consciousness such as reduced Awareness, inability to sustain attention	Level of attention not initially compromised
Altered cognition: memory, language, Disorientation, perceptual disturbance	Multiple cognitive impairments: language, motor Activities, agnosia, executive function
Caused by medical condition	Not explained by any medical condition
Evaluation: check medications, infections, CBC, Electrolytes, creatinine, glucose, liver function panel, cardiac enzymes, UA, CXR, ECG, pulse oximetry and/or ABG. Consider head CT and LP.	Evaluation: obtain thorough history from the patient and family members, physical exam (with focus on neurologic testing), MMSE, functional status, CBC, TSH, vitamin B12, electrolytes, VDRL, HIV. Consider neuroimaging and LP if onset <60, abrupt onset or rapid decline, or history of cancer or anticoagulant use

For more information on dementia, see page 292

INSOMNIA

- **Define**: inadequate sleep despite opportunities (3 episodes/week **for 3 months**) to obtain full sleep causing daytime impairment and there is no other disorder that is likely the cause. Has been associated with the development of CVD, T2DM, HTN (↑SBP during sleep, non-dipper).[394]
- Types
  - Short Term: <3 months
  - Chronic: >3 months of symptoms, 3x/week
  - Primary: present the whole life of patient
  - Secondary: developed, p/w sleepiness
- Treatment
  - **Inpatient**
    - You are not obligated to give a sleep aid if you think the patient is at high risk of becoming confused or altered. If you decide they can have one:
      - **Elderly**
        - Trazodone (Desyrel) 25-50 mg (max 150mg)
        - Mirtazapine 7.5mg PO x1

- **Any Age**
  - Temazepam (Restoril) 15-30 mg
  - Zolpidem (Ambien) 5-10 mg
  - Diphenhydramine (Benadryl) 25-50 mg (not a first-line choice)
  - Lorazepam (Ativan) IV 0.5-1 mg can be given to patients who are NPO.
  - Be cautious in elderly patients > 65. Would choose trazodone 25-50 mg in the elderly or Ambien. Avoid benzodiazepines and Benadryl.
  - If someone is delirious and agitated do not give sleep aid.
- **Outpatient**
  - Acute (<3 months) vs. Chronic (>3 months)
    - Rule out comorbid conditions (2/2 insomnia) such as depression, PTSD, anxiety, etc.
    - Rule out other causes of insomnia:
      - OSA (30-70%, more common in F), most validated tool is ESS
      - RLS
      - PLMS
      - Stress (psychological insomnia)
    - CBT is first line
    - Medication should also be used in conjunction with CBT (sleep hygiene, sleep restriction, stimulus control, etc.)
      - Behavioral Treatment
      CBT has been shown to have sustained beneficial effects up to 6 months past treatment per AHRQ.
        - *Sleep Hygiene* – maintain regular sleep schedule, avoid naps, avoid caffeine after lunch, avoid alcohol/tobacco/large meals near bedtime, adjust bedroom environment to be quiet, dark and cool.
        - *Stimulus control* – use bed only for sleep and sexual activity, go to bed only when sleepy, leave bed when unable to sleep and go to another room
        - *Relaxation* – progressive muscle relaxation, relaxation response
        - *Sleep restriction* – restrict time in bed to hours when sleeping, increase time in bed by 15-30m increments when sleep efficiency is >90%
  - Types
    - *Sleep Onset (SO)*
      - Ramelteon 8mg (30 min prior to bed-time)
      - Zaleplon 10mg QHS
      - Zolpidem 5-10 mg PO QHS prn insomnia
        - If hepatic impairment or elderly give 5 mg
      - Triazolam 0.25mg QHS (0.125mg if geriatric)
      - Lorazepam (Ativan) IV 0.5-1 mg can be given to patients who are NPO
    - *Sleep Onset and Maintenance (SO/SM)*
      - Suvorexant 10mg (5mg if other meds on board)
      - Lunesta 1mg PO QHS
      - Zolpidem ER 6.25mg
      - Temazepam (Restoril) 15 (7.5mg if geriatric)
      - Estazolam (ProSom) 1mg (0.5mg if low body weight)
      - Flurazepam 30mg (15mg if geriatric)
      - Vistaril 25-50 mg po or IM q HS prn
    - *Middle-of-Night Awakenings*
      - Zolpidem SL 3.5mg male/1.75mg female
    - *Sleep Maintenance (SM):*
      - Doxepin 6mg (3 mg if geriatric)
      - Zolpidem SL 3.5 male/ 1.75 female

- Safe in Elderly
  - Trazodone 25-50 mg QHS prn insomnia
  - Nefazodone 100mg QHS
  - Chloral hydrate 500-1000 mg PO QHS PRN
  - Restoril 15 mg po QHS prn
- Safe for Long-Term Use[395]
  - Trazodone (not recommended by VA)
  - Zolpidem
  - Zaleplon
  - Eszopiclone
  - Ramelteon
  - Doxepin
  - Suvorexant
- Off-Label
  - Antidepressants: trazodone, mirtazapine
  - Antipsychotics: quetiapine, olanzapine
  - Antihistamines: diphenhydramine, doxylamine
  - Herbs: melatonin

The medication classes with the strongest benefits have been eszopiclone, zolpidem, and suvorexant in the general adult population for global and sleep outcomes. Doxepin was shown to have the strongest evidence of effectiveness for global and sleep outcomes in adults >55. Ramelteon and benzos did very poorly.

Types and Treatment			
SO			
Zolpidem IR	Initial: 5mg		Take immediately before bedtime. Do not use unless have 7–8 h time in bed
Zolpidem SL	Initial: 5mg		
Zolpidem PO spray	Initial: 5mg (1 spray)		
Triazolam	Initial: 0.125mg Max:		
SO/SM			
Lunesta	Initial: 1mg Maximum: 2mg		Take immediately before bedtime.
SM			
Suvorexant	Initial: 10mg Maximum: 20mg		Take 30 min before bedtime. Starting dose 10 mg in elderly and maximum is 20 mg. It is contraindicated in narcolepsy patients. Concentration levels in elderly are higher by 15% compared with nonelderly
Doxepin	Initial: 3mg Maximum: 6mg		Take 30 min before bedtime. Do not take within 3 h of a meal it is contraindicated in untreated narrow-angle glaucoma, severe urinary retention
Middle of Night Awakenings			
Zolpidem ZST	Initial: 1.75mg		Must have at least 5 hrs of sleep left before taking
Zaleplon	Initial: 5mg		Take immediately before bedtime A high fat/heavy meal can delay absorption

SEDATION OF THE VIOLENT PATIENT

- **General**
  - Always call the police / hospital security in any Insafe situation
  - Pharmacologic restraints should be considered last resort

PSYCHIATRY

Pharmacologic management of a violent patient		
Oral	IM	IV (not recommended)
Lorazepam 1-2mg PO	Lorazepam 2-4mg IM	Benzodiazepine
Lorazepam 1-2mg PO + Haldol 1.5-3mg PO (if psychiatric context)	Lorazepam 2-4mg IM + Haldol 5-10mg IM (if psychiatric context)	Haldol

DEPRESSION

- **Work-up**[396,397, 398, 399]
    - TSH
    - OSA
    - Vitamin D
    - Bipolar depression
    - Medications: steroids, dopaminergic agents
    - EtOH
    - B12/folate
    - Post concussive symptoms
- **Screening**
    - PHQ-9
        - Scores ≥ 10 have highest sensitivity/specificity for MDD (50%)[400]
        - Interpretation:
            - 1-4: none
            - 5-9: mild
            - 10-14: moderate
            - 15-19: moderately severe
            - 20+: severe
    - Hamilton Depression Rating Scale
- **Co-Existing Anxiety**
    - Harder to treat depression with co-existing anxiety (STAR*D trial)
        - See page 602.
- **Treatment (see table on following pages)**
    - Phasic approach advised
        - *Acute phase* **(first 3 months)**
            - CBT +/- Rx
            - Continue to ↑ dosage q3-4wk until sx in remission. Full medication effect is complete in 4 to 6 weeks. Augmentation with second medication may be necessary.
            - F/u with patient within 2-4wof starting medication and q2wk until improvement and then monthly to monitor medication changes.
        - *Continuation phase* **(4-9 months)**
            - Regular visits to monitor for signs of relapse, q3-6mo if stable; depression rating scales should be used for objective data.
            - Once remission achieved, dosage should be continued for at least 6-9m to reduce relapse; CBT is also effective in reducing relapse (visits typically q2wk).
            - If/when drug discontinuation is considered, medications should be tapered gradually (weeks to months).
        - *Maintenance phase* **(9 months-d/c)**
            - Same as continuation phase above
    - Pharmacotherapy
        - *Based on Side Effect Profile*
            - Fatigue, amotivation: SNRI, bupropion

- Anxiety: SSRI
- Insomnia: trazodone, mirtazapine
- Concerned about libido: Wellbutrin
- *Augmentation*
    - For quicker initial effects: *use benzodiazepine* (see page 602)
    - To combat side effects:
        - Sexual s/e or ↓ energy → add Wellbutrin or T3-liothyronine
        - Concurrent anxiety → add Buspar (*STAR-D)*, gabapentin, pregabalin,
        - Insomnia → Remeron (↑sedation, ↑appetite), or hydroxyzine (↑sedation)
- *Options*
    - Watchful waiting
    - Psychopharmacology (see table on following page)
        - SSRI - Get baseline sodium and PLT
        - SNRI
            - ↑risk for HTN
        - Mirtazapine good for patients with both depression and insomnia
    - Psychotherapy
    - Referral to Psychiatrist
- **Combining Antidepressants**
    - Combining two antidepressants is not supported by high-level evidence.
    - Rationale is that targeting different receptors will have a synergistic effect.
    - Combinations
        - SSRI+bupropion (↓SSRI dose)
        - SSRI+mirtazapine (best evidence)
    - See table below for options
- **Switching Between Anti-Depressants[401]**
    - Multiple techniques exist, there is no consensus best option
    - Gradual antidepressant withdrawal reduces the risk of complications. If the washout period is not long enough (defined by half-life of the drug), introducing a new antidepressant can cause drug interactions leading to toxicity, particularly serotonin syndrome.
    - Conservative switch:
        - The first antidepressant is gradually reduced and stopped
        - There follows a drug-free washout interval of five half-lives of the first antidepressant
        - The new antidepressant is started according to its dose recommendation
    - Moderate switch:
        - The first antidepressant is gradually reduced and stopped
        - There follows a drug-free washout interval of 2-4 days
        - The new antidepressant is started at a low dose
    - Cross-taper switch:
        - The first antidepressant is quickly reduced and stopped over 1-2 weeks
        - The second antidepressant is introduced at a low dose after the first medication has been completely weaned off and then the second medication is slowly increased to the therapeutic dose
- **Treatment Resistant Depression**
    - Defined as treatment failure on 2 antidepressants
    - Approximately 50% of patients experience no response to treatment with a first-line antidepressant.
    - Clinicians have 4 broad pharmacologic strategies to choose from for treating antidepressant non responders:
        - Increasing the dose of the antidepressant when the patient has more than a partial response but needs a little more effect

- Switching to a different antidepressant advised if patient has **no** response to treatment
- Augmenting the treatment regimen with a non-antidepressant agent in a patient with only a **partial** response:
  - Antipsychotic agents: aripiprazole 2-5mg/d with goal 10mg/d but max 20mg/d[402], olanzapine (in combination with fluoxetine specifically)[403], quetiapine, and risperidone
  - Another antidepressant: **duloxetine, venlafaxine**
  - Other agents: **mirtazapine**, mianserin, and omega-3 fatty acids
  - Not well studied: bupropion, desipramine, mecamylamine, and testosterone
  - Advanced option includes ketamine drip[404]
    - Research has shown it to be a rapidly effective within hours of administration
      - Doses varied; m/c was 0.5mg/kg IV/IM
      - Patients with quickest response had a positive family history of alcohol dependence
    - Should only be administered by psychiatry
- **Discontinuation**
  - Treatment discontinuation is as high as 40% in the first 3 months
  - Longer tapers required for those medications with short half life
    - No official guidelines on the best taper method, options include:
    - Decreasing dose by 25% per week until DC of the medication
    - Decreasing dose by 25% per month or 12.5% per week to complete a 4 month w/d period
- **Acute Withdrawal Management**[405]
  - Symptoms start within 3 days and may last up to 3 weeks
  - Discontinuation Syndrome (DCS) symptoms are more likely after at least 5-8 weeks of therapy or those with a short half-life (such as paroxetine)
  - Those with short half-life may require 6-12-month tapers
    - Symptoms include dizziness, nausea, vomiting, fatigue, muscle aches/twitches, chills, anxiety, sensory abnormalities, and irritability
    - Symptoms may last 1-2 weeks
- **Monitoring**
  - PHQ-9
  - Follow up every 3 weeks for the first 3 months (first follow up should be a week later)

Pharmacologic treatment options for depression

Drug or Drug Class	Dosing	Side Effects	Precautions	Clinical Use
Selective serotonin reuptake inhibitors		Platelet dysfunction, GI side effects, xerostomia, insomnia, anxiety, agitation, asthenia, drowsiness, headache, sexual dysfunction, hyponatremia, rare serotonin syndrome or NMS. S/e typically resolve within the first week.	Suicidality, particularly in young adults. Avoid abrupt discontinuation, other serotonergic drugs and MAOI therapy. Drug interactions due to CYP450 metabolism	An option for first-line therapy. Use side effects to choose a specific agent
Citalopram (Celexa) *(6-8w duration req'd)*	Initial: 10mg Therapeutic: 20-40mg Max: 60mg <55 YO: Maximum 40 mg/d >55 YO: Maximum 20 mg/d	Dose-dependent QT prolongation Avoid in those with excessive sleep and apathy	Avoid if patient has active heart disease. Avoid with drugs that prolong QT interval. Maximum dose 20 mg qd with hepatic disease, age >60 years, poor metabolizers of CYP2C19 or receiving a CYP2C19 inhibitor. Caution with CrCl <20	Low rate of anxiety and activation (however co-existing anxiety does ↓ effectiveness of treatment as in STAR*D trial). ECG monitoring for doses > 40mg/d. Good for those with agitation and depression and those with GI sensitivity High doses (40mg; or 20mg if >60 YO) may cause conduction disturbances such as prolonged QT interval, Torsades.
Escitalopram (Lexapro) *(12-24w duration req'd)*	Initial: 10 mg qd. Therapeutic: 10-20mg Max: 20 mg qd if no response to 10mg after 6 weeks but limited evidence to support 20mg>10mg	CNS depression, Avoid in those with excessive sleep and apathy	Avoid if patient has active heart disease. Maximum dose 10 mg qd with hepatic disease, elderly. Caution with CrCl < 20	Low risk for drug interactions. **Low rate of anxiety and activation.** Better response than citalopram (iSPOT-D trial)

Pharmacologic treatment options for depression

Drug or Drug Class	Dosing	Side Effects	Precautions	Clinical Use
Fluoxetine (Prozac) *(4-49w duration req'd)*	Initial: 10mg x1week Therapeutic: 20-60mg Max: 80-100mg Weekly: 90 mg once weekly Consider dosing in AM or afternoon if patients complain of excessive arousal with PM dosing	Patient on several medications and/or frequent medication changes anticipated.	May need to decrease dose with hepatic disease. Significant inhibitor of CYP isoenzymes	Good for those with agitation and depression and those with GI sensitivity Long half-life. **Highest rate of anxiety and agitation.** Good for teenagers; low rate of discontinuation syndrome. Good for patients with excessive fatigue. Had better tolerability than SNRIs
Paroxetine (Paxil, Paxil CR) *(4-52w duration req'd)*	**Paxil** Initial: Start at 10mg x1week Therapeutic: 20-40mg Max: 60-80mg **Controlled-release** Initial: 12.5 mg qd in AM. Therapeutic: 5-62.5 mg qd (consider max 50mg in elderly/frail) Consider PM dosing if sedation reported with AM dosing	Tends to cause less agitation/insomnia (common with SSRIs); possesses some anticholinergic effects. Somnolence and nausea is dose-related. Short half-life, withdrawal effects common. Less nausea with CR formulation Avoid higher doses as they may cause anticholinergic effects (e.g. delirium).	Avoid with pregnancy. Decrease starting dose and maximum dose with hepatic disease, elderly, CrCl <60. Potent inhibitor of CYP2D6. May decrease efficacy of tamoxifen Half-life increased by 170% in elderly	More anticholinergic side effects than other agents; high rate of drowsiness; **highest association with weight gain of SSRIs** Less likely to produce initial anxiety and/or insomnia. **Highest sexual d/f s/e** **Highest rates of discontinuation syndrome**
Sertraline (Zoloft) *(8-49w duration req'd)*	Initial: 25mg Therapeutic: 50-200mg (50-150 is normally the target) Max: 200-300mg	Tends to initially **increase alertness.** patients with psychomotor retardation may benefit. Patients experience more GI distress (diarrhea) compared to other SSRIs.	May need to decrease dose with hepatic disease. Mild inhibitor of CYPs 2D6 and 3A4	Lowest incidence of weight gain among SSRIs Low risk for drug interactions. Initial activation and increased alertness desired
Serotonin-norepinephrine reuptake inhibitors		Platelet dysfunction, nausea, constipation, anorexia, weight loss,	Suicidality, particularly in young adults. Avoid abrupt	

Pharmacologic treatment options for depression

Drug or Drug Class	Dosing	Side Effects	Precautions	Clinical Use
Venlafaxine (Effexor, Effexor XR) *(8-16w duration req'd)*	Immediate-release: 37.5 mg. Goal: 75mg-375mg Max: 450mg Extended-release: 37.5mg to start; goal 75-225mg	xerostomia, insomnia, anxiety, asthenia, dizziness, drowsiness, headache, hypertension, tachycardia, hyperhidrosis, sexual dysfunction, hyponatremia, serotonin syndrome, rare NMS Similar to those common to all SSRIs with more nausea. **BP increases**, including sustained hypertension are dose dependent, with a linear dose response. Primarily functions as an SSRI at doses below 225 mg. Should not be combined with other SSRIs. High rates of withdrawal. Side effect profile similar to immediate release.	discontinuation. Avoid other serotonergic drugs and MAOI therapy Decrease initial dose by 50% with moderate hepatic disease. Decrease dose by 25%-50% if CrCl <70. Caution with CYP2D6 inhibitors Avoid in those with unstable BP as high doses (>225mg) can cause diastolic HTN	**High rate of nausea and vomiting.** May increase HR and BP, high rates of discontinuation syndrome Consider in those who fail an SSRI or with menopausal symptoms or comorbid anxiety. At higher doses (225mg) can help with chronic pain
Desvenlafaxine (Pristiq)	Initial: 50 mg qd Therapeutic: 50-100mg Max: 100mg higher doses do not increase efficacy and are associated with higher discontinuation rates and adverse effects. In patients with ESRD or severe renal impairment, use 50 mg every other day.	Major metabolite of venlafaxine with similar side effect profile. Side effects are similar to those to all SSRIs with more nausea. Can increase blood pressure as well as triglycerides and LDL cholesterol.	Maximum dose 100 mg qd with hepatic disease. If CrCl <50, maximum dose 50 mg qd. If CrCl <30, maximum dose 50 mg QOD	May increase BP; high rates of discontinuation syndrome
Duloxetine (Cymbalta)	Initial: 20 mg BID, may increase to 30 mg BID (or 60 mg QHS). If nausea is	Urinary retention, hepatotoxicity, musculoskeletal pain, muscle spasms	Avoid with hepatic disease, severe CKD, closed-angle glaucoma.	May increase BP Avoid in those with preexisting liver

Pharmacologic treatment options for depression

Drug or Drug Class	Dosing	Side Effects	Precautions	Clinical Use
	problematic, start with 20 or 30 mg once daily. Usual dose for pain is 60 mg/day. Doses of 120 mg/day appear safe but efficacy data fail to justify this dose. Max: 120mg	nausea (dose-dependent) and constipation most troublesome, but, unlike venlafaxine, does not appear to produce sustained hypertension. NOT TO BE PRESCRIBED if concurrent heavy alcohol use and/or evidence of chronic liver disease.	Substrate and moderate inhibitor of CYP2D6. Caution with diabetics	disease and/or heavy alcohol use; preexisting or treatment related anorexia, constipation, and/or other GI symptoms.
Tricyclic antidepressants	Due to sedation, bedtime dosing may be preferred	Drowsiness and other CNS side effects, anticholinergic side effects (such as constipation, xerostomia, urinary retention, visual impairment), orthostatic hypotension, ECG abnormalities, tremor, nausea, weight gain, sexual dysfunction	Suicidality, particularly in young adults. Avoid abrupt discontinuation, MAOI therapy. Decrease dose with hepatic disease, elderly. Caution with decreased GI motility, cardiac disease, closed-angle glaucoma, BPH, urinary retention, seizure disorder, thyroid disease, diabetes, sunlight	
Amitriptyline	25-50 mg qHS, up to 100-300 mg total daily dose, qHS or in divided doses			Most anticholinergic effects: -Constipation: ↑hydration, laxative -Delirium: assess other causes -Dry mouth: sugarless gum -Hesitancy: bethanechol -Visual chg: pilocarpine gtt -Orthostasis: fludrocortisone
Other				
Bupropion (Wellbutrin) *(12-14w duration req'd)*	Immediate-release: 200-450 mg/BID-TID Sustained-release (SRI): 150-400 mg/qd-bid. Extended-release (XL): 150-300 mg/d; maximum 450 mg	Dose-dependent seizures. Insomnia, dizziness, tremor, agitation, anxiety, confusion, weight loss, hyperhidrosis	Avoid with seizure disorder, eating disorder. Decrease dose with severe hepatic disease, moderate-severe CKD. Caution with mild-moderate hepatic disease. Inhibitor of CYP2D6 and substrate of CYP2B6	Commonly augmented with SSRI to ↓ fatigue, sexual s/e from SSRI (300mg dose req'd) Lowest rates of sexual side effects and weight gain

Pharmacologic treatment options for depression

Drug or Drug Class	Dosing	Side Effects	Precautions	Clinical Use
	qd. Aplenzin: 174-348 mg qd. Maximum 522 mg qd. Forfivo XL: Not for initial use. 450 mg qd			**Avoid high doses as it may precipitate seizures** Dry mouth: sugarless gum
Mirtazapine (Remeron)	Initial: 7.5mg qHS. Therapeutic: 15-30 mg/d Maximum dose: 60mg/d	Drowsiness, dizziness, nausea, vomiting, increased appetite, weight gain, constipation, xerostomia, rare agranulocytosis or severe neutropenia	Decrease dose with elderly, CrCl <40. Caution with seizure disorder, inhibitors of CYPs 2D6, 1A2, or 3A4	Can be augmented with SSRI to help ↓ sexual s/e and to help combat insomnia (↑sedation) and helps ↑ appetite. **Be aware of serotonin syndrome risk** More drowsiness; can **stimulate appetite** and cause weight gain (↑cholesterol reqd statin tx), quickest onset of action! Good in geriatric population for depression, weight loss, and insomnia symptoms
Trazodone (Oleptro)	Immediate-release: 150 mg total daily dose, given in divided doses. Maximum 400 mg total daily dose. Extended-release: 150 mg qHS, on an empty stomach. Maximum 375 mg qd	Drowsiness, dizziness, hypotension, anxiety, insomnia, xerostomia, constipation, nausea, blurred vision, priapism	Decrease dose with elderly, hepatic disease, potent CYP3A4 inhibitors. Caution with cardiac disease, CKD	Can be augmented with SNRI to ↑sedation but high risk for priapism Priapism Drowsiness

Side Effect Profile for SSRI and non-SSRI Medications

	Sexual dysfunct.	↑Weight	GI Toxicity	QTC prolonged	Insomnia	Sedation	Orthostasis	Anxiety	HA
SSRI									
Citalopram	⊕⊕	⊕	⊕	⊕	⊕	⊘		⊘	⊘
Escitalopram	⊕⊕	⊕	⊕	⊕⊘	⊕ ⊕	⊘		⊘	⊘
Fluoxetine	⊕⊕	⊕	⊕	⊕	⊕⊕	⊘		⊕	⊘
Fluvoxamine	⊕⊕	⊕	⊕	⊕	⊕	⊕⊕			
Paroxetine	⊕⊕⊕	⊕⊕	⊕	⊕	⊕	⊕⊕		⊕	⊕⊕
Sertraline	⊕⊕	⊕	⊕⊕	⊕	⊕⊕	⊕⊕		⊕⊕	⊕⊕
SNRI									
Desvenlafaxine	⊕⊕⊕	⊕⊘	⊕⊕	⊕⊘	⊕⊕	⊕	⊕⊘		
Duloxetine	⊕⊕⊕	⊕⊘	⊕⊕	⊕⊘	⊕⊕	⊕	⊕⊕⊘	⊘	⊘
Venlafaxine	⊕⊕⊕	⊕⊘	⊕⊕⊕	⊕⊘	⊕⊕	⊕	⊕⊕⊘	⊕	⊕
Other									
Wellbutrin	⊕⊘	⊕⊘	⊕	⊕	⊕⊕	⊘	⊕⊕	⊘⊘	⊘⊘
Mirtazapine	⊕	⊕⊕⊕	⊕⊘	⊕⊕	⊕⊘	⊕⊕⊕	⊕⊕⊘	⊘⊘	⊘⊘
Trazodone		⊕	⊕⊕⊕	⊕⊕	⊘⊘	⊕⊕⊕	⊕⊕⊕⊕		
Milnacipran	⊕⊘	⊕⊘	⊕⊕	⊕⊘	⊕⊘	⊕	⊕⊕⊘		
TCAs									
Amitriptyline			⊕	⊕⊕⊕	⊘	⊕⊕⊕		–	⊘⊘
Clomipramine			⊕⊕	⊕⊕⊕	⊕	⊕⊕		⊕	⊘
Nortriptyline			⊕	⊕⊕	⊕	⊕		⊕	⊘

PSYCHIATRY

Neuroleptic Malignant Syndrome Vs. Serotonin Syndrome		
	NMS[406]	SS[407]
Mental State	Confusion → Coma	Confusion → Coma
Vitals	Fever (>104), ↑HR, ↑BP	↑BP
Muscles	Rigid**	Unaffected
Neuro	Autonomic instability w/sweating, tremor	Sweating, Tremor, more GI symptoms of n/v/d**; ↑reflexes**
Labs	↑WBC	Nml WBC**
CPK	↑↑↑	Nml

ALCOHOLIC PATIENT

- **Banana Bag**[408]
  - Not all patients need a banana bag; especially be weary of providing this in a patient with alcoholic cardiomyopathy
  - Thiamine 100 mg IV + Folate 1 mg+ MVT 1 mg in 1 L NS. Continue this for 3-4 days.
    - Important to give Thiamine before giving any other IV Fluids with *glucose*
- **Labs**
  - Monitor PO4, Mg, and K for low levels
  - At risk for refeeding syndrome[409]
- **Delirium Tremens**[410]
  - Risk Factors: hx of DT, age>30, prolonged EtOH history, ↑ amount of days since last drink
  - Sx: hallucinations, disorientation, tachycardia, hypertension, low-grade fever, agitation, and diaphoresis

Progression of DT		
Phase	Last drink	Duration
Early *Tremulous* *Anxiety* *Palpitations* *Nausea* *Anorexia*	6-8 hours	1-2d
W/D seizure *Tonic/clonic*	6-48 hours	2-3d
Hallucinations *Visual* *Tactile* *Auditory*	12-48 hours	1-2d
DT ↑HR HTN ↑Temp Delirium Agitation	48-96 hours	1-5d

  - Labs to follow: Mg, K, PO4
  - Nursing: CIWA, seizure precautions

PSYCHIATRY

Medications for Alcohol Dependence		
Medication	Dose/Route/Frequency	Effect
Benzodiazepines		
Chlordiazepoxide	25-100mg PO/IV/IM q4-6h	↓severity of w/d, stabilized v/s, prevents seizures
Diazepam	5-10mg PO/IV/IM q6-8h	
Oxazepam	15-30mg PO q6-8h	
Lorazepam	1-4mg PO/IV/IM q4-8h	
B-blockers		
Atenolol	25-50mg PO daily	↓HR, ↓BP
Propranolol	10-40mg PO q6-8h	
Alpha-agonists		
Clonidine	0.1-0.2mg PO q6h	↓BP, fatigue
Prevention of Relapse		
Disulfiram	125-500mg PO daily	
Naltrexone	50mg PO daily	
Acamprosate	666mg PO TID	
Anti-psychotics		
Haldol	3-5mg q1h prn (double q30min for max 100-480mg)	Tx for severe agitation, hallucinations, delirium

- **Treatment**
  o Hydration: Plasmalyte or LR basal rate
  o Supplementation: **Thiamine** (50-100mg IV x 3d then 100mg PO), folate, MVI, replete electrolytes (K, Mg, PO4), fluids
    - Chronic thiamine deficiency can cause Wernicke's Encephalopathy and eventually Korsakoff if not replaced prior to giving any glucose.
      1. Other than EtOH, other causes of WE include chronic nausea/vomiting, malnutrition, bariatric surgery patients
  o Medications
    - Calculate Ativan requirement by this conversion (1mg Ativan for every 1 shot/beer day) is total requirement over 24-hour period
    - While trials have showed benefit in symptom triggered vs standing doses, patients with CIWA>15 +/- hx of complicated withdrawal may benefit from standing doses
      1. Ativan 2-4mg IV q1h or q2h with CIWA for breakthrough; shorter half-life; slower onset and preferred in COPD patients
      2. Diazepam 5-10 mg slow IV push q3-4h until calm, awake state (preferred choice esp. for rapid titration)
      OR
      3. Chlordiazepoxide (Librium) 25-100mg IV q3h (avoid in patients with marked liver disease) or 50-100mg PO. Longer duration of action can ↓ rate of breakthrough symptoms.
      4. Haldol 3-5mg q1h prn severe agitation/hallucinations/delirium (double q30min for max 100-480mg)
    - Drips:
      1. Versed
      2. Propofol
      3. Dexmedetomidine (rates <0.7mcg/kg/h) which can help decrease benzo doses[411]
      4. Avoid Ativan given risk for polyethylene glycol accumulation
    - Tapering
      1. After stability for 24 hours; convert to PO dosing and taper dose by 25% every day over 3-day period
- **Placement:**

- o Admit to telemetry
- o ICU referral:
  - Age >40 with medical comorbidities
  - Electrolyte deficiencies with ECG changes
  - Hemodynamic instability
  - Hyperthermia
  - Rhabdomyolysis
  - Need for IV benzodiazepines or drips

PTSD

- **Diagnosis**[412] - consists of re-experiencing trauma with distressing recollections, dreams, flashbacks, and/or psychological/physical distress; persistent avoidance of stimuli that might invite traumatic memories or experiences; and increased arousal.
- **Screening**
  - o Obtain trauma history
  - o DREAMS
    - Detached - With each event, the examiner should determine if the patient appears emotionally detached (called alexithymia), either from the event or in relationships with others. It may also manifest as a general numbing of emotional responsiveness.
    - Reexperiences - The patient reexperiences the event in the form of nightmares, recollections or flashbacks.
    - Event - The event involved substantial emotional distress, with threatened death or loss of physical integrity, and feelings of helplessness or disabling fear.
    - Avoids - The patient avoids places, activities or people that remind the patient of the event.
    - Month - The symptoms have been present longer than one month
- **Treatment**
  - o Nonpharmacologic therapy should always be initiated, many patients treated with psychotherapy will improve or recover.
  - o If pharmacologic therapy required, SSRI are considered first line therapy
    - Options include fluoxetine, paroxetine, sertraline, escitalopram, and fluoxetine
      - ▫ Help with ↓reexperiencing, avoidance/numbness, and hyperarousal
      - ▫ Consider combining with trazodone 50-200mg to counteract the insomnia s/e of SSRI
  - o Anti-adrenergic Agents
    - Help with nightmares, autonomic hyperactivity, hypervigilance, and startle reactions
    - Monitor BP
    - Prazosin 1mg/qHS x3d then ↑ 1mg/q3d until nightmares improve (max ~ 10mg)
    - Clonidine 0.2mg TID titrated from 0.1mg qHS
    - Propranolol and guanfacine also options
  - o Second generation anti-psychotics may be needed to treat comorbid psychotic-like features or anxiety refractory to other agents. Options include:
    - Clozapine (least often used, ↑weight), risperidone, olanzapine (↑weight, ↑DM risk), quetiapine, ziprasidone (weight neutral), and aripiprazole (weight neutral)
    - Patients started on 2nd generations should be monitored for the following (interval in parentheses)
      - ▫ BP (q12w, q1y)
      - ▫ BG (q12w, q1y)
      - ▫ Lipids (q12w, q1y)

- Weight Check (q4,8,12,18,24w)

ANXIETY DISORDER

- **Types**
  - Generalized anxiety disorder (GAD)
  - Panic disorder
  - Social anxiety disorder (SAD)

As Needed Treatment for Anxiety[413]			
Rx	Dosage	Peak Onset	Pearls
Short Acting			
Atarax	50-100mg QID	Fast	Good for elderly
Midazolam	0.5-1mg	0.5-1h	IV only
Intermediate Acting			
Alprazolam (Xanax)	0.25-0.5mg PO TID (therapeutic at 2-9mg)	0.7-1.6h	C/I Liver Dz
Clonazepam	0.25-1 mg po QHS (↑to 0.5mg prn after 3 days)	1-4h	
Lorazepam	1-1.5 mg PO/IV Q 4-6 h	1-1.5h	
Oxazepam	10-15mg	3h	Elderly Liver dz
Trazodone	50-100mg		3rd line agent
Temazepam	30mg	0.75-1.5h	½ life: 10-20h
Long Acting			
Librium	5-10mg TID	2-4h	½ life: 5-30h
Diazepam	2-10mg	0.25-2.5h	½ life: 20-50h
Flurazepam	30mg	0.5-2h	½ life: unknown

- **Augmentation with SSRI**
  - Best to use longer acting benzodiazepines.
  - Patients will likely experience rebound anxiety, insomnia, restlessness, tremor, sweating, agitation if taper is not done appropriately. These are more commonly seen if they were on the medication for >8 weeks.
    - Ensure patients are not concurrently using EtOH or stimulants
    - If withdrawal symptoms are noted, stay on current dose (or ↑ dose for 1-2 weeks longer) then continue taper at slower rate
  - The slower the taper, the better the adaptation to change will be tolerated
  - Avoid using for longer than 1-month, physiologic dependence can develop in 2 months.
  - Example Regimen
    - Fluoxetine 20mg + Clonazepam 0.5mg qHS (↑ to 1mg, split as 0.5 BID, after day 3) for 3 weeks then taper over 7 days
- **Pre-Procedure Anxiety**
  - Overview[414]
    Patients may experience anxiety in anticipation of or during procedures. In mild acute procedure anxiety, providing information on outcomes and realistic evaluations of the risks is often enough to decrease anxiety. Moderate to severe anxiety may require medications or psychotherapy to reduce distress and allow completion of the procedure.
  - Pharmacologic Treatment
    Give 30 to 90 minutes prior to surgery/procedure, benzodiazepines are preferred due to rapid onset and duration. Midazolam is IV preferred therapy, whereas diazepam is the PO preferred option. Some patients experience nonspecific symptoms for up to 24

hours after the administration of sedative meds. Advise the patient on this risk. Patients 60 should have a 50% reduction in the doses below.

Medications for pre-procedural anxiety management			
	PO	IV	Description
Midazolam		0.07 mg/kg 0.5-2mg IV	Best if IV will be established; rapid onset and short duration of action with amnestic properties
Diazepam	2-10mg	0.03-0.1 mg/kg	Onset: 15 min IV: 2-5 min Has rapid onset, short duration 15min prior to procedure; ↓by 50% if age>60 or on opioids
Lorazepam	1-2mg	0.02-0.04 mg/kg (1-4 mg per dose) PO: 2mg IV: 2-4mg	PO Onset: 15-30 min IV Onset: <10-15 min Favored if want to take well before procedure (>2 hrs. prior) and has intermediate onset and duration of action DOC if liver failure ** repeat with PO dose after 30 min if no effect
Alprazolam	0.05mg	N/A	Onset: 15-30 min

- **Benzodiazepine Taper**[415]
  o Commonly used if concurrently treating with SSRI for prolonged period
  o Often not required if benzo used for <1 month
  o Recommended taper durations

Example long taper of BZD		
Duration of use	Taper Length Recommendation	Comment
<6-8 weeks	May not be required	Depends on patient and their preference; may consider short taper if high dose was required or if you prescribed benzo with a short/intermediate half-life such as alprazolam or triazolam
8 weeks – 6 mo	Slow over 2-3 weeks	
6 mo – 1 year	Slow over 4-8 weeks	Go slow during latter half of taper
>1 year	Slow over 2-4 months	

  o Taper Regimens
    - **Slow (6 months)**

Alternate example of long taper	
Week	Dosage (mg/d)
1	Starting dose (i.e. diazepam 15mg/d)
2	↓ to 11mg
3	↓ to 8.5mg
4	↓ to 6mg
5	↓ to 4.75mg
6	↓ to 3.5mg
7	↓ to 2.5mg

8	↓ to 2mg
9	↓ to 1.5mg
10	↓ to 1mg
11	↓ to 0.75mg
12	↓ to 0.5mg
13	↓ to 0.25mg
14	Stop

- For patients who have been on the medication for >1 year, consider even slower taper by 10% a week
- **Fast (2-6 weeks)** [416]
    - *Example* #1 – decrease dose in half (1mg→0.5mg) for 7 days then QOD for 5 days then stop.
    - *Example #2* - calculate the total daily dose. Switch from short acting agent (alprazolam, lorazepam) to longer acting agent (diazepam, clonazepam) if necessary.
        - To start, decrease dose by 25% for first 2 weeks; continue decreasing by 25% q2w until lowest dose is reached
    - *Example #3* - decrease daily dose by 25% on weeks 1 and 2 then decrease by 10% a week until stopped.

Bibliography

[388] Journal of General Internal Medicine 1999;14:27.

[389] Der-Nigoghossian C et al: Status epilepticus — time is brain and treatment considerations. Curr Opin Crit Care 2019 Dec;25(6):638-646; Erkkinen MG, Berkowitz AL: A clinical approach to diagnosing encephalopathy. Am J Med 2019 Oct;132(10):1142-1147; Kimchi EY et al: Clinical EEG slowing correlates with delirium severity and predicts poor clinical outcomes. Neurology 2019 Sep 24;93(13):e1260-e1271; Moss MJ et al: Serotonin toxicity: associated agents and clinical characteristics. J Clin Psychopharmacol 2019 Nov/Dec;39(6):628-633; Sinha S et al: Wernicke encephalopathy-clinical pearls. Mayo Clin Proc 2019 Jun;94(6):1065-1072; Uzelac A: Imaging of altered mental status. Radiol Clin North Am 2020 Jan;58(1):187-197; Wilber ST, Ondrejka JE: Altered mental status and delirium. Emerg Med Clin North Am 2016 Aug;34(3):649-65; Zipser CM et al: Predisposing and precipitating factors for delirium in neurology: a prospective cohort study of 1487 patients. J Neurol 2019 Dec;266(12):3065-3075.

[390] Josephson SA, Miller BL. Chapter 25. Confusion and Delirium. In: Longo DL, Fauci AS, Kasper DL, Hauser SL, Jameson JL, Loscalzo J, eds. *Harrison's Principles of Internal Medicine*. 18th ed. New York: McGraw-Hill; 2012.

[391] Reuben DB, Herr KA, Pacala JT, Pollock BG, Potter JF, Semla TP. Dementia. In: Geriatrics At Your Fingertips: 2009.11th ed. New York: The American Geriatrics Society; 2009:54-59.

[392] Niforatos et al. CCJM. 2019:243-247.

[393] Imm et al. "Postoperative delirium in a 64-year-old woman." Cleveland Clinic Journal of Medicine. 2017 September;84(9):690-698.

[394] Abad, V. C., & Guilleminault, C. (2018). Insomnia in Elderly Patients: Recommendations for Pharmacological Management. Drugs & Aging. doi:10.1007/s40266-018-0569-8

[395] Riemann, D.; Spiegelhalder, K.; Espie, C.; Pollmächer, T.; Léger, D.; Bassetti, C.; van Someren, E. Chronic insomnia: Clinical and research challenges—An agenda. Pharmacopsychiatry 2011, 44, 1–14. Buysse, D.J. Insomnia. JAMA 2013, 309, 706–716. Krystal, A.D.; Durrence, H.H.; Scharf, M.; Jochelson, P.; Rogowski, R.; Ludington, E.; Roth, T. Efficacy and safety of doxepin 1 mg and 3 mg in a 12-week sleep laboratory and outpatient trial of elderly subjects with chronic primary insomnia. Sleep 2010, 33, 1553–1561. Michelson, D.; Snyder, E.; Paradis, E.; Chengan-Liu, M.; Snavely, D.B.; Hutzelmann, J.; Walsh, J.K.; Krystal, J.D.; Benca, R.M.; Cohn, M.; et al. Safety and efficacy of suvorexant during 1-year treatment of insomnia with subsequent abrupt treatment discontinuation: A phase 3 randomised, double-blind, placebo-controlled trial. Lancet Neurol. 2014, 13, 461–471. Mayer, G.; Wang-Weigand, S.; Roth-Schechter, B.; Lehmann, F.; Staner, C.; Partinen, M. Efficacy and safety of 6-month nightly ramelteon administration in adults with chronic primary insomnia. Sleep 2009, 32, 351–360. Roehrs, T.A.; Randall, S.; Harris, E.; Maan, R.; Roth, T. Twelve months of nightly zolpidem does not lead to dose escalation: A prospective placebo-controlled study. Sleep 2011, 34, 207–212. Krystal, A.D.; Erman, M.; Zammit, G.K.; Soubrane, C.; Roth, T. Long-term efficacy and safety of zolpidem extended-release 12.5 mg, administered 3 to 7 nights per week for 24 weeks, in patients with chronic primary insomnia: A 6-month, randomized, double-blind, placebo-controlled, parallel-group, multicenter study. Sleep 2008, 31, 79–90. Roth, T.; Walsh, J.K.; Krystal, A.; Wessel, T.; Roehrs, T.A. An evaluation of the efficacy and safety of eszopiclone over 12 months in patients with chronic primary insomnia. Sleep Med. 2005, 6, 487–495.

[396] McCarron et al. ACP Smart Medicine: Depression. May 2014.

[397] Armstrong, Carri.e. "APA Releases Guideline on Treatment of Patients with Major Depressive Disorder." *Am Fam Physician*. 2011 May 15;83(10):1219-1227.

[398] Lang, Michael. "Managing Depression in Primary Care." AudioDigest Volume 62 (16).

[399] Bostwick, Michael. A Generalist's Guide to Treating Patients With Depression With an Emphasis on Using Side Effects to Tailor Antidepressant Therapy. Mayo Clin Proc. 2010;85(6):538-550.

[400] Levis B et al. Accuracy of Patient Health Questionnaire-9 (PHQ-9) for screening to detect major depression: Individual participant data meta-analysis. BMJ 2019 Apr 9; 365:l1476

[401] Keks et al. "Switching and stopping antidepressants." Aust Prescr 2016;39:76–83.

[402] Nelson, J. C., Thase, M. E., Bellocchio, E. E., Rollin, L. M., Eudicone, J. M., McQuade, R. D., ... Baker, R. A. (2012). Efficacy of adjunctive aripiprazole in patients with major depressive disorder who showed minimal response to initial antidepressant therapy. International Clinical Psychopharmacology, 27(3), 125–133.

[403] Tohen et al. Olanzapine/fluoxetine combination in patients with treatment-resistant depression: rapid onset of therapeutic response and its predictive value for subsequent overall response in a pooled analysis of 5 studies. J Clin Psychiatry. 2010 Apr;71(4):451-62.

[404] Serafini et al. Curr Neuropharmacol. 2014 Sep; 12(5): 444–461.

[405] Ogle et al. "Guidance for the Discontinuation or Switching of Antidepressant Therapies in Adults." Journal of Pharmacy Practice 26(4) 389-396.

[406] Berman BD. "Neuroleptic malignant syndrome: a review for neurohospitalists." Neurohospitalist. 2011 Jan;1(1):41-7.

[407] Martin, Thomas G. "Serotonin Syndrome." Ann Emerg Med. 1996 Nov;28(5):520-6.

[408] Savel et al. "Alcohol Withdrawal in the ICU - Practice and Pitfalls." SCCM. 2010.

[409] Marinella MA. "Refeeding syndrome and hypophosphatemia." J Intensive Care Med. 2005 May-Jun;20(3):155-9.

[410] Shuk-Ling Wong et al. "Treatment of Delirium Tremends." USPharmacist.com

[411] Rayner et al. "Dexmedetomidine as adjunct treatment for severe alcohol withdrawal in the ICU." Annals of Intensive Care 2012, 2:12

[412] Vieweg, W. Victor R. et al. "Posttraumatic Stress Disorder: Clinical Features, Pathophysiology, and Treatment." The American Journal of Medicine , Volume 119 , Issue 5 , 383 - 390.

[413] Schneier, Franklin. "Social Anxiety Disorder." N Engl J Med 2006; 355:1029-1036.

[414] Donaldson et al. "Oral Sedation: A Primer on Anxiolysis for the Adult Patient." Anesth Prog. 2007 Fall; 54(3): 118–129.

[415] Lader, Malcolm, Andre Tylee, and John Donoghue. "Withdrawing benzodiazepines in primary care." CNS drugs 23.1 (2009): 19-34.

[416] Smith et al. Am J Psychiatry 1998; 155:1339-1345.

PERIOPERATIVE CARE

Perioperative Management of Warfarin 607
Bridging Anticoagulation 610
Perioperative Evaluation 616

PERIOPERATIVE MANAGEMENT OF WARFARIN

Warfarin Management Based on Stroke Risk

Risk[417]	Mechanical heart valve	Chronic AF	VTE	Bleeding risk	Recommendations
High	At least 1 of the following: Aortic valve prosthesis Mitral valve prosthesis (any) with risk factors for thromboembolism** Stroke or TIA within past 6 months May also include: Patients with a history of stroke or TIA more than 3 months before surgery and a CHA2DS2-VASc score < 5 Patients undergoing surgeries with high risk of thromboembolism	At least 1 of the following: Chad2 score of 5 or 6 Rheumatic mitral valve disease Stroke or TIA within past 3 months May also include: Patients with a history of stroke or TIA more than 3 months before surgery and a CHA2DS2-VASc score < 5 Patients undergoing surgeries with high risk of thromboembolism	At least 1 of the following: Severe thrombophilia VTE within past 3 months May also include: Previous thromboembolism during temporary vitamin k antagonist interruption Patients undergoing surgeries with high risk of thromboembolism	Very low	Dental: continue warfarin with an oral pro hemostatic agent or stop warfarin 2 to 3 days before procedure; INR of 2.0 dermatologic: continue warfarin and optimize local hemostasis cataract: continue warfarin
				Low	Stop warfarin 5 days before surgery and restart 12 to 24 hours postoperatively VTE prophylaxis and Therapeutic dose of LMWH before the procedure and beginning approximately 24 hours after the procedure
				High	Stop warfarin 5 days before surgery and restart 12 to 24 hours postoperatively VTE prophylaxis and therapeutic dose of LMHW before the procedure and beginning 48 to 72 hours after the procedure
Moderate	Aortic valve prosthesis (bileaflet) and at least 1 of the following: Age > 75 years AF CHF	CHA2DS2-VASc 3-4	At least 1 of the following: Active cancer Non severe thrombophilic condition Recurrent VTE	Very low	Dental: continue warfarin with an oral pro hemostatic agent or stop warfarin 2 to 3 days before procedure dermatologic: continue warfarin and optimize local hemostasis cataract: continue warfarin

Warfarin Management Based on Stroke Risk

Risk[437]	Mechanical heart valve	Chronic AF	VTE	Bleeding risk	Recommendations
	DM HTN Prior stroke or TIA		VTE within past 3 to 12 months	Low	Stop warfarin 5 days before surgery and restart 12 to 24 hours postoperatively Therapeutic dose of LMHW before the procedure and beginning approximately 24 hours after the procedure
				High	Stop warfarin 5 days before surgery and restart 12 to 24 hours postoperatively VTE prophylaxis and Therapeutic dose of LMHW before the procedure and beginning 48 to 72 hours after the procedure
Low	Aortic valve prosthesis (bileaflet) without thromboembolism risk factors**	No prior stroke or TIA and CHA2DS2-VASc Score ≤ 2	Single VTE occurred > 12 months ago and No other risk factors	Very low	Dental: continue warfarin with an oral pro hemostatic agent or stop warfarin 2 to 3 days before procedure Dermatologic: continue warfarin and optimize local hemostasis Cataract: continue warfarin
				Low	Stop warfarin 5 days before surgery and restart 12 to 24 hours postoperatively Do not bridge
				High	Stop warfarin 5 days before surgery and restart 12 to 24 hours postoperatively Do not bridge

** Atrial fibrillation, recent thromboembolism, LVEF <30%, hypercoagulable state, older generation thrombogenic valve, mechanical tricuspid valve, multiple mechanical valves

Perioperative Interruption of DOAC[818]

No medication on AM of surgery plus the # of days prior as indicated below

	Low Bleeding Risk		High Bleeding Risk		Neuraxial Anesthesia
Renal Function	GFR>50	GFR 30-50	GFR>50	GFR 30-50	
Dabigatran	1 day	2 days	2 days	3-4 days	5 days
Rivaroxaban	1 day	2 days	2 days	3 days	3 days
Apixaban	1 day	2 days	2 days	3 days	3 days
Edoxaban	1 day	2 days	2 days	3 days	3 days

Anticoagulation based on device

	Characteristics	Annual Risk of VTE	Recommendation
Mechanical heart valve, AF, or hx of VTE	No valvular prosthesis	Low (dental, colo)	Hold warfarin for 4-5 days before the procedure without bridge (grade 2C)
		Low (cataract, derm)	Continue warfarin perioperatively (grade 2C)
		High	Bridging with heparin or Lovenox (grade 2C) during cessation of warfarin 5 days prior to surgery (grade 1C) with last dose given 24 hours prior to surgery and resumption of Lovenox 12-24 hours after surgery (grade 2C) unless high bleeding risk surgery (see below) in which it should be delayed to 48-72 hours
		Moderate	
		Low	No bridging recommended (grade 2C)
	Bare metal coronary stent	High (within 6 months of placement)	Recommend deferring surgery for at least 6 weeks after placement of a bare-metal stent instead of undertaking surgery within these time periods however if absolutely necessary (grade 1C), continue ASA and Plavix (grade 2C) or delay for 30 days minimum
	DES	High (within 12 months of placement)	Recommend deferring surgery for at least 6 months (ideally 1 year) after placement of a drug-eluting stent instead of undertaking surgery within these time periods however if absolutely necessary (grade 1C), continue ASA and Plavix (grade 2C) and wait minimum of 3 months
	CAD	High/Moderate	Suggest continuing ASA around the time of surgery instead of stopping ASA 7-10 days before surgery (Grade 2C).
		Low	Suggest stopping ASA 7-10 days before surgery instead of continuation of ASA (Grade 2C).

Bridging *means enoxaparin, 1 mg/kg BID or 1.5 mg/kg QD, dalteparin 100 IU/kg BID or 200 IU/kg QD, | tinzaparin 175 IU/kg QD, IV UFH to attain aPTT 1.5- to 2-times the control aPTT*

PERIOPERATIVE CARE

Thromboembolism Risk stratification			
Mechanical Heart Valve	High	Any mitral valve prosthesis, caged-ball AV prosthesis, stroke/TIA <6mo ago	
	Medium	Bileaflet aortic valve with hx of any of: AF/CVA/TIA/HTN/DM/CHF/75y	
	Low	Bileaflet aortic valve without hx of above	
Atrial Fibrillation	High	CHA2DS2VASC ≥7	
	Medium	CHA2DS2VASC 5-6	
	Low	CHA2DS2VASC ≤4	
VTE	High	VTE<3m ago, severe thrombophilia	
	Medium	VTE 3-12m ago, heterozygous thrombophilia, recurrent VTE, active cancer	
	Low	VTE>12m ago	

High Risk for Bleeding

- Urologic surgery/procedures: TURP, bladder resection or tumor ablation, nephrectomy or kidney biopsy (untreated tissue damage after TURP and endogenous urokinase release)
- Pacemaker or ICD implantation (separation of infraclavicular fascia and no suturing of unopposed tissues may lead to hematoma)
- Colonic polyp resection, especially >1-2 cm sessile polyps (bleeding occurs at transected stalk after hemostatic plug release)
- Vascular organ surgery: thyroid, liver, spleen
- Bowel resection (bleeding may occur at anastomosis site)
- Major surgery involving considerable tissue injury: cancer surgery, joint arthroplasty, reconstructive plastic surgery
- Cardiac, intracranial or spinal surgery (small bleeds can have serious clinical consequences)

BRIDGING ANTICOAGULATION

- **Questions to ask**[419]
  1) Determine thrombo-embolic risk of patient via CHADS2VASC score
  2) Determine bleeding risk via HAS-BLED/ORBIT score
  3) Determine timing of stopping DOAC before an invasive procedure
  4) Consider any special considerations for invasive procedures such as neuraxial anesthesia and AF with ablation
  5) Consider when bridging therapy with heparin required
     *Heparin bridging has no clinical benefit in patients with a short period of perioperative DOAC interruption. If high thromboembolic risk and patient will require prolonged interruption however (>3 days), consider heparin bridge. See below for bridging for Warfarin (in most cases, it is **not** recommended).*
  6) Resume a DOAC after invasive procedure or surgery
     Almost all guidelines recommend resumption after 24-72h; consider restarting the night after surgery with a reduced dose (see table below).
- **Indications**
  o See tables below
- **Warfarin Management**
  o No Bridging
    - Warfarin should be withheld 5 days before the procedure to allow the INR to fall below 1.5.
    - Warfarin is restarted 12-24 hours after the procedure.
  o Bridging

- Bridging due to warfarin cessation not required in majority of patients as it unnecessarily ↑ risk of bleeding without benefit.
- Based on INR:
    - If INR 2-3, warfarin should be withheld 5 days before the procedure
    - If INR 2.5-4.5, warfarin should be withheld 6 days before and consider 1-2mg of Vitamin K if INR remains elevated 1-2 days before surgery
- LMWH:
    - *Pre-procedure*
        - Bridging begins 36 hours after last dose of warfarin at therapeutic dose of 1mg/kg BID or dalteparin 200U/kg daily
            - BID dosing: hold evening dose prior to surgery
            - Daily dosing: ½ dose is giving the morning of surgery
        - **Stop 24 hours prior to surgery** and resume 48-72 hours after if high risk for bleeding, otherwise 24 hours.
        - Check INR on AM of surgery, goal <1.5
    - *Post-procedure*
        - If low risk bleed, restart 24 hours postop
        - If high risk bleed, consider prophylactic dose for 1-3 days then therapeutic dose after
        - Check INR daily and stop LMWH when INR ≥ 2
- UFH:
    - *Pre-procedure*
        - Goal aPTT of 1.5-2x control
        - Started when the INR falls below 2 (usually 36 hours after last warfarin dose).
        - **Stop 4 hrs prior to surgery**
        - Heparin is stopped 4 to 6 hours before the procedure.
        - Restarted as soon as bleeding stability permits, goal 12-24 hours
            - Heparin is discontinued when the INR reaches therapeutic levels.
    - *Post-procedure*
        - If low risk bleed, restart 24 hours postop
        - If high risk bleed, consider prophylactic dose for 1-3 days then therapeutic dose after
        - Check INR daily and stop LMWH when INR ≥ 2

PERIOPERATIVE CARE

Bleeding risk stratification for invasive procedures

Minimal risk of bleeding	Low to moderate risk of bleeding	High risk of bleeding
• Tooth extraction (1-3 teeth) • Periodontology • Simple endoscopy without biopsy • Superficial surgery (e.g. abscess incision or minor dermatologic procedures (small superficial excision) • Cataract procedure • Double J stent insertion	• Endoscopy with simple biopsy • Prostate or bladder biopsy • Coronary angiography • Simple abdominal hernia repair • Anal surgery • Gynecologic surgery: simple total laparoscopic hysterectomy • Orthopedic surgery: hand surgery, arthroscopy • Pacemaker or cardioverter-defibrillator implantation	• Neuraxial anesthesia Intracranial surgery • Thoracic surgery • Cardiac surgery • Complex abdominal or gynecological cancer surgery • Major orthopedic surgery to include joint replacement • ENT cancer surgery or specific surgery requiring good hemostasis (e.g. cochlear implant or thyroid surgery) • Liver and kidney biopsy • Transurethral prostate or bladder resection • Extracorporeal shockwave lithotripsy Infected pacemaker lead extraction (↑↑risk of cardiac tamponade) • Robotic surgery

ACC Recommendations on Anticoagulation in AF

Bridging Advised	Uncertain	No Bridging Advised
• Mechanical aortic valve with any risk factor (atrial fibrillation, previous thromboembolism, left ventricular dysfunction, a hypercoagulable state, older generation thrombogenic valves, a mechanical tricuspid valve, or multiple valves) • Mechanical mitral valve • Stroke within 6 months of surgery • Caged-ball or tilting disc aortic prosthesis • Atrial fibrillation and multiple stroke risk factors (eg, $CHADS_2 \geq 5$, $CHA_2DS_2\text{-VASc} \geq 7$) or thromboembolic event due to AF in last 3 months • VTE within 3 months of surgery • Severe thrombophilia (protein C/s deficiency, antiphospholipid abs)	• Mechanical heart valve with AF or VTE history with moderate risk for thromboembolism	• Bileaflet aortic valve with no risk factors (see column to right) • Dental procedures (stop warfarin 2-3 days prior to procedure) • Continue warfarin without cessation in dermatology and cataract procedures

Thromboembolism Risk Categories with Anticoagulation Cessation Recommendation

	High	**Moderate**	**Low**
Mechanical Heart Valve	• Cardiac valve replacement surgery • CHADS<5 but prior stroke >3mo prior to surgery • Carotid endarterectomy • Major vascular surgery • Any mitral valve prosthesis • Caged-ball or tilting disc aortic valve • Recent stroke or TIA (<6 mo)	• Bileaflet aortic valve prosthesis **and** one or more of the of following risk factors: atrial fibrillation, prior stroke or transient ischemic attack, hypertension, diabetes, congestive heart failure, age >75)	• Bileaflet aortic valve prosthesis without atrial fibrillation and no other risk factors for stroke
Atrial Fibrillation	• CHADS ≥6 • Recent (<3 mo) stroke or TIA • Rheumatic valvular heart disease	• CHAD 4-5 • Prior stroke or TIA > 3 mo ago	• CHAD 2-3 • No prior stroke or TIA
VTE	• Recent (within 3 mo) VTE • Severe thrombophilia	• Non severe thrombophilia (heterozygous factor V, prothrombin) • VTE in last 3-12 mo • Active cancer	• VTE > 12 mo previous and no other risk factors

Thromboembolism Risk Categories with Anticoagulation Cessation Recommendation

		High	Moderate	Low
Anti-coagulation Management	**High Bleeding Risk Procedure**	**Warfarin** • Give last dose 6 days prior to operation and bridge with LMWH or UFH. • Resume 24 hours post operatively **DOAC** • Give last dose 3 days prior (extend to 4-5 days if high risk bleeding procedure) to operation and resume 2-3 days after	**Warfarin** • Give last dose 6 days before operation, determine need for bridging by clinician judgment and current evidence, resume 24 hours postoperatively **DOAC** • Give last dose 3 days prior to operation*, resume 2-3 days postoperatively	**Warfarin** • Give last dose 6 days before operation, bridging not recommended, resume 24 hours postoperatively **DOAC** • Give last dose 3 days prior to operation*, resume 2-3 days postoperatively
	Low Bleeding Risk Procedure	**Warfarin** • Give last dose 6 days before operation, bridge with LMWH or UFH, resume 24 hours postoperatively **DOAC** • Give last dose 2 days prior to operation*, resume 24 hours postoperatively	**Warfarin** • Give last dose 6 days before operation, determine need for bridging by clinician judgment and current evidence, resume 24 hours postoperatively **DOAC** • Give last dose 2 days prior to operation*, resume 24 hours postoperatively	**Warfarin** • Give last dose 6 days before operation, bridging not recommended, resume 24 hours postoperatively **DOAC** • Give last dose 2 days prior to operation*, resume 24 hours postoperatively

Example propositions for perioperative management of DOACs

Bleeding risk of invasive procedure		Dabigatran		Rivaroxiban-Apixiban-Edoxaban	
		Low bleeding risk	High bleeding risk	Low bleeding risk	High bleeding risk
Preoperative interruption No bridging (except patients	CrCl ≥50 ml/min	Last dose 24-36h before surgery	Last dose 2-3 days before surgery	CrCl >30: ≥ 1 day CrCl 15-29: ≥36h CrCl <15: ≥2 days	CrCl >30: ≥2 days CrCl <30: ≥ 3 days
	CrCl 30-50 ml/min	Last dose 2 days before surgery	Last dose 4-5 days before surgery		

with high risk of TE)	For very high-risk procedure (neuraxial anaesthesia)	Dabigatran: Last dose 5-7 days before surgery (5 days if CrCl >50; 7 days if less) Rivaroxaban: 3 days Apixaban: 3-5 days Edoxaban: 3 days		
Resumption after invasive procedure or surgery		Resume on day after surgery at 150mg BID	Resume 2 days after surgery at 150mg BID	Resume on day after surgery at 10mg/d	Resume 2 days after surgery at 10mg/d
		Prophylactic dose of LMWH, UFH or fondaparinux minimum 6 h after invasive procedure or surgery if venous thromboprophylaxis is indicated For neuraxial anesthesia with indwelling catheter: Resumption with LMWH or UFH until indwelling catheter is out			

ACC Recommendations on Warfarin Management in AF

Thromboembolic Risk Category (see page 613)	Bleeding Risk Category	Recommendation
Low (CHA2DS2VASC < 4) without prior CVA/TIA/DVT/PE	All levels	Stop Vit K antagonists without bridging
Moderate (CHA2DS2VASC 5-6)	High Risk	Stop Vit K antagonists without bridging
	No significant bleeding risk (no h/o stroke or TIA)	Bridging should not be considered
	No significant bleeding risk **with history of stroke or TIA**	Bridging should be considered
High (CHA2DS2VASC > 7)	All levels	Bridging should be considered in patients with TIA/CVA/PE/DVT in last 3 months
	High bleeding risk	Clinical judgement

PERIOPERATIVE CARE

PERIOPERATIVE EVALUATION

Figure. Perioperative evaluation of patient with possible CAD risk

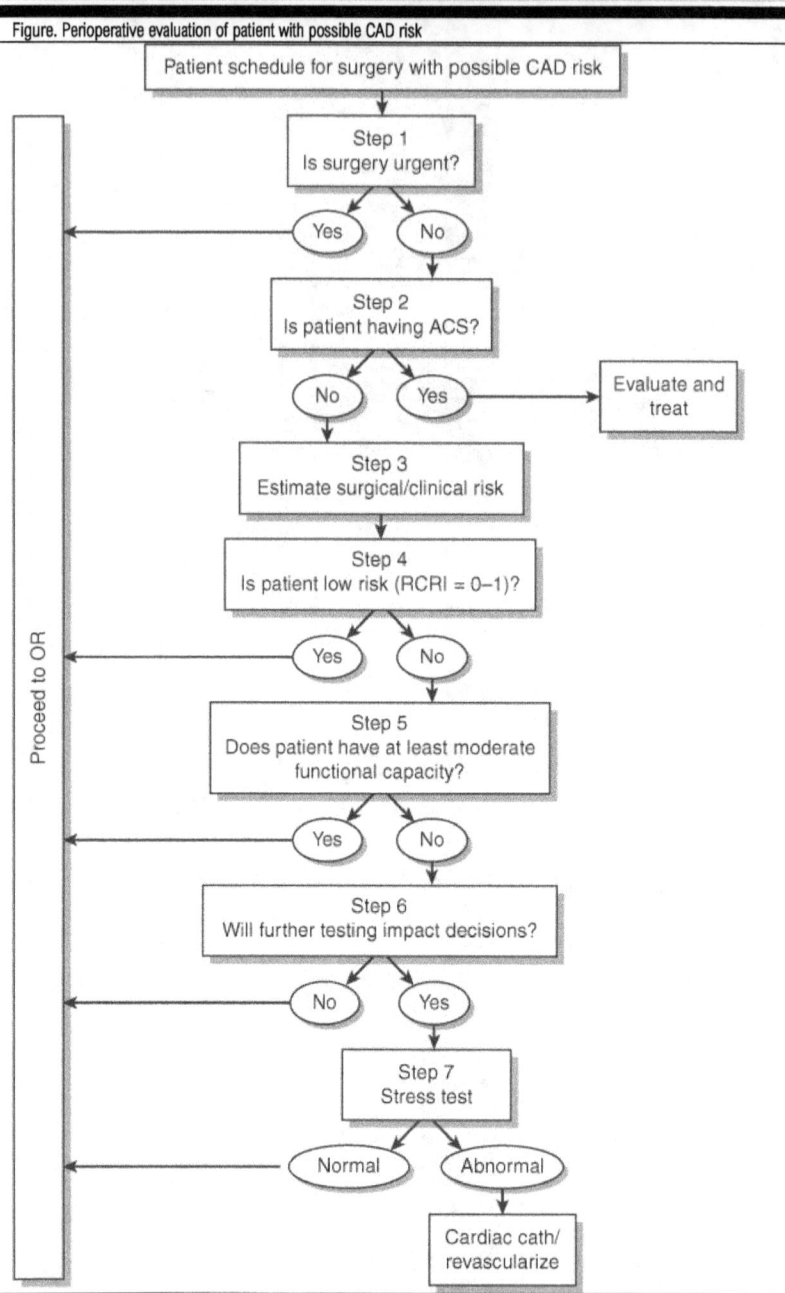

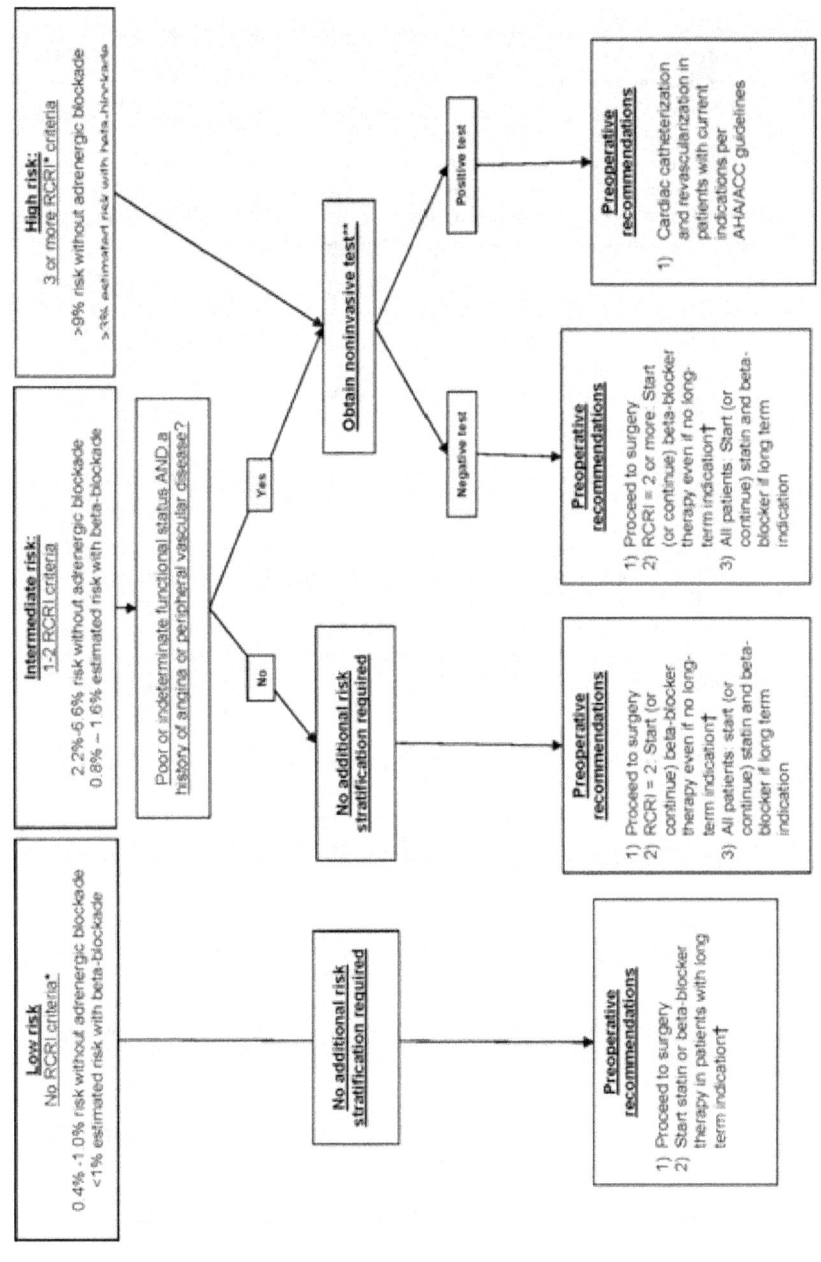

PERIOPERATIVE CARE

- **General**[420,421]
  - Goal is to assess and optimize risk (or lower the risk as much as possible)
  - Not needed for: emergency surgery, patients without active cardiac conditions undergoing a low risk surgery, or those with no active cardiac conditions or symptoms with good exercise capacity.
  - Can use any surgical calculator (RCRI, ACS-NSQIP, or MICA)
    - ACS-NSQIP best for **medically complex patients**
    - RCRI is the oldest and has been externally validated for predicting major adverse cardiac events. It may **overestimate** the risk for low risk surgical procedures and **underestimate** the risk for major vascular surgeries. Best for high-risk procedures.
    - MICA may perform best at identifying **high risk** patients
  - Evaluate for risk of OHS and RH failure

The most notable significant risk factors	
CHF	H/o stroke/TIA
CAD	Advancing age
Type of surgery	ASA physical status classification
Elevated preoperative Cr	Dependent functional status
Diabetes	HTN
Emergency surgery	

  - The essential elements of a preoperative evaluation include reviewing overall health and underlying conditions, including pregnancy; exercise tolerance; reaction to previous anesthesia and surgery; and use of medications, tobacco, alcohol, and illicit drugs from the patient's history and physical examination. These results should guide laboratory testing, and healthy patients having minor procedures may need no testing. In patients at elevated cardiac risk with poor functional status, noninvasive cardiac testing should be considered only if the results are likely to change management.
- **Functional Status**
  - Duke Activity Score Index (DASI) > METS assessment in predicting postoperative events
- **Type of Surgery** - see page 623 for risk classifications
- **Questions to ask**
  - HPI - Last meal
  - Medical History – ask about any known medical conditions (esp. thyroid, OSA, CHF, HTN, ACS, cirrhosis, DM), bleeding history, ACS
  - Surgical History - complications from prior surgeries, ICD placement
  - Family History – ensure no history of malignant hyperthermia that affects susceptible patients under anesthesia and is heritable. Another condition to consider is pseudocholinesterase deficiency which affects succinylcholine duration and may require extended postoperative ventilation.
  - Allergies – be aware of any that may be important from an anesthesia standpoint
  - Social –
    - Currently smoking? Airway and secretion management can become more difficult in smokers. Recommend smoking cessation 30 days prior to surgery.
    - Alcohol Consumption or Drug Abuse? - Drinkers have an increased tolerance to many sedative drugs (conversely, they have a decreased requirement if drunk), and are at an increased risk of hepatic disease, which can impact the choice of anesthetic agents.

PERIOPERATIVE CARE

Perioperative Medication Management

Medication	When to stop	When to restart (risk based on bleeding)
ASA	Primary Prophylaxis: 6 days Secondary Prophylaxis: see below	24 hours
NSAIDs	5 half-lives In general, 1-4 days	24 hours
Cilostazol	2 days	24 hours
Coumadin	5 days (normal INR)	24 hours
Heparin	4 hours	2 hours
LMWH	Prophylactic: 12 hours Therapeutic: 24 hours	Low risk: 4 hours Medium/High: 12 to 24 hours
Plavix	7 days	12-24h
Prasugrel	7-10 days	12-24h
Ticagrelor	5 days	12-24h
Dabigatran	4-5 days (6 days if impaired GFR)	24 hours
Rivaroxaban	5 days	24 hours
Apixaban	3-5 days	24 hours
Ginsing	1-2 weeks	Inconclusive
Biologics	4 weeks prior, surgery when next dose due	After surgery
Methotrexate	Continue through	N/A
Beta Blocker	Continue through; starting as a new rx prior to surgery is controversial	N/A

- **Medication Management**
  o Hold: hyoscyamine, NSAIDs (stop 5 half-lives prior in high-risk procedures/typically 1-4 days), herbals/ vitamins/ supplements (x7 days prior), TNF-alpha (x1-2 half-lives prior; appx 4 weeks but typically do surgery at the start of the next cycle), warfarin (x5 days prior, pre-op goal INR <1.5, re-start 12-24 hours post-op), NOACS (x2-3 days prior, re-start post-op when hemostasis achieved), oral/injectable non-insulin diabetic medications (x1-2 days prior), P2Y12 inhibitors (i.e. Plavix) 7 days and restarted within 12-24 hours, Lithium, Estrogen, Levodopa/Carbidopa
  o Individualize: Opioids, Methotrexate, Aspirin (continue if prior PCI or CVA recently, otherwise hold 5-7 days prior if high bleeding-risk surgery and re-start 8-10d after surgery per *PEP Trial*, also hold even in patients with *concern for* VTE)[422], DAPT (can stop after minimum 6 months after ACS regardless of management, minimum 6 months after DES, minimum of 6w after BMS)
  o Continue: alpha blockers, beta blockers (if hypotense, dose reduction preferred to discontinuation), calcium channel blockers, nitrates, vasodilators, statins, acetaminophen, antacids, Plaquenil, SSRIs, benzos, antipsychotics, basal insulin (consider 25-50% dose reduction in DM2), thyroid hormone, clonidine, pulmonary medications
  o Start: beta-blockers (may be started in pts with +myocardial ischemia on preoperative testing if it can be started at least 1-2 weeks prior to surgery (never start same day of surgery)), statins (undergoing vascular surgery if indicated by GDMT)
  o Controversial – diuretics (consider holding), ACEi/ARBs (**in most cases -- continue**, can hold if concern for intra-op hypotension for 24 hours before non-cardiac surgery and restart on POD#2, *VISION*), beta blockers (consider starting in those with intermediate-high risk MI based on perioperative risk stratification or 3+ RCRI risk factors)
    - Continuing ACE inhibitor treatment before noncardiac nonvascular surgery is associated with a greater frequency and duration of intraoperative hypotension, but does not increase the incidences of AKI, MACE, death, nor hospital length of stay.[423]
    - Diuretics typically held the AM of surgery to avoid electrolyte imbalances
  o Bridging: see page 609
  o DOAC: see page 614
  o Stents: see page 626

PERIOPERATIVE CARE

- Steroids
  - If patient was on suppressive doses and came off the steroid <1 year from surgery, or if 5-20 mg/d prednisone for >3 weeks in prior 3 months:
    - Consider cosyntropin stim testing if moderate to severe surgery stress expected
      - Can also obtain fasting cortisol (<5 concerning for suppression)
    - If on <5mg of daily prednisone or any dose for <3 weeks, then continue current dose through surgery
    - Minor surgery: no additional steroid
    - Moderate surgery: 50 HCT IV preoperatively and 25mg IV q8h for 24 hr
    - Major surgery: 100 HCT IV and 50mg IV q8h for 24 hours
  - Steroids Indicated in:
    - Primary adrenal insufficiency, cushingoid features, and/or >20 mg/d prednisone for >3 weeks in prior 3 months
  - If steroids will be continued, keep home dose and...
    - Surgical stress minor (i.e. outpt proc), rec hydrocortisone (HDC) 25 mg IV x 1d
    - Stress moderate (i.e. orthopedic surg), rec HDC 50-75 mg IV x 1- 2d
    - Stress severe (i.e. CABG), rec HDC 100 mg IV x 1 f/b 50 mg IV q6 hrs. x 2-3d
- DVT Prophylaxis (focusing on THA, TKA, HFx)
  - Use SCDs
  - Enoxaparin 30mg SQ BID starting 12-24h post operatively x 5 weeks
  - Rivaroxaban 10mg/d starting 6-8h post operatively or can do only 5 days and then replace with ASA 81mg/d for 30 days
  - Dabigatran 220mg/d with first dose given as 110mg 4 hours post op
  - Apixaban 2.5mg BID 12 hours post op
- Diabetes
  - Hospital
    - *Before Surgery* - BS goal 140(pre-meal)-180 (random) mg/dL
    - *Evening before surgery* - If insulin-dependent → reduce evening glargine by 20%
    - *Morning of Surgery*
      - Preoperative glucose levels of <200 mg/dL on the day of surgery is ideal for elective surgery (also a goal of HgA1c of <8% is ideal)
      - If surgery <2 hours
        - Patient on oral diabetes medications only → simply hold the day-of medication and plan for morning surgery
      - If surgery >4 hours
        - Use continuous IV insulin with rate = current glucose / 100
        - Monitor glucose hourly
        - Always have D51/2NS running concurrently with insulin (separate IV) at 100cc/hr.
        - If on 70/30 give half the total morning dose the day of surgery as intermediate acting
        - Start D51/2NS with 40meQ of K at 100cc/hr.

Perioperative Glucose Management[424]

Situation	Changes Recommended
Basal QHS + Premeals = 50/50 with no hypoglycemic episodes	Full basal dose given (75% dose if experiencing hypoglycemic episodes)
Basal QAM + Premeals = 50/50 with no hypoglycemic episodes	75% of basal dose in AM
Premixed insulins (70/30 NPH)	Two Options 1. Switch to regimen of long acting and short acting independent of one another and follow above instructions 2. Take 50% of normal NPH (short acting) morning dose (and if BID then 25% of previous evening dose) and give concomitant D5W and routine BS checks
Preprandial insulin	Stop doses on the AM of surgery
Oral hypoglycemic for T2DM	1. Hold sulfonylurea or secretagogue on day of procedure and resume when tolerates NL diet 2. Hold metformin for safety concern the day of procedure and resume 48 hr post-op if renal function normal or near normal 3. Can continue TZDs
Sliding scale insulin	Used to correct for BS>200 mg/dL
Fluids	D5W with 1/2NS @ 50cc/hr
Short acting insulin	Hold AM of surgery
Non-insulin injectables	Hold AM of surgery
Intermediate acting insulin (NPH)	25% of PM dose prior to surgery and 50-75% of dose in AM of surgery
Insulin pump	Consider consulting endocrinology; can remove/turn off pump and switch to basal + nutritional insulin

- *Perioperative insulin management*
    - *Preoperative glucose levels of <200 mg/dL on the day of surgery is ideal for elective surgery (also a goal of HgA1c of <8% is ideal)*
    - Maintain BG **100-180 mg/dL** to prevent dehydration/ketosis, promote wound healing, optimize leukocyte function, avoid hypoglycemia.
    - Start 5 gm/hr glucose infusion (i.e. D51/2NS + 20 mEq KCl @ 100 mL/h).
    - Can start IV regular insulin (1 unit/h) and adjust for goal or, if surgery is minor and patient's glucose is well-controlled, give 50% of usual SC insulin (if NPH) in the AM of surgery and supplement with regular insulin q4-6 hr to achieve goal.
- *Transitioning from IV to SQ*
    - Ideal patients are off pressors, stable IV insulin rates (past 6-8h), stable glucose levels (110-180) and are clinically stable
    - Use the average infusion rate to determine the total daily dose or TDD (ie, 2 units/h x 24 h/d = 48 units/d).
        - Take appx 50% of this value for the basal dose if patient on tube feeds or some other form of nutrition. Take 80% of this value for the basal dose if the patient was NPO.
        - If the patient was NPO while on the drip, this TDD will basically be their pure basal dose
        - Ensure that the basal insulin overlaps the IV insulin by 2-4 hours
    - *Post Operatively*
        - Continue Lantus/glargine at 80% of home dose and use scheduled aspart q6h until eating and then provide with meals and at bedtime
        - If unknown insulin dose, then use the 50/50 rule for long/short acting but calculate based on 0.5U/kg *(RABBIT-2)*
- **Diagnostics**

- o EKG – indicated in patients with acute or new cardiac symptoms, arrhythmia, PAD, know CAD undergoing medium to high risk surgery; routine age-directed EKGs no longer advised. Patients undergoing a low risk procedure (see page 623), regardless of CAD history, do not require an EKG.
- o CXR – acute symptoms suggestive of COPD (worsening from baseline), age ≥ 70 with no CXR in last 6 months
- o TTE – not advised in asymptomatic individuals; patients with known murmur, new murmur, symptoms of new or worsening CHF, or known valvular disease should have performed perioperatively. Those with known CHF, *consider* repeat TTE if older than 1 year.
- o CBC – if high estimated blood loss, consider if >65 years old
- **Pulmonary Consult Consideration**
  - o Patients with chronic but not active COPD do not require further therapy
  - o Therapies for pulmonary hypertension should not be discontinued preoperatively
  - o Low albumin (<3.5) best predictor of perioperative pulmonary complications

Step 1	Step 2	Step 3	Step 4
Is the procedure an emergency? If so, proceed to OR. If not, proceed to step 2	For elective/urgent surgeries, Does the patient have ACS? If so, treat accordingly, if not, proceed to step 3	Estimate the risk of MACE using one of various calculators. Recommend first calculating the **NSQIP** or **Bilimoria** to get an accurate estimate of the chance of a very serious event. While this is an accurate picture, its incomplete in regard to potential cardiac complications given what they defined as cardiac history (more catastrophic were only included). Then, use another calculator to obtain a broader assessment of cardiac risk, such as **RCRI**.	Low risk (MACE<1%) then no further testing and proceed to surgery. If risk >1%, proceed to step 5
Step 5	Step 6	Step 7	
Assess functional capacity (METS), if ≥ 4 then proceed without further testing, if <4, then continue to Step 6	If <4 METS and further testing will not impact decision making, proceed to surgery or alternative tx. Otherwise, continue to step 7	If <4 METS and further testing **will** change treatment, then perform pharmacologic stress testing and revascularize pending results	

Step by Step Non-Cardiac Surgery Perioperative Evaluation[425,426]

Step 1: Establish the urgency of surgery. Many surgeries are unlikely to allow for a time-consuming evaluation
- <u>Emergent</u>: loss of life, limb, or eyesight in 6 hrs of no surgery
- <u>Urgent</u>: loss of life, limb, or eyesight within 24 hours if no surgery
- <u>Time-Sensitive</u>: delay of 1-6 weeks for further evaluation would negatively affect outcome
- <u>Elective</u>: delay for up to 1 year safe

Step 2: Assess for active cardiac conditions (following are highest risk)
- Unstable coronary syndromes including severe angina (without intervention)
- Recent MI (b/w 7-30 days ago)
- Decompensated CHF
- Significant arrhythmia (ventricular)
- Severe valvular disease (esp. severe AS)
- Clinical risk factors for coronary artery disease (CAD)
- Preexisting, stable CAD (also known as chronic coronary syndrome)
- Diabetes mellitus
- Prior CVA or TIA
- CKD
- Poorly controlled HTN (SBP<180+DBP<110 are acceptable)
- Abnormal ECG (i.e. LVH, LBBB, ST-T wave abnormalities)
- Age >70 years
- CHF

Reschedule Surgery if.....
Recent MI (7-30d) with ischemia, class 3-4 angina, decompensated CHF, high grade AV block, critical AS with symptoms.

Step 3: Determine the surgery-specific risk

High (Reported cardiac risk often greater than 5%; any procedure with MACE risk >1%)
- Emergent major operations, particularly in the elderly
- Aortic and other major vascular surgery
- Peripheral vascular surgery
- Anticipated prolonged surgical procedures associated with large fluid shifts and/or blood loss
- Major abdominal surgery and prolonged procedures with large fluid shifts or blood loss (duodenopancreatic, liver resection, bile duct surgery, perforated bowel, total cystectomy)
- Esophagectomy
- Pneumonectomy
- Adrenal resection
- Carotid endarterectomy surgery
- Endovascular aneurysm repair (stents/coils)
- Neurologic or orthopedic, major (hip and spine surgery)

- Urologic (prostate) or gynecologic, major
- Head and neck surgery
- Intraperitoneal and intrathoracic surgery
- Orthopedic surgery
- Renal transplant

Low (any procedure with MACE risk < 1%)
- Endoscopic procedures
- Superficial procedure
- Cataract surgery
- Breast surgery
- Dental
- Orthopedics, minor
- Urologic, minor (TURP, TURBT)
- Thyroid
- Reconstructive, cosmetic

Step 4: Assess the patient's functional capacity

Poor functional capacity (<4 METs) is associated with an increased risk of perioperative cardiac events. Exercise testing is the gold standard, but functional capacity can be estimated by patient self-report. Examples of activities that are at least of moderate functional capacity (>4 METs) include: climbing one to two flights of stairs or walking a block at a brisk pace. Patients with a functional capacity of >4 METs without symptoms can proceed to surgery with relatively low risk.
>If unclear METS, can do pharmacologic stress test if it will change your plan (class IIa)

Can use the website **whyiexercise.com** to estimate METS however the Duke Activity Status Index (DASI) and NT-proBNP are better predictors of adverse outcomes as METS alone underclassifies risk
>A lower DASI predicated primary outcome of death or MI when METS, CPEX did not

Step 5: Estimate the patient's perioperative risk.

This is one of the most controversial steps. In general, no one calculator is superior to another. Instead, using a combination of two may be beneficial. Consider starting with the NIS-QIP or Bilimoria to get an idea of major, severe cardiac events. These do not give a broad enough picture however (only major events), therefore do a secondary calculation using the RCRI.

The history, PE, and ECG will help identify risk factors and can be used to determine/estimate the perioperative risk of adverse cardiac events. Example factors include history of: ischemic heart disease, heart failure, CVA/TIA, IDDM, SCr≥2. The risk will determine whether surgery should proceed without further cardiovascular testing or not. You can use one of the following calculators to determine this risk:

RCRI	NS-QIP	MICA	GSCRI
Indication – MI/cardiac arrest, CHB, pulmonary edema **during admission (do not use for post-operative risk)**	*Indication* – MI/cardiac arrest **within 30 days** after surgery and can predict length of stay.	*Indication* - MI/cardiac arrest **within 30 days** after surgery	*Indication* – Specifically for geriatric patients >65

When to use – Best for higher risk procedures, and high risk patients. **Pearls** – May over-estimate risk of post-operative cardiac events **except** in geriatric patients (>65) where it underestimates. Easier to use.	**When to use** – High risk patients: use this when patients are undergoing a low-risk procedure or those with an expected LOS of ≤ 2 days. **Pearls** – Made specifically for surgeons. As with the MICA, very good at predicting cardiac event within 30 days of surgery. Underestimate cardiac events in patients at **elevated** risk per ACC/AHA. Did not perform well specifically with head and neck surgery patients.	**When to use** – Best to use for high risk patients (can use RCRI to determine) who are undergoing a low or intermediate-risk procedure or those with an expected LOS of ≤ 2 days. **Pearls** – Most reliable in selecting **higher risk patients**. Incorporates newer laparoscopic surgeries. Uses same variables as the NS-QIP. Underestimate cardiac events in patients at **elevated** risk per ACC/AHA.
		When to use – Patients >65 have a higher risk of cardiac complications post operatively. This is to be used specifically for this population. **Pearls** – Most accurate for geriatric patients

Step 6: Now based on the risk you calculated, determine if you need to do any further evaluation:

Low	High
RCRI: ≤1 risk factors MACE<1%	(see risk factors from Step 2) RCRI: >1 risk factors ACS NSQIP >1% MACE>1%
Patients with 0 clinical risk factors are at low risk (<1% risk of cardiac events) and may proceed to surgery without further testing.	Patients with ≥3 clinical risk factors are at high risk of adverse cardiac events (>5%), particularly when undergoing vascular surgery. In this population, stress testing may provide a better estimate of cardiovascular risk and may be considered if knowledge of this increased risk would change management.

PERIOPERATIVE CARE

- **Considerations**
  - Stable CAD/Chronic Coronary Syndrome - *COURAGE Trial* – PCI can safely be deferred in pts with stable CAD even in those with significant inducible ischemia and MV involvement provided medical tx is instituted and maintained
  - Positive Stress Test
    - Need to intervene with CABG/PCI:
      - Angioplasty only: 2-week delay of surgery
      - CABG: delay surgery 2 weeks
      - **BMS**: 1 month minimum but push for 6 weeks, ideal 12 months if low risk bleed; ASA lifetime delay surgery 2 weeks. BMS are riskier than DES in first 6 months of placement.
      - **DES**: 6 months minimum; ideally for 12 months if low risk bleed; lifelong ASA; delay surgery 3-6 months (can consider stopping after 3 months if further delay in surgery holds greater risk than benefit from preventing stent thrombosis)
  - Cardiac Stents – see page 609
  - Repair of hip fractures should be done within 48 hours if possible
  - Myocardial infarction (NSTEMI) – 6 month delay minimum in surgery
- **Diagnostics**
  - Labs

Guideline-directed labs to consider prior to elective noncardiac surgery	
Hgb	Major blood loss or symptoms of anemia
PLT	h/o bleeding diathesis, myeloproliferative dz, liver dz, thrombocytopenia
PT	h/o bleeding diathesis, liver dz, malnutrition, recent or long term ABx, warfarin use
PTT	Heparin use, bleeding diathesis, controversial but may consider in intracranial and spine surgery regardless of PMHx
Electrolytes	Renal insufficiency, CHF, diuretics
BUN/SCr	CKD, HTN, DM, cardiac dz
Glucose	DM, obesity
LFT	Cirrhosis, suspected acute hepatitis
UA	LUTS, instrumentation of the GU tract
ECG	Known CAD, DM, uncontrolled HTN, CKD
CXR	Sx of active pulmonary disease
T&S	If large amount of blood loss expected
BNP	Risk stratification for anyone with risk factors or ≥65 years old (per CCS 2016 guidelines)
HCG	Females of childbearing age
proBNP	BNP or N-terminal fragment of proBNP (NT-proBNP) should be measured before surgery in patients who are ≥65 years of age, are 45-64 years of age with significant cardiovascular disease, or have a Revised Cardiac Risk Index score ≥1.
TROP	Recommended daily for 48-72h after surgery in patients with an elevated NT-proBNP/BNP measurement before surgery or if there is no NT-proBNP/BNP measurement before surgery, in those who have an RCRI score ≥1, age 45-64 years with significant cardiovascular disease, or age ≥65 years.

  - Pacemaker Management
    - If patient is pacemaker dependent, the device should be reprogrammed to an asynchronous mode (e.g., VOO, DOO) for the surgery. If no cardiologist available, consider applying a magnet.
    - Anti-tachycardia functions of an ICD will typically need to be programmed off for surgical procedures in which electrocautery may cause interference with device function, leading to the potential for unintentional discharge.
    - Consultation with an EP is recommended if there is uncertainty regarding the perioperative management of a device.
  - Who needs TTE
    - Current CHF symptoms
    - Prior CHF with worsening sx
    - Dyspnea of unknown cause

- Murmur on examination suggestive of severe valvular disease
- ECG: in patients with hx CAD/PVD, arrhythmia, structural heart disease undergoing moderate to high risk surgery; may not alter preoperative decision making but provides a useful baseline in the event of postoperative complications
- Imaging
  - CXR: if signs and sx of pulmonary dz or hx cardiopulm dz w/ new or unstable symptoms
  - C-spine: patient with RA obtain flexion and extension films
- **Who requires cardiology consultation?**
  - Moderate or greater valvular stenosis/regurgitation
  - Cardiac implantable electronic disease
  - pHTN
  - Congenital heart disease
- **What if I have a patient undergoing major vascular surgery?**
  - Use the AHA/ACC guidelines, which feature a complex algorithm that is based on functional capacity, clinical predictors, and procedure-specific risks (see reference below).
  - Delay surgery and proceed to direct treatment/risk reduction if patient has a major clinical predictor of postoperative cardiac complication. Noninvasive testing may not be helpful here because of the high rate of false negatives. Major clinical predictors are defined as:
    - Unstable coronary syndromes (recent MI, unstable or severe angina)
    - Decompensated CHF
    - Symptomatic or uncontrolled arrhythmias (such as symptomatic ventricular arrhythmias, SVT with uncontrolled rate, high grade AV block)
    - Severe valvular disease
- **What are defined as cardiac complications?**
  - Hard end-points: MI, cardiovascular death (by MI, arrhythmia, heart failure).
  - Soft end-points: non-fatal arrhythmia, CHF/pulmonary edema, ischemia.
- **Postoperative Atrial Fibrillation**
  - Postoperative AFib is associated with outcomes similar to those of nonsurgical nonvalvular AFib.
  - Patients should be started on anticoagulation after calculating bleeding risk and CHA2DS2VASC2 score.
- **Perioperative MI after Non-Cardiac Surgery (MINS)**
  - Usually presents atypically (without chest pain). Look for ↓BP, pulmonary edema, altered mental status (especially in elderly patients), and arrhythmia.
  - Usually occurs within the first 2 days of surgery and carries a high mortality.
  - Patients experiencing MINS and given dabigatran 110mg PO BID x2y had lower major vascular complication than those who did not. *(MANAGE)*
- **How can you reduce cardiac risk?**
  - Consider a lower risk alternative to the planned type of operation.
  - Consider using epidural or spinal anesthesia.
  - Correct, modify, and optimize the management of co-morbid medical conditions.
  - Recent MI: delay surgery for 6 months; if the surgery is semi-elective, fully evaluate/optimize from cardiac standpoint and wait at least 6-12 weeks.
  - CHF: optimize and avoid over-diuresis (patient should not be orthostatic)
  - Aortic stenosis: in general, treatment based on symptoms (syncope, CHF, angina). If the patient has symptoms, evaluate fully (obtain echocardiogram, rule out other causes of symptoms). However, if the patient has no symptoms (make sure they are active enough to produce symptoms), then proceed with surgery. This even applies to patients who have severe AS. Patient with critical AS and without symptoms should only undergo procedures that are truly necessary.

PERIOPERATIVE CARE

- o Use perioperative beta-blockers - Only use if: pt already using β-Blocker, Pt with known CAD, need additional tx for HTN, RCRI>1
- o Consider adding statin if using beta-blocker
- o Only control hypertension if >180/110
- **Medications**
  - o *Essential medications*: beta blockers, clonidine, CCB
  - o *Medications to withhold*: ACEi, ARB, diuretics AM of surgery. NSAIDs stopped 1 week prior to surgery
  - o Stop ASA/Plavix 7 days prior to surgery
  - o NSAIDS: 3-5 days prior to surgery
  - o HRT: ok if DVT ppx used post-op
  - o The decision to hold diuretics/ARB/ACEi in AM of surgery due to risk of refractory ↓BP should be made on a case by case basis. However, in some studies, worse outcomes were noted in patients who experienced perioperative ↓BP.
  - o Continue beta blockers (don't start on day of surgery if not on, *POISE*, but can consider if intermediate/high risk at least 1 week before surgery)
  - o Continue statins; those not on them but at-risk, and undergoing vascular or intermediate risk surgery (with RFs) may benefit from starting statin preoperatively
- **Take home points**
  - o When to do stress test:
    - 1) poor/unknown fxl status
    - (2) >=3 risk predictors
    - (3) major vascular surgery
    - (4) results will change management
    - Chest pain in past week and symptoms are class 3/4
  - o When to skip stress test:
    - Pt had stress test in past 2 years and asymptomatic
    - PCI/CABG in past 5 years and remains asx
  - o If patient is cleared state: **"Pt is optimized medically and there are no further additional recommended tests necessary"**
  - o It is often helpful to give an estimate of the percentage risk of cardiac complications (see above, by risk class) so that the surgeons can make the most educated decision regarding whether or not to proceed with surgery.

Bibliography

[417] Wigle et al. Updated Guidelines on Outpatient Anticoagulation. Am Fam Physician. 2013;87(8):556-566.
[418] Moll. Stephan. "New insights into treatment of venous thromboembolism." Hematology 2014.
[419] Dubois et al. "Perioperative management of patients on direct oral anticoagulants." Thrombosis Journal. 2017. 15:14.
[420] Cohn SL. Preoperative Evaluation for Noncardiac Surgery. Ann Intern Med. ;165.
[421] Cohn et al. "2019 Update in perioperative cardiovascular medicine." CCJM: 86(10). 2019.
[422] N Engl J Med 2014; 370:1494-1503
[423] Hollmann C, Fernandes NL, Biccard BM. A systematic review of outcomes associated with withholding or continuing angiotensin-converting enzyme inhibitors and angiotensin receptor blockers before noncardiac surgery. Anesth Analg 2018; 127(3):678–687.
[424] Dobri et al. "How should we manage insulin therapy before surgery?" Cleveland Clinic Journal of Medicine. 80(11). November 2013.
[425] Alexandra Dretler MD, Dominique Williams MD, Mark Gdowski MD, Pavat Bhat MD, Rajeev Ramgopal MD, eds. 2016. Washington Manual® of Medical Therapeutics, The - 35th Ed.
[426] UCSF Hospitalist Handbook 2002

TOXICOLOGY

Alcohol Withdrawal 630
Urine Drug Testing 635
Overdose 637

ALCOHOL WITHDRAWAL

Effects of various concentrations of alcohol	
Concentration (mg/100cc = mg/dL)	Effect
30-50	Measurable impairment of motor skills
50-100	Reduced inhibitions, excitant effect
100-150	Loss of co-ordination and control
150-200	Drunkenness; nausea, ataxia
200-350	Vomiting, stupor, possible coma
350+	Respiratory paralysis, ?death

- **General**[427,428,429]
  - Symptoms that occur due to abrupt cessation of EtOH in a patient who has previous heavy use. Symptoms often start within 6-24h, peak at 72h, and diminish within 5-7d of abstinence.
  - Patients with high use prior to admission, consider prophylactic Librium (standing orders+prn)
- **Physical Exam/Diagnosis**
  - Initial Withdrawal Symptoms (minor withdrawal; onset 6-8 hours after last drink):
    - Tachycardia, hypertension, ↑body temperature, tremulousness, anxiety, nausea/vomiting, headache, diaphoresis, and palpitations
      - Patients taking beta blockers, or alpha-2 agonists may display blunted vital signs.
    - Alcohol Hallucinations (onset 12-24 hours after last drink):
    - 7–8% of patients with AWS
    - Tactile hallucinations common, visual less likely
    - Auditory hallucinations possible (sometimes persecutory)
    - May present with tremors and other withdrawal symptoms, though some do not
    - Normal sensorium
  - Withdrawal Seizures (12-48h after last drink)
    - Generalized tonic-clonic, though often isolated, short in duration, short post-ictal period
    - 1/3 of patients with withdrawal seizures will progress to delirium tremens
  - Delirium Tremens (begins 3 days after withdrawal symptoms start; lasts up to 8 days):
    - Criteria for DTs include ≥2 of the criteria for AWS and rapid-onset, fluctuating disturbances in orientation, memory, attention, awareness, visuospatial ability, or perception.
      - Diagnosis requires autonomic instability

Example CIWA Protocol		
CIWA Score	Lorazepam IV	Oxazepam (Serax) IV
	Recommended for patients with compromised hepatic function/hepatic encephalopathy, geriatric, high risk for respiratory depression/over sedation	For patients with history of withdrawal seizures or seizure disorder, need for a smoother withdrawal (fewer withdrawal symptoms, less breakthrough or rebound symptoms), or if withdrawal symptoms are not controlled on lorazepam
0-9	None	None
10-15	2mg	2.5mg

TOXICOLOGY

16-21	2mg	2.5mg
22-30	4mg	5mg
31-45	4mg	7.5mg
>45	Continuous IV Ativan	10mg
PRN breakthrough	1mg between scheduled doses	5mg between scheduled doses

- **Labs**
  - Carbohydrate Deficient Transferase (can detect EtOH use in past 2 weeks)
  - CBC, CMP, LFTs, Coags, ETOH level, Urine Tox
    - Monitor K, Mg, PO4, and Glucose specifically
- **Imaging**
  - CNS imaging should be considered in patients with AMS
- **Orders**
  - **CIWA order set available**
    - CIWA Score
      - < 8 = not yet in withdrawal
      - > 8 = withdrawing
      - > 25 = needs monitoring
    - When to Start The CIWA-Ar
      - What the client's history indicated a likelihood of withdrawal reaction-large amounts over a long period of time, history of withdrawal symptoms, and last drink within the past 12 hours. If history not evident, observe informally until symptoms occur-not all people develop withdrawal symptoms.
    - When to Stop The CIWA-Ar/Discharge Criteria
      - When the score is <10 after 3 consecutive assessments.
  - Elevate HOB > 30 degrees
  - Suction PRN orally
  - Thiamine 200mg (if DTs, then 500mg BID for 3 days) until resuming normal diet
  - MgSO4 2gm
  - VS q15min
- **Supportive Treatment**
  - NS+Banana Bag initially
  - Vitamin Supplements: Thiamine 100mg IV x3d, Folic Acid 1mg, & MVI PO when tolerating
  - Promethazine 12.5mg IV Q4H for nausea/vomiting
  - Benzodiazepines Regimens
    - Diazepam 10-20mg IV or PO q1h or q4h prn
    - Diazepam 5mg IV (if prn, repeat 10min later, then 10mg 10min later prn, etc.)
    - Ativan 2-4mg IV/IM/PO q15-20m prn, after 16mg administered and if delirium is still severe, administer 8mg bolus IV then 10-30mg/hr
    - Ativan 1-4mgIV q5-15m prn –or- 1-40mg IM q30-60m prn
  - Haldol (for uncontrolled agitation or hallucinations)
    - 0.5-5.0mg IV or IM q30-60m prn for severe agitation NOT TO EXCEED 20mg
    - 0.5-5.0mg PO q4h up to 30mg
- **Treatment**
  - Schedule Ativan/Serax if hx of complicated withdrawals
  - **Calculating Ativan Requirement**
    - Total # mg's in a day = # shots/beer
    - Use above to then calculate requirement per hour
  - Long-Acting/Prophylactic/Scheduled Therapy
    - *Best for preventing seizures (pt's with known DT's, seizures)*
      - Chlordiazepoxide [Librium]) – 10-25mg IV q6h based on severity of EtOH use

TOXICOLOGY

- Always have prn ativan on board
- Avoid if known marked liver disease
  - Short-Acting
    - *Used in elderly or when other conditions make you fearful of having prolonged sedation*
    - *Preferable in patients with known hepatic disease*
    - Serax 15-45 mg PO with Ativan 2mg Q6-8 hr
      - If in acute w/d, order Serax **scheduled** AND PRN to be given for CIWA > 8
      - If only h/o abuse without acute w/d symptoms, can order Serax PRN for CIWA >8
    - Valium 10mg PO Q6-8 hr x 24h, then 5mg PO TID-QID
  - Delirium Tremens
    - Thiamine 100mg IV BID for 3 days (if known Wernicke's, then 500mg IV qd or TID for 3 days)
    - MVI
- **Long term management (outpatient)**
  - Consider d/c to outpatient treatment facility for further management
  - Available medication-assisted treatments for EtOH cessation include acamprosate (666mg PO TID), naltrexone (50mg/d PO; 380mg IM q4w), and disulfiram (250mg daily PO)

History: duration and quantity of alcohol intake, time since last drink, previous episodes of alcohol withdrawal, concurrent substance use, preexisting medical and psychiatric conditions, prior detoxification admissions, prior seizure activity, living situation, social supports, stressors, triggers

Physical: VS (fever, tachycardia, tachypnea, hypertension), **CIWA** (see below), **MSE** (arousal, orientation, hallucinations), **HEENT** (diaphoresis, scleral icterus), **CV** (arrhythmias, M/R/G), evaluate s/sx of liver failure (ascites, varices, caput medusae, asterixis, palmar erythema), neuro (nystagmus, tremor, seizure activity)

Include assessment of conditions likely to *complicate*, *exacerbate*, or *precipitate* alcohol withdrawal: arrhythmias, CHF, CAD, dehydration, GI bleeding, infections, liver disease, pancreatitis, neurologic deficits.

Clinical Institute Withdrawal Assessment (CIWA) of Alcohol Scale

- Nausea and vomiting 0–7 (0, none; 4, intermittent; 7, constant nausea: frequent dry heaves/vomiting)
- Tremor 0–7 (0, none; 4, moderate; 7, severe; even with arms not extended)
- Paroxysmal sweats 0–7 (0, none; 4, beads of sweat; 7, drenching sweats)
- Anxiety 0–7 (0, none; 4, moderate; 7, acute panic state)
- Agitation 0–7 (0, none; 4, moderately restless; 7, constantly thrashing about or pacing)
- Tactile disturbances 0–7 (0, none; 4–7 for hallucinations; 1–3 for pruritus or paresthesias)
- Auditory disturbances 0–7 (0, none; 4–7 for hallucinations; 1–3 for increased sensitivity)
- Visual disturbances 0–7 (0, none; 4–7 for hallucinations; 1–3 for increased sensitivity)
- Headache 0–7 (0, no headache; 4, moderate; 7, extremely severe)
- Orientation 0–4 (0, fully oriented; 1, cannot do serial additions or is uncertain about date; 2, disoriented to date but within 2 calendar days; 3, disoriented to date by >2 days; 4, disoriented to place or person)

Mild withdrawal—CIWA 0–7 onset 5–8 hours after cessation or significant decrease in consumption: anxiety, restlessness, agitation, mild nausea, decreased appetite, sleep disturbance, facial sweating, mild tremulousness, fluctuating tachycardia and hypertension, possible mild cognitive impairment

Moderate withdrawal—CIWA 8–14 onset 24–72 hours after cessation: marked restlessness and agitation, moderate tremulousness with constant eye movement, diaphoresis, nausea, vomiting, anorexia, diarrhea

Severe withdrawal/delirium tremens—CIWA 15–30 onset 72–96 hours after alcohol cessation: marked tremulousness, fever, drenching sweats, severe hypertension and tachycardia, delirium

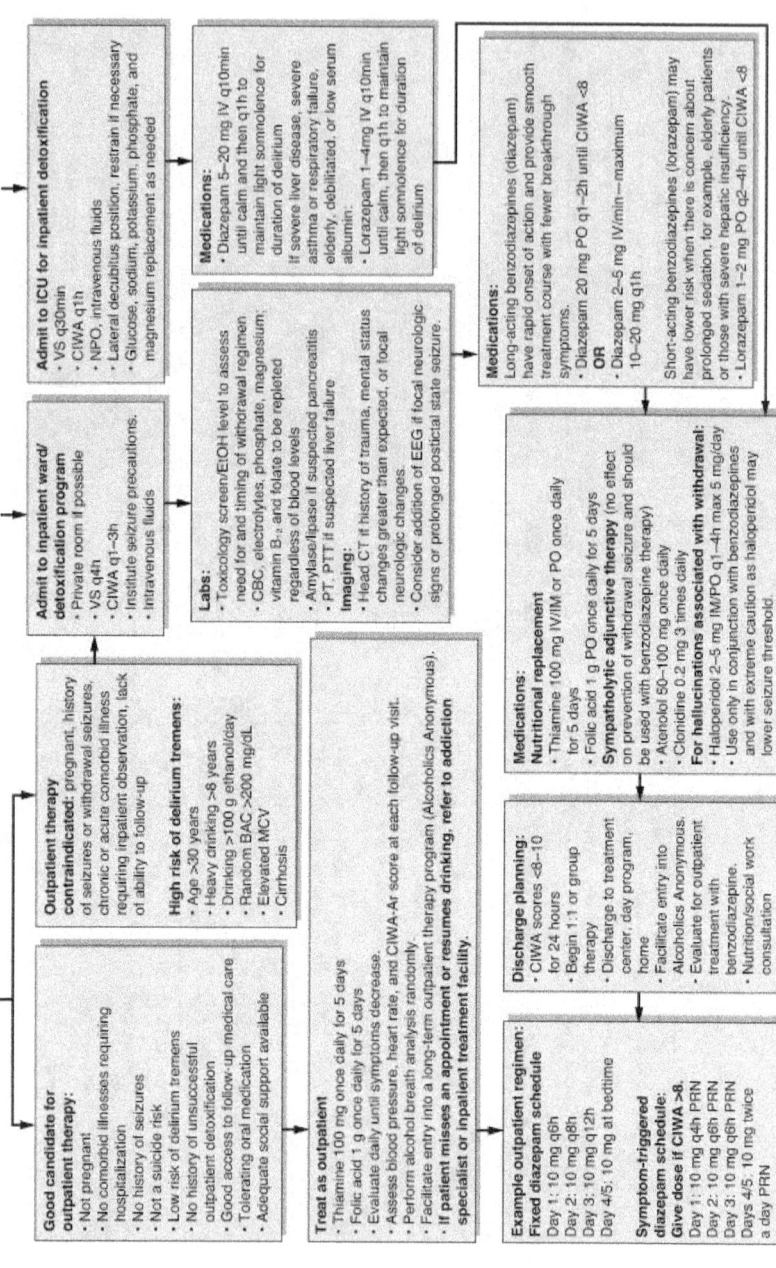

URINE DRUG TESTING

- **Pearls**
  - Fentanyl does not show up on standard 5-item UDS testing
- **General Information**[430,431,432]
  - Specimens collected in the early morning have the highest concentration and therefore will contain higher levels of the drug.
  - Adulteration or dilution of the urine specimen should be suspected if the pH is less than 3 or greater than 11 or the specific gravity is less than 1.002 or greater than 1.030.
  - Urine drug testing for marijuana is based on THC's main metabolite 11-nor-delta-9-tetrahydrocannabinol-9-carboxylic acid.
    - Detection of marijuana can occur in the urine for greater than 30 days after cessation among chronic users, whereas single exposure to marijuana in nonusers typically can be detected in the urine only up to 72 hours.
    - Medications reported to cross-react with cannabinoid immunoassays include proton pump inhibitors (PPIs), nonsteroidal anti-inflammatory drugs (NSAIDs), and efavirenz.
- **Confirmatory Testing**
  - The basic principle of confirming a positive drug test is to retest the same urine sample with a different type of test. Gas chromatography / mass spectrometry (GC / MS) is the procedure generally accepted by the scientific community for the confirmed identification of drugs of abuse.

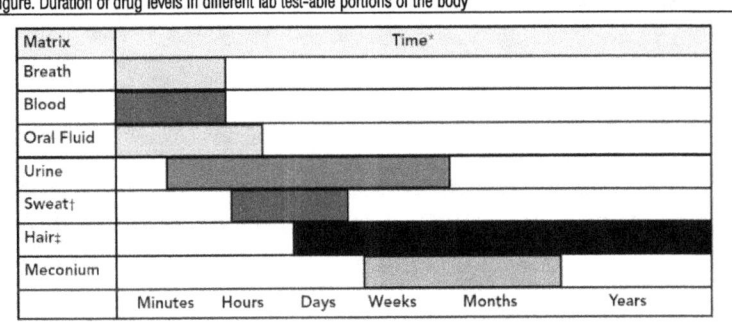

Figure. Duration of drug levels in different lab test-able portions of the body

TOXICOLOGY

Approximate Drug Detection Time in the Urine

Drug	Urine	Hair	Saliva	Sweat
Alcohol	7-12 h	N/A	24h	N/A
Amphetamine	2d	Up to 90d	1h-2d	7-14d
Methamphetamine	2d	Up to 90d	1h-2d	7-14d
Barbiturate				
Short-acting (e.g., pentobarbital)	1d	Up to 90d	N//A	N/A
Long-acting (e.g., phenobarbital)	3 wks.			
Benzodiazepine				
Short-acting (may not detect alprazolam, clonazepam, or lorazepam)	3 d	Up to 90d	N//A	N/A
Long-acting (eg, diazepam)	30 d			
Cocaine metabolites	2-4 d	Up to 90d	1-36h	7-14d
Marijuana				
Single use	3 d	Up to 90d	Up to 24h	7-14d
Moderate use (4 times/wk.)	5-7 d			
Chronic use (daily)	10-15 d			
Chronic heavy smoker	>30 d			
Opioids				
Codeine	2-4d	Up to 90d	1-36h	7-14d
Heroin (morphine)	2-3d	Up to 90d	1-36h	7-14d
Hydromorphone	2-4 d	Up to 90d	1-36h	7-14d
Methadone	3 d			
Morphine	48-72 h	Up to 90d	1-36h	7-14d
Oxycodone	2-4 d			
Synthetic cannabinoids				
Single use	72 h			
Chronic use	>72 h			
Synthetic cathinone	Variable			

TOXICOLOGY

OVERDOSE

- Poison control hotline: 1-800-222-1222
- Charcoal 1g/kg with sorbitol for unknown exposures, coma cocktail (see page 438)

Medications associated with overdose

Substance	Symptoms	Labs/Work-up	Treatment
Acetaminophen	N/V with asymptomatic period with abdominal pain, n, v, and jaundice	>150 ug/dl after 4 hours LFTs ↑ @ 12 hours, peak 4-6 hours (AST and ALT > 10,000) Obtain acetaminophen levels 4 hours post-acute ingestion to plot below Use Rumack-Matthews nomogram to dictate treatment in patients with acute treatment when time of ingestion is <u>known</u> and has been validated for use only up to 24 hours after ingestion	

	Treatment
	Charcoal if within 30 minutes of presentation
	
	NAC
	Time Known Ingestion
	1. Plot the APAP concentration onto the Rumack-Matthew nomogram.
	2. If the level will not return before 8 hours from the time of ingestion, begin NAC pending the level.
	3. If the level plots above the 150 (mg/mL) treatment line, begin NAC.
	4. Two regimens equally effective and if patient is above the treatment line in R-M nomogram within 8 hours of ingestion:
	   a. 140 mg/kg load then 70 mg/kg q4h x 15-20 doses
	   b. 150 mg/kg IV over 15min followed by 50 mg/kg over the next 4 hours @ 12.5 mg/kg/h and then 100mg/kg over the next 16 hours (@ 6.25 mg/kg/h)
	
	Time Unknown Ingestion
	1. Obtain serum APAP level and serum AST and ALT levels.
	2. If APAP is less than 10 mg/mL and the AST and ALT are normal, no treatment is necessary.
	3. If either the APAP level is detectable more than 10 mg/mL or either the AST or ALT are elevated more than the reference range and not otherwise explained, begin NAC treatment.
	4. Continue NAC until APAP is less than 10 mg/mL and the AST and ALT have peaked and are improving and there are no other signs of hepatic dysfunction, including INR of 1.3 or less.		

Anticholinergics	Flushing, dry skin, mydriasis, AMS, fever	↑HR, BCx, Ucx, ABG, HCG, ECG	If presenting <1h, use activated charcoal Physostigmine 0.5-2.0mg slow IV push if hemodynamically unstable otherwise no antidote may be needed
ASA	n/v, tinnitus, GI bleed	Anion gap metabolic acidosis ↑ serum salicylate	Active. charcoal NaHCO3 to goal pH 7.4-7.5 Hemodialysis
Beta Blocker	Nonspecific, look at vitals for evidence	↓BP, ↓HR, ECG with ↑PR, ↑K, ↑QRS, ↓glucose	IVF bolus Atropine 1mg IVP Glucagon 5mg IV bolus for BP<90 then infusion of 75-150mg/kg/h CaCl 10-20cc of 10% in central line
Benzodiazepine	CNS depression, slurred speech, ataxia, AMS	FS, ECG, HCG	Do not use activated charcoal <u>Intoxication</u>: Flumazenil 0.2mg IV over 15s repeated after 45s and again each subsequent minute until sedation reversed

TOXICOLOGY

Medications associated with overdose

Substance	Symptoms	Labs/Work-up	Treatment
			(max 1mg) Overdose: Flumazenil 0.2mg IV over 30s, 0.3mg after 30s if no response and up to 0.5mg each subsequent 30s interval to total dose 3mg
Cholinergics	Garlic like odor exposure	N/A	Atropine 0.5-2mg IV up to 5mg IV q15min if severe Pralidoxime 2g at 0.5g/min
Lithium	Altered MS, tremor, hyperreflexia, vomiting, diarrhea	↑lithium level	NaHCO3 to urine Volume replacement Dialysis if level >4 mEq/L
SSRI	Somnolence, agitation	--	Supportive
TCA	Dilated pupils, dry mouth, tachycardia, ileus, urinary retention	Widened QRS AV block	Activated charcoal NaHCO3 3 amps (50 mg/50 mL) in 1 L D5W at 2–3 mL/kg/h Lidocaine
Methanol	Altered MS Seizures Visual disturbance, Blindness	Anion gap metabolic acidosis with elevated osmolar gap	Within 1-2 hours = gastric lavage >50mg/dL = immediate hemodialysis (>50 mg/dl) IV fomepizole Folic acid 50-100mg q4-24h
Opiates	Myosis, ↓RR	N/A	Dosing: - IV/SQ: Narcan 0.4mg (can do 0.2mg initially if patient is opiate naïve) repeated q3-5 minutes - Intranasal: 4.0mg intranasal repeated q3-5 minutes until effect. - Drip: often done in patients on methadone; use 2/3 of total effective dose of naloxone per hour (typically 0.25-6.25mg/hr) and provide ½ of that bolus dose about 15 minutes after starting the drip to prevent a drop in naloxone levels
Ethylene Glycol	Oxalate crystals in urine Fluorescence of urine in woods lamp	Anion gap metabolic acidosis Elevated osmolar gap	Within 1-2 hours = gastric lavage Severe = immediate hemodialysis (>20 mg/dl) IV fomepizole

TOXICOLOGY

Bibliography

[427] Frank J. Domino, MD, ed. 2014. 5-Minute Clinical Consult - 22nd Ed. Philadelphia, PA. Lippincott Williams & Wilkins Health. ISBN-10: 1-4511-8850-1, ISBN-13: 978-1-4511-8850-9. STAT!Ref Online Electronic Medical Library. https://online.statref.com/Document.aspx?fxId=31&docId=200. 8/12/2013 2:38:53 AM CDT (UTC -05:00).

[428] Long D, et al, The emergency medicine management of severe alcohol withdrawal, American Journal of Emergency Medicine (2017).

[429] Frank J. Domino, MD, Jeremy Golding, MD, FAAFP, Mark B. Stephens, MD, Robert A. Baldor MD, FAAFP, eds. 2019. 5-Minute Clinical Consult - 27th Ed. Philadelphia, PA. Lippincott Williams & Wilkins Health.

[430] Moeller, Karen E. et al. "Clinical Interpretation of Urine Drug Tests." Mayo Clinic Proceedings. Volume 92, Issue 5, 774 – 796.

[431] Hadland et al. "OBJECTIVE TESTING – URINE AND OTHER DRUG TESTS." Child Adolesc Psychiatr Clin N Am. 2016 Jul; 25(3): 549–565.

[432] Urine Drug Screening: Practical Guide for Clinicians Moeller, Karen E. et al. Mayo Clinic Proceedings, Volume 83, Issue 1, 66 - 76

WOMENS HEALTH

Abnormal Uterine Bleeding..................641
Polycystic Ovarian Syndrome (PCOS)..................643
Menopause..................644
Contraception..................645
Emergency Contraception..................651
Menorrhagia..................652

ABNORMAL UTERINE BLEEDING

Contributor: Loren Walwyn-Tross, MD

- **Overview**[433,434]
    - Normal Menstrual Cycle
        - 5 Days: average duration of menstrual flow
        - 21-35 days: duration of avg menstrual cycle
        - 5- 80cc
    - Physiology Review
        - Anterior pituitary release LH and FSH → FSH leads to ovarian production of estrogen and proliferation of the endometrium while LH surge leads to ovulation.
        - The corpus luteum produces progesterone which stabilizes the endometrium
        - The loss of estrogen leads to sloughing of the endometrium
- **Types**
    - Acute – heavy bleeding warranting intervention to prevent further loss
    - Chronic – abnormal volume of bleeding, regularity, or timing present for 6 months
- **Causes**
    - Non-pregnant vs. Pregnant
        - Non-pregnant: menses, DUB, leiomyoma, polyp, trauma
        - Pregnant: threatened abortion, spontaneous abortion, ectopic pregnancy
    - Structural – polyps, adenomyosis, leiomyoma, malignancy, ovarian cyst, PCOS, liver dz
    - Non-structural – coagulopathy, ovulatory dysfunction, endometrial, iatrogenic, unknown, eating disorder, thyroid d/o, medications (antiepileptics, antipsychotics)
- **Evaluation/History**
    - Age of menarche
    - Menstrual bleeding pattern
    - Bleeding severity
    - Pain
    - Medical conditions
    - Surgical hx
    - Medications
- **Exam**
    - Pelvic exam
- **Labs**
    - HCG, TSH, PRL
    - CBC, COAG, G/C
- **Imaging**
    - TV ultrasound
    - Saline infused sonohysterography
    - MRI

WOMENS HEALTH

Acute Bleeding	Chronic Bleeding
Conjugated equine estrogen 25mg IV q4-6h x24h with IV anti-nausea medications	Ibuprofen 800 mg q8h or naproxen 500 mg initially then repeat 3-5 h later, then 250-500 mg BID
Monophasic 35-mg estrogen-containing OCP (i.e. Sronyx, Provera 20mg) TID for 7 d, then 1 tablet daily	Monophasic 30- to 35-mg estrogen containing OCP daily with or without inert pills
Medroxyprogesterone 20 mg or norethindrone 20 mg TID for 7d	Medroxyprogesterone 5-10 mg or norethindrone 5-10 mg daily
Tranexamic acid 10 mg/kg IV (maximum, 600 mg per dose) or 1.5 g orally every 8 h for 5d	Depot medroxyprogesterone 150 mg subcutaneously q 3 mo
	Levonorgestrel 19.5- to 52-mg intrauterine devices for 5 y (19.5-mg LNG IUS is a slightly smaller device)
	Etonogestrel subdermal implant x 3 y
	Tranexamic acid 1.5 g orally TID for 5 d with menses

- **Management**
  See table above as well as options below
  - Ovulatory
    - Levonorgestrel-releasing intrauterine system 20mcg per 24 hours
    - Medroxyprogesterone acetate 10mg PO TID for 21 days/month
    - TXA 1.3g PO TID for 5 days/month
    - Ibuprofen 600-1200mg/d 5 days
    - Naproxen 550-1100mg/d 5 days
  - Anovulatory
    - Combined OCP with 20-35mcg of ethinyl estradiol-monophasic
    - Medroxyprogesterone 10mg/d x14d

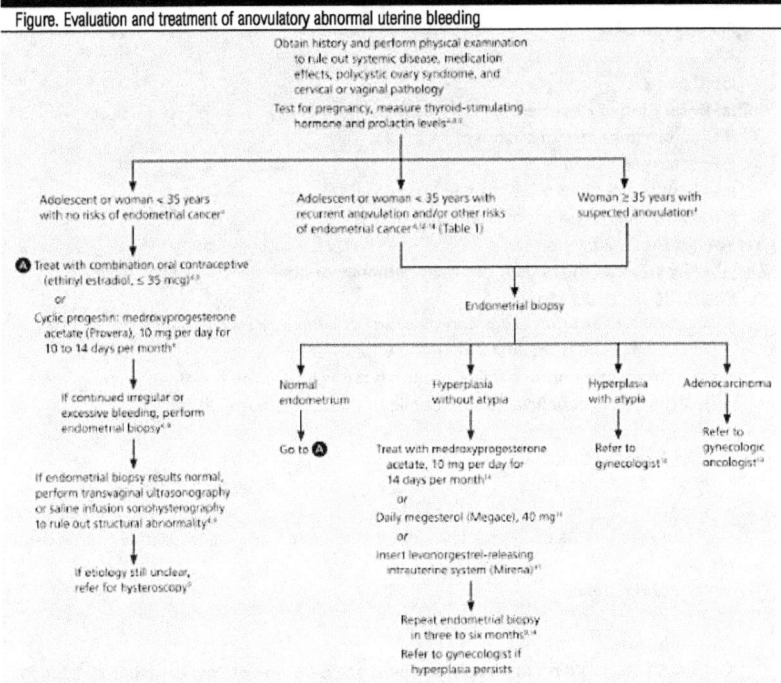

Figure. Evaluation and treatment of anovulatory abnormal uterine bleeding

POLYCYSTIC OVARIAN SYNDROME (PCOS)

- **Pearls**[435]
  - Etiology is unknown
  - Associated with hirsutism, obesity as well as an increased risk of diabetes mellitus, cardiovascular disease, and metabolic syndrome
  - Affects 5–10% of women of reproductive age
  - Usually presents with menstrual irregularities and hyperandrogenism
  - Pelvic US is not required to make the diagnosis but is recommended in patients with high suspicion for androgen-secreting tumors
  - OCPs and weight loss is the preferred treatment
- **Clinical Exam**
  - Pts often present with menstrual disorder (amenorrhea to menorrhagia) and infertility
  - May have associated hirsutism and acne along with male pattern blood loss
- **Differential**
  - Hypothalamic amenorrhea 2/2 stress, weight loss, exercise
  - Obesity
  - ↓T4
  - ↑PRL
  - Cushing's
- **Diagnosis**
  - Clinical or biochemical evidence of hyperandrogenism
  - Anovulation or oligo ovulation
  - PCO on US
- **Labs**

- FSH, LH, TSH, DHEAS
- Fasting glucose
- A1c
- Lipid panel
- **Initial Evaluation of Hirsutism**
  - R/O common causes of hirsutism
    - s/e to medication
  - If only mild, consider cosmetic treatment or OCP
  - If moderate/severe, perform AM testosterone
- **Treatment for PCOS**
  Dictated by whether the patient desires pregnancy or not
  - Wishes to become pregnant
    - Clomiphene or other drugs can be used for ovulatory stimulation
      - Clomiphene is the first-line therapy for infertility
    - Metformin can improve menstruation but has little or no benefit in treating infertility; it is beneficial for metabolic or glucose abnormalities
    - Weight loss
  - Does not desire pregnancy
    - Medroxyprogesterone acetate, 10 mg daily orally for the first 10 days of each month
    - If contraception is desired, a low-dose combination oral contraceptive can be used
  - Weight loss
- **Treatment of Hirsutism**
  - OCP
  - Anti-androgens
    - CPA 50-100 mg/d on menstrual cycle on day 5-15 with ethinyl estradiol 20-35 mcg on day 5-25
    - Spironolactone 100-200mg/d (divided BID)
    - Finasteride 2.5-5mg/d

MENOPAUSE

- **Defined** - physiologic event characterized by loss of ovarian activity and permanent cessation of menses, diagnosed after **12 consecutive months** of amenorrhea.[436,437]
- **Symptoms** (typically last 4-10 years)
  - Hot flashes
  - Night sweats
  - Insomnia
  - Vaginal atrophy
  - Sexual dysfunction
- **Labs**
  - Not typically obtained but can be used to stage menopause
  - Estradiol (<20 pcg/mL may indicate menopause)
  - FSH (>30-40 miu/mL)
- **Treatment**
  - Vasomotor symptoms best treated with systemic therapy; genitourinary symptoms (vaginal atrophy) can be treated with topical therapy
  - Stroke risk is lower in transdermal hormonal preparations vs. PO therapy
  - Duration advised not to exceed past 65 years of age (ACOG) or less than 5 years (AACE, ACE)
    - Vasomotor Symptoms

- Hormonal Therapy (<60 YO, within 10 years of menopause, moderate to severe sx severity)
  - Conjugated estrogen 0.625mg/day (Premarin) or micronized 17-beta-estradiol 1mg/day (can give transdermal as well)
  - When stopping therapy, taper over last 3-5 years; if cannot taper d/t persistent bothersome sx, consider transdermal therapy or minimize dose and try extended duration
  - Medroxyprogesterone acetate 2.5mg/day or micronized progesterone 100mg/day
- Non-Hormonal (>60 YO, >10 years from menopause, h/o CVA, ACS, PE, breast CA, CVD, VTE)
  - SSRI
    - Paroxetine 10-25mg/d (avoid if taking tamoxifen)
    - Paroxetine salt 7.5mg/d
    - Escitalopram 10-20mg/d
    - Others with less supportive data: citalopram 10-20mg/d and fluoxetine 20mg/d
  - SNRI
    - Venlafaxine 37.5-75mg/d
    - Desvenlafaxine 75mg daily or BID
  - Gabapentin 300mg QHS (up to 900mg in divided doses)
  - Pregabalin 75-150mg BID
  - Nonpharmacologics:
    - CBT
    - Black cohosh (not superior to placebo)
    - Hypnosis
- Genitourinary Symptoms (vaginal dryness, painful sex)
  - If no systemic symptoms, can use topical lubricants only (water or silicone based) or local conjugated vaginal hormone creams
  - If using hormonal therapies in patients with history of breast cancer, consider Oncology consult and using the lowest dose possible
- *Mild symptoms* - respond to CBT or behavioral modification
- *Moderate symptoms* - may require pharmacologic intervention (SSRI if contraindication to systemic estrogen (i.e. h/o breast CA, CVD, endometrial CA, liver dz, h/o clots), systemic hormones if no contraindication)
  - Intact uterus → use estrogen+progesterone
  - S/p hysterectomy → can use estrogen alone
- Unopposed estrogen should never be used in women with an intact uterus (add progestin)

CONTRACEPTION

Contributor: Dr. Natasha Pyzocha

- **Pearls**[438,439]
  - Breastfeeding – progestin only is safe; avoid restarting combined hormone pills until 6 weeks post-delivery (alternative option is barrier method)
  - Start PNV at visit if patients are sexually active and in child-bearing age
  - Decrease estrogen content if want to decrease bleeding amount during periods
- **PMHx That May Alter Management**
  With the below conditions, if present, consider non-hormonal options or progestin-only contraception

WOMENS HEALTH

- - Severe decompensated cirrhosis
  - Migraines with aura (will worsen)
  - CAD risk factors (Uncontrolled HTN >160/100, smoker, DM)
  - Active smoker (↑risk for thrombosis) - >35 pack year history smoking >15 cig/d
  - Breast/Endometrial/HCC/Cervical cancer history
  - Recent surgery
  - DM
- **Permanent Contraception**
  - Vasectomy vs tubal ligation (not necessarily 100%)
  - Hysterectomy
    - 99% effective with side effects including scrotal pain/epididymitis
  - Neither is easily reversed
- **Initiating Contraception**
  - Quick Start Method
    - First day of LMP <5 days ago → start today
    - First day of LMP >5 days ago → do HCG and initiate therapy with condom use concurrently for 1 week
- **Common side effects from contraception**
  - HA/nausea/mastalgia – likely due to estrogen excess; try dosing QHS vs. using a low estrogen pill (understand this ↑↑ risk for breakthrough bleeding)
  - Hirsutism/acne/weight gain – likely due to progestin and/or androgen excess; try changing to 3rd generation progestin
  - Mood changes or ↓ libido – due to progestin excess; as above, change to 3rd gen progestin
  - Breakthrough bleeding – often multifactorial in causes; first rule out other causes such as polyps or infection, consider changing to continuous cycle treatment or chest to triphasic preparation
  - Amenorrhea – get a pregnancy test and if negative, reassure patient but if they desire a period then ↑ estrogen content or chose a progestin with ↑endometrial activity such as 1mg norethindrone to 5mg

Contraception Options Based on MOA

	Combined OCP	Progestin Only	Vaginal Ring	Patch	Nexplanon	IUD	Depo-Provera
MOA	Inhibits ovulation with estrogen and progestin	Thickens mucus in cervix to prevent sperm from attaching, may stop ovulation	Prevents ovulation with estrogen and progestin	Prevents ovulation with estrogen and progestin	Prevents ovulation Progestin only	Copper: spermicide and disrupts implantation. Mirena: progestin and disrupts implantation	Prevents ovulation as a progestin only
Efficacy (perfect use)	93%	93%	93%	93%	99.9%	99.2%	96%
S/E	Blood clots, MI, CVA	**Irregular bleeding**	Blood clots, MI, CVA Vaginal discharge	Blood clots, MI, CVA	Irregular bleeding Headaches Weight gain Mood changes	Irregular bleeding Migration possible ↑ risk for PID	Irregular bleeding ?weight gain (5#)
Notes	Needs to be taken every day to be effective!	Good for breastfeeding moms Needs to be taken daily	3 weeks on, **1 week off** Good if can't remember to take pills	New patch qweek then no patch on 4th week Not effective if >200#	Lasts 3 years Reversible Expensive $$$ Good if can't remember to take pills	Mirena: lasts 5 years Copper: lasts 10 years Best for stable monogamous relationships	Lasts 12 weeks May take up to 18 months for fertility to return Reversible osteopenia
Example Options	**Sronyx** Yaz Ortho Tri Cyclin **Seasonique** Loestrin	Minipill Nor-QD Nexplanon (see right)	NuvaRing	Ortho evra		Copper Mirena	Depo-Provera

Contraception Options Explained[440]

IUD

- Very effective, no maintenance; good option for women who desire to avoid pregnancy for >3 y; avoids estrogen exposure
- <u>Contraindications</u>: Uterine distortion, active pelvic infection (wait 3 mos. before insertion), women w/ ↑risk for STIs, pregnancy, unexplained uterine bleeding, active cervical/endometrial CA; not contraindicated in adolescents/young adults or nulliparous women

Name	Dosing	Info	Side Effects/C/I	Effectiveness	Pearls
ParaGard	N/A	Stable monogamous relationship with low risk for STD; <1% failure rate	Heavy or painful periods, iron deficiency anemia, severe distortion of uterine cavity, copper allergy or Wilson disease, active pelvic infection	10-12 years	Heavier menses Contains copper Can be used for 10 years
Mirena				5 years for Kyleena 3 years if Skyla Liletta and Mirena are effective up to 7 years	Lighter bleeds/Amenorrhea Irregular bleeds and spotting in first month are common Risk for ectopic pregnancy **place during start of menses because cervical os is largest**
Copper				10 years	Releases copper continuously into uterine cavity, interferes w/ sperm transport, prevents fertilization;

Injectable

Name	Dosing	Info	Side Effects/C/I	Effectiveness	Pearls
Nexplanon	Placed subdermally in upper arm, approved for 3 years, effective to 4 years		Overweight Psych history Hx of HA Planned pregnancy in the next year (~delayed return of fertility)	3 years	Reversible with rapid return of fertility upon removal Placed @ start of menses S/E: irregular bleeds, weight gain, HA, depression, emotional lability

Oral

- Monophasic (Yaz) vs Multiphasic (Ortho Tri Cyclin)
- Estrogen dose varies from 10mcg, 20mcg, 25, 30, 50 (goal is <35mcg)
- Cyclic vs Continuous Dose (21:7, 24:3, 84:7, 365 days)
- Combined pill: stops ovaries from releasing egg/monthly; small chance of blood clots, CVD. Should not be used if >30YO+smoke. May cause irreg. bleeds
- Progestin only: thickens mucous and may stop ovarian release of egg; may cause irregular bleeding

Initiation:
- Quick start – preferred method; take first dose as soon as prescription filled
- 1st day start – take first pill on 1st day of period
- Sunday start – take first pill on Sunday after period begins

Pattern of use:
- Cyclic (21 active pills → 7 hormone free pills)
- Extended cycle regimen (e.g., 84 active pills → 7 hormone-free pill)
- Continuously

Combination / Extended Cycle			
Seasonique 20 mcg E/0.1mcg P	1 tab x91d, repeat Take 84 levonogestrel+ethinyl estr tabs then 7 ethinyl estradiol tabs	Only 4 periods/year	N/A
Lybrel 20 mcg E/90mcg P	1 tab/d	Continuous so **no** periods	0.15mg levonogestrel 30mcg estradiol Q3M periods
Ortho Tri-Cyclen	1 tab x28d, repeat		No breakthrough period, used continuously 18mcg ethinyl estradiol1 Decreases acne
Combination Monophasic			
Sronyx	1 tab x 28d, repeat		20mcg estradiol
Yaz	1 tab x 28d, repeat		20mcg estradiol Decreases acne

Micronor (Minipill)	1 tab/d	Progestin only; taken daily by mouth with no off week			Safe for women who are breast-feeding (should not reduce milk supply). Patients should start taking the pill two weeks after delivery.
Patch					
Ortho-Evra	20 μg EE, 150 μg norelgestromin; apply q1wk for 3 weeks then 1 week off	Apply to buttock, abdomen, upper arm, or upper torso	Hx of skin pathology Wt>195lb Hx of CVA/TIA	1 week	92% effective 1x each week x 3 weeks and stop on 4th week
Xulane	Single patch changed weekly for 3wk then off for 1 wk (for withdrawal bleed)				Efficacy depends on user compliance
IM					
Depo-Provera	N/A	N/A	Hx of osteoporosis Desire to become pregnant quickly (delay in 18 months after cessation)	3 months	97% effective Irregular bleeds in first few months; amenorrhea common after 1 year of use
Ring					
Nuvaring	15 μg EE, 150 μg etonogestrel; flexibleplastic ring inserted by pt; intravaginal x 3 wk, removed x 1 wk; new ring every month	Patient desires low doses of hormones	Hx of vaginal discharge or UTI	3 weeks	92% effective 1 ring q 3 weeks Higher risk for UTI
Barrier					
Condom	N/A	Reversible; STD prevention	N/A		85% effective in males 80% effective in females
Diaphragm with spermicide		See above			80% effective

EMERGENCY CONTRACEPTION

- Refer patients to not-2-late.com[441,442]
- Regimen should be used as soon as possible after sex but appear to have some efficacy through at least 4 to 5 days after sex (some studies say no more than 72 hours).
- Neither regimen has any contraindications.
- The most commonly used oral emergency contraceptive regimen is the **progestin-only pill**, which consists of 1.5 mg of levonorgestrel (see table below).
- The levonorgestrel regimen is labeled for use for up to 72 hours after unprotected sex but is best used as soon as possible after unprotected sex
- **The copper IUD is the most effective option**
- Patients should have STI screen
- Pregnancy test if no menses in 3-4 weeks
- The most effective method of emergency contraception is the copper intrauterine device, which almost eliminates the risk of pregnancy resulting from recent unprotected sex and can be used for ongoing contraception for at least 10 years. It is contraindicated if active cervicitis or PID is present.
- If starting routine contraception after, start after the next menstrual period and use a barrier method in the interim
- You can also use a different dose of a number of brands of regular birth control pills. While these are not sold specifically as emergency contraceptive pills, they have been proven safe and effective for preventing pregnancy in the few days after sex. You take the first dose as soon as possible (up to 120 hours after you have sex without using birth control, your birth control failed, or you were made to have sex against your will. You take the second dose **12 hours later.**

Name	Formulation	Timing of Use from Intercourse Date	Access	FDA
Aftera	1 tablet	Up to 3 days	OTC	Y
After Pill	1 pill	Up to 3 days	OTC	Y
Copper IUD (most effective)	N/A	Up to 5 days (? up to 10)	Office visit	N
OCP	Variety	Up to 5 days	Office visit	Y
Ulipristal acetate (Ella) (best pill option)	1 tablet (30 mg)	Up to 5 days	Office visit	Y
Yuzpe (EE 200mcg; Norg 2mg)	200mcg ethinyl estradiol 2mg norgestrel/1mg LNG	Up to 3 days	Office visit	Y

MENORRHAGIA

- **Defined**[443] - widely defined as menstrual blood loss (MBL) of 80 mL or more per cycle based on the research undertaken by Hallberg et al. in the 1960s
- **Risks** – ↑↑ risk for iron deficiency anemia; 20% of patients will have underlying coagulation disorder (ask if family history of heavy bleeding, ask if heavy bleeding since menarche)
- **Assessment**
    - Menstrual History – cycle length, duration of menses, passage of clots or flooding, how frequently changing tampons, symptoms of anemia. History of irregular bleeding should ↑ suspicion for uterine pathology
    - Quality of life – limitations at work, exercise, social functions
    - Bleeding history
- **Causes** – those that are underlined can be distinguished through imaging/visualization or histology
    - Polyps
    - Adenomyosis
    - Leiomyoma
    - Malignancy
    - Hyperplasia
    - Coagulopathy
        - Von Willebrand disease (13% prevalence) – ask about bleeding with brushing teeth, tooth extraction, post-partum, epistaxis, bruising, excessive bleeding with minor lacerations
        - Platelet Function Disorders (PFD)
    - Ovulatory dysfunction
    - Endometrial
    - Iatrogenic
    - Other/Not classified
- **Labs**
    - Obtain HCG to r/o pregnancy, ectopic, etc.
    - CBC
    - Iron panel
    - PT/PTT
    - TSH/PRL
    - HFP if suspecting liver disease
- **Imaging**
    - Pelvic US to r/o lesions
- **Treatment Options**

Treatment modalities for menorrhagia

Other	Hormonal	Hemostatic	Surgical
NSAIDS – first line therapy with success in up to 46% of patients by directly acting on prostaglandin levels. Treatment should only be for 5 days. Options include naproxen and diclofenac	*Oral progestin's are most commonly prescribed for menorrhagia. Oral therapy for 21 continuous days (starting on day 5 of cycle) can reduce menstrual related blood loss. Higher satisfaction scores in patients are seen with the levonorgestrel-releasing IUD* • Progestin-releasing IUD – the most common is levonorgestrel-releasing IUD which is a good option if females want to maintain a form of contraception. Major s/e are spotting, pain. • Combined Hormonal Contraception – another good option if form of contraception remains desired. Major s/e were related to the hormones themselves. The only FDA approved form is estradiol valerate and dienogest (Natazia). This form is contraindicated in women with a h/o migraines w/aura, VTE, breast cancer. • Cyclic oral Progestogens – short-phase which are administered for <14 days; poor evidence.	• TXA – effective in stopping bleeding but does not affect the actual cycle itself. • DDAVP – specifically indicated for heavy bleeding in women with mild history of inherited coagulopathy.	Endometrial ablation

Bibliography

[433] Armstrong C. ACOG guidelines on noncontraceptive uses of hormonal contraceptives. Am Fam Physician. 2010;82(3):288-295. doi:10.1097/AOG.0b013e3181cb50b5.

[434] Mamach et al. "Evaluation and Management of Abnormal Uterine Bleeding." Mayo Clin Proc. 2019;94(2):326-335.

[435] Polycystic Ovary Syndrome (Persistent Anovulation). In: Papadakis MA, McPhee SJ, Bernstein J. eds. Quick Medical Diagnosis & Treatment 2018 New York, NY: McGraw-Hill; . http://accessmedicine.mhmedical.com/content.aspx?bookid=2273&sectionid=178303475. Accessed March 25, 2018.

[436] ACOG Practice Bulletin No. 141: Management of menopausal symptoms. (2014, January). Retrieved from https://www.ncbi.nlm.nih.gov/pubmed/24463691

[437] Pinkerton, JoAnn V. N Engl J Med 2020; 382:446-455

[438] Contraceptive Use, Centers for Disease Control and Prevention, http://www.cdc.gov/reproductivehealth/unintendedpregnancy/usmec.htm. 11Sept2015.

[439] Kiefer et al. "Pocket Primary Care."

[440] Raymond EG, Cleland K. Emergency contraception. *N Engl J Med* 2015;372:1342-1348. doi:10.1056/NEJMcp1406328.

[441] Raymond EG, Cleland K. Emergency contraception. *N Engl J Med* 2015;372:1342-1348. doi:10.1056/NEJMcp1406328.

[442] Practice Bulletin No. 152: Emergency Contraception. Obstet Gynecol. 2015;126(3):e1-11.

[443] Davies, Joanna et al. "Heavy menstrual bleeding: An update on management." Thrombosis Research. Volume 151 , S70 - S77.

UROLOGY

Hematuria 656

BPH 657

Testicular Pain 658

Overactive Bladder 659

Urinary Incontinence 661

HEMATURIA

- **Diagnosis**[444]
  - Amount
    - Gross Hematuria (Visible)
      1. Females, consider menses
      2. Confirm with urine dipstick testing
      3. Seen with ARF and can be confirmed with renal biopsy; etiology often ATN, IgA nephropathy, and lupus nephritis
      4. Recommend cystoscopy (see below)
    - Microscopic (≥3 RBC/HPF)
      1. Always repeat dipstick finding
      2. If confirmed, do microscopic analysis
         - Look for dysmorphic RBCs, casts, proteinuria → findings suggestive of glomerular disease. These findings may warrant concurrent nephrology consultation.
         - If above not found, continue to *Imaging*.
  - Type
    - Painless/Asymptomatic (in those >35 YO)
      1. R/O benign causes: infection, menstruation, vigorous exercise, trauma
      2. Obtain good history → tobacco use, chemical exposures (aniline dye), irritative voiding symptoms which are all suggestive of malignant cause
      3. Obtain CMP to measure GFR → r/o intrinsic kidney disease
      4. Next step is to do urology consult for cystoscopy (ages 35+) to r/o malignancy
         - May obtain multiphase CT urography w/w-o contrast to evaluate renal parenchyma to r/o mass (MRI alternative if CT contraindicated d/t dye)
         - Alternative is renal US with retrograde pyelogram
      5. If workup so far is negative, may need to obtain cytology
      6. If workup is completely negative, do yearly UA
    - Painful
      1. Consider kidney stone
- **Imaging**
  - CT Urography – unexplained persistent hematuria (no infection or glomerular source)
  - Cystoscopy – done with gross hematuria unless active UTI
  - If unable to do CTU, then consider MR Urogram or retrograde pyelogram
- **Etiologies**
  - Prostatitis
  - Glomerulonephritis
  - Kidney stone
  - Urinary tract malignancy (confirmed with IVP)
  - BPH
  - Bladder cancer

Figure. Hematuria algorithm

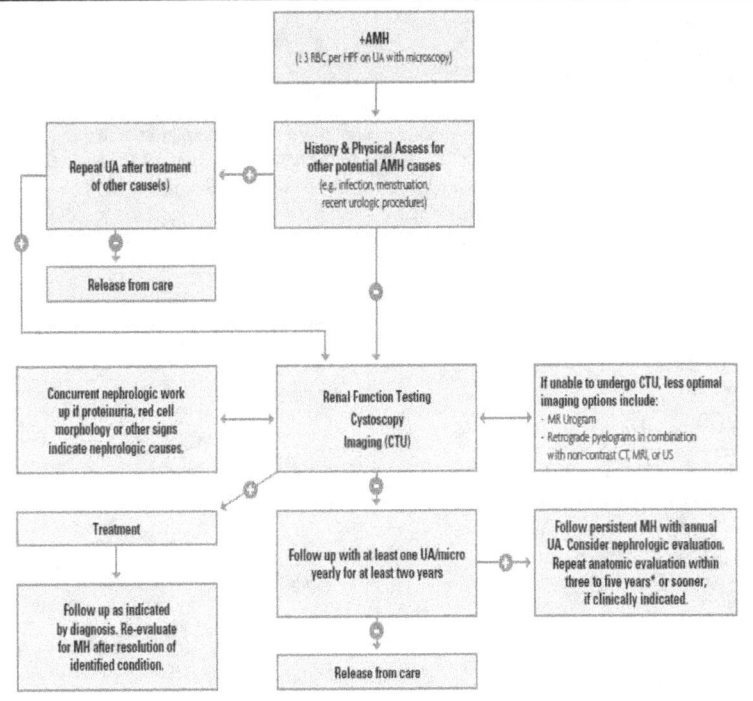

BPH

- **Symptoms**[445]
    - Obstructive: weak stream, strain to void, hesitancy, incomplete emptying, post-void dribbling
    - Irritative: frequency, urgency, incontinence, nocturia
- **Examination/DRE**
    - Size: large or not
    - Shape: irregularities, nodules (both are bad)
    - Texture: firm, soft/spongy (bad), hard (bad)
- **Labs**
    - UA: r/o UTI, hematuria
    - SCr: r/o hydronephrosis
    - PSA[446]
        - <3 → routine f/u
        - 3-7 ng/dl → repeat PSA weeks later and if remains >3 then TRUS
        - >7 ng/dl → TRUS and Urology consult
        - If ↑PSA and low %free PSA think cancer
- **Indications for Urology Referral**
    - Moderate to severe sx
    - PSA>7 (for TRUS-guided prostate biopsy without further testing)
    - Persistent gross hematuria

- Urinary retention
- Renal insufficiency 2/2 to BPH
- Recurrent UTI
- Bladder calculi
- **Symptom Assessment**
  - IPSS
    - An important part relates to quality of life ("If you were to spend the rest of your life with your urinary condition just the way it is now, how would you feel about that?") as this can tailor how aggressively (if at all) the treatment should be approached.
    - Scores 8-20 are moderate; >20 are severe
- **Treatment**

BPH Treatment

	Drugs	Time req'd	S/E
α_1-antagonists *First line therapy; works quickly to relax prostate and the bladder neck smooth muscle tone. Take QPM d/t orthostatic potential*	Selective Tamsulosin 0.4-0.8mg Silodosin 8mg Nonselective Terazosin 1-20mg Doxazosin 1-8mg Alfuzosin 10mg	~1 week	Nonselective have highest risk of orthostatic ↓BP ED Dizziness Syncope
After one year of combined alpha and 5a therapy, can consider stopping alpha-blocker[447]			
5α-reductase Inhibitors *Work gradually to reduce prostate size over multiple months. Use if patient has obstructive sx and ↑prostate*	Finasteride 5mg Dutasteride 0.5mg	2-6 months	Act on anatomic component by reducing conversion of testosterone→DHT which ↓growth ED Abnormal ejaculation
Anti-muscarinic	Selective Darifenacin 7.5-15mg Solifenacin 5-10mg Nonselective Trospium 20mg BID Oxybutynin 2.5-20mg Tolterodine 2-4mg	12 weeks	Constipation Dry mouth/Dry eyes Headache

- **Non-pharmacologic**
  - Scheduled voiding q3h
  - Avoid excessive evening fluid intake

TESTICULAR PAIN

Differential Diagnosis

Diagnosis	Description	Clinical features	Risk Factors	Treatment
Acute epididymitis	Infection from retrograde spread of organism (chlamydia or gonorrhea) via the vas deferens; gradual onset of pain and swelling	Marked scrotal swelling and pain, urethral discharge, irritative symptoms; heaviness; pain into spermatic cord and flank (posterior	Sexually active men younger than 35, heavy physical strain	<35: Ceftriaxone 250mg IV x1 + Doxycycline 100mg PO BID x10d >35:

		testes); +Prehn sign; +/- fever, chills		Levofloxacin 500mg/d x10d or Ofloxacin 300mg/d x10d
Cellulitis	Non-necrotizing infection, inflammation of skin and SQ tissue; expands over 6-36 hours	Local erythema, pain, swelling; no fluctuance; usually lower extremity; +/- fever, chills, malaise	H/o venous insufficiency, IVDA, open wounds, DM, trauma, obesity	PCN
Fournier's gangrene	Necrotizing fasciitis of perineal, perianal, genital areas; can spread up to 3cm/h; high mortality	Sudden, intense pain out of proportion to PE; severe swelling, erythema, bullae, tissue crepitus, eventual necrosis	Males 5-70; impaired immunity, esp DM; urogenital trauma	IV fluids ER transfer for possible surgical intervention; initiate ABx such as ciprofloxacin and clindamycin or amp/sulb or Zosyn. Consider vanco to cover MRSA
Scrotal abscess	Collection of pus in dermis and deeper tissues; often at hair follicle; grows over 4-14d; +/- multiple in one area	Local swelling, pain, warmth, erythema; round or conical nodule; fluctuance; +/- drainage; +/- fever, chills, malaise	H/o DM, shaving, IVDA, therapeutic injections, HIV, immunosuppression	
Testicular torsion	Testicle rotates, twisting the spermatic cord and reducing blood flow to the scrotum	Sudden, severe pain; high-riding testicle, erythema, swelling; +/- nausea, vomiting; painful urination; absent cremasteric reflex	Prepubertal boys (12-16); direct trauma; h/o cryptorchidism	ER transfer for surgical intervention

OVERACTIVE BLADDER

- Diagnosis[448,449]
    - Overactive bladder (OAB) is a clinical diagnosis characterized by the presence of bothersome urinary symptoms. OAB symptoms consist of four components: urgency, frequency, nocturia, and urgency incontinence.
    - Urgency is defined as the complaint of a sudden, compelling desire to pass urine which is difficult to defer." Urgency is considered the hallmark symptom of OAB.
    - Urinary frequency: traditionally, up to seven micturition episodes during waking hours has been considered normal
    - Nocturia is the complaint of interruption of sleep one or more times because of the need to void.
    - Urgency urinary incontinence is defined as the involuntary leakage of urine, associated with a sudden compelling desire to void.
- Mimickers
    - OAB also must be distinguished from other conditions such as polydipsia. In OAB, urinary frequency is associated with many small volume voids. Frequency that is the result of polydipsia and resulting polyuria may mimic OAB; the two can only be distinguished with the use of frequency-volume charts. In polydipsia, urinary frequency occurs with normal or large volume voids and the intake is volume matched.
    - Cystitis
    - Bladder pain syndrome

- Endocrine: DM, CDI, Cushing's syndrome
- Renal: CRF, relief of urinary tract obstruction, chronic pyelonephritis, NDI, Fanconi syndrome
- Iatrogenic: Diuretic therapy, alcohol, lithium, tetracyclines
- Metabolic: Hypercalcemia, potassium depletion
- Psychological: PPD or CWD
- Other causes: Sickle cell anemia, pulmonary and systemic venous thromboembolism (PSVT).

- **History**
  - Rule out co-morbid conditions such as neurologic disease (stroke, MS), mobility deficits, DM, fecal motility disorders, h/o recurrent UTIs, pelvic cancer
- **Questionnaires**
  - Urogenital Distress Inventory
  - UDI-6 Short Form
  - Incontinence Bladder Questionnaire
- **Exam**
  - Abdominal exam (look for suprapubic distention)
  - LE edema
  - GU exam to r/o pelvic floor dysfunction or prolapse
  - Perianal skin breakdown
- **Diagnostics**
  - Urinalysis (r/o UTI and hematuria)
  - Urine culture (r/o infection; need at least 100k CFU)
  - Post-void residual volumes (want <300cc; that or more is defined as urinary retention)
- **Advanced**
  - Urodynamics
  - Cystoscopy
  - Diagnostic renal and bladder US
- **Treatments**
  Most treatments can improve symptoms but will not always eliminate them
  - Nonpharmacologic
    - Behavioral Therapy
    - Bladder training
    - Bladder control strategies
    - Pelvic floor muscle training
    - Fluid management
  - Pharmacologic
    - Primary
      - Tolterodine ER (better tolerated) 2mg, 4mg BID or daily
      - Oxybutynin IR 5, 10, 15mg BID/TID/daily
      - Fesoterodine 4, 8mg daily
      - Solifenacin 5, 10mg daily
      - Mirabegron 25, 50mg/d
      - Trospium 60mg/d
    - Second Line Therapy
      - Anti-muscarinic (avoid in patients with glaucoma, impaired gastric emptying, h/o urinary retention)
      - Oral β-3 adrenoreceptor agonists

URINARY INCONTINENCE

- **Types**
  - Urge
  - Stress
  - Mixed
- **Differential Diagnosis**
  - Atrophic vaginitis
  - Prolapse
  - Bladder cancer
  - Dysfunctional voiding
  - Diabetes
  - Urethral obstruction
  - Interstitial cystitis
  - Urinary tract infection
  - Neurogenic bladder
  - Vulvodynia/vestibulitis
- **Transient Causes**
  - Delirium (UI can be secondary to acute delirium)
  - Infection
  - Atrophic vaginitis
  - Pharmacologic
  - Psychological (depression)
  - Excessive urine production (diabetes, hypercalcemia, CHF, peripheral edema ? polyuria ? incontinence)
  - Restricted mobility (patient cannot get to toilet fast enough)
  - Stool impaction (can cause UTI, overflow UI, fecal incontinence)
- **Exam**
  - Women → pelvic
  - Men → digital rectal
  - Also do neurologic exam to r/o MS, PD
- **Labs**
  - UA, culture, VB12, Ca, glucose
- **Orders**
  - Postvoid residual volume
    - Post void residual (PVR) testing, by catheterization or ultrasound, is recommended in current guidelines for evaluation of incontinence
    - High quality evidence from randomized trials is not available to support this recommendation, which is based on expert opinion
    - A PVR of less than 50 ml is considered adequate emptying, and a pvr greater than 200 ml is considered inadequate and suggestive of either detrusor weakness or obstruction
    - Treatment of coexisting conditions (eg, treatment of constipation, stopping medications with antimuscarinic action) may reduce PVR
  - Timed voids
- **Treatment**

Treatment
Urge
• Bladder training (void on schedule during day i.e. q2h and suppress urges between)
• Strength training (pelvic floor)
• May be combined with biofeedback.

- Behavior modification: ↓fluid intake by 25%, pelvic floor muscle training (Kegel), ↓caffeine intake, scheduled voids (q2-3hr)
- Antimuscarinic therapy
    o Aim to use ER formulations to ↓s/e
    o Oxybutynin IR 2.5-5mg BID-QID / ER 5-20mg/d / patch 3.9mg 2x/week
    o Tolterodine IR 1-2mg BID / LA 2-4mg/d
    o Solifenacin 5-10mg/d
    o Mirabegron 25-50mg/d
    o Trospium chloride 20mg/BID / XR 60mg/d

Stress

Pelvic muscle exercises (Kegel exercises) are recommended for urge, stress, and mixed incontinence. The following regimen can be performed: 3 sets of 8 to 12 slow-velocity contractions sustained for 6 to 8 seconds each, performed 3 or four 4 a week and continued for at least 15 to 20 weeks.

Bibliography

[444] Diagnosis, Evaluation and Follow-Up of Asymptomatic Microhematuria (AMH) in Adults: AUA Guideline Algorithm (2012)

[445] TheCurbSiders.com

[446] Sarma et al. "Benign Prostatic Hyperplasia and Lower Urinary Tract Symptoms." NEJM. 2012. 367: 248-257.

[447] Matsukawa Y et al. Effects of withdrawing α1-blocker from combination therapy with α1-blocker and 5α-reductase inhibitor in patients with lower urinary tract symptoms suggestive of benign prostatic hyperplasia: A prospective and comparative trial using urodynamics. J Urol 2017 Oct; 198:905.

[448] Sarma, RVSN. "Algorithmic Approach for the Diagnosis of Polyuria." Accessed December 21, 2017. < http://www.apiindia.org/medicine_update_2013/chap69.pdf>

[449] "Diagnosis and Treatment of Non-Neurogenic Overactive Bladder (OAB) in Adults: AUA/SUFU Guideline." AUA/SUFU Guideline: Published 2012; Amended 2014.

NUTRITION/DIET

Inpatient Diets	664
Body Weight Calculations	666
Labs Associated with Nutrition	666
Hyperlipidemia	667
Hypertriglyceridemia	672
Nutritional Requirements	674

INPATIENT DIETS

Inpatient Diet Options

Diet	Guidelines	Indications
Regular	Adequate in all essential nutrients All foods are permitted Can be modified according to patient's food preferences	No diet restrictions or modifications
Mechanical Soft	Includes soft-textured or ground foods that are easily masticated and swallowed	↓ Ability to chew or swallow. Presence of oral mucositis or esophagitis. May be appropriate for some patients with dysphagia
Pureed	Includes liquids as well as strained and pureed foods	Inability to chew or swallow solid foods. Presence of oral mucositis or esophagitis. May be appropriate for some patients with dysphagia
Full Liquid	Includes foods that are liquid at body temperature Includes milk/milk products <u>Can provide approximately</u>: 2500–3000 mL fluid 1500–2000 Cal 60–80 g high-quality protein <10 g dietary fiber 60–80 g fat per day	May be appropriate for patients with severely impaired chewing ability. Not appropriate for a lactase-deficient patient unless commercially available lactase enzyme tablets are provided
Clear Liquid	Includes foods that are liquid at body temperature Foods are very low in fiber Lactose free Virtually fat free Can provide approximately: 2000 mL fluid 400-600 Cal <7g low-quality protein <1g dietary fiber <1g fat/day This diet is inadequate in all nutrients and should not be used >3d without supplementation	Ordered as initial diet in the transition from NPO to solids. Used for bowel preparation before certain medical or surgical procedures. For management of acute medical conditions warranting minimalized biliary contraction or pancreatic exocrine secretion.
Low-fiber	Foods that are low in indigestible carbohydrates Decreases stool volume, transit time, and frequency	Management of acute radiation enteritis and inflammatory bowel disease when narrowing or stenosis of the gut lumen is present
Carbohydrate controlled diet (ADA)	Calorie level should be adequate to maintain or achieve desirable body weight Total carbohydrates are limited to 50–60% of total calories Ideally fat should be limited to ≈30% of total calories	Diabetes mellitus
Acute renal failure	Protein (g/kg DBW) 0.6 Calories 35–50 Sodium (g/day) 1–3 Potassium (g/day) Variable Fluid (mL/day) Urine output + 500	For patients in renal failure who are not undergoing dialysis

Renal failure/hemodialysis	Protein (g/kg DBW) 1.0–1.2 Calories (per kilogram DBW) 30–35 Sodium (g/d) 1–2 Potassium (g/d) 1.5–3 Fluid (mL/d) Urine output + 500	For patients in renal failure on hemodialysis. Confirm placement on CXR at R atrium
Peritoneal dialysis	Protein (g/kg DBW) 1.2–1.6 Calories (per kilogram DBW) 25–35 Sodium (g/d) 3—4 Potassium (g/d) 3–4 Fluid (mL/d) Urine output + 500	For patients in renal failure on peritoneal dialysis
Liver failure	In the absence of encephalopathy do not restrict protein In the presence of encephalopathy initially restricted protein to 40–60 g/d then liberalize in increments of 10 g/d as tolerated Sodium and fluid restriction should be specified based on severity of ascites and edema	Management of chronic liver disorders
Low lactose/lactose free	Limits or restricts mild products Commercially available lactase enzyme tablets are available on the market	Lactase deficiency
Low fat	<50 g total fat per day	Pancreatitis Fat malabsorption
Fat/cholesterol restricted	Total fat >30% total calories Saturated fat limited to 10% of calories <300 mg cholesterol <50% calories from complex carbohydrates	Hypercholesterolemia
Low-sodium	Sodium allowance should be as liberal as possible to maximize nutritional intake yet control symptoms "No-added salt" is 4 g/d; no added salt or highly salted food; 2 g/d avoids processed foods (ie, meats) <1 g/d is unpalatable and thus compromises adequate intake	Indicated for patients with hypertension, ascites, and edema associated with the underlying disease

NUTRITION/DIET

BODY WEIGHT CALCULATIONS

- Males: 106lb for the first 5ft + 6lb for each additional inch
  - (48kg for the first 152.4cm + 1.1kg for each additional cm)
- Females: 100lb for the first 5ft + 5lb for each additional inch
  - (45kg for the first 152.4cm + 0.9kg for each additional cm)

LABS ASSOCIATED WITH NUTRITION

- **BUN:** reflects protein intake and hydration
- **SCr:** reflects muscle breakdown

- **General Recommendations**
  - Provide calories of 30-35 cal/kg current weight (adjust if obese)
    - ↑ Calorie foods: butter, sour cream, etc.
  - Provide a high protein diet (1.5-2.0 g/kg)
  - ↑fluid to promote wound healing (30-40 cc/kg) → should match caloric intake
- **Vitamins**
  - MVI
  - Wound Healing
    - Vitamin C
    - Arginine (general, C/I if patient septic) and Glutamine (GI) → Juven supplement here at Tripler
    - Zinc 220mg x 14d
- **Tube Feeds**
  - Start at 20-30 mL/hr and advance 10-20 mL/hr x 4-6hrs or as tolerated to goal rate
  - Types
    - Pivot 1.5 – high protein with arginine and glutamine
    - Two Cal HN – high calorie may require additional fluids
    - Nepro – good for dialysis patients
  - Goal rate
    - (Total calories needed per day / 24 hours) / calories per mL of formula
  - Flushing
    - Determine the patient's total fluid needs (free water deficit: see pg 690)
    - Determine the amount of free water provided by tube feeding formula (free water content x total volume of tube feeds = free water provided)
    - This gives you:
      Fluid needs – Free water from formula = volume of free water flushes required
    - Divide the above into 3-4 boluses per day
- **Oral Supplements**
  - Ensure Plus 8oz
  - ProCel (1 scoop)
  - ProMod
  - Supershake
  - Juven
  - Carnation Instant Bfast 8oz
- **TPN**
  - Indication – patient unable to use gut at goal feeds within 5 days of admission
  - Risks
    - Trauma, hematoma, pneumothorax when inserting PICC
    - Hyperglycemia

1. BS should be monitored q4h for first 48hrs then daily
2. Do a UA BID
3. Should be started at slow rate (40-60cc/hr) due to the risk of hyperglycemia (if occurs with glycosuria, should be suspicious for underlying sepsis)
    - Sepsis from line infection
    - Refeeding syndrome – electrolyte abnormalities seen in a patient with severe protein malnutrition (↓PO4, ↓K, and ↓Mg).
- Labs
    - Ca/Mg/PO4
    - LFT weekly
    - INR weekly
    - UA and BS as above
- Initiating
    - Start enteral tube feeding at full strength formula at 20 cc/hr
    - ↑rate by 10-20 cc/hr every 6-8 hours to get to goal rate
- Estimating Needs
    - Ideal Body Weight (IBW)
        1. Energy: 25-30 kcal/kg (aim for 25 cals/kg)
        2. Protein: 1.0-1.8 g/kg (aim for 1.5)
        3. Lipids: 30-70 g/day
- Weaning Off
    - Enteral feeding → If patient receiving TF at 50% goal then ↓TPN to 50% and continue weaning as tolerated
    - PO intake → once patient tolerating 50% of needs then ↓TPN to 50% goal and wean off

HYPERLIPIDEMIA

- **Risk Calculation**[450,451,452]
    - Pooled co-hort 10 year risk (ASCVD risk calculator)
- **Intermediate Risk Patients (ASCVD 5-20%)**
    - Intermediate risk patients that are asymptomatic with no history of CAD should have either (1) coronary artery calcium scoring or (2) hsC-RP done to determine level of risk factor modification
    - Concerning Factors
        - LDL≥160 or non-HDL>190
        - HTN
        - Family history of premature CAD
        - CAC>300
        - Albumin/Cr >30 mg/g
        - Smoking
        - hs-CRP≥2
- **Secondary Causes**
    - Untreated hypothyroidism, nephrotic syndrome, renal failure, cholestasis, acute pancreatitis, pregnancy, polycystic ovarian disease, excess alcohol use, treatment with estrogens/oral contraceptives, antipsychotic agents, glucocorticoids, cyclosporine, protease inhibitors, retinoids, and beta blockers
- **LDL vs. Non-HDL-C**
    - While LDL is still bad, Non-HDL-C is considered a better predictor of absolute risk for development of cardiovascular disease as it encompasses all bad cholesterol factors.
    - Non-HDL-C is calculated as CHOL-HDL

NUTRITION/DIET

- Rough goals:
    - Very high risk (known CVD): <100; LDL<70
    - High risk (traditional risk factors; high ASCVD score, high CAC): <130; LDL<100
- **Goals**
    - LDL reduction of 100 points or 50% from baseline or non-HDL-C remains >130

Goal lipids based on risk factors			
Risk Category	LDL goal	ApoB	Non-HDL Goal
Extreme risk (Known CAD plus progressive CAD, T2DM, CKD 3/4, FH, or premature CAD in family)	<55	<70	<80
Very high risk (known CAD + comorbidities, CVA, TIA)	<70	≤80	<100
High Risk Risk equivalents (10-year risk >20%) • Male > 45YO or Female > 55YO • Smoker • HTN • HDL < 35 • DM • Family hx of CAD	<100	<130	<90

Non-HDL is calculated by subtracting total cholesterol from HDL

Management of Elevated TG		
Classification	Serum TG	Additional Treatments
Normal	<150	
Borderline High	150-199	↓Weight, ↑activity
High	200-499	Intensify LDL therapy or add nicotinic acid or fibrate*
Very High	>500	Prevent pancreatitis by lowering TG; low fat diet, ↓weight, ↑activity, and TG lowering drug (fibrate or nicotinic acid). Once level <500, focus on LDL

*fibrate recommended by Endocrine Society

- **Pharmacotherapy**
    - Unless allergy exists, start with **statin therapy**
    - If above goal metrics are not met with maximally tolerated statin alone:
        - Assess statin adherence
        - ↑lifestyle exercise
        - In very high risk patients:
            - Consider adding **ezetimibe or PCSK9 inhibitor**
- **Statins**
    - Types
        - *Hydrophilic*
            - Atorvastatin (liver metabolized → avoid if pt on multi meds; used if high-dose statin therapy req'd); long acting → rx in AM
            - Fluvastatin (liver metabolized → avoid with concurrent warfarin use); short acting → rx in PM
            - Rosuvastatin (liver metabolized → avoid with concurrent warfarin use; used if high-dose statin therapy req'd' d); long acting → rx in AM
            - Pravastatin (renally metabolized → good if pt. taking multiple medications but not considered 'high' dose statin therapy) ; short acting → rx in PM
            - Pitavastatin – less potential for interactions compared with other statins
        - *Lipophilic*

- Lovastatin (liver metabolized → avoid if pt on multi meds)
- Simvastatin (liver metabolized → avoid if pt on multi meds)

Choosing Statin Intensity	
High Intensity	Moderate Intensity
• Clinical ASCVD and Age≤75 • LDL≥190 • DM + Age 40-75+10 year risk ≥ 7.5% • 10 year risk ≥ 7.5%**	• Clinical ASCVD and Age>75 • Type 1 or Type 2 Diabetes Mellitus (10 year risk <7.5%) • Any patient with 10 year risk 5-7.5%

**or moderate-intensity
Newer researchers are suggesting higher thresholds feeling that ASCVD risk calculator is inappropriately starting statins in patients at low risk without a longterm CVD benefit (suggest threshold of >14% in men 40-49 and 21% if 70-75, and >17% in women of any age).[453]
(see flow chart on following page)

Statin Therapy Options (dose in parenthesis was used in RCTs)		
High Intensity	Medium Intensity	Low Intensity
Daily dosage lowers LDL-C by approximately ≥ 50% on average Dose in AM	Daily dosage lowers LDL-C by approximately 30% to 50% on average; dose in PM	Daily dosage lowers LDL-C by < 30% average. Dose in PM
Atorvastatin 40 (80) mg Rosuvastatin 20 (40) mg	Atorvastatin, 10 (20) mg Rosuvastatin (5) 10 mg Simvastatin 20-40 mg Pravastatin 40 (80) mg Lovastatin 40 mg Fluvastatin XL 80 mg Fluvastatin 40 mg BID Pitavastatin 2-4 mg	Simvastatin, 10 mg Pravastatin, 10-20 mg Lovastatin, 20 mg Fluvastatin, 20-40 mg Pitavastatin, 1 mg

- Effects
  - ↓LDL
    - Lovastatin
    - Pravastatin
  - Normal LDL and underlying CAD
    - Simvastatin
  - ↓LDL with underlying CAD
    - Atorvastatin

Management of Elevated TG			
Genetic Name and Dosage	Avg. Expected LDL ↓	Clinical Studied Dosages	Starting mg
Rosuvastatin 10,20, 40mg	55-60%	20mg	10mg
Atorvastatin 20,40, 80mg	42-54%	10mg	20mg
Simvastatin 20, 40, 80	30-50%		40mg
Lovastatin 20, 40, 80, 60ER	39-40%	40mg	40mg
Pravastatin 20, 40, 80mg	30-37%	40mg	40mg
Fluvastatin SR80mg	35%		

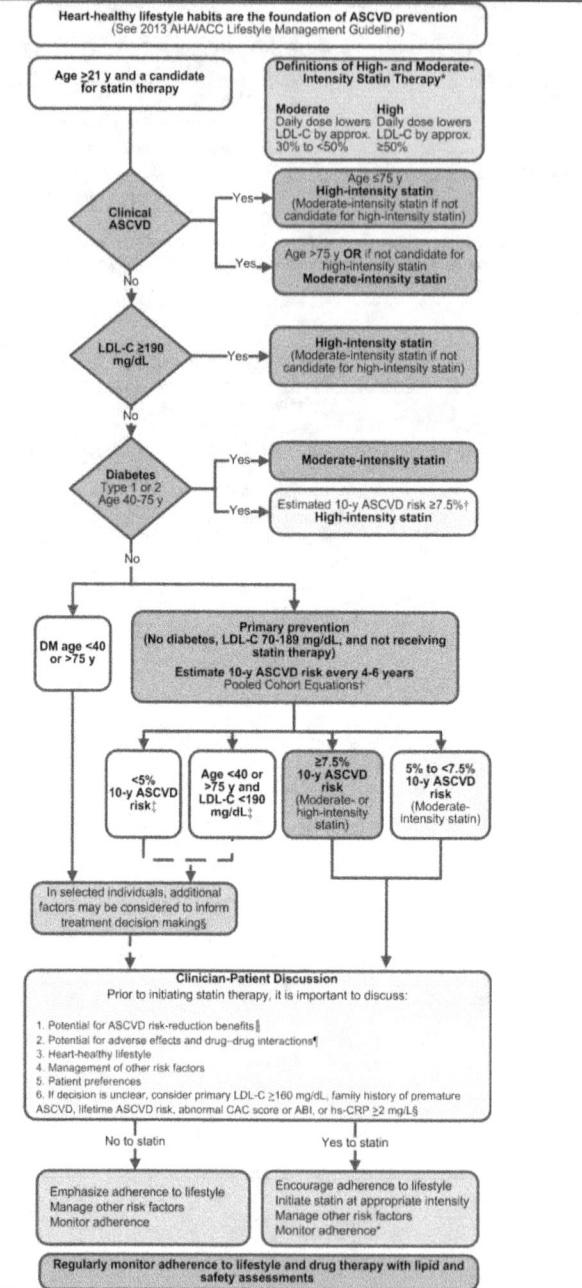

Figure. Statin implementation based on risk factors

NUTRITION/DIET

Classes of Cholesterol-Lowering Drugs

Drug class	Cholesterol	LDL	HDL	Triglycerides	Side effects
Bile acid–binding resins	↓20%	↓10% to 20%	↑3% to 5%	Neutral or ↑	Unpalatability, bloating, constipation, heartburn
Nicotinic acid	↓25%	↓10% to 25%	↑15% to 35%	↓20% to 50%	Flushing, nausea, glucose intolerance, abnormal liver function test
Fibric acid analogs	↓15%	↓5% to 15%	↑14% to 20%	↓20% to 50%	Nausea, skin rash
HMG-CoA reductase Inhibitors	↓15% to 30%	↓20% to 60%	↑5% to 15%	↓10% to 40%	Myositis, myalgia, elevated hepatic transaminases
Omega-3-Fatty Acids	↔	↔	↔	↓ (unknown %)	Low but large amount (4g/d) required

Statin alternatives

Medication (trial)	MOA	Indication	Dose
Ezetimbe (IMPROVE-IT)	Reduces cholesterol absorption in the small intestines	Adjunct to diet for patients not reaching LDL goal (<70) with statin alone (may reduce CHOL by 25%), LDL by 25%. Combine with simvastatin 20-40mg/d	10mg/d
Colesevelam (LRC-CPPT)	Bile acid sequestrant	Adjunct to diet exercise **combined with statin and ezetimibe** when LDL remains high and TG ≤300	Colesevelam 6 tablets PO daily or 3 tablets PO BID (3.8g/d)
Cholestyramine	Bile acid sequestrant	↓LDL by 9%, ↑HDL by 4% Adjunct to diet exercise combined with statin and ezetimibe when LDL remains high and TG ≤300	16g/d
Alirocumab (ODYSSEY) Evolocumab (FOURIER)	PCSK9 inhibitor	Adjunct to diet **if ezetimibe not enough** or it was not tolerated. Lowers LDL by 45% when added to statin	Alirocumab 75m SQ q2w (up to 150mg) Evolocumab 140mg SQ q2w (up to 420mg qmonth)
Fenofibrate	Fibric acid analogs	**Only used if TG≥500** Lowers LDL by 20% and increases HDL by 11%. Does not lower risk of non-fatal MI, CVA, or CV death in diabetics. Consider in patients with TG>500	145mg/d
Niacin	Nicotinic acid	Good option if patient cannot take a statin Avoid in diabetics Not as potent as fenofibrate Raises HDL the most Can cause chemical hepatitis No mortality benefits Increases risk of statin myopathy	>1500mg/d

- **Side Effects**
  - Any statin intolerance should be evaluated with:
    - TSH
    - Vitamin D level
      - Assessing and treating low vitamin D levels (25-hydroxyvitamin D; less than 32 ng/mL) may be worth considering before starting or restarting a statin in patients who develop muscle pain while taking a statin. Supplementation with vitamin D2 (ergocalciferol) supplements (from 50,000 units to 100,000 units per week) advised for Vitamin D levels <10 mg/mL, can use cholecalciferol for levels between 20-30 mg/mL at 400mg U daily.
        - A retrospective chart review found that replenishing vitamin D before a statin re-challenge in previously intolerant patients increases statin tolerability and adherence.
    - Drug interactions
      - Statins with highest interactions with other drugs: simvastatin, lovastatin, and atorvastatin
  - Can try every other day or once-weekly dosing (atorvastatin, rosuvastatin)
  - Non-Statin Options:
    - Ezetimibe/Fenofibrate combination
    - PCSK9 inhibitor (i.e. Evolocumab)
  - Myalgias
    - Tx by switching to lipophilic, changing to QOD dosing, adding coenzyme Q10 (poor data) or vitamin D[454]
      - Lowest myalgia risk: pravastatin, lovastatin, pitavastatin
    - Check CPK, UA to r/o rhabdomyolysis
  - Elevated LFTs
  - GI intolerance
  - Monitoring
  - Obtain lipid panel 6 weeks after starting therapy
  - Then obtain every 6-12 months from then on out

HYPERTRIGLYCERIDEMIA

- It is often caused or exacerbated by uncontrolled diabetes mellitus, obesity, and sedentary habits
- **Causes/Types**
  - Type I
    - Rare disorder
    - Severe elevations in chylomicrons and extremely elevated triglycerides, always reaching well above 1000 mg/dL and not infrequently rising as high as 10,000 mg/dL or more.
    - Caused by mutations of either the lipoprotein lipase gene (LPL), which is critical for the metabolism of chylomicrons and very low-density lipoprotein (VLDL)
  - Type IIb
    - Classic mixed hyperlipidemia (high cholesterol and triglyceride levels), caused by elevations in low-density lipoprotein (LDL) and VLDL.
  - Type III
    - AKA dysbetalipoproteinemia,
    - Typically, patients with this rare condition have elevated total cholesterol (range, 300 600 mg/dL) and triglyceride levels (usually >400 mg/dL; may exceed 1000 mg/dL),
  - Type IV

- Abnormal elevations of VLDL, and triglyceride levels are almost always less than 1000 mg/dL.
- Serum cholesterol levels are normal.
  o Type V
    - Triglyceride levels are invariably greater than 1000 mg/dL, and total cholesterol levels are always elevated.
    - The LDL cholesterol level is usually low.
- **Symptoms**
  o Hypertriglyceridemia is usually asymptomatic until triglycerides are greater than 1000-2000 mg/dL (i.e. pancreatitis).
  o Signs and symptoms may include the following:
    - GI: Pain in the mid-epigastric, chest, or back regions; nausea, vomiting
    - Respiratory: Dyspnea
    - Dermatologic: Xanthomas
    - Ophthalmologic: Corneal arcus, xanthelasmas
- **Diagnostics**
  o Lipid analysis
  o Chylomicron determination
  o Fasting blood glucose level
  o TSH level
  o Urinalysis
  o Liver function studies

Pharmacologic treatments when TG>500 (or as high as 866)			
Medication (trial)	Dose	LDL/HDL/TG effect	Other
Fenofibrate	Nanocrystal: 145mg/d Micronized: 200mg/dinner	↓LDL: 20% ↑HDL: 11% ↓TG: 54.5%	Consider in CV patients with high TG but low HDL. Combine with statin
Ometa-3-Fatty Acids (REDUCE-IT)	4g/d	↑LDL: 44% ↑HD: 9.1% ↓TG: 45%	Safe to use with statins May increase AFib/flutter
Gemfibrozil	1200mg/d	↑HDL: 9% ↓TG: 41%	More s/e than fenofibrate No effects to LDL Avoid concurrent statin use No mortality benefit
Niacin	>1500mg/d	↓LDL: 8% ↑HDL: 23% ↓TG: 24%	Not as potent as fenofibrate Raises HDL the most Can cause chemical hepatitis No mortality benefits Increases risk of statin myopathy

- **Management**
  o Nonpharmacologic – diet, exercise, Mediterranean diet, smoking and EtOH cessation, consider stopping any estrogen containing OCP
  o Pharmacologic - many physicians use drugs to reduce the triglyceride level only when the level exceeds 866 mg/dL. Main indications for pharmacologic therapy are prevention of pancreatitis and lowering of cardiovascular risk; goal is TRG < 500.
    - **Statins – recommend high dose such as atorvastatin 80mg and rosuvastatin 20mg; best if TRIG<500 and LDL is elevated. Should be taken at bedtime**
      □ Takes up to 2 weeks to see result, maximum 8 weeks. Safe to re-test lipid results in 2 months.

NUTRITIONAL REQUIREMENTS

- Caloric needs can be determined by one of two means: the Harris–Benedict BEE and the "rule of thumb" method.
- A patient's caloric needs can be calculated by the following methods:
- **Harris–Benedict BEE**
  - For men:
    - BEE = 66.47 + 13.75 (**w**) + 5.00 (**h**) − 6.76 (**a**)
  - For women:
    - BEE = 655.10 + 9.56 (**w**) + 1.85 (**h**) − 4.689 (**a**)

  where **w** = weight in kilograms; **h** = height in centimeters; and **a** = age in years.

  - After the BEE has been determined from the Harris–Benedict equation, the patient's total daily maintenance energy requirements are estimated by multiplying the BEE by an activity factor and a stress factor.

  > Total energy requirements = BEE x Activity factor x Stress factor

  Use the following correction factors:

Activity Level	Correction Factor
Bedridden	1.2
Ambulatory	1.3
Minor operation	1.2
Skeletal trauma	1.35
Major sepsis	1.60
Severe burn	2.10

  - **"Rule of Thumb" Method**
    - Maintenance of the patient's nutritional status without significant metabolic stress requires 25–30 Cal/kg body weight/d.
    - Maintenance needs for the hypermetabolic, severely stressed patient or for supporting weight gain in the underweight patient without significant metabolic stress requires 35–40 Cal/kg body weight/d.
    - Greater than 40 Cal/kg body weight/d may be needed to meet the needs of severely burned patients.

Bibliography

[450] Sharma M, Ansari MT, Abou-setta AM, Soares-Weiser K, Ooi TC, Sears M, et al., Systematic Review: Comparative Effectiveness and Harms of Combinations of Lipid-Modifying Agents and High-Dose Statin Monotherapy. Ann. Int. Med. 2009;151.

[451] Gotto AM Jr. Management of lipid and lipoprotein disorders. In: Gotto AM Jr, Pownall HJ, eds. Manual of lipid disorders. Baltimore: Williams & Wilkins, 1992.

[452] Ahmed SM et al. Management of Dyslipidemia in Adults. Am Fam Physician. 1998 May 1;57(9):2192-2204, 2207-8.

[453] Yebyo et al. Ann Intern Med. 2019.
[454] Kang JH, Nguyen QN, Mutka J, Le QA. Rechallenging statin therapy in veterans with statin-induced myopathy post vitamin D replenishment. J Pharm Pract. 2016 Oct 24. pii: 0897190016674407. [Epub ahead of print]

FLUIDS

Fluid Calculations 677
IV Fluids 678

FLUID CALCULATIONS

- **Body fluid composition:**
  - Total Body Water = 0.6 x wt (kg) for males|0.5 x wt (kg) for females
    - Extracellular fluid (ECF) = 0.2 x wt (kg)
    - *Intravascular* = 1/3 ECF
      - Interstitial = 2/3 ECF
      - Intracellular fluid (ICF) = 0.4 x wt (kg)
- **Maintenance Fluids**
  - Generic
    - Weight in kg + 40 = hourly rate
  - 24HR Requirements
    - **100/50/20 RULE**
      1. Administer 100 mL/kg/day for the first 10 kg of weight
      2. Add 50 mL/kg for the next 10 kg
      3. Add 20 mL/kg for each kg over 20kg
  - Hourly Requirements
    - **4/2/1 RULE**
      1. Administer 4 mL/kg/hr. for the first 10 kg
      2. Add 2 mL/kg/hr. for the next 10 kg
      3. Add 1 mL/kg/hr. for each kg over 20
      4. Maintenance Fluids
- **Fluid deficit ml/hr**
  - (Pre-illness weight in kg - illness weight in kg)/24
  - 1 kg of weight lost = 1 L of fluid lost
- **Figure out IV rate:**
  - Maintenance dose + Fluid deficit to get Total Deficit in ml/hr
  - Give ½ of Total deficit over 1st 8 hours
  - If gave any boluses, subtract them from this number.
  - Give 2nd ½ of Total Deficit over next 16 hours
- **Decide what IV fluid to give:**
  - Hypovolemic: NS
    - Postural ↓BP, dry mucous mems, flat neck veins, skin tenting
  - Euvolemic: NS
    - Hypervolemic: D5W at KVO or Hep lock
    - Tachypnea, moist MM, crackles, JVP >3cm above sternal angle, taut skin, S3,
  - **Look at BUN: Cr ratio:**
    - Ratio less than 12 = volume depletion
  - Check Ins/Outs
    - Human: 140 mEq/L Na^+, 103 mEq/L Cl^-, 4 mEq/L K^+, 5 mEq/L Ca^{++}, 2 mEq/L Mg^{++}, 25 mEq/L $HCO3^-$, pH 7.4, Osmolality 290 mOsm/L

IV Solutions					
Solution	pH	Contents (1L)	Osmolality mOsm/L (nml 240-340)	Type	
D5W	5	5g dextrose	252	Isotonic – hypotonic in body	
0.9NaCl	5.7	154 mEq Na 154 mEq Cl	308	Isotonic	
Ringers Lactate	5.8	147 mEq Na 4 mEq K 4 mEq Ca	308-324	Isotonic	

FLUIDS

Fluid	pH	Composition	Osm	Tonicity
Lactated Ringers	6.6	155 mEq Cl 130 mEq Na 4 mEq K 3 mEq Ca 109 mEq Cl 28 mEq NaLa	273	Isotonic
0.45 NaCl	5.6	77 mEq Na 77 mEq Cl	154	Hypotonic
3% NaCl	5.0	513 mEq Na 513 mEq Cl	1026	Hypertonic
5% NaCl	5.8	855 mEq Na 855 mEq Cl	1710	Hypertonic
10% Dextrose	4.3	10g dextrose	505	Hypertonic
D5¼NS	4.4	5g Dextrose 34 mEq Na 34 mEq Cl	406	Hypertonic
D5½NS	4.4	5g Dextrose 77 mEq Na 77 mEq Cl	406	Hypertonic
D5NS	4.4	5g Dextrose 154 mEq Na 154 mEq Cl	560	Hypertonic
D5LR	4.9	5g Dextrose 130 mEq Na 4 mEq K 3 mEq Ca 109 mEq Cl 28 mEq NaLa	525	Hypertonic
0.9NS + 150 mEQ NAHCO3		Na 308 K 0 Cl 0 HCO3 50	616	Very hypertonic

** 50g of dextrose is rapidly metabolized therefore does NOT contribute to tonicity

IV FLUIDS

- **For Most Patients**
  - <u>Maintenance Fluids</u>*: "4/2/1 Rule" = [4 ml/hr for first 10 kg wt] + [2 ml/hr for next 10 kg] + [1 ml/hr for every 1 kg over 20 kg]
  - <u>Deficit</u>: (Hrs NPO x Maintenance)
  - <u>Insensible Loss</u>: 3-15 cc/hr
  - <u>Trauma</u>: Replace 1 cc of EBL with 3 cc of isotonic IVF
  - **Parkland Formula*** for burn patients: wt (kg) x TBSA% x 4cc LR over 24 hr.
    Give ½ first 8 hours, second ½ over next 16 hours.
    *Common: (wt) (% TBSA) (3cc LR) over 24 hours

Electrolyte Requirements		
	Adults	**Children**
Na	80-120 mEq/day	3-4 mEq/kg/day or per 100 ml fluid
K	50-100 mEq/day	2-3 mEq/day or per 100 ml fluid
Cl	80-120 mEq/day	3 mEq/day or per 100 ml fluid
Glucose	100-200 g/day	100-200 mg/kg/hr
	The protein-sparing effect is one of the goals of basic IV therapy. The administration of at least 100 g of glucose/d reduces protein loss by more than one-half. Virtually all IV fluid solutions supply glucose as dextrose (pure dextrorotatory glucose).	
PO4	7-10 mmol/1000kcal	
Mg	20 mEq	
Ca	1-3 gm/d	

Specific Replacement Fluids

Gastric Loss (Nasogastric Tube, Emesis):	D51/2NS with 20 mEq/L (mmol/L) potassium chloride (KCl)
Diarrhea:	D5LR with 15 mEq/L (mmol/L) KCl. Use body weight as a replacement guide (about 1 L for each 1 kg, or 2.2 lb, lost)
Bile Loss:	D5LR with 25 mEq/L (1/2 ampule) of sodium bicarbonate mL for mL
Pancreatic Loss:	D5LR with 50 mEq/liter (1 amp) HCO3 mL for mL
Burn Patients:	Use the Parkland: (% body burn) x (body weight in kg) x 4 mL or "Rule of Nines" Formulas:

PAIN MANAGEMENT

Pain Management 681
Conversion Factors for Opioids 687

PAIN MANAGEMENT

- **General Approach**
  - Characterize pain: nociceptive vs neuropathic
  - Multi-modal therapy: PT+pharmacologic+BH
  - Utilize hot packs, lidocaine patches, capsaicin cream
  - Concurrent AKI or CKD are contraindications to morphine use
- **Risk Stratify**
  - SOAPP-R score is a system used to rate patient as high risk for addiction
- **Medications**
  - Always aim for non-opiate therapy
  - Avoid NSAIDs in decompensated cirrhosis
  - Determine risk for GI bleed:
    - *Risk Factors*
      1. Age>65
      2. H/o complicated GI ulcer
      3. High dose NSAID therapy hx
      4. Concurrent ASA/steroid/anticoagulant use
    - *Score*
      1. Low risk: no risk factors
      2. Moderate risk: 1-2 risk factors
      3. High risk: >2 or h/o previously complicated ulcer
  - Consider
    - Nociceptive: acetaminophen 1g q8h + ketorolac 15mg q6h as standing orders
      1. Can use naproxen 500mg BID or ibuprofen 400mg TID instead of ketorolac in patients with GIB risk
    - Neuropathic: pregabalin or gabapentin
    - Morphine is **contraindicated** in patients with ESRD (or GFR<30) due to rapid accumulation that can occur.
- **Chronic Opiate Patients**
  - Ensure sole provider in place
  - Create pain contract
  - Address opiate induced constipation at every visit
  - Q12M evaluate:
    - ECG for QT prolongation
    - Random UDS
    - Chronic opiate panel
- **Example Inpatient Opiate Regimen**
  - Use combination of long acting + short acting options
    - Long Acting
      1. Percocet 5/325 1-2 tabs PO q3h PRN (1 tab for mild-mod pain < 5/10; 2 tabs for mod-severe pain > 5/10)
      Hydrocodone/Acetaminophen (Norco) 5/325mg 1 tab PO q4h PRN mild to moderate pain (< 5/10)
      Hydrocodone/Acetaminophen (Norco) 5/325mg 2 tabs PO q4h PRN moderate to severe pain (> 5/10)
    - Short Acting
      1. Morphine Sulfate 4-8mg IV q1-2h PRN
      2. Dilaudid .5-1.5mg IV q2h PRN
  - Review after 24 hours, add up total daily dose of morphine given to determine PO dosing

PAIN MANAGEMENT

- Calculate how many mg of opioid pt is using in 24 hrs → convert that amt to Opioid (SR) by 1/2
- Add a rescue doses (IR) of same opioid if possible - should be~10-20% of total daily opioid dose
  1. **Example**
     - 10mg oxycodone 6 times/day = 60mg oxycodone in 24 hrs
     - Equivalent SR Oxycodone = Oxycontin 30mg q12h
     - Add opioid rescue dose – Oxycodone 5- 10 mg q4h prn

Pain Management by Administration Type

Method	Type	Medication
IV/IM	Opioids	Fentanyl 25-100 mg/kg q30-60 min
		Hydromorphone 0.2-2 mg q4-6h
		Meperidine 25-50 mg q3-4h
		Morphine 1-10 mg q2-6h *(avoid in AKI/CKD)*
	NSAIDs	Ketorolac 30-60 mg loading then 15-30 mg IV q6h MAX 5 days
		Rofecoxib 50mg MAX 5 days
	Mixed	Butorphanol 20 mg/kg
		Nalbuphine 0.25 mg/kg
Oral	Acetaminophen	Acetaminophen 325mg-650g q4-6h max 3250mg/day
	NSAIDs	Ibuprofen 400-800mg PO q6-8h
		Naproxen 250-500 mg PO q8-12h
		Meloxicam 7.5-15mg PO daily
		Rofecoxib 50mg QDx5d then 25mg QD
	Cox-2 inhib	Celecoxib 400 mg x1 then p12h 200mg BID
	Opioid/non Combination	Acetaminophen/propoxyphene Napsylate (Darvocet) q4-6h
		Acetaminophen/oxycodone (Percocet) q4-6h
		Acetaminophen/codeine (Tylenol with codeine) q4-6h
		Acetaminophen/hydrocodone (Vicodin) q4-6h
	Opioids	Hydrocodone 5-10 mg q4-6h
		Morphine 10-30 mg q3-4h *(avoid in AKI/CKD)*
		Oxycodone 5 mg q3-6h
	Other	Acetaminophen 325-1000mg q4-6h
Transdermal	Opioids	Fentanyl patch 25-100 mcg/h q12h
Intranasal	Opioids	Fentanyl 1.5-2 mcg/kg q1-2h divided per nostril
		Midazolam 0.3mg/kg (max 1cc/nostril)
		Ketamine 0.5-1mg/kg (unknown max)
Topical	N/A	Diclofenac 1% gel (2-4g QID)
		Diclofenac 1.3% patch (1 patch @ 180mg BID)
		Lidocaine 5% patch (1-3 patches applied daily)
		Fentanyl 12-25mcg/h q72h
		Capsaicin (thin layer to area QID)
		EMLA 20g applied for 4h (onset 1h)
Non Pharm	N/a	Heat/cold therapy, massage, TENS relaxation, hypnosis, acupuncture, biofeedback

Pain Management by Pain Type

Type	Prescription
Neuropathic Pain	- Gabapentin 300 mg PO QHS to TID prn pain (max 3600mg)
	- Pregabalin 50mg PO TID (max 300mg)
	- Duloxetine 30mg PO daily (max 60mg/d)
	- Venlafaxine ER 37.5mg PO daily (max 225mg/d)
	- Amitriptyline 25mg PO QHS (max 200mg/d)
	- Nortriptyline 25mg PO QHS (max 150mg/d)
	- Capsaicin 0.075% topical QID
	- Lidocaine patch 4% - Apply patch to painful area. Patch may remain in place for up to 12 hours in any 24-hour period. No more than 1 patch should be used in a 24-hour period.

PAIN MANAGEMENT

Nociceptive Muscle pain/Spasm	•	General
		○ Flexeril IR 5mg TID x 3 weeks (max 30mg)
		○ Flexeril ER 15mg daily
		○ Baclofen 5mg TID (max 80mg)
		○ Robaxin 1-1.5mg PO TID to QID x48-72h then 500-700 mg PO TID to QID (max 8g/d)
	•	Acute/Severe Pain
		○ Valium IM 2-10mg PO TID-QID; 5-10mg IV/IM
		○ Zanaflex 4mg daily→TID q6h
Cancer related pain	•	Mild → Tylenol, NSAID
	•	Moderate → Codeine, Hydrocodone, or Tramadol + above
	•	Severe → Short acting (Morphine or Hydromorphone) and calculate to long acting (fentanyl patch or oxycodone) and give short acting for break through
	•	Fentanyl Patch Conversion
		○ Morphine 2mg PO/day = Fentanyl 1mag/hr TSD
		○ Percocet (9 tabs/day) = Fentanyl 25mag TSD
		○ Lortab (9 tabs/day) = Fentanyl 25mag TSD
		○ Tylenol #3 (9 tabs/day) = Fentanyl 25mag TSD

Local Anesthetics					
Medication	Onset	Duration (without epi)	Duration (with epi)	Max dose (without epi)	Max dose (with epi)
Lidocaine 1%	Rapid	0.5-2h	1-6h	300mg	500mg
Bupivicaine (0.5%)	Slow	2-4h	4-8h	2.5mg/kg	3mg/kg
Mepivicaine 1.5%	Rapid	2-3h	2-6h	5mg/kg	7mg/kg
Ropivicaine (0.5%)	Medium	3h	6h	2-3mgkg	2-3mg/kg

Pain Management (Nociceptive) by Severity

	Name	Dosage	Onset	Duration	Timing/Interval	Other
Mild	Tylenol	650mg-1g (Max 3250mg/day (2 g per day in patients with liver disease)	30min-1hour		PO q4-6h prn mild pain	Check LFTs
	ASA (Bayer)	325-650 mg			PO q4h (max 3.9 g/day)	
	Ibuprofen (Advil, Motrin)	600mg PO			Q6h (max 1.2g/day)	
	Naproxen (Aleve)	220-440 PO initially then 220			Q8-12h (max 600mg/day)	
	Tramadol (Ultram)	50-100mg	1 hour	3-6 hours	q6 hrs x' max 400 mg/day	
	Celecoxib	100-200mg			PO q12h	
Moderate	Opioid+NSAID/Acetaminophen					
	Toradol (IV/IM NSAID)	15-30mg IV/IM	10 min		q6h MAX 5d (120mg/day)	
	Hydrocodone 5mg/acetaminophen 325mg (Vicodin)	1-2 tab po			Q4 hours prn	
	Neurontin	300-1200mg			TID	
	Morphine	15-30 mg PO q3-6h 2-10 mg IV/IM/SQ	30 min 5-10min	3-6 hours 3-6 hours	q3-4h	Avoid morphine in AKI or CKD; instead use hydromorphone
	Morphine ER (MS Contin)	PO: 30 mg IV: 10 mg	30-90min	8-12h	q12h	
	Percocet	Mild: 1 5/325 tab PO q3h prn			q6 hours PO	

Pain Management (Nociceptive) by Severity

	Name	Dosage	Onset	Duration	Timing/Interval	Other
	Percocet	Severe: 2 10/325 tab PO q3h				
	Norco	Mild: 5/325 Mod: 10/325	30-60 min	4-6 hours	q3-4h	
	Codeine	RR: 120mg q4-6h CR: 50-300mg q12h	1-1.5 hours	4-6 hours		
Topical Agents						
	Lidoderm	1 patch for 12 hours daily				Apply to intact skin, cover most painful area
	Capsaicin cream	3-4x/day x 2 months				
Opioid/Epidural/Periph Nerve Block						
	Fentanyl	TD: 12-25 mcg/h IV: 100mcg	TD: 12-24h IV: immediate	TD: 72 hours IV: 30m-1 h	q1-2h	
	Demerol	0.5mg IV			q2-3 hours	5x stronger than morphine and can lower seizure threshold
	Oxymorphone SR	20/40/60mg		48 hours		
Severe	Dilaudid	IV: 0.2-1.5mg PO: 2-4mg	IV: 5-15min PO: 15-30min	IV: 4-6 hours PO: 4-6 hours	IV: Q2-4H PRN PO: Q4H PRN	5-6x stronger than morphine
	Meperidine	25-100 mg iv/im/subq (1-1.8mg/kg)	2 hours	2-4 hours	Q4H	Max 150mg
	Methadone	Start 5-10mg PO	30-60m	>8 hours	Q8-12H	Can accumulate in adipose → delayed toxicity; pretreatment

Pain Management (Nociceptive) by Severity

Name	Dosage	Onset	Duration	Timing/Interval	Other
					ECG req'd to evaluate for prolonged QT
Oxycodone IR 5/325	Mild pain - 5 mg Mod pain - 10 mg	15-30m Peak @60m	3-6 hours	4 hours	Morphine can be given rectally, or as a liquid, **avoid in renal failure**. Do not crush CR/ER tablets
Oxycodone ER 5/325	10-20 mg	1 hour	8-12 hours	q12h	
Oxycontin	10-30mg PO	4-5 hours	<12 hours	q4-6h	
Morphine IR (tab, liquid)	0.1mg/kg (up to 15mg) IM/SQ/slow IV	15-30 min (peak @ 60)	O: 4 hours IV: 3-4 hours	Q4H prn	Morphine can be given rectally, or as a liquid, **avoid in renal failure**. Do not crush CR/ER tablets
Morphine ER (tab)		2-4 hours	8-12 hours	Q12h	Patients should be taking at least 60 PO morphine equivalents before starting; need 3 days after placement to assess benefit before adjusting; **safest in renal failure**
Fentanyl IV	0.35-0.5 mcg/kg	IV: 1-2min	IV: 2-4 hours	Q30min – q1h	
Fentanyl IR (lozenge, buccal)	Unknown	5-15min	4 hours	Q6H	
Fentanyl ER (patch)	Unknown	12-18 hours	72 hours		
Ketamine	IV Initial: 0.1 to 0.5 mg/kg bolus; followed by 0.83 to 6.7 mcg/kg/minute (equivalent to 0.05 to 0.4 **mg/kg/hour**)				Patients should be taking at least 60 PO morphine equivalents before starting; need 3 days after placement to assess benefit before adjusting; **safest in renal failure**

CONVERSION FACTORS FOR OPIOIDS

Narcotic analgesic conversions

Oxycontin	Morphine ER	Fentanyl Patch	Methadone
10mg BID	15mg BID		2.5mg TID to 5mg BID
20mg BID	30mg BID	25mcg/hr	5mg TID to 10mg BID
40mg BID	60mg BID	25mcg/hr	5mg QID to 10mg BID
60mg BID	30mg 3 tabs BID	50mcg/hr	5mg QID to 10mg TID
80mg BID	60mg 2 tabs BID	75mcg/hr	10mg TID to 10mg QID

Long Acting Opioids

Drug	Duration	Dose
Buprenorphine Patch 5/10/20mcg/hr	72 hrs	120 mcg
		240 mcg
		480 mcg
Fentanyl ER 25mcg/hr	72 hrs	600 mcg
Hydromorphone SR 8/12/16 mg	24 hrs	8/12/16 mg
Methadone 5/10 mg	72 hrs	15/30 mg
Morphine ER 15/30/60/80/90/100 mg	48 hrs	30/60/90...
Oxymorphone SR 10/15/20/40 mg	48 hrs	20/40/60
Oxycodone SR 10/20/40/80	48 hrs	" "

Opioid Conversion

Morphine q4h	Morphine MR BID	Oxycodone q4h	Oxycontin BID	Fentanyl patch (q3d)
5mg	20mg	2.5mg	10mg	25mcg
10mg	30mg	5mg	20mg	25mcg
15mg	50mg	10mg	30mg	25mcg
20mg	60mg	12.5mg	40mg	25-50mcg
30mg	90mg	20mg	60mg	50mcg
40mg	120mg	25mg	80mg	50-75mcg
50mg	150mg	35mg	100mg	75mcg
60mg	180mg	40mg	120mg	100mcg
70mg	200mg	45mg	130mg	125mcg

** Oxycodone is 1.5x stronger than Morphine

- PCA
  - Dilaudid PCA: Adult naive: load 0.2mg; demand 0.2mg, lockout 10min, 4hr limit 4.8mg
- Pain Contract
  - Medication is for patient only
  - Will take as directed
  - Will only fill at one pharmacy
  - Will not accept controlled substances from any other physician
  - Will come to office for monthly refills
  - Will be held to random drug testing

Figure. Adult acute pain management in the opioid naïve patient

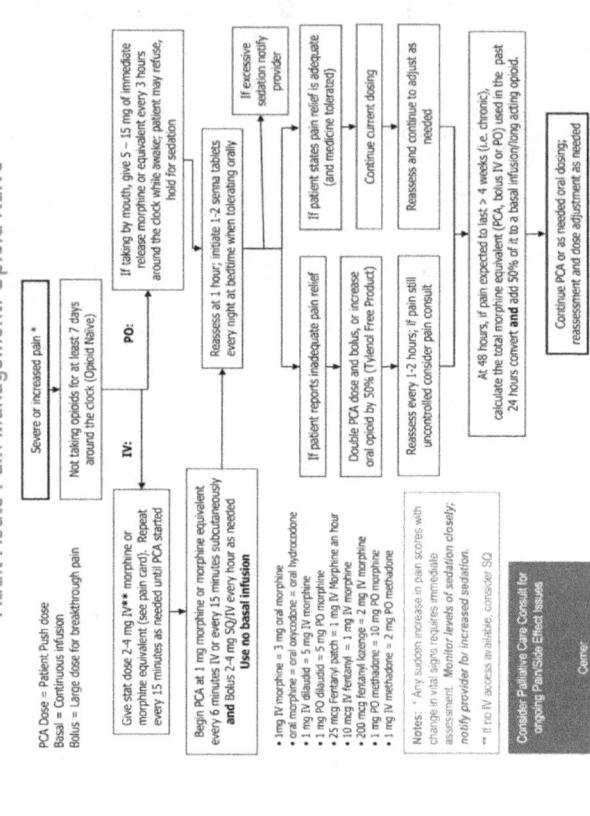

Figure. Adult acute pain management in the opioid tolerant patient

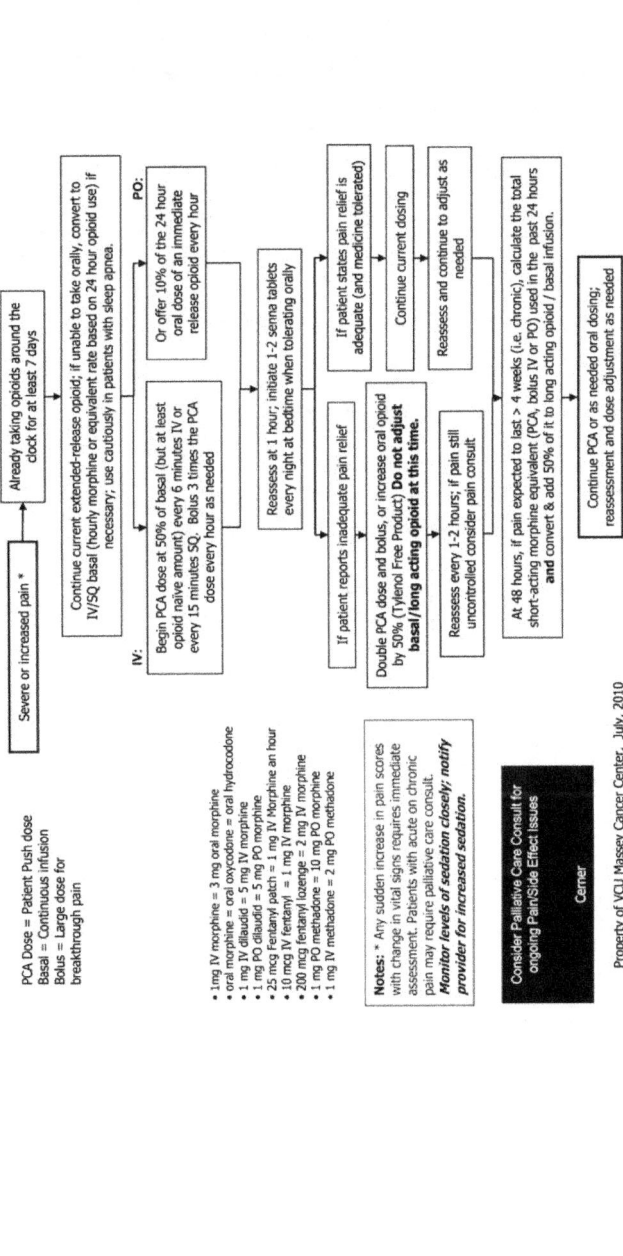

FORMULAS

Electrolytes

Na+ (corrected for hyperglycemia):
Corrected Na+ = measured Na+ + [(glucose − 100) x 0.024].

Ca++ (corrected for hypoalbuminemia):
Corrected Ca++ = [(4 − serum albumin) x 0.8] + measured Ca++.

Free Water Deficit:
Body water deficit in L = wt. (kg) x † x [(plasma Na − 140)/140]
where † = 0.5 for males and 0.4 for females.

Osmolality:
Calculated Serum Osm = (2 x Na+) + (glucose / 18) + (BUN / 2.8) + (EtOH / 4.6)
{normal 270–290}

Osm gap = measured Osm − calculated Osm {normal < 10}.
>10 is abnormal: caused by renal failure, methanol, ethylene glycol,
sorbitol, mannitol, isopropanol, radiocontrast dye.

Anion Gaps
- Serum AG = [Na+] − [Cl-] − [HCO3] {normal 10-14}.
    - Corrected AG (for hypoalbuminemia):
      Corrected AG = serum AG + [(4 − serum albumin) x 2.5]   OR   albumin x 3
- Delta Gap (DAG) = (AG − 12) + HC03 {normal 23–30}.
    - DAG >30: concomitant metabolic alkalosis (excessively high HCO3).
    - DAG <23: concomitant non-AG metabolic acidosis (excessively low HCO3).
- Urine AG = U[Na+] + U[K+] − U[Cl-]
  NH4+ is the major unmeasured cation, so a strongly negative UAG suggests high urine NH4+.
    - Urine AG <0: GI HCO3 loss.
    - Urine AG >0: Renal HCO3 loss (RTA).

Critical Care

- **Oxygenation Index**
  Calculates oxygenation index, useful for predicting outcome especially in pediatric patients.
  (F_iO_2 * Mean Airway Pressure) / P_aO_2
- **King's College Criteria for Acetaminophen Toxicity**
  Provides lab-based recommendations for who should be immediately referred for liver transplant after acetaminophen overdose.
    - Lactate > 3.5 mg/dL (0.39 mmol/L) 4 hrs after early fluid resuscitation?
    - pH < 7.30 or lactate > 3 mg/dL (0.33 mmol/L) after full fluid resuscitation at 12 hours
    - INR > 6.5 (PTT > 100s)
    - Creatinine > 3.4 mg/dL (300 μmol/L)
    - Grade 3 or 4 Hepatic Encephalopathy?
    - Phosphorus > 3.75 mg/dL (1.2 mmol/L) at 48 hours
- **Hemodynamics**
  Pulse Pressure = SBP − DBP (normal 30-40)
  Cerebral Perfusion Pressure = MAP − ICP (normal 60-100)

Nephrology

- **CrCl**
  [(140-age) x Wt in kg] / (Serum Cr x 72) (For ♀: result x 0.85)
  Medications are dosed based on creatinine clearance, not GFR.

- **FeNa**
  [(UrineNa x PlasmaCr) / (PlasmaNa x UrineCr)] x 100
  - <1% = prerenal; >2% = intrinsic renal etiology (ATN)
  - for FeUrea (pts on diuretics), substitude Urea for Na in equation
  - FeUrea <30% = prerenal; >50% = intrinsic (ATN)

Pulmonology

- **Minute Volume**
  $MV = V_T \times RR$
- **Tidal Volume**
  $V_T = V_A + V_D$
  D = deadspace volume
  A = alveolar volume
- **Ratio of physiologic dead space over tidal volume**
  Typically used in those with known respiratory disease and septic patients with pulmonary dysfunction
  $$\frac{V_D}{V_T} = \frac{PaCO2 - P_{Expired\ CO2}}{PaCO2}$$

ELECTROLYTES

PHOSPHATE

Low Phosphate Treatment

Symptoms of Low PO4: Myopathy, weakness, confusion, red cell hemolysis

If K+ <4.0 mEq/L

PO₄ 1-2 mg/dl	Peripheral: 30 mmol KPO4 (contains 44mEq of K+) in 500aa NS over 6 hrs
	Central: 30 mmol KPO4 (contains 44mEq of K+) in 100aa NS over 6 hrs
	Enteral: Use equivalent neutraphos packets (1 packet = 8mmol PO4; 7mmEq Na, 7mmEq K+) → 3 packets
PO₄ <1 mg/dl	30 mmol KPO₄ (contains 44mEq of K+) q6h x 2
	Check labs 1 hour after completion of last bag

If K+ >4.0 mEq/L

PO₄ 1-2 mg/dl	30 mmol NaPO₄ (contains 44mEq of K+) in 250aa NS over 6 hrs
PO₄ <1 mg/dl	30 mmol NaPO₄ (infused over 6 hrs) q6h x 2
	Check labs 1 hour after completion of last bag
	Enteral: Use equivalent neutraphos packets (1 packet = 8mmol PO4; 7mmEq Na, 7mmEq K+)

High Phosphate Treatment (ESRD)

Steps to follow	
1	Restrict dietary intake by 900mg/d
	If Ca < 9.5: calcium carbonate or acetate
	If Ca > 9.5: Sevelamer or Lanthum
2 (if PO4 remains high despite #1)	Check PTH and If PTH>300pg/mL then
	PO4<5.5 & Aa <9.5: Vitamin D analog
	PO4<5.5 & Aa >9.5: Cinacalcet
	PO4>5.5: Cinacalcet

- **Goals In Dialysis Patients:**
    - Ca: 8.4-9.5 mg/dL
    - PO4: 3.5-5.5 mg/dL
    - PTH: 150-300

HYPOMAGNESEMIA

- **Etiology** – m/c due to renal or GI losses
    - Increased excretion - Alcoholism, DM, renal tubular disorders, hypercalcemia/hypercalciuria, hyperaldosteronism, Bartter's syndrome, excessive lactation, marked diaphoresis, diarrhea/vomiting
    - Reduced intake/malabsorption - starvation, bowel bypass/resection, TPN w/o Mg, chronic diarrhea

- Medications: thiazides & loop diuretics, aminoglycosides, amphotericin B, cisplatin, pentamidine, Fl poisoning, cyclosporin.
- Other - acute pancreatitis, low Albumin, Vit D therapy
- **Symptoms**
  - Lethargy, weakness, ↓ mentation, nausea, vomiting, tachyarrhythmias, hypocalcemia, and hypokalemia.
- **Diagnostics**
  - Labs: CMP w/Mg, 24hr urine Mg, consider Mg retention test, LFTs, amylase/lipase if suspect pancreatitis
  - ECG/tele: prolong PR, QT, QRS and arrhythmias
  - Consider calculating functional excretion of Mg:

    $FE_{Mg} = U_{Mg} \times P_{SCr} \times 100$

    $(0.7 \times S_{Mg}) \times U_{SCr}$

    $Fe_{Mg} > 2\%$ drugs such as diuretics, aminoglycosides, or cisplatin.

    $Fe_{Mg} < 2\%$ extrarenal causes
- **Treatment**
  - Beware, SE Oral magnesium = Diarrhea (can be used to your advantage if pt constipated...)
  - If pt has chronic Mg deficiency, give daily supplement
  - Infuse each gram over 1 hour; Milk of Magnesia provides the most elemental Mg then MgCl is the second-best option. PO options include MgOH tablet 400-800mg daily or MOM 24% concentrate susp 10cc (1001 mg of elemental Mg/82 mEq)

Treatment of Hypomagnesemia	
Level	Treatment
>= 1.8 mEq	1gm MgSO4 IV or 400mg PO TID of MgOH
1.4-1.8	2gm MgSO4 IV in 100cc of D5W or NS over 2 hours or 800mg PO MgOH
<1.4	4gm MgSO4 IV in 250cc of D5W or NS over 4 hours

HYPERCALCEMIA

- **Symptoms**[455,456,457]
  - Neuromuscular - somnolence, confusion, depression, psychosis, coma, muscle weakness
  - Gastrointestinal - constipation, anorexia, nausea, abdominal pain, peptic ulcer disease, pancreatitis
  - Renal- ↓ ability to maximally concentrate urine, polyuria, polydipsia, nephrolithiasis, nephrocalcinosis, renal failure
  - Cardiovascular - hypertension, short QT interval, arrhythmias, digitalis sensitivity
  - Skeletal - osteoporosis, fracture, bone pain
- **Differential**
  - Vitamin A/D overdose
  - Iatrogenic
  - Thyroid (bone turnover)
  - Addison's (adrenal failure)
  - Milk alkali syndrome
  - Immobilization / Infection (think TB, histoplasmosis)
  - Neoplastic (think lymphoma, leukemia, SCC)
  - Medications (thiazides, lithium, theophylline)
  - Rhabdomyolysis
  - AIDS

ELECTROLYTES

- o Hyperparathyroidism
- o Sarcoidosis
- o Paget's
- **Orders**
  - o Restrict dietary Calcium to 400 mg/day, push PO fluids
  - o Vitals Q 4 hours; Seizure precautions; I&Os
- **Imaging**
  - o CXR, ECG, mammogram
- **Labs**
  - o Total and ionized Calcium, PTH, CMP, Phosphate, Mg level, PSA, CEA, 24 hour urine Calcium and Phosphate
- **Classifications**
  - o <u>Asymptomatic</u> (Calcium < 12 mg/dL)
    - No immediate therapy required
    - Hold any diuretics
    - Avoid volume depletion
    - ↑activity
  - o <u>Moderate</u> (calcium 12-14 mg/dL)
    - No immediate treatment unless symptomatic
    - *See below*
  - o <u>Severe</u> (>14; symptomatic)
    - Aggressive IVF (NS) and more as below

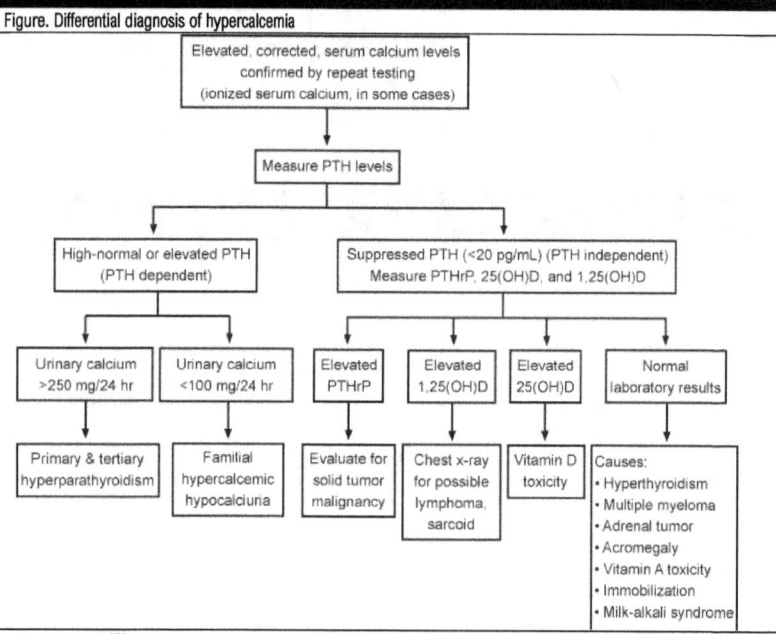

Figure. Differential diagnosis of hypercalcemia

- **Treatment**[458]
  - o <u>Immediate</u>
    - Fluids first
      1. 1-2 L of <u>0.9% saline</u> over 1-4 hours until no longer hypotensive, then saline diuresis with 0.9% saline infused at 200-500 cc/hr **AND**

- Calcitonin (Calcimar) 4-8 IU/kg IM Q 12 hr **OR** 2-4 IU/kg SQ Q 6-12 hours (effective only for 48 hrs)
- Lasix 20-100 mg IV Q 4-12 hours
    1. *Only if patient does not respond initially to fluids above and concern for hypervolemia (CHF)*
    2. Maintain urine output of 200ml/hr, Monitor serum Na, K, Mg
- Pamidronate 60-90 mg IV over 2-24 hrs in patients with hypercalcemia 2/2 malignancy
- Prednisone 50-100mg/d can be considered
- Dialysis is employed if cannot safely give fluids due to severe renal failure or HF
  - Long-Term
    - Bisphosphonate (take 2-4 days for full effect) and act to inhibit osteoclast function and bone resorption **but can worsen renal function**.
        1. Zoledronic Acid 3-4mg over 15-30 minutes – has the best efficacy compared to other bisphosphonates but is usually **reserved for malignancy** with **renal insufficiency (Cr Cl <35)**
        2. Etidronate (Didronel) 7.5 mg/kg/day in 250 ml of normal saline IV infusion over 2 hours. May repeat in 3 days
        3. Pamidronate (Aredia) 60 mg in 500 ml of NS infused over 4 hours **OR** 90 mg in 1 L of NS infused over 24 hours x 1 dose
        4. Denosumab is used for patients who do not respond to above bisphosphonates
    - Surgery – asymptomatic hypercalcemia is treated if patients have a serum level > 1mg/dL over normal, osteoporosis, GFR<60, and are less than 50 years old

HYPOCALCEMIA

- **Etiology** – either due to deficiency in parathyroid hormone or vitamin D
- **Differential**
  - Hypoparathyroidism
  - Parathyroid hormone resistance
  - Vitamin D deficiency or resistance
  - CRF
  - Hungry bone syndrome
  - Pancreatitis
  - Multiple blood transfusions (due to citrate)
  - PO4
  - Osteoblastic metastasis
  - Bisphosphonates
  - Calcitonin
- Symptoms
  - Paresthesias, Chvostek's sign, laryngospasm, bronchospasm, carpopedal spasm, tetany, seizures, ↑ICP
  - Bradycardia, ↑QT
- **Confirmation**
  - Check serum albumin
    - Serum Ca decreases by 0.2 mmol/L or 0.4mEq/L for every 1 g/dL decrease in serum albumin

$$\text{Corrected Ca} = (\text{Measured Ca}) + \{(4.0 - \text{albumin}) \times 0.8\}$$

- Check Mg to ensure concurrent ↓Mg not present

Magnesium level and intervention	
>7.5mmEq	Do Nothing
0.85-1	Check iCa... IV Replacement - If >0.8mMol/L → Do Nothing - If <0.8, give 1gm Calcium Gluconate in 50cc D5W over 30 minutes or 2g in 100cc over 1 hour in D5W Oral Replacement - Calcium carbonate 1250-2500mg (500-1000mg elemental Ca) PO TID-QID
<0.85	3 grams Calcium Gluconate IV in 100 mL of D5W or NS over 2 hours

- **Treatment**
  - Goals: >8.5 or ionized 1
  - Replacement:
    - **Ca Gluconate 1-2 amps in 100cc 1-2 h** (1 amp =1g = 4.65 mEq)
    - Calcium Chloride in Central IV only (3x stronger)
    - PO: Ca carbonate/citrate 500-1000mg PO TID plus daily supplement of Ca+Vit D (600mg/400IU) BID
  - Symptomatic Hypocalcemia
    - CaCl 10% (270 mg Ca/ 10 ml vial) give 5-10 ml slowly (or skin will slough) over 10 min or dilute in 50-100 ml of D5W and infuse over 20 min, repeat Q 20-30 min if symptomatic, or hourly if asymptomatic. Correct hyperphosphatemia before hypocalcemia **OR**
    - Calcium Gluconate 20 ml of 10% solution IV (2 vials) (90mg elemental Ca/10 ml vial) infused over 10-15 minutes, followed by infusion of 60 ml of Ca gluconate in 500cc of D5W (1 mg/ml) at 0.5-2.0 mg/kg/hour
    - Common in **blood transfusions** in patients with renal or hepatic impairment. *See page 313.*
- **Chronic Hypocalcemia:**
  - Ca Carbonate with Vitamin D (Oscal-D) 1-2 tab PO tid OR
  - Ca Carbonate (Oscal) 1-2 tabs PO tid OR
  - Ca Citrate (Citracal) 1 tab PO Q 8 hour or Extra Strength Tums 1-2 tabs PO with meals
  - Vitamin D2 (Ergocalciferol) 1 tab PO daily
  - Calcitriol (Rocaltrol) 0.25mcg PO daily, titrate up to 0.5-2.0 mcg

HYPERKALEMIA

- **Etiology**[459]
  - Consider hemolysis, sepsis (metabolic acidosis), hypoaldosteronism
- **Hospitalize** those with K>6.5 or >5.5 with concurrent EKG signs, AKI, AEHFrEF
- **IV Fluids:** D5NS at 125 cc/hr

ELECTROLYTES

Treatment options for Hyperkalemia

Agent	Mechanism	Dosage	OOA	Duration
Calcium gluconate (10%)	Direct antagonism Membrane stabilization	30cc (or 10cc of calcium chloride 30%)	1-3min	30-60min
Hypertonic Saline* (if ↓Na)	Membrane stabilization	50-250cc	5-10min	2 hours
Sodium Bicarbonate (consideration if pH≤7.2 with HCO3 ≤20)	Redistribution	1 mEq/kg IV over 1-5min; 150 cc/hr; at least 3 amps HCO3;	5-10min	2 hours
Glucose/Insulin	Redistribution	50 cc (50g) D50W with 10U regular insulin IV then D10W 1L with regular insulin 25-50U @ 250cc/hr	30min	4-6 hours
Albuterol/Xopenex (typically added if K>6.5) Risk of SVT and AF; caution in cardiomypathy	Redistribution	2U neb over 5 min up to 20mg	30min	2 hours
Kayexalate	↑ Elimination	15-30g/d or 30-50g/rectum up to q6h	2-3 hours	4-6 hours
Lasix (Typically only done if concurrent fluid overload)	↑ Elimination	40-80mg IV repeat prn	Varies with start of diuresis	Until diuresis present
Fludrocortisone* (known aldosterone deficiency)	↑ Elimination	0.1mg or higher (up to 0.4-1mg/d for chronic use)	N/A	N/A
Lokelma	Binds to K exchange	5mg PO/qod→titrate up to max 15g/d	1-2h	
Patiromer	Polymer exchange resin	8.4g/d w/food titrate weekly up to 25.2g/d	7h	24h

- **Identification:**
    - EKG considered with:
        - New ↑K>6
        - K>5.5 with unstable condition (AKI, shock, AEHFrEF)
    - Earliest sign is an ECG with peaked T waves with a narrow base best seen in leads II, III, V2-V4
        - *Don't be fooled: other causes for peaked T waves include acute myocardial infarction, early repolarization, and LVH*
    - Other signs include a shortened QT interval and ST depression
    - PR interval widening and QRS widening will later be seen
    - The last sign is often a disappearance of the P wave with QRS widening into a sinusoidal pattern
- **Labs:** CBC, CMP, Mg
    - UA, Urine SpG, Urine Na and Cr, 24-hour Urine K
    - Monitor ICU panel q2h
- **Other Source:**
    - STAT ECG, recheck BMP; consider holding ACEI/ARB
    - Immediate Tx for ECG changes with measures that work quickly by shifting K+ into cells:
        - Calcium gluconate 1 amp
        - 2 amps D50 + 10 unit's regular insulin IV over 15 mins
        - Albuterol nebs (20 mg neb over 15 min)
        - HCO3 gtt 150cc/hr
    - Give additional agents to decrease total body store of K+:

- Kayexalate 30 g PO (repeat Q 2 hours until BM) or retention enema
    - **this is not an FDA approved use**
  - Dialysis if necessary- contact nephrology, consider placing trialysis catheter or mahuker
- **Treatment**
  - Goal K 4-4.5
  - See table above
  - Stop RAAS medications
  - Hospitalized patients need:
    - Cardiac membrane stabilization with calcium gluconate
    - Insulin/glucose and/or albuterol (combination given If K>6.5)
      - Inhaled salbutamol (10mg) as affective as 10U if insulin dextrose
    - Consider hypertonic NaHCO3 in patients with severe AGMA
    - RRT if ESRD or severe AKI
    - Loop diuretics adjunct if fluid overload present
  - Outpatient management includes:
    - Frequent K monitoring
    - K+ binders
    - Consider loop diuretics if fluid overload present
    - Temporary discontinuation of RAAS medications

HYPOKALEMIA

- **Etiology**[460]
  U_K Gradient = Urine Potassium (meq/L) × 100 [(mg × L)/(dL × g)] ÷ Urine Creatinine (mg/dL)
  - Urinary potassium concentration is low (< 20 mEq/L) 2/2 extrarenal loss and inappropriately high (> 40 mEq/L) with renal losses
    - U_K >40 mEq/L: kidney potassium wasting: ↑aldosterone, RVS HTN, Cushing, diuretics, RTA, interstitial nephritis
    - U_K <20 mEq/L: extrarenal losses: diarrhea, vomiting, laxatives
    - Potassium shift into cells: ↑insulin, alkalosis, beta agonists, trauma

- **Work-up**
  1) $\underline{TTKG} = \dfrac{Urine_K}{Plasma_K} / \dfrac{Urine_{osm}}{Plasma_{osm}}$
     1. TTKG > 4 = renal or endocrine defect with ↑ distal K secretion
     2. TTKG < 2 = extrarenal cause
  2) Check 24 hr urine K
     3. UK > 30 mmol/day suggests renal losses
     4. UK < 25 mmol/day suggests extrarenal losses
- **Guide**
  - Estimated mEq KCl needed = $\dfrac{\text{Desired K-Measured K}}{\text{Serum SCr}} \times 100$
  - If SCr < 1, then assume SCr = 1

IV Replacement	
Central line:	20 mEq/hr max rate
Peripheral line:	10 mEq/hr max rate
K>4 mEq/L	Give Nothing

ELECTROLYTES

K 3.5-4.0 mEq/L	Peripheral: 20 mEq KAl over 2 hours
	Central: 20 mEq KAl over 1 hours
K 3.1-3.4 mEq/L	Peripheral: 40 mEq KAl over 4 hours
	Central: 40 mEq KAl over 2 hours
K 2.5-3.0 mEq/L	Peripheral: 60 mEq KAl over 6 hours
	Central: 60 mEq KAl over 3 hours
K <2.5 mEq/L	Peripheral: 80 mEq KAl over 8 hours
	Central: 80 mEq KAl over 4 hours
Enteral Replacement (KCl)	
K>4 mEq/L	Give Nothing
K 3.5-4.0 mEq/L	20 mEq KCl
K 3.1-3.4 mEq/L	40 mEq KCl
K 2.5-3.0 mEq/L	40 mEq KCl now then 20mEq in 2 hours
K <2.5 mEq/L	40 mEq KAl now then another 40mEq in 2 hours, consider IV replacement

- **Acute Therapy**
    - K Lyte 50 mEq Po x 1
    - K flash: 40 mEq KCl with 25 cc Lidocaine 1% in NS at 125 cc/hr
    - KCl 20-40 mEq in 100 cc saline infused IVPB over 2-4 hours
        - **OR** Add 40-80 mEq to 1 L of IV fluid and infuse over 4-8 hours
    - KCl elixir 40 mEq PO tid (in addition to IV)
        - Max total dose 100-200 mEq/day (3mEq/kg/day)
- **Chronic Therapy:**
    - Micro-K 10 mEq tabs 2-3 tabs PO tid after meals (40-100 mEq/day) **OR**
    - K-Dur 20 mEq tabs 1 PO bid-tid
- **Hypokalemia with Metabolic Acidosis:**
    - Potassium citrate 15-30 ml in juice PO QID after meals (1 mEq/ml)
    - Potassium gluconate 15 ml in juice PO QID after meals (20 mEq/15 ml)
- **Extras:** ECG, dietetics consult
- **Labs:** CBC, Mg, CMP
    - UA, Urine Na and Cr, 24 hour urine K+
- **Other Source**
    - Preferred to do PO replacement up to 40 mEq as more can cause GI upset
    - Preferred to do IV replacement if patient sx or has ECG changes
        - Max IV rate
            - Peripheral line = 10 mEq/hr
            - Central line = 20 mEq/hr
    - Add 10 mEq K+ for every 0.1 mEq K+ above 3.0
    - Add 20 mEq K+ for every 0.2 mEq K+ below 3.0
        - Ex: if K is 2.8 and want to correct to 4.0, you need (20x1)+(10x10)=120 mEq
    - For urgent replacement give PO liquid or IV
    - If pt has renal failure, cut dose by 1/2
    - If pt extremely low, most K+ you can give at one time is "40mEq PO and 40 mEq IV over 4 hours"

Sliding Scale	
Potassium Level	IV or PO Replacement
3.7-3.8	20 mEq KCl
3.5-3.6	40 mEq KCl
3.3-3.4	60 mEq KCl
3.1-3.2	80 mEq KCl
<3.0	100 mEq KCl

ELECTROLYTES

- **Immediate Treatment Indications**
  - Hepatic Encephalopathy (often 2/2 use of loop diuretics)
  - Cardiac arrythmia (stabilize with calcium gluconate first)
  - Ventilatory failure

HYPONATREMIA

- **Pathophysiology**[461,462,463]
  - Based on volume status:
    - Hypovolemic (decreased total body water with greater decrease in sodium level)
    - Euvolemic (increased total body water with normal sodium level)
    - Hypervolemic (increased total body water compared with sodium).11
  - Osmolality refers to the total concentration of solutes in water (osmolarity is concentration per kg).
    - Effective osmolality is the osmotic gradient created by solutes that do not cross the cell membrane.
    - Plasma osmolality is maintained by strict regulation of ADH and thirst.
      - If plasma osmolality increases, ADH is secreted and water is retained by the kidneys
      - If plasma osmolality decreases, ADH also decreases, resulting in diuresis of free water and a return to homeostasis.
- **Step by Step Approach**
  (also see flow chart at end of section)
  - Must get labs
    - Serum osmolarity
      - Hyper: >295
      - Iso: 285-295
      - Hypo: <280
    - Urine Na
    - Urine Cl
    - Urine Osmolarity (estimate by taking last 2 #'s of SG and multiply by 30)
    - Serum Uric Acid
    - FE_{Uric} to rule out reset osmostat
    - ICUP to look at glucose and albumin
    - UA to look for excess protein
    - Consider
      - Lipid panel
      - AM Cortisol (euvolemic patients may have adrenal insufficiency)
      - TSH (euvolemic patients may have hypothyroidism, particularly myxedema coma)
  - Rule out pseudohyponatremia
    - ↑Lipids → often seen with PBC; tx with statin
    - ↑Protein → tx with chemo (r/o MM)
    - ↑Glucose (DKA, Gluc>400) → tx with fluids, IV insulin
    - ↑TG
  - Determine fluid status
    - *Hypervolemic* – hx of CHF, cirrhosis, or nephrotic syndrome. Significant edema, JVD. S3 gallop auscultated.
    - *Euvolemia* – no evidence of fluid overload of dehydration. U_{Na}>30, $U_{Osmolarity}$>300
    - *Hypovolemia* – recent or chronic use of diuretics, UA with ↑SG, orthostatic ↓BP /tachycardia, poor cap. refill, MM dry. U_{Na}<20 (may be ↑ in contraction alkalosis d/t vomiting for which you use U_{Cl}<20), $U_{Osmoloarity}$>500

ELECTROLYTES

- **Lab assistance**
  - 3 most accurate tests are
    (1) spot urine sodium
    (2) FENa
    (3) FEUrea / FECr
  - Spot Urine Na
    - U_{Na} > 20: euvolemia/SIADH, hypovolemia (unless contraction alkalosis)
    - U_{Na} < 20: hypovolemia (elevated if ARF present)
    - Most hypovolemic patients avidly reabsorb sodium resulting in ↓ urine sodium concentration.
    - Concurrent contraction alkalosis will lead to low U_{Na}, use U_{Cl} instead which should be low in these circumstances of hypovolemia
    - Helps differentiate SIADH from CSW as well
    - Average urinary sodium in hypovolemic patients: 18.4 mEq/L, compared with 72 mEq/L in euvolemic patients
    - If initial sodium is equivocal, give patient 1L 0.9%NS and recheck U_{Na} and Uosm. ↑ urine osmolarity seen in SIADH, low UOsm seen with hypovolemia.
  - FE_{Na} and FE_{Urea} – see below
    - Recent diuretics? Yes, then do FE_{Urea}, if not do FE_{Na}
    - FE_{Urea} <=35% - prerenal (hypovolemia)
    - FE_{Na} <= 1% - prerenal (hypovolemia)
  - Urine Osmolarity
    - Determine the kidneys capacity to dilute urine
    - U_{osm} < 100 : dilute urine due to appropriate suppression of ADH; hypervolemic state

Evaluation of Hypotonic (S_{Osm}<275 mOsm/kg) Hyponatremia based on Volume Status

	Definition	Differential	Labs/Management	Treatment
Hypervolemia	U_{Osm} >100 U_{Na}>20 mmol/L then think renal failure U_{Na}<20 mmol/L then nephrotic syndrome, cirrhosis, CHF	• Heart failure (HF) • Cirrhosis • Nephrotic syndrome • Renal failure (glomerular filtration rate [GFR] < 5 mL/min)	• Serum albumin, UA, BUN, SCr, spot Prot/SCr ratio, PT/PTT, LFTs • Imaging: CXR, TTE	• Fluid restriction (1-1.5L), treat as below • Sodium restriction of 40mEq/day • Optional: Furosemide 40-80 mg IV/PO daily-BID • If symptomatic, then use hypertonic saline • Treatment of asymptomatic hyponatremia in CHF has not been shown to improve mortality

Euvolemia	U_{Osm} <100 (PP, Beer potomania)
	
	U_{Osm}>100: SIADH, diuretic induced, rest osm, adrenal insufficiency, hypothyroidism, reset osmostat
		• Syndrome of inappropriate **antidiuretic hormone** (SIADH) ~ m/c cause, 40%
		   ◦ Must rule out thyroid or adrenal source with normal cortisol and TSH
		   ◦ CNS: trauma, hemorrhage, CVA, infection, vasculitis
		   ◦ Pulmonary: TB, pneumonia, empyema, COPD
		   ◦ Malignancy: small cell, pancreatic, lymphoma, thymoma
		   ◦ Drugs: Chlorpropamide, vincristine, vinblastine, cyclophosphamide, carbamazepine, morphine, SSRI, TCAs, HCTZ
		   ◦ Cancers (eg, pancreas, lung)
		   ◦ CNS disease (eg, cerebrovascular accident, trauma, infection, hemorrhage, mass)
		   ◦ Pulmonary diseases (eg, infections, respiratory failure)
		   ◦ Drugs: Thiazides, Vasopressin, Chlorpropamide, Carbamazepine, NSAIDs, TCAs, Opiates
		• Hypothyroidism
		• Reset Osmostat
			• Check urine osmolarity (estimate = 35 x last 2 digits of SG on UA), TSH, EtOH, K, cortisol
			• Primary adrenal insufficiency
			   ◦ ↓Na /↑K/↑Ca/↓cortisol
			• Beer potomania/ Psychogenic polydypsia
			   ◦ Urine osmolarity << 100 mOsm/L
			• SIADH or Cerebral Salt Wasting
			   ◦ Urine osmolarity >= 300 mOsm/L with ↑FENa
			• SIADH:
			   ◦ U_{Na}>20
			   ◦ S_{UA}<4mg/dL
			   ◦ ↑FE_{Na}
			   ◦ Uric acid low
			   ◦ Low anion gap
			   ◦ Low urea
				Beer Potomania
				• If mild sx or asx: NPO for 24 hours, fluid restriction (1L), no IV fluids.
				• If sx: D5½/2NS bolus of 500cc repeated until sx resolve goal increase of 2 mEq/L/h in 2h then when sx resolve, follow steps above.
				
				Others
				• NPO
				• Fluid restrict 1l/d
				• Oral NaCl tablets (TID)
				
				Primary Polydipsia
				• If mild sx or asx: fluid restrict to 1L and monitor Na q4h
				• If sx: hypertonic saline @ 1cc/kg/hr (can combine with furosemide 20mg IVP if Uosm>500) to decrease total fluid load) until sx resolve (goal ↑ 2mEq/L/h for 2h but <10

Evaluation of Hypotonic (S_{OSM}<275 mOsm/kg) Hyponatremia based on Volume Status

	Definition	Differential	Labs/Management	Treatment
		o Suspect in patient with mild hyponatremia (>125) where the Na remains stable despite changes in fluids and salt intake. o Can differentiate from SIADH by giving a water load (10cc/kg IV) and within 4 hrs, 80% of water load will be urinated (whereas in SIADH it will be mostly retained) • Psychogenic polydipsia • Beer Potomania (↓protein to allow for adequate H2O excretion; normal kidney function) • Secondary adrenal insufficiency • Exercise-associated hyponatremia • Psychogenic Polydipsia o U_{Na}<30		mEq/L in 24h) monitoring Na q2h. After sx resolve then fluid restrict to 1L as above • Optional: Conivaptan (Vaprisol) 20 mg IV over 30 minutes once, followed by a continuous infusion of 40 mg over 24 hours for 4 days (if PO formulation desired, use Tolvaptan 15mg/d)
Hypovolemia	U_{Osm}>100 U_{Na}<10 but U_{Cr}>10: vomiting, diarrhea, 3rd space/resp/skin loss U_{Osm}>100 Urine Na>20: Diuretics, CSW, RTA, Partial obstruction	• Salt and water loss with free water replacement • Severe diarrhea with free water ingestion • Large burns with free water replacement • Third-spacing with free water replacement • Renal disease • Diuretics • Salt-wasting nephropathy	SCr Lactate	• Concept is that with vessels contracted d/t ↓BP, ADH is released causing dilution. With resuscitation, vessels expand and no ADH is released often resulting in large diuresis. Thiazide Diuretic Cause? • Fluid restrict to 1L • Salt tablets 3g TID • Treat hypokalemia CSW • Replete with NS • Consider fludrocortisone 0.1-0.2mg PO BID

Evaluation of Hypotonic (S_{osm}<275 mOsm/kg) Hyponatremia based on Volume Status

Definition	Differential	Labs/Management	Treatment
			- Check Na q4h GI Losses (U_{Na} < 20 d/t contraction but U_{Cl}>20) - Give 0.5-2 L of **0.9% NS** over 1-2 hours until no longer hypotensive, then 0.9% NS at 125 ml/hr **OR** 100-500 ml of 3% hypertonic saline over first 4 hours and titrate to avoid ↑ of more than 12 mEq/L/day

Comparison of Laboratory Findings in SIADH with CSW

	SIADH	CSW
Intravascular volume contraction	No	Yes
Serum sodium	↓	↓
Urine sodium	↑	↑↑
Urine volume	N or ↓	↑
Endocrine		
Plasma ADH	↑	N or ↑
Plasma aldosterone	↓	N or ↑
Plasma renin	↓	N or –↓
Plasma ANP	↑	↑
Urea nitrogen, serum	N or ↓	↑
Serum uric acid	↓	N or ↑

- **Pearls**
    - Diuretics on board – consider diuretic induced hyponatremia (hypovolemic)
    - Hyperkalemia with Hypocalcemia and Hypoglycemia – think adrenal insufficiency
    - Urine osmolarity <= 100 consider PP
    - Don't forget to correct potassium as well!
    - Fluid restriction goal is 500cc below total UOP in a day (typically patients will urinate 1.5L/d therefore we choose 1L for restriction)
    - Patient glucose or lipids highly elevated consider pseudohyponatremia
    - General labs: urine lytes, serum osmolarity, TSH, AM cortisol, urine osmolarity

- **Replacing Sodium**
    1. <u>First correct sodium for any hyperglycemia present</u>

    > Corrected = Measured sodium + 0.024 * (Serum glucose - 100)

    2. <u>Determine if symptomatic or not</u>
        - Severe/Acute: nausea with vomiting, headache, lethargy, pulmonary edema, obtundation, seizures, coma
        - Mild/Chronic: fatigue, nausea, dizziness, gait disturbances, forgetfulness, muscle cramps
    3. <u>Determine the speed of correction</u>
    http://www.mdcalc.com/sodium-correction-rate-in-hyponatremia/
        - **Acute**[464]
            - *No established guidelines*
            - ≤10 mmol/L in 24 hours
            - 12-14 mmol/L in 48 hours
            - 14-16 mmol/L in 72 hours
        - **Chronic**
            - ≤12 mmol/L in first 24 hours
            - ≤18 mmol/L in first 48 hours
        - **Asymptomatic**
            - Increase ↑ S_{Na} @ 0.5 mEq/hr and/or 10 mEq/day or desired Na x wt in kg
        - **Symptomatic**
            - <u>Mild symptoms</u> (see above) – ↑ S_{Na} up to 1.0 mEq/L/hr for 4 hours then decrease rate to ↑ S_{Na} 6 mEq/20h for total increase in 24h of 10 mEq
            - <u>Severe symptoms</u> (see above) - ↑ S_{Na} 1.5-2 mEq/L/hr for 3-4 hours then ↓ rate to achieve 12 mEq/L/day
    4. Order ICU Panel Q2H for first 24 hours

5. Goal correction is for Na to be 120-130 mEq/L
6. Calculate the sodium deficit

> Na deficit = Weight x 0.6 (target S_{Na} − current S_{Na})

7. Determine the best fluid replacement and amount to give:

IVF Composition						
Fluid	Na+	K+	Cl-	HCO₃	Other	Osmolality
3%NS	513	-	513	-	-	1026
Plasma	142	4	104	27	29	306
NS	154	-	154	-	-	308
D₅W	-	-	-	-	-	278
D₅1/2NS	77	-	77	-	-	421
1 amp NaHCO₃	50	-	-	50	-	100
20 mEq KCl	-	20	20	-	-	40

First you want to determine how much free water the patient will excrete (if any) based on what fluids you give. If you give a fluid that is hypotonic to their current status, they will retain fluid. To calculate the fluid osm, multiple the sodium content of the fluid by 2 (NS = 154 x 2; 3% is 513 x 2). The "-1" is for the 1L of fluid given.

$$\frac{\text{Fluid osm}}{\text{Urine osm}} - 1 = \text{amount of free water excreted}$$

A negative number means the patient will **retain** fluid whereas a positive is how much is **excreted**.

8. Determine Infusion Rate based on what fluid you chose above

$$\text{Change in Serum Na/Liter of Infusate} = \frac{\text{Infusate [Na] - Serum [Na]}}{\text{Total Body Water + 1}}$$

Note: TBW = Weight in kg x 0.5 in women, 0.6 in men
The 1 in the denominator accounts for the liter of fluid infused.

- Remember in the equation above, the infusate for NS it would be 154 and hypertonic would be 513
- The equation will give you the total change in sodium expected if you give the entire bag of fluid, based on that, divide it by 1000 (size of fluid bag) to determine how many cc's will be equivalent to 1 mEq of sodium change.
- Based on if they are acute or not, you will need to do the math to determine how much to give in 4 hours, then how much to give for the remaining 20 hours.

9. Consider addition of diuretic if treating with hypertonic saline and large Uosm (>500)
10. If too high of correction, switch to D5W and after you are able to then correct, then turn off fluids
    - If want to reverse, add DDAVP 1-2 mcg IV or IM q6h
    - If right rate, keep going

Figure. Evaluation of hyponatremia

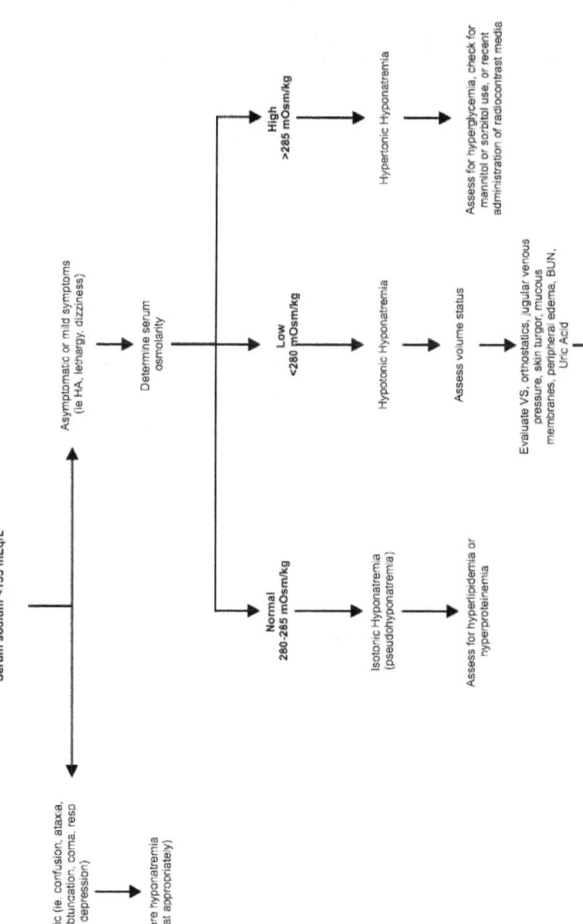

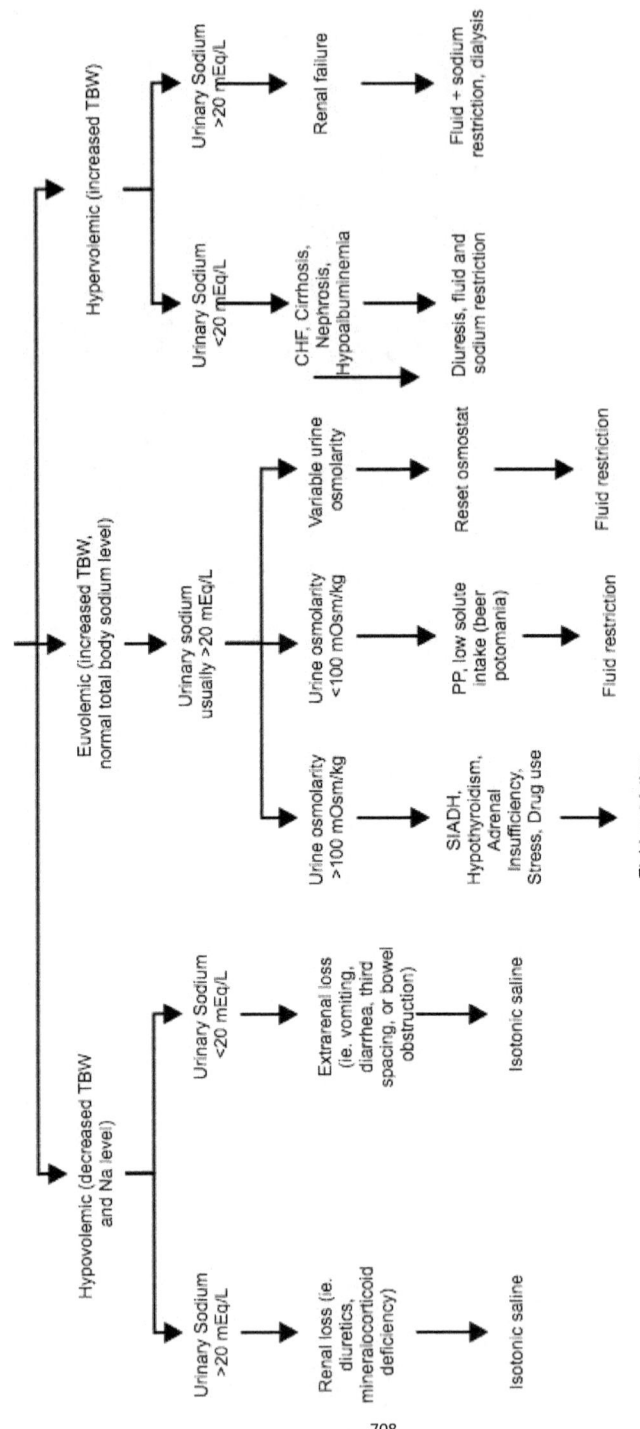

HYPERNATREMIA

- **Definition** - Serum Na is greater than 145 mmol/L.
- **Pathology** - Signs and symptoms are similar to that found in patients with hyponatremia and are due to intracellular dehydration, as high plasma osmolality causes large fluid shifts out of cells.
- **Pearls**
  o Patients who can drink water, should be able to protect themselves against hypernatremia. Thus, in elderly, consider dementia, diarrhea, or inability to obtain water as potential causes.
  o When correcting hypernatremia, think about not only the water the patient must have lost to get to their current sodium (free water deficit), but also their ongoing losses including urine output.
- **Differential**
  o Impaired water intake: urine osmolality > 700 mOsm/L
    - Neurologic disease (e.g., dementia, delirium, coma, stroke)
    - Water unavailable (i.e., desert conditions)
    - Osmotic diuresis with impaired water intake
  o Hyperosmolar hyperglycemia
  o Post obstructive diuresis
  o Rare etiologies
    - DI (if associated with ↓ water intake)
    - Neurogenic DI (↓ADH production)
    - Nephrogenic DI (ADH resistance)
    - Long-term lithium ingestion
- **Evaluation**
  o See polyuria work-up on page 547
- **Treatment**
  o Hypovolemic
    1. Determine how much sodium is elevated relative to target (as a percentage)

       (Current Na / Target Na) / Target Na

    2. Multiply above by the total body water:

       TBW: (% Body Water x Body Weight) x [(Current Na - Target Na)/Target Na]

       % body water = 60% for healthy men / 50% for healthy women / 45% for elderly

    3. Calculate the ongoing fluid losses, how much free water the patient is losing daily as you replete:

       Ongoing losses = Urine volume x (1- (Urine Na + Urine K) / serum Na)

       Or use the following:
       o For first 1L urine, ignore.
       o For urine output (UOP) between 1-3L, assume half of this UOP is lost free water.
       o Assume all UOP beyond 3L is completely lost as free water.

4. **Add the results from the two formulas above** to determine the target water intake for the following hospital day. Divide this number by 24 to determine hourly goal of free water (or D5W).
   - Correction should be no faster than 0.5-1mmol/hour → goal 4-6 mmol/24 hours
     o Calculate fall in serum sodium depending on fluid chosen above
       - D5W = 0 mEq sodium = "0"
       - 0.45NS = 77 mEq = "77"
       - TBW = (0.5 x wt. kgs)
   - Failsafe: infuse at 1-2cc/kg/hr

Bibliography

[455] McPhee, SJ. Current Medical Diagnosis and Treatment 2010. 49th Edition.
[456] Carroll et al. "Evaluation of Hypercalcemia." AFP. May 1, 2003: 67(9)
[457] 61-Year-Old Man With Hypercalcemia and Generalized Lymphadenopathy Egan, Ashley M. et al. Mayo Clinic Proceedings, Volume 0, Issue 0.
[458] Maier et al. "Hypercalcemia in the Intensive Care Unit: A Review of Pathophysiology, Diagnosis, and Modern Therapy." J Intensive Care Med published online 15 October 2013.
[459] Kovesdy, Csaba. "Management of Hyperkalemia: An Update for the Internist." The American Journal of Medicine (2015) 128, 1281-1287
[460] Adopted from the ICU Book (Tripler)
[461] Spasovski et al. "Clinical practice guideline on diagnosis and treatment of hyponatraemia." Eur J Endocrinol March 1, 2014 170 G1-G47
[462] Gardner DG. Chapter 24. Endocrine Emergencies. In: Gardner DG, Shoback D.eds. *Greenspan's Basic & Clinical Endocrinology, 9e.* New York, NY: McGraw-Hill; 2011
[463] Braun et al. "Diagnosis and Management of Sodium Disorders: Hyponatremia and Hypernatremia." Am Fam Physician. 2015;91(5):299-307.
[464] Sterns et al. "The Treatment of Hyponatremia." Seminars in Nephrology. 29(3) May 2009

ABBREVIATIONS

Ab ......antibody
AACG......acute angle closure glaucoma
ABC ......airway, breathing, and circulation
ABG ......arterial blood gas
ABx......antibiotics
ACEi ......angiotensin-converting enzyme inhibitor
ACS ......acute coronary syndrome
ADH ......antidiuretic hormone
AF ......atrial fibrillation
AFB ......acid-fast bacillus
Ag ......antigen
AIDS ....acquired immunodeficiency syndrome
AKI ......acute kidney injury
ALKP ......alkaline phosphatase
ANA ......antinuclear antibody
ANCA ...antineutrophil cytoplasmic antibody
APTT ....activated partial thromboplastin time
ARB ......angiotensin II receptor blocker
ARDS ...acute respiratory distress syndrome
AS ......aortic stenosis
AST ......aspartate transaminase
ATN ......acute tubular necrosis
AV ......atrioventricular
BAL ......bronchoalveolar lavage
BKA ......below-knee amputation
BNP ......brain natriuretic peptide
BP ......blood pressure
BPH ......benign prostatic hyperplasia
CA ......cancer
CABG ...coronary artery bypass graft
CI ......contraindications
CKD ......chronic kidney disease
CMV ......cytomegalovirus
CNS ......central nervous system
C/f......concerning for
C/o......complaining of
COPD ......chronic obstructive pulmonary disease
CPAP ....continuous positive airway pressure
CPR ......cardiopulmonary resuscitation
CRP ......c-reactive protein
CSF ......cerebrospinal fluid
CT ......computed tomography
CVA ......cerebrovascular accident
CVP ......central venous pressure
CXR ......chest x-ray
DAPT....dual antiplatelet therapy
D/C......discharge
DM ......diabetes mellitus
DVT ......deep venous thrombosis
ECG......electrocardiogram
EEG ......electroencephalogram
EMG ......electromyogram
ERCP ......endoscopic retrograde cholangiopancreatography
ESR ......erythrocyte sedimentation rate
FEV1 ......forced expiratory volume in 1st sec
FiO2 ......partial pressure of O2 in inspired air
FFP ......fresh frozen plasma
FHx......family history
FLQ ......fluoroquinolone
FSH ......follicle-stimulating hormone
FVC ......forced vital capacity
g ......gram
G6PD ....glucose-6-phosphate dehydrogenase
GCS ......Glasgow Coma Scale
GDMT....Guideline directed medical therapy
GFR ......glomerular filtration rate
GGT ......gamma-glutamyl transferase
Hgb ......hemoglobin
HbA1c ..glycated hemoglobin
Hct ......hematocrit
HCV ......hepatitis C virus
HDL ......high-density lipoprotein
HIV ......human immunodeficiency virus
H/o......history of
HoTN......hypotension
HSV ......herpes simplex virus
IBD ......inflammatory bowel disease
ICD ......implantable cardiac defibrillator
ICP ......intracranial pressure
ICUP....ICU panel / Metabolic Panel
IDDM ......insulin-dependent diabetes mellitus
INR ......international normalized ratio
IVC ......inferior vena cava
JVP ......jugular venous pressure
K ......potassium
kg ......kilogram
L ......liter
LA......left atrium of the heart
LAD ......left axis deviation on the ECG
LBBB ...left bundle branch block
LDH ......lactate dehydrogenase
LDL ......low-density lipoprotein
LFT ......liver function test
LH ......luteinizing hormone
LMN ......lower motor neuron
LMWH ..low-molecular-weight heparin
LOC ......loss of consciousness
LP ......lumbar puncture
LUQ ......left upper quadrant
LV ......left ventricle of the heart
LVH ......left ventricular hypertrophy
MAP ......mean arterial pressure
MCV ......mean cell volume
mcg......microgram
mg ......milligram
MI ......myocardial infarction
mmHg... millimeters of mercury
MRCP ...magnetic resonance cholangiopancreatography
MRI ......magnetic resonance imaging
MRSA ...methicillin-resistant Staph. aureus
MS ......multiple sclerosis
MSM ...men who have sex with men
NA......not applicable
NIDDM .non-insulin-dependent diabetes mellitus
NOAC...non-vitamin K oral anticoagulant
NSAID ..non-steroidal anti-inflammatory drug
OCP ......oral contraceptive pill
PaCO2 ...partial pressure of CO2 in arterial blood
PaO2 ......partial pressure of O2 in arterial blood
PCI......percutaneous coronary intervention
PCR ......polymerase chain reaction
PE ......pulmonary embolism
PEEP ....positive end-expiratory pressure
PET ......positron emission tomography

ELECTROLYTES

PMH/PMHx .....past medical history
PRN......as needed
PSA ......prostate-specific antigen
PSHx....past surgical history
PTH ......parathyroid hormone
PTT ......prothrombin time
PTX......pneumothorax
PUD.....peptic ulcer disease
PVD ......peripheral vascular disease
RA.......right atrium of the heart
RAD .....right axis deviation on the ECG
RBBB ...right bundle branch block
RBC ......red blood cell
RCT ......randomized controlled trial
RDW ....red cell distribution width
RUQ .....right upper quadrant
R/O ......rule out
RTA......renal tubular acidosis
RV ....right ventricle of heart
RVF ......right ventricular failure
RVH ......right ventricular hypertrophy
S1, S2 ....first and second heart sounds
SC ....subcutaneous
s/e ....side-effect
SIADH ..syndrome of inappropriate anti-diuretic hormone secretion
SL ....sublingual
SLE ......systemic lupus erythematosus
SOB ......short of breath
SpO2 ....peripheral oxygen saturation (%)
STD/I ...sexually transmitted disease/infection
SVC ......superior vena cava
SVT ......supraventricular tachycardia
T2DM...type 2 diabetes mellitus
T3 ....tri-iodothyronine
T4 ....thyroxine
TFT ......thyroid function test
TIA ......transient ischemic attack
TIBC ....total iron-binding capacity
TPN ......total parenteral nutrition
TSH ......thyroid-stimulating hormone
TTP ......thrombotic thrombocytopenic purpura
U ....units
UC ....ulcerative colitis
UMN .....upper motor neuron
URT ..upper respiratory tract
US....ultrasound
UTI ......urinary tract infection
VF ....ventricular fibrillation
V/Q ....ventilation/perfusion scan
VTach ....ventricular tachycardia
VTE ......venous thromboembolism
WBC ....white blood cell

APPENDIX

COMMON OUTPATIENT TREATMENTS

Bloating
- Nexium 20mg daily
- Simethicone 40-360 mg after meals and QHS prn
- Dicyclomine
- Probiotics (Lactobacillus)

Indigestion
- Maalox 30 ml PO Q 4 hours prn indigestion
- Avoid in dialysis pts
- CaCO3 (Tums) 2 tablets PO
- Safe in dialysis pts
- Zantac 150 mg PO BID prn indigestion
- GI Cocktail (Benmalid 15cc; combo of Maalox, viscous lidocaine, Benadryl), give with Toradol 15mg

Dry Eyes
- Liquitears (1-2 drops into eye(s) prn to relieve sx)
- HCMP (1-2 drops per eye prn q6h or qhs)
- Tears Naturale (1-2 drops into eye(s) prn to relieve sx)
- Fish oil
- Polyvinyl alcohol 1.4% 1 drop OU q4h prn
- PEG/PG 0.4/0.3% (Systane) 1 drop OU q4h prn
- Lacri Lube ophthalmic ointment thin ribbon to both eyes Q6H

Hiccups
- Baclofen 10mg po Q8H prn.
- Chlorpromazine 25mg po Q6H prn.
- Metoclopramide 10mg PO or IV Q6H prn

Mucolytics
- Mucomyst
- Pulmozyme
- NAC

Nausea/Vomiting
- Alcohol pads (smelling)
- Zofran 4 mg IV Q 4 hours prn nausea
- Phenergan 25 mg IV/IM or 50mg PO Q 4 hours prn N/V
  - Use lower doses in elderly d/t increase side effects
  - Watch for dystonic reactions and restlessness
- Reglan 10 mg IV/PO Q 6 hours prn N/V
  - Avoid in bowel obstruction or diarrhea b/c stimulates gut motility
  - Consider risk of Extrapyramidal Symptoms
    - Given Benadryl concurrently to ↓ risk
  - Document you discussed risk with patient
  - If EPS develops, give Cogentin
- Tigan 250 mg po TID/QID or 200 mg IM/PR q 6-8h
- Compazine 10 mg IM/IV/PO/PR Q 6 hours prn Nausea
- Scopolamine 1.5mg patch behind ear q3d
- Meclizine 25 mg PO 4 times daily
  - For N/V d/t motion sickness & vertigo
- Zyprexa 10mg QHS – used by heme/onc

Oral Ulcers
- Triamcinolone 0.1% dental paste

Pruritis
- Benadryl 25-50 mg PO/IV Q 4 hours
  - Avoid or reduce dose in elderly

ELECTROLYTES

- Hydroxyzine 25-100 mg PO/IM Q 6 hours
  - Avoid in elderly, can't be given IV
- Cholestyramine 4g BID-TID
- Ursodiol

Secretions

- Atropine ophthalmic solution 1% 2gtts SL Q4H prn
- Glycopyrrolate (Robinul) 0.4mg IV Q6H prn
- Scopolamine patch 1.5mg behind the ear Q3days

Hemorrhoids

- Medical management (e.g., stool softeners, topical over-the-counter preparations, topical nitroglycerine), dietary modifications (e.g., increased fiber and water intake), and behavioral therapies (sitz baths) are the mainstays of initial therapy. [465]
- Rubber band ligation
- Sclerotherapy
- Infrared coagulation (IRC)
- Cryotherapy
- Sitz bath
- Topical hydrocortisone 10mg/zinc acetate 10mg rectal suppository
- Hydrocortisone 25mg rectal
- Hydrocortisone 2.5% cream
- Topical nifedipine 0.3% BID x12w
- Topical lidocaine 1.5% BID x12w
- Topical mineral oil+Petrolatum+phenylephrine

SUTURING

Wound closure timelines

Location	Suture type	Technique	Removal
Scalp	3-0/4-0 nylon or polypropylene	Interrupted in galea, tight single layer in scalp, use horizontal mattress to control bleeding	7-12 d
Ear	5-0 vicryl/dexon in perichondrium	Close perichondrium with interrupted Vicryl; use nylon for skin	3-5 d
Eyebrow	4-0/5-0 vicryl (SQ) 6-0 for skin	Layered	3-5 d
Eyelid	6-0 nylon	Single-layer horizontal mattress or simple interrupted	3-5 d
Lip	4-0 vicryl (mucosa) 5-0 vicryl (muscle) 6-0 nylon (skin)	Must close three layers if involving lip; all others do 2 layers	3-5 d
Perioral	4-0 vicryl	Single interrupted or horizontal mattress if muscularis of tongue involved	N/A
Face	6-0 nylon (skin) 5-0 vicryl (SQ)	Simple interrupted for single layer but use layered closure for full-thickness lac	3-5 d
Trunk	4-0 vicryl (SQ, fat) 4-0/5-0 nylon (skin)	Single or layered closure	7-12 d
Extremity	3-0/4-0 vicryl (SQ, muscle) 4-0/5-0 nylon (skin)	Single-layer interrupted or vertical mattress Use a splint if over a joint	10-14 d
Hand/Foot	4-0/5-0 nylon	Single-layer closure Use simple interrupted or horizontal mattress sutures Use a splint if over a joint	7-12 d
Nail	5-0 vicryl	Ensure you maintain even edges Allow sutures to dissolve	N/A

QUALIFYING FOR HOME OXYGEN

- Conditions

- o Physician determines patient suffers from severe lung disease or hypoxia-related symptoms that may improve with oxygen:

Diagnoses Qualifying for Home Oxygen
COPD
Interstitial Lung Disease
Cystic Fibrosis
Bronchiectasis
Pulmonary malignancy
Pulmonary Hypertension
CHF c/b cor pulmonale
Erythrocytosis
Impaired cognition
Nocternal Restlessnes
AM Headaches

- o **Diagnostic Requirements**
Patient's arterial blood gas indicates a need for oxygen:
  - Continuous Oxygen
    - □ PaO2 < 55 mmHg or O2 sat < 88% at rest
    - □ PaO2 56-59 mmHg or O2 sat ≥ 89% AND dependent edema suggesting CHF OR pulmonary hypertension/cor pulmonale (measured PA pressure, echocardiogram, P pulmonale on ECG→P wave > 3 mm in leads II, III, or aVF)
  - Nocturnal oxygen therapy only if
    - □ PaO2 < 55 mmHg or O2 sat < 88% while asleep AND PaO2 > 56 mmHg or O2 sat > 89% while awake
    - □ PaO2 ↓ > 10 mmHg, Resting PaO2 ≤ 59 mmHg or O2 sat ↓ > 5% from waking to sleeping or SaO2 ≤ 89% AND cor pulmonale or erythrocytosis (HCT>55%)
  - Exercise oxygen therapy only if:
    - □ PaO2 < 55 mmHg or O2 sat < 88% during activity for a patient with PaO2 > 56 mmHg or O2 sat > 89% during the day at rest, and it is documented that use of oxygen improves hypoxemia with exercise
  - Alternative treatment measures have been tried or considered and have failed

MUSCULOSKELETAL INJECTIONS

Supplies		
Medication	**Dosage**	**Description**
Methylprednisolone	40mg/mL	Intermediate acting
		May cause more injection site pain
		May form crystals if mixed with lidocaine
		Preferred use with soft tissue injections d/t solubility
Triamcinolone (Kenalog)	40mg/mL	Recommended for joints d/t insolubility
Lidocaine	0.5% (5mg/mL)	Recommended
	1.0% (10mg/mL)	Rapid acting
	2.0% (20mg/mL)	Lasts 30 minutes
		With epinephrine prolongs effect and decreases bleeding
Bupivacaine (Marcaine)	0.25% (2.5mg/mL)	Slower onset (takes 30 min for full effect)
	0.5% (5mg/mL)	Duration >8h
Sodium bicarbonate	8.4% (9ml/1mL)	Helps decrease burn from lidocaine

Injection Cheat Sheet		
Use steroid "in suspension"; syringe should be luer-lock tip		
Location	**Supplies**	**Description/Other**
Knee	5cc syringe	Medial approach

ELECTROLYTES

	4cc 1% lidocaine 1cc 40mg Triamcinolone 22g x 1.5" needle Ethyl chloride for topical	Locate the insertion of the tendon of quadriceps femoris into the proximal patella, follow 1/3 of the way around the medial border of the patella and insert the needle 2cm below this parallel to the horizontal axis Performed q3-4m Lateral approach Find the equator of the patella (the middle line) and inject to the upper outer rim in a medial direction
Shoulder	Glenohumeral Injection 5cc syringe 4cc 1% lidocaine 1/2cc 40mg Triamcinolone 22g x 1.5" needle Subacromial Injection 5cc syringe 2cc 1% lidocaine 1/2cc 40mg Triamcinolone 22g x 1.5" needle	Indications: tendonitis, OA, impingement, bursitis Glenohumeral Posterior approach recommended Subacromial space is target Trace spine of scapula laterally to angle of acromion, 2cm down Angle 15° up with injection towards ipsilateral coracoid Subacromial (pain @ lateral shoulder near deltoid; painful arc) Lateral approach recommended Hands resting on lap, neck and shoulder relaxed Inject @ 2cm below midpoint of lateral edge of acromion
Trigger Finger	3cc syringe 1/2cc 1% lidocaine 1/2cc 40mg Triamcinolone 22g x 1.5" needle	First identify the MCP joint crease at the base of the palm side of the finger to be injected. Pick a point 1-2 centimeters proximal to the MCP crease and exactly in the midline of the affected finger. Advance the needle through the skin at an angle perpendicular to the surface of the palm. Once you have entered the tendon (confirm by having patient slowly flex and extend finger which should cause needle to rock). Start the push medication in as you slowly pull out needle, when it starts to freely flow, you will be out of the tendon and the medication will be safe to finish. You do not want to inject into the tendon itself!
Trigger Point	5cc syringe 2cc 0.25% Bupivacaine (or 2% lidocaine) 2cc Sodium Chloride 25g x 1.5" needle	Inject 1ml into each trigger pt TTP with referral pattern pain No steroid needed
Elbow	3cc syringe 1cc 1% lidocaine 1/2cc 40mg Triamcinolone 22g x 1.5" needle	Mostly lateral injections Injection with patient lying down and elbow flexed + internally rotated onto chest
Trochanteric Bursa	5cc syringe 4cc 1% lidocaine 1cc 40mg Triamcinolone 18g-22g x 2" needle	Patient lies on unaffected side with hip flexed 90 degrees to help with the ID of painful site Inject needle perpendicular to ground Hit bone, then retract and inject (medication must be delivered to the surface of the lateral femur; there will be some resistance)

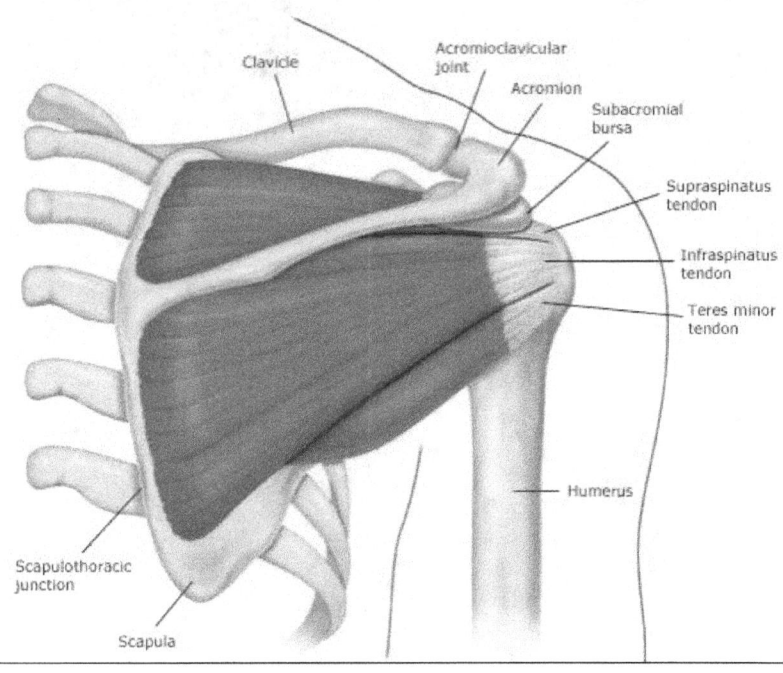

Figure. Posterior shoulder anatomy

Figure. Steroid injection into shoulder

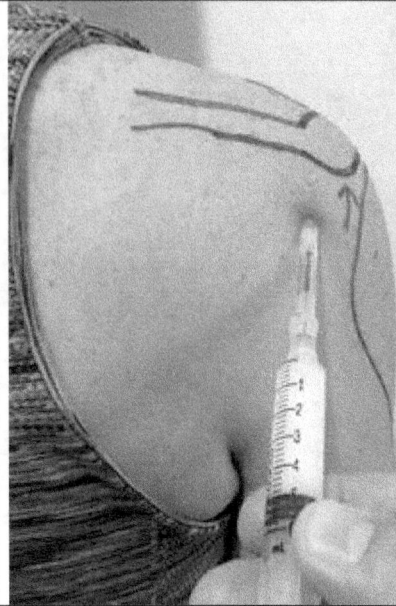
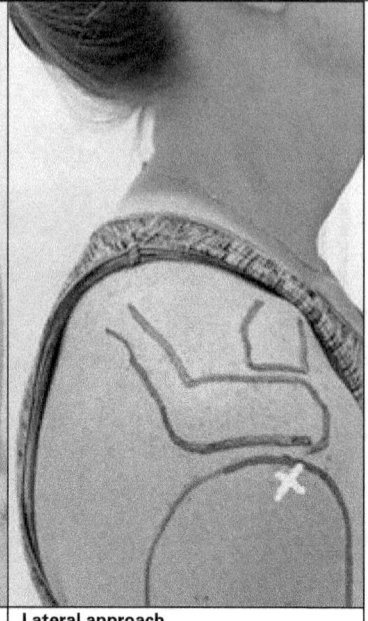

Posterior approach (entry point is 1-2 cm inferior and medial to the posterior-lateral corner of the acromion. Needle angled upward until contacting the acromion then walk under the acromion to enter the subacromial space; needle will be about 2cm deep)	**Lateral approach** (needle is angled upward 45 degrees until the tip touches the edge of the acromion; then walk the needle along the undersurface as you are lowering the needle inferiorly; needle will be about 1cm deep)

Figure. Steroid injection into knee via lateral approach

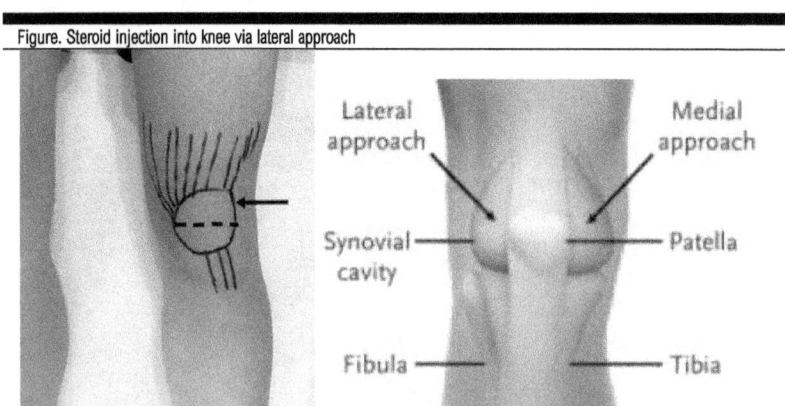

USPSTF SCREENING RECOMMENDATIONS

Age	18	21	24	25	35	40	45	50	55	59	65	70	74	75	80
UPSPSTF screening recommendations															
HIV infection												if at increased risk			
Hepatitis B viral infxn															
Syphilis															
TB															
Chlamydia and Ghonorrea	if sexually active														
Cervical cancer		Pap smear q3y, or q5y with HPV cotest starting at 30													
Hyperglycemia						if overweight or obese									
Hepatitis C viral infxn			if at high risk											if at high risk	
Colon CA								if born between 1945-1965							
Breast CA								biennial screening (depends on society)							
Lung CA									if 30 pack years and current or former smoker (within past 15y)						
Osteoporosis								if ≥9.3% 10 year FRAX risk			starting at 65				
AAA											if ever smoker				
Vaccinations															
Zoster									2 doses of RZV 2-6mo apart regardless of history						
HPV women	through age 26														
HPV men	age to 21														
PCV13											starting @ 65, 1 dose if not prev. received f/b PPSV23 1 year later				
PPSV23											If PCV13 req'd, start there. PPSV23 1 year after PCV13				
Influenza	yearly														

	normal risk, men only
	men only with risk factors
	Normal risk men and women
	with risk factors, men and women
	with risk factors, women only
	normal risk, women only

PCV13/PPSV23 Specific High Risk Populations
- Chronic heart disease (except HTN)
- Chronic lung disease
- Chronic liver disease
- EtoH abuse
- T2DM or IDDM
- Cigarette smoking
- Chronic renal failure
- Nephrotic syndrome

ELECTROLYTES

Pneumonia vaccinations compared[466]

≥65 Years Old

Pneumovax 23	Prevnar 13
Asplenia	*Shared Decision making for the following conditions:*
Hemoglobinopathy (i.e. SSD)	
Congenital or acquired immunodeficiency	Asplenia
Cancer (e.g., leukemia, lymphoma, MM)	Hemoglobinopathy (i.e. SSD)
HIV	Congenital or acquired immunodeficiency
CKD or nephrotic syndrome	Cancer (e.g., leukemia, lymphoma, MM)
Organ transplant	HIV
Immunosuppression (corticosteroids ≥14 days)	CKD or nephrotic syndrome
CSF leak	Organ transplant
Cochlear implant	Immunosuppression (corticosteroids ≥14 days)
Heart disease (CHF, cardiomyopathy)	CSF leak
Pulmonary disease (COPD, emphysema, or asthma)	Cochlear implant
Diabetes	
Alcoholism	
Cigarette smoking	
Chronic liver disease	

19-64 Years Old

Pneumovax 23	Prevnar 13
Asplenia	Asplenia
Hemoglobinopathy (i.e. SSD)	Hemoglobinopathy (i.e. SSD)
Congenital or acquired immunodeficiency	Congenital or acquired immunodeficiency
Cancer (e.g., leukemia, lymphoma, MM)	Cancer (e.g., leukemia, lymphoma, MM)
HIV	HIV
CKD or nephrotic syndrome	CKD or nephrotic syndrome
Organ transplant	Organ transplant
Immunosuppression (corticosteroids ≥14 days)	Immunosuppression (corticosteroids ≥14 days)
CSF leak	CSF leak
Cochlear implant	Cochlear implant
Heart disease (CHF, cardiomyopathy)	
Pulmonary disease (COPD, emphysema, or asthma)	
Diabetes	
Alcoholism	
Cigarette smoking	
Chronic liver disease	

Give vaccinations 1 year apart if patient will receive both

- **Preventive services covered by Medicare**[467]
  - Vaccinations: influenza (yearly), PCV-23 (x1), hepatitis B (series)
    - PCV-13 only advised in high risk groups
  - BMD: q2y
  - CV screening: lipid q5y, AAA
  - CRC screening
  - Glaucoma: yearly
  - DM: q2y
  - Mammography: yearly after 40yo
  - Pap testing: q2y
  - Prostate CA: DRE, PSA

TOBACCO DEPENDENCE

- **General**
  - Quitting smoking by age 50 cuts the risk of a smoking-related death in half and quitting by age 30 almost completely negates it.

- o Nicotine patches are contraindicated at the time of acute coronary syndrome, malignant arrhythmia, CHF exacerbation, pregnancy.
- **Treatment Options by Success Rate**[468,469]
  - o Highly nicotine-dependent smokers may require initial therapy for 6 months or longer. Some individuals may require low-dose maintenance therapy for years.

Smoking Cessation Options

Therapy	Indications	Prescription	Instructions	Side Effects
Chantix	No effect on weight gain	- Days 1-3: 0.5 mg/day. Days 4-7: 0.5 mg twice a day. - Day 8+: 1 mg twice a day. - Use 6 months (safe up to 12m)	- **Start 1-4 weeks before quit date.** - Take with food and a tall glass of water to minimize nausea. - Quit date can be flexible, from 1 week to 3 months **after** starting drug. - Dual action: relieves nicotine withdrawal and blocks reward of smoking. - May require >4w to reach peak effect	Nausea, insomnia, abnormal dreams, neuropsych sx?
Patch	Helps to **prevent** cravings from occurring	<u>If smoking ≥10 cigarettes/day</u> - 21-mg/day patch for the first 4-6 weeks then taper by 7mg at 2wk intervals <u>If smoking <10 cigarettes/day</u> - 14-mg/day patch for the first 4-6 weeks then taper by 7mg at 2wk intervals	- **Start high then decrease over 8-10 weeks** - Apply a new patch each morning to dry skin. - Rotate application site to avoid skin irritation. - May start patch before or on quit date. - Can add prn gum, lozenge, inhaler, or nasal spray to patch to cover situational cravings.	- Skin irritation - Insomnia - Vivid dreams (patch can be removed at bedtime to manage insomnia or vivid dreams)
Patch+Nortryptiline		(OFF LABEL) 75-100mg/d for 12-14wk	Good if co-morbid depression present	↑QT interval, drowsiness, dry mouth
Wellbutrin SR	Good option if concurrent psychiatric disease; less weight gain. Combine with NRT (patch) for best results	- 150 mg/day for 3 days, then 150 mg twice a day - Use 3-6 months or longer if h/o depression	**Start 1-2 weeks before quite date.** May lessen post-cessation weight gain while drug is being taken.	Insomnia, dry mouth, seizures, neuropsych sx?

Gum			
Often used in conjunction with patch (>14 weeks of therapy) to treat **sudden** urges	<ul><li>If 1st cigarette is ≤30 minutes of waking: 4 mg.</li><li>If 1st cigarette is >30 minutes of waking: 2 mg.</li><li>Use ≥3 months.</li><li>Patients are instructed to use 1 piece of gum every 1-2 hours for the first 6 weeks and then reduce their use to 1 piece every 2-4 hours for the next 3 weeks and finally to 1 piece every 4-8 hours for the 3 weeks after that.</li><li>In highly dependent smokers, the 4-mg gum is superior to the 2-mg gum.</li><li>Because about 50% of the nicotine in gum is absorbed, a smoker who is on a fixed schedule of 10 pieces per day will receive a daily nicotine dose of about 10 mg with the 2-mg gum and 20 mg with the 4-mg gum.</li></ul>	<ul><li>Chew briefly until mouth tingles, then 'park' gum inside cheek until tingle fades. Repeat chew-and-park each time tingle fades. Discard gum after 30 minutes of use.</li><li>Use ~ 1 piece per hour (Max: 24/day).</li><li>Can damage dental work and be difficult to use with dentures.</li><li>No food or drink 15 minutes prior to use and during use.</li></ul>	Mouth soreness, dyspepsia

MEDICAL CODING/BILLING

Established Patient

Face to Face Time	History			Exam	Medical Decision Making (MDM)
	HPI	ROS	PFSH		
99213 (15 minutes)	Brief (1-3 elements or status of 1-2 chronic conditions)	Problem Pertinent (1 system)	N/A	Expanded Problem Focused (2-7 body areas or organ systems)	Low Complexity
99214 (25 minutes)	Extended (4+ elements or status of 3+ associated chronic conditions)	Extended (2-9 systems)	Pertinent (1 of 3)	Detailed (2-7 body areas or organ systems)	Moderate Complexity
99215	Extended (4+ elements or status of 3+ associated chronic conditions)	Complete (10+ systems)	Complete (2 of 3)	Comprehensive (8+ organ systems or complete exam of single system)	High Complexity

E&M Tool

Time
- Face-to-face Time: total length of encounter

History

Elements of HPI
- Location
- Quality
- Severity
- Duration
- Timing
- Content
- Modifying Factors
- AS&S

Elements of ROS

Exam

Exam (Organ Systems)
- Constitutional
- HEENT
- Cardiovascular
- Respiratory
- Gastrointestinal

MDM

To qualify for a given type of MDM, 2 of the 3 elements in the table must be met or exceeded

Elements of MDM	Level of Complexity			
	Straight-forward	Low	Moderate	High

Constitutional	GI
HEENT	GU
CV	MSK
Resp	Skin
Endocrine	Psych

Elements of PFSH
Medications, allergies, injuries, surgeries
Family diseases, medical events
Marital status, living arrangements, IVDA

Exam (Body Areas)
Genitourinary	HEENT
MSK	Chest
Skin	Abdomen
Neurologic	Genitalia, groin, buttocks
Psych	Back, including spine
	Each extremity

	Minimal	Limited	Multiple	Extensive
Number of diagnoses or management options	Minimal (1 dx)	Limited (2 dx)	Multiple (3 dx)	Extensive ($\geq$4 dx)
Amount and/or Complexity of Data to be Reviewed	Minimal or none ($\leq$1 data pt)	Limited (2 data pts)	Moderate (3 data pts)	Extensive ($\geq$4 data pts)
Risk of Complications and/or Morbidity/Mortality	Minimal	Low	Moderate	High

- >50% face to face time with the patient and/or family spent in counseling and/or coordination of care, including time spent with parties who have assumed responsibility for patient's care
- the nature/extent of the counseling and/or coordination of care

New Patient

History & Exam	99203	99204	99205
Components Required: 2 of 3			

		Required
Chief Complaint		
HPI	1-3 elements	≥4 elements (or ≥3 chronic dz)
ROS	2 systems	≥10 systems
PMHx/PSHx	1 element	≥3 elements
Examination	1 detailed system + 1 brief system (≥12 elements)	8 systems or 1 complete single system (comprehensive)

Medical Decision Making		
Risk of complications +/- M&M	Low	Moderate	High
Diagnosis/Treatment	Low	Moderate	High
Typical Time (minutes)	30	45	60

Duration of the visit does not control the LOS to be billed unless >50% of the face-to-face time or more than 50% of the floor time (for inpatient service) is spent providing counseling or coordination of care.

In-patient

Admission Visit		Daily Visit		Consultation	
Time (min)	Code	Time (min)	Code	Time (min)	Code
30	99221	15	99231	20	99221
50	99222	25	99232	40	99222
70	99223	35	99233	55	99223

Observation Status (24h)		Discharge Day Management		Admin/Discharge Same Day	
Code		Time (min)	Code	Time (min)	Code
99218		≤30	99238		99234
99219		>30	99239		99235
99220		99217 for observation discharge			99326

Others

Prolonged Services (outpatient)

99354	Prolonged evaluation and management (E/M) or psychotherapy service(s) (beyond the typical service time of the primary procedure) in the office or other outpatient setting, with direct patient contact beyond the usual service; 30 minutes beyond usual time.
99357	+30 min thereafter
Medical Team Conference	
99366	With interdisciplinary team of health care professionals, face-to-face with patient and/or family, 30 minutes or more; **participation by nonphysician** qualified health care professional
99367	With interdisciplinary team of health care professionals, face-to-face with patient and/or family, 30 minutes or more; **participation by physician**
Preventive Medicine Services	
99385	Age 18-39; initial comprehensive preventive medicine E/M
99386	Age 40-64; initial comprehensive preventive medicine E/M
99387	Age ≥65; initial comprehensive preventive medicine E/M
99395	Age 18-39; periodic comprehensive preventive medicine re-evaluation and management of established patient
99396	Age 40-64; periodic comprehensive preventive medicine re-evaluation and management of established patient
99397	Age ≥65; periodic comprehensive preventive medicine re-evaluation and management of established patient
Transition from Inpatient to Outpatient	
99495	Includes communication (direct contact, telephone, electronic) with the patient/caregiver within 2 business days of discharge from an inpatient hospital setting; medical decision-making of at least moderate complexity during service period; and face-to-face visit within **14 calendar** days of discharge
99496	Includes communication (direct contact, telephone, electronic) with the patient and/or caregiver within 2 business days of discharge from an inpatient hospital setting; medical decision-making of high complexity during the service period; and face-to-face visit, within **7 calendar** days of discharge
Telephone Services	
99441	Telephone E/M service provided by a physician or other qualified health professional who may report E/M services provided to an established patient, parent, or guardian not originating from a related E/M service provided within the previous 7 days nor leading to an E/M service or procedure within the next 24 hours or soonest available appointment; 5-10 minutes of medical discussion
99442	11-20min

99443	21-30min

Online Evaluation

99444	Online E/M service provided by physician or other qualified health care professional who may report E/M services provided to an established patient or guardian, not originating from a related E/M service provided within the previous 7 days, using the Internet or similar electronic communications network

Modifiers

-25	Significant, separately identifiable E/M service by the same physician or other qualified health care professional on the same day of the other service. *Example: patient comes in for knee pain, OA is diagnosed, decide to do intraarticular steroid injection.*
-59	Distinct procedural service
-95	Synchronous telemedicine service
-GC	Used with CPT code to show involvement of a resident or fellow

Supervised Resident Visits

- The attending physician does not need to copy the history. Acceptable language might be "I saw and evaluated the patient. I agree with the findings and the plan of care as documented by the resident." or "I was present during the history and physical. I discussed the case with the resident and agree with the findings and plan as documented by the resident."
- Remember to use GC modifier

Bibliography

[465] Davies et al. "Diagnosis and Management of Anorectal Disorders in the Primary Care Setting." Prim Care. 2017 Dec;44(4):709-720.
[466] Clinical Resource, *Pneumococcal Vaccination in Adults: Who Gets What and When? Pharmacist's Letter/Prescriber's Letter.* September 2019.
[467] Heidelbaugh et al. JFP. 2008: 57(11).
[468] Lande et al. "Nicotine Addiction Treatment & Management." Medscape.
[469] Bornemann et al. "Smoking cessation: What should you recommend?" J Fam Pract. 2016 January;65(1):22-29B.
Icons in TOC used under Creative Commons License from Pixabay.com

INDEX

4

4-f-pcc, 318

A

A1c. See hga1c
A-a gradient, 495
Abcd2 score, 454
Abdominal compartment syndrome, 64
Abdominal film, 366
Abdominal pain by location, 29
Abnormal uterine bleeding, 641
Acd, 309
Acetaminophen toxicity criteria, 690
Acetominophen overdose, 637
Acid base, 531
Acid-base compensations, 489
Acidosis
    Metabolic, 534
    Respiratory, 534
Acls
    Abcd survey, 80
    Asystole, 80
    Bradycardia, 80
    Medications, 79
    Pea, 81
    Torsades de pointes, 82
    Vfib, 82
    Wpw, 82
Acne, 19
Acs
    Anticoagulation with afib, 190
    Posterior infarction, 149
    Rv infarction, 147
Acute coronary syndrome, 176
Acute kidney injury, 536
Acute myocardial infarction
    Angina, defined, 176
    Minoca, 167
    Universal classification of mi, 183
Acute myocardial infarction
    Defined, 178
    Supply/demand mismatch, 179
Acute pancreatitis, 60
    Complications, 65
    Management, 62
    Monitoring, 64
    Ranson, 61
    Scoring, 61
        Apache, 61
        Bisap, 61
Acute renal failure, 536
Adenosine, 79
Adrenal incidentaloma, 235
Adrenal insufficiency, 206
Adult nutrition
    Associated labs, 666
    Inpatient diet, 664
Agitation, 585
Agma, 532
Aivr, 144
Alcohol withdrawal, 599, 630
Alcoholic patient, 599
Alkalosis
    Metabolic, 534
    Respiratory, 534
Allergic rhinitis, 557
Altered mental status, 411
Alzheimers dementia, 292
Ambien, 589
Amiodarone, 79
Ams, 411
Ana, 579
Ana pattern, 578
Anaphylactic reactions, 323
Anaphylaxis, 525
Anemia, 305
    Acd treatment, 309
    B12 deficiency, 309
    Ckd, 545
    Epo, 545
    Folate deficiency, 309
    Icd labs, 307
Anemia of chronic disease, 307
Anemia of chronic inflammation, 307
Angina
    Defined, 176
    Stable, 177
    Stable, risk assessment, 169
    Unstable, 176
    Unstable, risk assessment, 170
Angina, defined, 167
Angiotensin ii, 126
Anion gap
    Elevated, 534
    Low, 536
    Nagma, 534
Anion gaps, 690
Ankle/foot pain differential, 388
Anticoagulation
    Acs and afib post pci, 190
    Atrial fibrillation bridging, 612
    Doac, 228
    Dvt, 347
    Perioperative cessation, 614
    Recurrent vte, 347
    Stents, 201
    Vte, 342
Antiphospholipid abs, 342
Anxiety disorder, 602
    As needed treatment, 602
    Augmentation for ssri, 602
    Pre-procedural, 602
Aortic aneurysm, 177
Apixaban, 344
Apthous ulcers, 713
Aptt, 324, 325
Ards, 523
Ascites
    Child-turcotte-pugh scoring, 31
    Labs, 30
    Meld score, 32
    Refractory, 32
    Saag, 31
    Tips, 33
    Treatment, 32
Ascvd, 167, 667
    High risk conditions, 171
    Very high risk, 171
Aspiration pneumonia, 135
Aspiration pneumonia, 93
Asthma, 472
    Exacerbation, 479
    Refractory, 478
    Treatment based on severity, 480
    Treatment,acute, 479
    Treatment,chronic, 474
Asthma exacerbation, 479
Atopic dermatitis, 25
Atrial arrhythmias, 142
Atrial fibrillation
    Antiarrhythmics, 224
    Anticoagulation, 225
    Has bled, 226
    Valvular, definition of, 226
Atrial fibrillation
    Cha2ds2-vasc, 226
    Outpatient treatment, 223
    Rvr, 222
Atrial fibrillation

Anticoagulation post pci, 190
Atrial fibrillation, 221
Atrial flutter, 142
Atropine, 79
Autoantibody profile, 579
Avnrt, 145
Avrt, 145

B

B12 deficiency, 309
Back pain, 376
Bacteremia, 99
Billing. See medical coding
Bipap, 519
Birth control, 645
Bisphosphonates, 238
Bladder pressures, 64
Bleeding disorders, 324
Bleeding time, 325
Bloating, 713
Blood transfusion, 314
  Blood products, 319
  Specialized transfusions, 315
Bms, 201
Body weight calculations, 666
Bowel obstruction, 66
Bph, 657
Bradycardia, 81
Breast cancer screening, 313
Bundle branch block, 146
Bupivicaine, 683

C

Ca chloride, 79
Ca gluconate, 79
Cacs, 169
Cad, 167, 609
Caloric requirements, 674
Cam, 584
Cancer screening
  Breast, 313
  Lung, 500
Capacity, 582
Cardiac index, 504
Cardiac resynchronization therapy, 166
Cardiac stress testing, 172
Cardiogenic shock, 527
Cardiogenic shock, 527
Cardiomyopathy, 205
Cardiorenal syndrome, 165
Cbc, 304
Ccta, 169
Cellulitis, 98, 105
Centor criteria, 562
Centromere, 578
Cervical cancer, 719
Chest pain, 176
  Atypical, 183
  Differential, 178
  Nstemi, 183
  Risk assessment, 184
  Stemi, 183
  Unstable angina, 183
Child-turcotte-pugh scoring, 31
Cholelithiasis, 33, 34
Chronic kidney disease, 543
Chronic obstructive pulmonary disease, 480
Cirrhosis
  Complications, 37
  Decompensated, 38
  Hepatic encephalopathy, 38
  Labs, 36
  Management, 38
  Sbp, 39
  Variceal prophylaxis, 36
Ciwa protocol, 630
Ciwa score, 631
Ciwa score, 631
Ckd, 543
Clabsi, 334
Clostridium difficile, 107
Clostridium difficle
  Diagnosis, 107
  Prevention, 109
  Recurrent, 108
  Treatment, 110
Code cart medications, 79
Code status, 16
Colonoscopy prep, 58
Colonscopy, 44
Coma, 438
Coma cocktail, 439
Common cold, 559
Concussion, 413
Conductive hearing loss, 567
Confrontation testing, 405
Congestion, 563
Congestive heart failure, 150
  Assessment, 151
  Diagnosis, 151
  Hfpef, 165
  Hfref, 156
  Nhya stages, 150
  Primary prevention, 166
  Treatment, 154
    Medications, 159
Conjunctivitis, 353
  Bacterial, 354
  Viral, 354
Constipation, 339
Contraception
  Options, 648
Contraception, 645
Contraception
  Emergency, 651
Contrast induced nephropathy, 540
Copd, 480
Copd
  Air travel, 488
Chronic treatment, 482
Diagnosis, 481
Exacerbation, 488
  Abx, 489
  Diagnostics, 489
  Steroids, 489
  Treatment, 490
  Gold criteria, 483
  Labs, 481
  Treatment, 485
Corneal abrasion, 352, 357
Coronary artery calcium score, 169
Coronary artery disease, 167
  Primary prevention, 171
  Secondary prevention, 171
Coronary artery diseasegorithim for treatment approach to cad
  Treatment approach, 169
Coronary calcium score, 169
Coronary cta, 169
Cough
  Asthma, 462
  Gerd, 462
  Uacs, 462
Cpap, 519
Cpap vs bipap, 520
Cranial nerves, 405
Crrt, 541
Crt, 166
Cryoprecipitate, 317, 321, 327
Cushing's disease, 235
Cva
  1-3-6-12 rule, 454
  Abc/2 method, 454
  Bleeding after tpa, 448
Cvp, 503
Cxr, 360
Cystitis. See urinary tract infections

D

Dabigatran, 345
Death requiring autopsy/medical examiner, 14
Deceased, 13
Declaring patient deceased, 13
Delirium, 582
  Common symptoms, 584
  Prophylaxis, 587
  Vs. Dementia, 587
Dementia, 292
  And pyschosis, 295
  Rapid onset, 296
  Rapidly progressive, 298, 322
  Treatment, 299
  With behavioral disorder, 295
Depression, 590

Acute withdrawal, 592
Augmentation with benzo, 591
Medication discontinuation, 592
Monitoring, 592
Treatment, 593
Treatment resistent, 591
Dermatomes, 403
Des, 201, 609
Dexa, 237
Diabetes insipidus, 547
Diabetes mellitus, 244
    Insulin titration, 266
Diabetes mellitus
    Combination agents, 255
    Injectable agents, 248
    Oral agents, 247
    Sglt2 vs. Glp1, 248
Diabetes mellitus
    Po medications, 249
Diabetes mellitus
    Medications compared, 254
Diabetes mellitus
    Combination medications, 255
Diabetes mellitus
    Ordering supplies, 258
Diabetes mellitus
    Inpatient care, 258
Diabetes mellitus
    Gestational, 258
Diabetes mellitus
    Microvascular vs macrovascular, 259
Diabetes mellitus
    Preventive interventions, 259
Diabetes mellitus
    Insulin management, 263
Diabetes mellitus
    Insulin, 265
Diabetes mellitus
    Insulin sensitivity ratio, 266
Diabetes mellitus
    Insulin sliding scale, 266
Diabetes mellitus
    Preoperative insulin, 621
Diabetes mellitus
    Iv insulin to sq, 621
Diabetic ketoacidosis
    Dka vs. Hhs, 267
    Labs, 267
    Management, 272
    Monitoring, 267
    Treatment, 270
        Fluids, 270
        Insulin, 271
        K, 270
Diarrhea
    Acute, 44
        Bacterial causes, 46
    Chronic, 49
        Differential, 50
        Labs, 51
        Treatment, 52

Etiologies, 45
Inflammatory, 45
Labs, 49
Management, 49
Noninflammatory, 45
Osmolar gap, 50
Red flags, 49
Stool osmolarity, 50
Diarrhea treatment, 339
Diastolic heart failure, 165
Dic, 326
Differential diagnosis, 11
Digoxin, 223
Diruetic resistence, 155
Discharging patients, 15
Disk herniation, 377
Disseminated intravascular coagulation, 326
Diverticulitis
    Treatment, 53
Dka, 267
Dlco, 467
Doac, 228
    Perioperative cessation, 614
    Perioperative interruption, 609
    Reversal agents, 227
    Table of options, 228
Dobutamine, 126
Dopamine, 79, 125
Dry eyes, 713
Dvt, 340
Dvt prophylaxis, 347
Dyspepsia, 67, 713
Dyspnea, 12, 463

E

Early repolarization, 149
Ebv, 561
Echocardiography, 367
Edoxaban, 345
Effusion
    Knee, 386
    Pleura, 496
Ekg, 140
    Axis deviation, 141
    Sinus arrhythmia, 142
    Sinus bradycardia, 142
    Sinus tachycardia, 141
Electrolytes, 690
    Goals in dialysis patients, 692
    Hypercalcemia, 693
    Hyperkalemia, 696
    Hypernatremia, 709
    Hypocalcemia, 695
    Hypokalemia, 698
    Hypomagnesemia, 692
    Hyponatremia, 700
    Phosphate, 692
    Requirements, 678
    Sodium
        Fena, 691

        Feurea, 691
Emesis, 713
Empiric antibiotic management, 88
End of life management, 301
Endocarditis, 127
Epididymitis, 658
Epinephrine, 79, 125
Epo, 545
Erectile dysfunction, 241
Etoh, 599
Extubation criteria, 516
Eye pain, 352
Ezetimbe, 671

F

Fenofibrate, 671
Feurea, 539
Fever of unknown origin (fuo), 103
Ffp. See fresh frozen plasma
Fibrinolytic agents, 198
Folate deficiency, 309
Framingham/atp iii risk score, 167
Frax, 238
Free water deficit, 690
Fresh frozen plasma, 317
Fresh frozen plasma, 321
Frontotemporal dementia, 292
Full fever workup, 103

G

Gait types, 427
Gca, 419
Gerd, 67
Gi bleed
    Admission criteria, 55
    Labs, 56
    Lower, 55
    Management, 58
    Upper, 54
Gi cocktail, 713
Glomerular disease, 551
Glomerulonephritis, 552
Gout, 570
Graft-vs-host disease, 324
Gram negative
    Cocci, 87
    Rods, 87
Gram positive
    Cocci, 87
    Rods, 87
Gram stain interpretation, 88
Graves disease, 278

H

H. Pylori treatment, 70

Headache
  Er cocktail, 424
Headaches, 417
  Acute treatment, 424
  Cluster, 420
  Cocktail, 421
  Differential, 420
  Menstruation related, 423
  Migraine, 421
  Preventative, 425
  Tension, 420
Hearing loss, 565
Heart failure, 150
Heart failure, 150
Heart score, 170
Hematuria, 656
Hemodynamic monitoring in the icu, 503
Hemolytic anemia, 308
Hemolytic anemia, 328
Hemolytic reactions, 322
Hemophilias, 325
Hemorrhagic strokes, 450
Hemorrhoids, 714
Heparin induced thrombocytopenia, 328
Hepatic encephalopathy
  Grading, 37
Hepatic encephalopathy, 38
  Treatment, 38
Hepatitis b, 74
Hepatorenal syndrome, 40
Herpes zoster, 355
Hfpef, 165
Hfref, 156
Hga1c, 245
Hhs, 275
Hiccups, 424, 713
Hip arthroplasty, 347
Hit. See heparin induced thrombocytopenia
Hospitalized
  Hcap, 132
Hypercalcemia, 693
Hypercoagulable state, 342
Hyperkalemia, 696
Hypernatremia, 709
Hypertension, 207
  Essential, 207
  Goals, 208
  Hypertensive crisis, 217
  Hypertensive emergency, 216
  Hypertensive urgency, 216
  Medications, 212
  Resistent, 219
  Secondary, 207
  Treatment, 208
Hyperthyroidism, 277
  Causes, 278
Hypertriglyceridemia, 669, 672
Hypertrophy, 146
Hypocalcemia, 695
Hypoglycemia, 277
Hypokalemia, 698
Hypomagnesemia, 692
Hyponatremia, 700
Hypotension, 205
Hypothyroidism, 281
Hypovolemic shock, 527
Hypoxia, 494

I

Ibs, 40
Ibw, 124
Ich, 450
Ild, 490
Impingement, 392, 395
Implantable cardioverter-defibrilltor, 166
Inbutation
  Rapid sequence intubation steps, 510
Incontinence, 661
  Mixed, 661
  Stress, 661
  Urge, 661
Indigestion, 713
Initial vent settings, 520
Injections (steroid), 715
Insomnia, 587
Insulin
  Iv to sq, 621
  Perioperative management, 621
  Preoperative management, 621
  Split mixed human regimen, 263
Insulin initiation, 263
Interstitial lung diseases, 490
Intubation
  Neuromuscular blockade agents, 513
  Pain medications, 508
  Rapid sequence intubation, 516
  Sedation medications, 506
  Vent settings, 513
Intubationii, 504
Intubationii, 504
Ipf, 492
Iron deficiency anemia, 309
Iron panel, 307
Iron, iv replacement, 310, 311
Iron, oral replacement, 309
Irradiated blood. See blood transfusion
Irritable bowel syndrome, 40
Ischemic heart disease, 167
Iv fluid replacement, 679
Iv fluids, 678
  Maintenance, 677

J

Joint aspiration labs, 574
Joint fluid analysis, 386
Joint pain, 573
  Approach, 573
  Aspiration labs, 574
  Broad assessment, 577
  Differential, 575
  Exam findings, 574
  Labs, 576
  Monoarthritis, 574
  Polyarticular, 575
J-point elevation, 149

K

Ketamine, 682
Kidney stone, 553
Knee arthroplasty, 347
Knee effusion, 386
Knee examination, 378
Knee injection, 715
Knee pain, 378

L

Lactate, 122
Lbbb, 147
Lbp, 376
Leg pain, 390
Leg pain differential, 390
Leukoreduced blood. See blood transfusion
Lewy body dementia, 292
Lidocaine, 683
Liver associated enzymes, 71
  Causes, 73
  Hepatitis b panel, 74
  Labs, 74, 75
  Marked, 73
  Mild, 73
  Moderate, 73
Local analgesia, 683
Loss of consciousness. See syncope
Lower gi bleeds, 55
Lumbar puncture, 112
  Csf evaluation, 113
  Labs, 112
Lunesta, 589
Lung cancer screening, 500
Lung volumes, 467

M

Map, 504
Mcmurray's test, 379
Mcv, 307
Mdd, 590

Mechanical ventilation, 517
Medical coding, 724
Medications
  Abx, 88
  Acls, 79
    Afib, 83
    Asystole, 80
    Bradycardia, 81
  Acs
    Anticoag, 201
  Afib, 222
  Agitation, 585
  Alcohol withdrawal, 600
  Anxiety, 602
  Asthma, 474
  Atrial fibrillation, 222
  Atrial flutter, 143
  Benzo+ssri, 602
  Bloating, 713
  Bph, 657
  Cellulitis, 106
  Chf, 159
  Cholesterol lowering, 671
  Contraception, 648
  Copd exacerbation, 490
  Copd,chronic, 485
  Delirium, 585
  Doac, 228
  Dry eyes, 713
  Empiric antibiotics, 91
  Ezetimibe, 171
  Gp2b3a, 198
  Hemorrhoids, 714
  Hfpef, 165
  Hiccups, 713
  Hypertension, 212
  Hypertensive emergency, 218, 220
  Incontinence, 661
  Indigestion, 713
  Insulin, 263, 265
  Intubation, 506
  Iron replacement, 310
  Lasix drip, 164
  Meningitis, 115, 116
  Nausea, 713
  Noac, 228
  Osteoporosis, 238, 239
  P2y12, 198
  Pain management, 684
  Pci, 196
  Pcsk9, 171
  Pharyngitis, 563
  Pneumonia, 132
  Ppi, 68
  Pre-procedural, 603
  Pruitis, 713
  Rhinitis, 558
  Rsi, 510
  Sleep, 587
  Snri, 594
  Spironolactone, 164
  Ssri, 593
  Statins, 669
  T2dm, 249
  Tcas, 596
  Testosterone replacement, 242
  Ua/nstemi, 188
  Uti, 117
  Vomiting, 713
Meld score, 32
Meningitis, 102, 112
  Causes, 115
  Csf findings, 114
  Demographic, 116
  Gram stain interpretatin, 88
Menopause, 644
Menorrhagia, 652
Metabolic acidosis, 534
Metabolic acidosis
  Chronic, 536
Metabolic alkalosis, 534
Metabolic alkalosis, 532
Metabolic syndrome
  Triglycerides, 668
Mgso4, 79
Migraine
  Treatment, 424
Migraine headaches, 421
Mild cognitive impairment, 301
Mini-cog, 294
Mmse, 294
Moca, 294
Monoarthritis, 574
Monoarticular arthritis, 574
Mucolytic, 713
Mucolytics
  Copd, 487
Mucositis, 339
Murmurs, 203
Musculoskeletal exam
  Knee, 378
  Shoulder, 391
Musculoskeletal injections, 715
Muscuoskeletal exam
  Back, 376
Myocardial infarction
  Type 1, 183
  Type 2, 183
  Type 3, 183
  Type 4a, 183
  Type 4b, 183
  Type 5, 183

N

Nafld, 75
Nagma, 532
Naloxone, 439
Narrow complex tachycardia, 82
Nasal congestion, 563
Nausea, 339, 713
  Gi cocktail, 713
Needle stick, 12
Nephritic range proteinuria, 551
Nephrolithiasis, 553
Nephrotic range proteinuria, 551
Neurogenic cough, 462
Neuroleptic malignant syndrome, 599
Neurological exam, 404
Neuromuscular blockade agents, 513
Neuromuscular blockers, 123
Neutropenia, 331
Neutropenic fever, 332
Nicotine abuse, 720
Noac, 228
  Perioperative cessation, 614
  Perioperative interruption, 609
Noacs for vte, 345
Norepinephrine, 125
Nstemi, 183
Nucleolar, 578

O

Obstructive sleep apnea, 502
Ocp, 645
Ogilvie's, 66
Ogtt, 245
Opiate-induced constipation, 42
Opthalmology referral indications, 353
Orthostatic hypotension, 407
Orthostatics, 413
Osmolality formula, 690
Osteoporosis, 236
Overactive bladder, 659
Overdose, 637
Oxygen, 714
Oxygen
  Home, qualifying diagnoses, 496
Oxygenation index, 690

P

P2y12 inhibitors, 198
Pacemaker basics, 229
Pain, 681
  Abdominal pain, 29
  Cancer, 683
  Conversion factors for opioids, 687
  Example inpatient opiate regimen, 681
  Muscle spasm, 683
  Neuropathic, 682
  Pain contract, 687
  Pca, 687
  Pharmacologic options, 684
Pancreatitis, 60
Pap smear, 719
Paracentesis labs, 30
Parkinson's disease, 427
Parkland formula* for burn patients, 678
Passed out. See syncope

Pcsk9 inhibitor, 171, 201, 671
Pcwp, 504
Pe, 340
Peak pressure, 518
Peptic ulcer disease, 69
Pericarditis, 177
Perioperative
   Bleeding risk by procedure, 612
Perioperative evaluation
   Cardiac, 616
Perioperative evaluation
   Bridging anticoagulation, 610
   Doac interruption, 609
   High risk bleeding, 610
   Vte risk, 610
   Vte risk per valve type, 613
   Warfarin, 607
Perioperative evaluation
   Surgical operative risks, 623
Perioperative evaluation
   Tte, 626
Perioperative evaluation
   Ekg, 627
Perioperative evaluation
   Medication management, 628
Perioral dermatitis, 25
Periperative stress testing, 175
Peripheral neuropathy, 429
Pfps, 383
Pft's, 465
Pharyngitis, 560
Phenazopyridine, 117
Phenylephrine, 125
Pheochromocytoma, 235
Phosphate, 692
Pituitary incidentaloma, 284
Plantar fasciitis, 389
Plateau pressure, 518
Platelets, leukocyte, 321
Pleural effusion, 496
   Analysis, 497
   Lights criteria, 497
Pleural effusions
   Transudative vs. Exudative, 497
Pneumonia, 102, 129
   Aspiration, 93, 135
   Cap, 132
   Diagnostic workup, 129
   Hap, 134
   Mdr risk factors, 130
   Treatment, 132
Pocus, 368
Poison control, 637
Polyarthritis, 575
Polyarticular arthritis, 575
Polycystic ovarian syndrome, 643
Polyuria, 547
Post catheterization, 200
Posterior infarction, 148
Prediabetes, 246

Pregnancy
   Agitation, 586
   Hypertension, 211
   Vte, 343
Preoperative evaluation, 616
Pressors, 125
Preventive medicine screening, 719
Pronator drift, 405
Proteinuria
   Nephritic range, 551
   Nephrotic range, 551
Pruitis, 713
Psi, 130
Psychosis
   Due to dementia, 295
Pt, 324, 325
Ptsd, 601
Pulmonary capillary wedge pressure, 504
Pulmonary embolism, 340
Pulmonary embolism, 340
Pulmonary embolus, 177
Pulmonary nodule, 499
Pvc, 143
Pyelonephritis, 120
Pyuria, 117

R

Raiu, 279
Ranson, 61
Rapid shallow breathing index, 523
Rbbb, 147
Rbc morphology, 305
Rbc transfusion, 315
Reflux, 67
Renal tubular acidosis, 535
Resistant hypertension, 219
Respiratory acidosis, 534
Respiratory acidosis, 532
Respiratory alkalosis, 534
Respiratory alkalosis, 532
Reticulocyte count, 308
Revised geneva, 341
Rheumatologic labs, 578
Rhinosinusitis, 559
Rivaroxaban, 344
Romberg, 406
Rta, 535
Rv infarction, 147
R-wave progression, 149

S

Saag, 31
Sbp, 39
Schistocytes, 305
Scrotal pain, 658
Scvo2, 504

Seborrheic dermatitis, 25
Secondary hypertension, 207
Secretions, 714
Sedation of violent patient, 589
Seizure, 430
Sensorineural hearing loss, 567
Sensory/motor deficits, 429
Sepsis, 121
   Rapid fluid infusions, 122
   Treatment, 122
Septic shock, 527
Serotonin syndrome, 599
Shock, 526, 527
   Cardiogenic, 527
   Hypovolemic, 527
   Septic, 527
Shortness of breath, 12
Shortness of breath, 463
Shoulder examination, 391
Shoulder injection, 716
Siadh, 705
Significance of ana pattern, 578
Silent thyroiditis, 278
Sinusitis, 102, 559
Skin biopsy, 26
Sleep aids, 587
Sleep apnea, 502
Solitary thyroid nodule, 278
Sore throat, 563
Speckled, 578
Spherocytes, 305
Spinal stenosis, 376
Spirometry, 466
Spn, 499
Ssri, 593
   Side effect profiles, 598
Stasis dermatitis, 25
Statin
   Treatment based on intensity, 670
Statin induced liver damage, 74
Statins
   Alternatives, 671, 673
   Choosing intensity, 669
   Options, 669
Status epilepticus, 433
Stemi, 183, 194
Stents
   Bms, 201
   Des, 201
Stents, coronary, 201
Steroids
   Dermatology, 19
   Potency/conversion, 285
Stone analysis, 553
Stool osmolarity, 50
Strep pharyngitis, 561
Stress test
   Perioperative, 175
Stress testing, 172
Stroke, 439
   Bp management, 446
   Imaging, 444
   Intracerebral hemorrhage, 450

Management, 444
Secondary prevention, 453
Subarachnoid hemorrhage, 451
Thrombolytic, 446
Treatment, 450
Types, 439
Vascular territory, 443
Workup, 440
Supplemental oxygen, 495
Supplemental oxygen, 714
Supportive care of oncology patients, 339
Supraventricular tachycardia, 145
Susceptibility interpretation, 88
Suturing, 714
Svr, 504
Svv, 503
Syncope, 407
Synovial fluid analysis, 574
Systemic vascular resistance, 504
Systolic heart failure, 156

T

Taco, 324
Target cells, 305
Tbi, 413, see concussion
Testicular pain, 658
Testosterone replacement therapy. See sexual dysfunction
Tha, 347
Thalassemia, 307
Thoracentesis, 496
Thrombin time, 325
Thrombophilia work-up, 325
Thyroid
  Hyperthyroidism, 277
  Hypothyroidism, 281
Thyroid nodule, 286
Thyroid storm, 278
Tia, 454
Tips, 33
Tka, 347
Tobacco abuse, 720

Torsades de pointes, 82
Tpa, 446
Tpn, 666
Trali, 323
Transfusion, 314
Transfusion associated circulatory overload (taco), 324
Transfusion related acute lung injury, 323
Transient ischemic attack, 454
Tremor
  Essential, 428
  Parkinsons, 428
Trigger finger injection, 716
Trigger point injection, 716
Triglyceride elevation treatment, 668
Troponin
  Causes of elevation, 178
  Interpretation, 178, 180
Tube feeds, 666

U

Uds, 635
Umn vs. Lmn, 429
Unresponsive patient, 438
Upper gi bleeds, 54
Urinary tract infections, 116
Urine ag, 690
Urine anion gap, 535
Urine drug testing, 635
Urosepsis, 97
Urticaria, 323
Usa, 183
Uspstf screening recommendations, 719
Uti. See urinary tract infections
  Esbl, 118

V

V/q mismatch, 495
Vaccination schedule, 719
Variceal bleed, 39
Variceal prophylaxis, 36

Vasopressin, 79, 126
Vasopressors, 123, 125
Vasovagal syncope, 407
Venous thromboembolism, 340
Vent, 517
  Acpc, 518
  Acvc, 518
  Adjusting, 520
  Auto-peep, 520
  Bi-level, 519
  Common settings by condition, 522
  Failure to wean, 523
  Generic initial settings, 520
  Modes, 518
  Peak pressure, 518
  Plateau pressure, 518
  Pressure support, 519
  Simv, 518
  Weaning modes, 523
  Weaning predictors, 516
Vent modes, 514
Vent settings, 513
Ventricular arrhythmias, 143
Ventricular fibrillation, 145
Ventricular hypertrophy, 146
Ventricular tachycardia, 144
Vertigo, 456
Vitamin b12 deficiency, 309
Vitamin d deficiency, 288
Vomiting, 339, 713
Vte, 340
Vwd, 325

W

Water deprivation testing, 547
Weaning parameters, 523
Weber / rinne testing, 566
Weber/rinne, 566

X

Xr
  Abdomen, 366
  Chest, 360

www.ingramcontent.com/pod-product-compliance
Lightning Source LLC
Chambersburg PA
CBHW071147230426
43668CB00009B/870